Plant Based Medicines: Novel Perspectives

Plant Based Medicines: Novel Perspectives

Editor: Elise Morrison

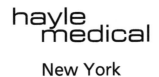

New York

Hayle Medical,
750 Third Avenue, 9th Floor,
New York, NY 10017, USA

Visit us on the World Wide Web at:
www.haylemedical.com

ISBN 978-1-64647-597-1 (Hardback)

Cataloging-in-Publication Data

Plant based medicines : novel perspectives / edited by Elise Morrison.
       p. cm.
Includes bibliographical references and index.
ISBN 978-1-64647-597-1
1. Medicinal plants. 2. Botany, Medical. 3. Materia medica, Vegetable. 4. Plants, Useful. I. Morrison, Elise.
QK99.A1 P53 2023
581.634--dc23

Contents

Preface

The majority of medicines presently in use have their origins in plant sources. Plant-derived compounds contain immunomodulatory properties that make them appropriate for use in drug development. Plant polysaccharides including açaí fruit, ganoderma lucidum and cordyceps sinensis exhibit immunostimulatory or immunomodulatory properties. Flavonoids which include flavonones, isoflavone, xanthones, flavones and flavonols are found in nearly all plants and have a variety of bioactive qualities. Proteins derived from certain herbs are utilized as natural protein supplements for convalescent patients. Additionally plant-based drugs such as silymarin derived from the seeds of silybum marianum is utilized to treat liver disease, and artemisinin derived from the seeds of artemisia annua is utilized to treat multidrug-resistant malaria. Alkaloids are being repurposed as nitric oxide activators to aid in the prevention of atherosclerosis and obesity. This book is a valuable compilation of topics, ranging from the basic to the most complex advancements in the field of plant based medicines. Those with an interest in this field would find it helpful.

Significant researches are present in this book. Intensive efforts have been employed by authors to make this book an outstanding discourse. This book contains the enlightening chapters which have been written on the basis of significant researches done by the experts.

Finally, I would also like to thank all the members involved in this book for being a team and meeting all the deadlines for the submission of their respective works. I would also like to thank my friends and family for being supportive in my efforts.

Editor

A Comprehensive Comparative Study for the Authentication of the *Kadsura* Crude Drug

Jiushi Liu[1,2], Xueping Wei[1,3], Xiaoyi Zhang[1,2], Yaodong Qi[1,3], Bengang Zhang[1,3], Haitao Liu[1,2]* and Peigen Xiao[1,2]

[1] Institute of Medicinal Plant Development, Chinese Academy of Medical Sciences, Peking Union Medical College, Beijing, China, [2] Key Laboratory of Bioactive Substances and Resources Utilization of Chinese Herbal Medicine (Peking Union Medical College), Ministry of Education, Beijing, China, [3] Engineering Research Center of Traditional Chinese Medicine Resources, Ministry of Education, Beijing, China

*Correspondence:
Haitao Liu
htliu0718@126.com

The stems and roots of *Kadsura* species have been used as the folk medicine in Traditional Chinese medicine (TCM) and have good traditional efficacy and medicinal application with a long history. Among these species, *K. coccinea*, *K. heteroclita* and *K. longipedunculata* are the most widely distributed species in the regions of south and southwest China. Owing to their similar appearance, the crude drugs are often confusedly used by some folk doctors, even some pharmaceutical factories. To discriminate the crude drugs, haplotype analysis based on cpDNA markers and ITS was firstly employed in this study. Generic delimitation, interspecific interrelationships, and the identification of medicinal materials between *K. longipedunculata* and *K. heteroclita* remained unresolved by the existing molecular fragments. The original plant could be identified through the morphological character of flower, fruit and leaf. However, in most situation collectors have no chance to find out these characters due to lack of reproductive organs, and have no experience with the minor difference and transitional variation of leaf morphology. The chemical characterization show that the chemometric of chemical composition owned higher resolution to discriminate three herbs of *Kadsura* species. In conclusion, this integrative approach involving molecular phylogeny, morphology and chemical characterization could be applied for authentication of the *Kadusra*. Our study suggests the use of this comprehensive approach for accurate characterization of this closely related taxa as well as identifying the source plant and confused herbs of TCM.

Keywords: *Kadsura*, morphology, molecular markers, chemical characterization, identification

INTRODUCTION

Traditional Chinese medicine (TCM) is widely accepted in the health care system, and has made a significant contribution to prevention and treatment of human diseases. This extensive use warrants safety measures and so TCM drug safety monitoring and quality control are becoming increasingly important tasks to guarantee the safety and efficacy of TCM treatments (Chen et al., 1999). However, the use of substitute products and confused materials still aggravate the chaotic situation in clinical application. It is important to find a reliable way for distinguishing them from each other (Li et al., 2015).

Kadsura belongs to the economically and medicinally important family Schisandraceae and eight species mainly distributed in the southwest and southeast in China (Saunders, 1998; Wu et al., 2008). In China, the stems and roots of genus *Kadsura* are commonly used as folk medicines and 5 species of genus *Kadsura* are documented in the official Pharmacopoeia and folk record (GuangXi Zhuang Autonomous Region Health Department, 1992; Guangdong Food and Drug Administration, 2004; FuJian Food and Drug Administration, 2006; Chinese Pharmacopeia Commission, 2015). The stems of *K. heteroclita*, *K. longipedunculata* and *K. coccinea* are the most widely used in south China which have good traditional efficacy and medicinal application with a long history, and often used confusedly in clinical application. Numerous phytochemical and pharmacological studies have been carried out and focus on its health benefits (Liu et al., 2014). There are differences in clinical efficacy between the three crude drugs. *K. heteroclita* was used for the treatment of rheumatic arthralgia. *K. longipedunculata* was used for the treatment of irregular menstruation. *K. coccinea* was used for the treatment of gastric and duodenal ulcer. Owing to their similar appearance, these crude drugs are often confusedly used by some folk doctors, even some pharmaceutical factories. There is an urgent need to find a reliable, accurate way for distinguishing three *Kadsura* crude drugs (Liu et al., 2012).

In order to identify this kind of medicine herbs by molecular sequences, Zhou et al. chose psbA-trnH for distinguishing eight species. Although they found a stabilized single nucleotide polymorphism (SNP), SNPs as potential tool to distinguish *Kadsrua* crude drugs could not be further analyzed because of poor samples of *K. heteroclite* (Zhou et al., 2016). Combination of ITS + psbA-trnH + matK + rbcL as the most ideal DNA barcode for discriminating the medicinal plants of Schisandra and *Kadsura*, nonetheless, degree of species resolution was lower among the closely related species, and exposed *K. heteroclita* and *K. longipedunculata* could not be discriminated by four commonly used DNA barcodes (Zhang et al., 2015). Molecular identification of TCM is objective, more accurate, and easier to perform than traditional identification methods, and has successfully been applied to identify medicinal plants (Kress et al., 2005; Chen et al., 2010; de Boer et al., 2015). However, previous studies of DNA barcoding have not effectively resolved the problem of identifying three crude drugs of the *Kadsura*. In this study, we try to identify three crude drugs by haplotype analysis based on cpDNA and ITS markers.

The high selectivity and sensitivity of UPLC-QTOF/MS has been successfully applied to the metabolite analysis and identification of complex compounds in herbal materials (Song et al., 2013; Yao et al., 2013; Cubero-Leon et al., 2014). There are few researches in investigated chemical profiles of *Kadsura* species for the safety and efficacy, and the comparative analysis on chemical composition of these *Kadsura* herbs is needed. Bioactivity-based characteristics are good quality indicators too, as they are pharmacologically relevant (Liu et al., 2017). Analysis on main chemical components disparity in three medicinal materials could guarantee the clinical uses the medicine the rationality, the security and the validity.

Adequately considering samples representativeness and experiments economy, we therefore started multi-populations survey in twenty populations covering five provinces including Hunan, Guangxi, Guizhou, Chongqing and Sichuan provinces and in reproductive stage at summer and autumn from June 2016 to December 2017. The overall aim of this study was to explore the usefulness of an authentication approach to three crude

TABLE 1 | Samples of *K. longipedunculata*, *K. coccinea*, and *K. heteroclita*.

No.	Species	Voucher number	Sources
S1	*K. longipedunculata*	2015082801	Nanchuan, Chongqin
S2	*K. longipedunculata*	2015082903	Emei, Sichuan
S3	*K. longipedunculata*	2015090604	Guiyang, Guizhou
S4	*K. longipedunculata*	2015090801	Leishan, Guizhou
S5	*K. longipedunculata*	2015090804	Baojing, Hunan
S6	*K. longipedunculata*	2015090807	Xingan, Guangxi
S7	*K. coccinea*	2015082901	Jinxiu, Guangxi
S8	*K. coccinea*	2015083101	Jinxiu, Guangxi
S9	*K. coccinea*	2015090502	Emei, Sichuan
S10	*K. coccinea*	2015091601	Guiyang, Guizhou
S11	*K. coccinea*	2015092304	Huaihua, Hunan
S12	*K. coccinea*	2015092704	Xingan, Guangxi
S13	*K. heteroclita*	2015091201	Jianhe, Guizhou
S14	*K. heteroclita*	2015091803	Baojing, Hunan
S15	*K. heteroclita*	2015091804	Jinxiu, Guangxi
S16	*K. heteroclita*	2015092104	Jinxiu, Guangxi
S17	*K. heteroclita*	2015092105	Nanchuan, Chongqin
S18	*K. heteroclita*	2015091201	Emei, Sichuan

TABLE 2 | The main morphology characters of *K. coccinea*, *K. heteroclita* and *K. longipedunculata*.

	K. coccinea	*K. heteroclita*	*K. longipedunculata*
Petiole	0.9–3 (–4.1) cm	0.7–2.9 cm	0.6–1.7 (–3) cm
Leaf blade	elliptic to rarely ovate; papery to leathery; margin entire or rarely denticulate; apex acute; shortly acuminate, or rarely obtuse	ovate-elliptic to elliptic; papery to subleathery; margin entire or denticulate; apex acute to acuminate	elliptic to rarely ovate-elliptic or obovate-elliptic; papery to leathery; secondary veins 4–8 on each side of midvein; margin subentire, denticulate, serrulate, or serrate; apex shortly to long acuminate
Staminate	stamens 10–50; staminodes generally present at apex of torus	stamens 40–74; staminodes absent	stamens 26–54; staminodes absent
Fruit	6–10 cm; apocarps red to purplish red	2.5–4 cm; apocarps red	1–3.5 cm; apocarps red, purple, or rarely black
Stem	black or brown; lenticel, no suberinlamellae	brown;older stems phellem layer thickness, longitudinal split	slender

drugs of the *Kadsura* complex using cpDNA and ITS markers, morphology, and UPLC-QTOF/MS chemical profiling. We want to compare the genetic polymorphism of haplotypes and analyze their population difference for the taxa in the *Kadsura* species, and distinguish chemotypes of the species complex by comparing their UPLC-QTOF/MS chemical profiles using chemometric data analysis.

MATERIALS AND METHODS

Plant Materials

There are morphological differences between the three species to discriminate them during flower or fruit stages of life cycles. For the sake of sampling accuracy, we therefore started multi-populations survey in reproductive stage at summer and autumn from June 2016 to December 2017. The *Kadsura* samples were collected in the main areas in China: Hunan, Guangxi, Guizhou, Chongqing and Sichuan provinces. In total 52 samples of *K. coccinea, K. heteroclita* and *K. longipedunculata* were collected directly from wild region. The 52 leaves dried using silica gel for DNA extraction and stored at 4°C until use. And 18 the stems dried in the shade for UPLC-MS analysis (**Table 1**).

DNA Extraction, PCR Amplification and Sequencing

Total genomic DNA was extracted from silica gel-dried leaves by using the Plant Genomic DNA Kit (Tiangen Biotech, Beijing, China) following the manufacturer's instructions. Three cpDNA gene markers, matK,rbcL,psbA-trnH and one nrDNA ITS, were separately amplified for each individual by using the primers and protocol of Guo et al. (2015). Sanger sequence reactions were carried out using the DYEnamic ETDye Terminator Cycle Sequencing Kit (Amersham Pharmacia Biotech) and sequenced on ABI 3730XL genetic analyzer (Applied Biosystems, CA, United States).

Network Analysis of Haplotypes

The DNA sequences were aligned using the program Clustal X v.1.83 (Thompson et al., 1997) and manually adjusted in BioEdit v. 7.0.9 (Hall, 1999). Voucher and GenBank accession numbers were listed in the **Supplementary Table S1**. A network of the cpDNA haplotypes (chlorotypes) was constructed using NETWORK 5.0.0.1 (Bandelt et al., 1999), with a default parsimony connection limit of 95% and each insertion/deletion (indel) treated as a single mutation event.

Sample Preparation and UPLC-QTOF/MS Conditions

HPLC-grade acetonitrile (Merck KGaA, Darmstadt, Germany) and formic acid (Fisher Scientific, NH, United States) were utilized for UPLC analysis. Pure water (18.2 MΩ) for UPLC analysis was obtained from a Milli-Q system (Millipore, MA, United States). All other chemicals were of analytical grade.

Kadsura samples (0.5000 g, 65-mesh) were accurately weighed and extracted with 25 mL methanol by ultrasonication (35 kHz)

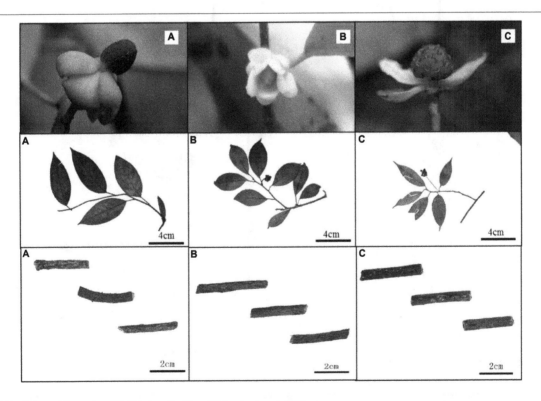

FIGURE 1 | Morphology of *K. coccinea* **(A)**, *K. heteroclita* **(B)** and *K. longipedunculata* **(C)**.

for 30 min. After centrifugation at 10,000 × *g* for 10 min, the supernatant was stored at 4°C and filtered through 0.22 μm membrane prior to injection into the UPLC system.

A Thermo Scientific™ Dionex™ UltiMate™ 3000 Rapid Separation LC (RSLC) system performed UHPLC separations using the gradient conditions as follows. Mobile phase A was water and mobile phase B was acetonitrile; both A and B contained 0.1% formic acid. The conditions were optimized as follows: 0–3 min, 2–20% B; 3–4.5 min, 20–75% B; 4.5–6.5 min, 75–100% B; 6.5–15 min, 100% B; 15–15.5 min, 100–5% B; 15.5–17 min, 5% B. The column was a HSS T3 column (2.1 mm × 100 mm, 1.7 μm, waters) operated at 45°C. The flow rate was 300 μL/min and the injection volume was 2 μL.

A Thermo Scientific™ Q Exactive™ hybrid quadrupole Orbitrap mass spectrometer equipped with a HESI-II probe was employed. The HESI-II spray voltages were 3.7 kV for positive mode, the heated capillary temperature was 320°C, the sheath gas pressure was 30 psi, the auxiliary gas setting was 10 psi, and the heated vaporizer temperature was 300°C. Both the sheath gas and the auxiliary gas were nitrogen. The collision gas was argon at a pressure of 1.5 mTorr. The parameters of the full mass scan were as follows: a resolution of 70,000, an auto gain control

target under 1×10^6, a maximum isolation time of 50 ms, and an m/z range 150–1500. The calibration was customized for the analysis of Q Exactive to keep the mass tolerance of 5 ppm. The LC-MS system was controlled using Xcalibur 2.2 SP1.48 software (Thermo Fisher Scientific), and data were collected and processed with the same software.

UPLC-QTOF/MS Data Analysis

UPLC-QTOF/MS data for *Kadsura* samples were analyzed to identify potential discriminant variables. Peak finding, alignment and filtering of ES raw data were carried out using Xcalibur 2.2 SP1.48 software (Thermo Fisher Scientific). The parameters used were as follows: retention time (tR) of 0.5–10.5 min, mass of 150–800 Da, retention time tolerance of 0.05 min, and mass tolerance of 0.02 Da. Three replicate samples collected from each geographic location were used (*n* = 3). A total of three, 114 variables were used to create the model. The resulting data was analyzed by heatmap analysis with MetaboAnalyst, which is a web-based tool for visualization of chemometrics (Deng et al., 2014). And principal component analysis (PCA) and partial least squares discriminant analysis (PLS-DA) were applied to discriminate three *Kadsura* species

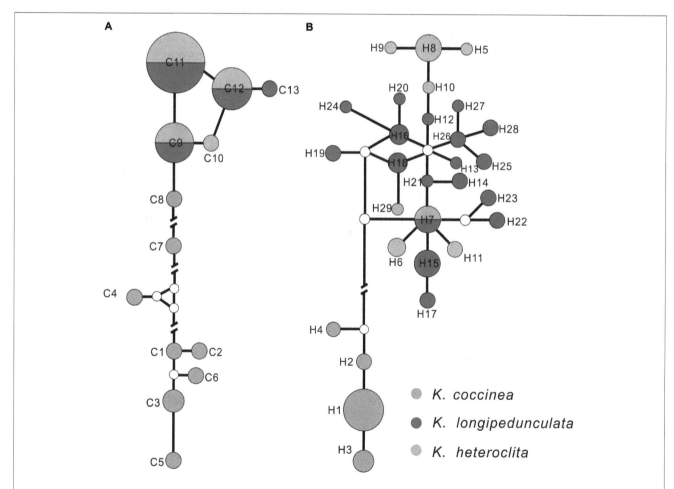

FIGURE 2 | Networks of the cpDNA **(A)** and ITS **(B)** haplotypes constructed by using NETWORK 5.0.0.1. The sizes of the circles in the network are proportional to the observed frequencies of the haplotypes.

TABLE 3 | Tentatively identified compounds from *K. longipedunculata*, *K. heteroclita*, and *K. coccinea*.

No.	t_R(min)	Mean measured mass [M+H]$^+$ m/z	Theoretical exact mass [M+H]$^+$ m/z	Error (ppm)	Fragments m/z	Formula	Identification	Reference
1	4.25	445.1861	445.1862	−0.22	355.1545, 337.1440, 323.1283	$C_{24}H_{28}O_8$	kadsumarin A	Kuo et al., 1999
2	4.34	419.2073	419.2070	0.72	269.1542, 234.1409, 206.1096	$C_{23}H_{30}O_7$	gomisin H	Li et al., 1985
3	4.35	415.1390	415.1393	−0.72	291.1385, 273.1279, 247.1123	$C_{22}H_{22}O_8$	kadsurindutin H	Ma et al., 2009
4	4.37	433.1866	433.1862	0.92	313.1440, 279.1385, 253.1229	$C_{23}H_{28}O_8$	kadangustin L	Gao et al., 2012
5	4.41	433.2219	433.2226	−1.62	415.2044, 384.1856, 369.1677	$C_{24}H_{32}O_7$	schisandrin	Sun et al., 2011
6	4.45	387.1809	387.1808	0.26	297.1491, 279.1385	$C_{22}H_{26}O_6$	gomisin M1	Han et al., 1992
7	4.59	625.2071	625.2074	−0.48	317.0814, 291.0657	$C_{36}H_{32}O_{10}$	angustifolin A	Chen et al., 1998
8	4.76	505.1870	505.1862	1.58	321.1127, 295.0970	$C_{29}H_{28}O_8$	interiotherin A	Chen et al., 1998
9	4.87	431.2070	431.2070	0.00	251.1436, 225.1279	$C_{24}H_{30}O_7$	schisanlignone A	Liu et al., 1991
10	5.15	415.1758	415.1757	0.24	295.1334, 269.1178	$C_{23}H_{26}O_7$	kadsulignan L	Liu and Li, 1995
11	5.18	389.1974	389.1964	2.6	357.1719	$C_{22}H_{28}O_6$	gomisin J	Chen et al., 2006
12	5.28	459.2017	459.2019	−0.44	339.1596, 321.1491, 308.1412	$C_{25}H_{30}O_8$	ananolignan A	Yang et al., 2011
13	5.42	581.2385	581.2387	−0.34	458.1941, 308.1412, 290.1307, 277.1229	$C_{32}H_{36}O_{10}$	kadangustin E	Gao et al., 2008
14	5.61	417.1556	417.1549	1.68	327.1232, 291.1021	$C_{22}H_{24}O_8$	kadoblongifolin B	Liu et al., 2009
15	5.73	637.2645	637.2649	−0.63	517.2226, 394.1780, 376.1675, 350.1518, 336.1362	$C_{35}H_{40}O_{11}$	schisantherin J	Liu and Pan, 1991
16	6.15	483.2022	483.2019	0.62	423.1808	$C_{27}H_{30}O_8$	heteroclitin D	Chen et al., 1992
17	6.21	537.2115	537.2125	−1.86	415.1545, 316.1099	$C_{30}H_{32}O_9$	gomisin C	Chen et al., 1992
18	7.57	499.2329	499.2332	−0.60	379.1909	$C_{28}H_{34}O_8$	heteroclitin B	Chen et al., 1992
19	7.65	485.2181	485.2175	1.24	425.1964	$C_{27}H_{32}O_8$	kadsulignan J	Liu et al., 2009
20	7.95	607.2181	607.2179	0.33	517.1862, 394.1933, 360.1878, 346.1722	$C_{33}H_{34}O_{11}$	kadsuphilol L	Shen et al., 2009

by the EZinfo 2.0 software (Masssart et al., 1998; Xia et al., 2012).

RESULTS

Morphology

The variation of morphological traits in the *Kadsura* is relatively complex and the *Kadsura* in relationship was near with each other. There are still some morphological differences among three species. We observed main morphology characters (male flower, fruit shape, stem and leaf listed in **Table 2**) of *K. coccinea*, *K. heteroclita* and *K. longipedunculata* by specimens and natural populations, and established morphological basis to identify three *Kadsura* species. The morphology of male flower, fruit shape, stem and leaf are an important basis of identifying *Kadsura* (**Figure 1**). In most situations, collectors have no chance to find out these characters because of comparatively short flower and fruit time or lack of these organs in some habits and young individuals. Minor difference and transitional variation of leaf morphology make it difficult for those inexperienced collectors to identify. It is important to find a reliable, accurate way for distinguishing three crude drugs.

Haplotypes Network

The alignment of the combined three cpDNA fragments were designated 13 haplotypes (C1–C13) including 52 variable characters, and ITS were designated 29 haplotypes (H1–H29) with 49 variable characters. *K. coccinea* occupied eight private chloroplastic haplotypes (**Figure 2A**; C1–C8), while *K. longipedunculata* and *K. heteroclita* shared the three main haplotypes (C9, C11, and C12), two rare haplotypes C10 and C13 were fixed by *K. heteroclita* and *K. longipedunculata*, respectively. In the ITS haplotypes network (**Figure 2B**), *K. coccinea* occupied four private haplotypes which were quite different from the others (H1–H4). 17 haplotypes were fixed in *K. longipedunculata*, and seven haplotypes in *K. heteroclita*. Only one H17 was shared by *K. longipedunculata* and *K. heteroclita*. H17 was one of the main haplotypes of ITS and it was the center of the "star-like" haplotypes network of *K. longipedunculata* and *K. heteroclita*. It was obviously to see that both cpDNA markers and ITS can distinguish *K. coccinea* from *K. longipedunculata* and *K. heteroclita* clearly. However, the phylogenetic relationship between *K. longipedunculata* and *K. heteroclita* are quite closely related, their haplotypes are star-like and they shared the main haploptypes in both cpDNA markers and ITS (**Supplementary Table S2**).

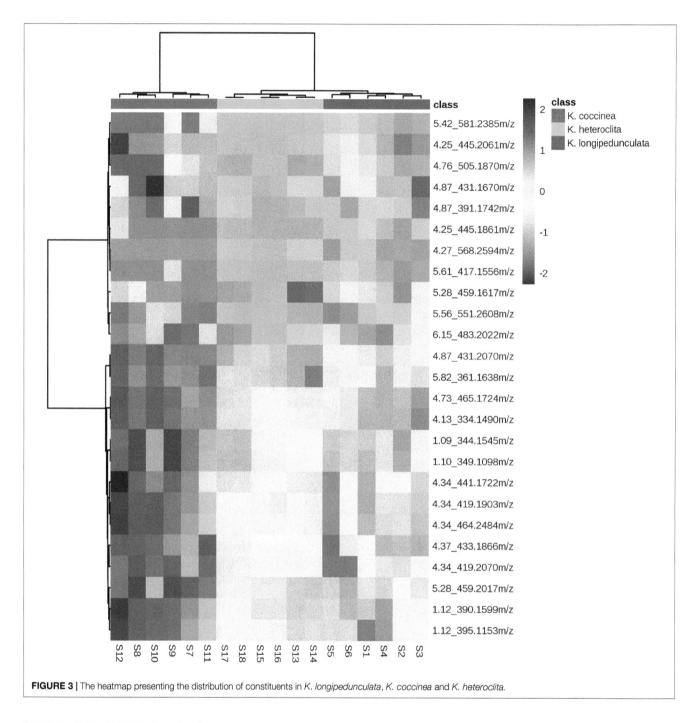

FIGURE 3 | The heatmap presenting the distribution of constituents in *K. longipedunculata*, *K. coccinea* and *K. heteroclita*.

UPLC-QTOF/MS Analysis

Twenty compounds were tentatively identified by elucidating the retention time (min), parentions $[M+H]^+$, MS/MS fragmentation pattern and calculated molecular formula of each peak, and by matching above data with those reported previously (**Table 3**). For example, schisandrin, in the low energy spectrum, the protonated adduct ion $[M+H]^+$ at m/z 433.1866. Further confirmation of schisandrin was provided by the high-energy function. At m/z 415.2115 was detected the fragment identified as $[M-H_2O+H]^+$ and at m/z 384.1932 we assigned a fragment due to the further loss of methoxy group corresponding to

$[M-H_2O-OCH_3+H]^+$. It was identified to schisandrin based on the parent and characteristic fragmentions information.

As depicted in **Figure 3**, we can observe that: (a) the chemical components of three *Kadsura* species were very different by the heatmaps, and the components of *K. longipedunculata* were close to *K. heteroclita*. (b) Among all the identified compounds, kadangustin L, gomisin H, and ananolignan A have a relatively high concentration in *K. coccinea*, while showing low levels in the *K. heteroclita* and *K. longipedunculata*. While kadangustin E, kadsumarin A, interiotherin A and kadoblongifolin B are present mainly in the *K. longipedunculata*, followed by the

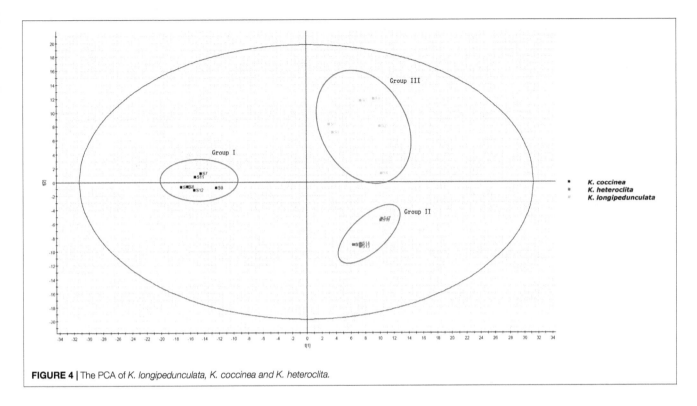

FIGURE 4 | The PCA of *K. longipedunculata*, *K. coccinea* and *K. heteroclita*.

K. heteroclita and limited concentratins in the *K. coccinea*. Previous studies have suggested that these compounds are found in high concentrations in *K. heteroclita*, which is supported by our results (Liu et al., 2014).

The two-component PCA model cumulatively accounted for 46.04% of the variation (PC1, 36.43%; PC2, 9.61%). The PCA score plot shows that these three species were obtained the very good separation. Group I was formed by *K. coccinea*, Group II consisted of *K. heteroclita* and Group III was formed by *K. longipedunculata* (**Figure 4**).

The PLS–DA model performed well in classifying the three species of *Kadsura*, and group I was far away from the group II and III (**Figure 5A**). A total of six credible and significant markers were determined to facilitate discrimination of these groups by the S-plot of PLS-DA. The identities of six potential markers were tentatively assigned (**Figure 5B**). The components correlated with these six ions were tentatively identified as isomers of kadsumarin A, gomisin H, kadangustin L, interiotherin A, kadangustin E, and kadoblongifolin B. The marker compounds could be used to distinguish the three plant species, as the ion intensities of kadsumarin A, kadoblongifolin B, and interiotherin A in *K. heteroclita* and *K. longipedunculata* was higher than in *K. coccinea*. Marker gomisin H and kadangustin L could be detected in *K. coccinea*, which was higher than in the other two species (**Figure 6** and **Supplementary Data Sheet S1**).

DISCUSSION

The three *Kadsura* species distribute widely in tropical or subtropical evergreen forests of south of Yangtze River in

China. In fact, there are morphological differences between the three species to discriminate them during flower or fruit stages of life cycles. For the sake of sampling accuracy, we therefore started multi-populations survey in reproductive stage at summer and autumn from 2016 June to December 2017. Adequately considering samples representativeness and experiments economy, we chose following survey and sampling strategy. 80 individuals were observed in twenty populations covering five provinces including Hunan, Guangxi, Guizhou, Chongqing and Sichuan provinces, while 45 leaves samples were collected for DNA barcoding experiment and 18 stems samples were used for metabolites analysis, in which samples of each species included ten individuals (DNA test) and six individuals (Chemical test) from different populations.

Morphology

As mentioned above, we usually discriminate the three species by the shape of staminate flower torus, the size and shape of fruits, the length of fruit stalk and leaf shape. For example, the shape of staminate flower torus of *K. coccinea* is conical, *K. heteroclite* is elliptical and *K. longipedunculata* is spherical. The size of fruit is *K. coccinea* (6–10 cm) > *K. heteroclita* (2.5–4 cm) > *K. longipedunculata* (1–3.5 cm). These identifying characteristics also were record in FRPS and FOC (Academiae Sinicae Edita, 2004; Flora of China Edita, 2013). When we surveyed in wild populations, these morphological characters were very valuable to discriminate them. In spite of obvious differences between reproductive organs, in most situation collectors have no chance to find out these characters due to comparatively short flower and fruit time or lack of these organs in some habits and young individuals. In addition, leaf

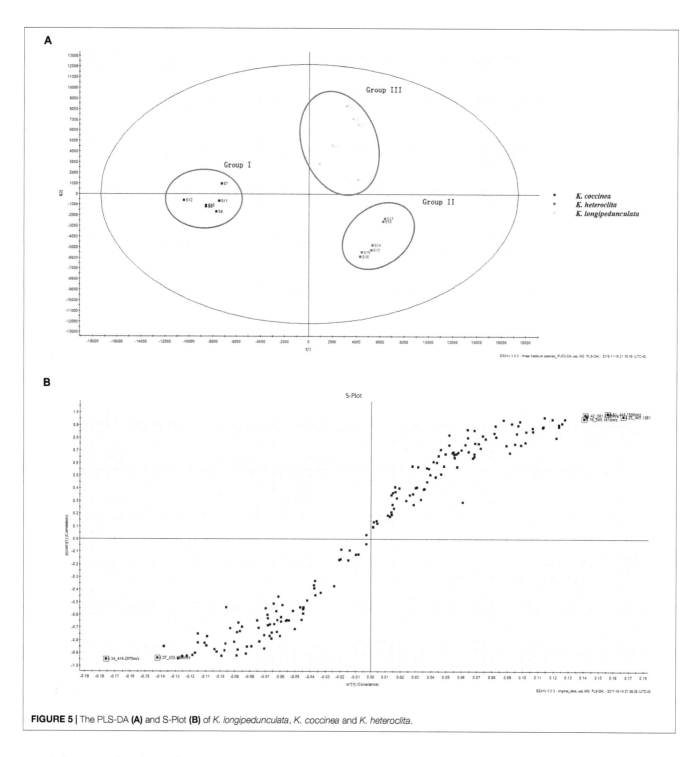

FIGURE 5 | The PLS-DA **(A)** and S-Plot **(B)** of *K. longipedunculata*, *K. coccinea* and *K. heteroclita*.

morphology may be observed through whole growth period, minor difference and transitional variation between species make difficult for those inexperienced collectors. Consequently this leads to collection uncertainty for the three crude drugs, and confusedly mixed application often occurs in present research and clinic use. Nowadays a popular solution is to extract DNA fragments from dried materials, and then conducts DNA barcoding or SNPs analysis (Kress et al., 2005; Chen et al., 2010).

DNA Sequence

In our study, haplotype analysis based on cpDNA and ITS markers can distinguish clearly *K. coccinea* from *K. longipedunculata* and *K. heteroclita*, but can't distinguish *K. longipedunculata* and *K. heteroclite*. Haplotype analysis is suitable for the study of closely related species and genetic diversity of intraspecific species by molecular biology methods. However, it does not show any advantage to delimit the boundary between *K. longipendunculata* and *K. heteroclita*.

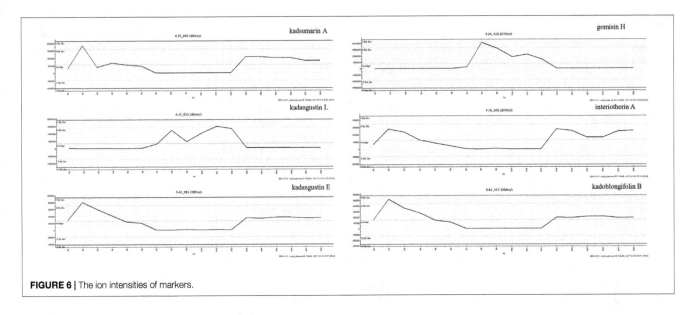

FIGURE 6 | The ion intensities of markers.

Haplotypes of *K. longipedunculata* and *K. heteroclita* shared the main haploptypes in both cpDNA markers and ITS. MatK,rbcL,psbA-trnH and ITS are the four suggested DNA barcode in plant (CBOL Plant Working Group, 2009). The cpDNA is characterized by its evolutionary conservatism, matrilineal inheritance, and lack of recombination (Wolfe et al., 1987). However, the complicated relationship such as the potential hybridization, reticulate evolution and gene introgression may further intersify the difficulty of species identification in closely related species of the *Kadsura*. The existing DNA barcode have not effectively resolved the problem of identifying *K. longipedunculata* and *K. heteroclita*.

Chemical Characteristics

Three herbs differ from their metabolite profiles including lignan based chemometric analysis. Heatmap analysis, PCA analysis and PLS-DA showed the chemical constituents of three kinds of medicinal materials differed significantly. We summarized the chemical constituents of *Kadsura* and found that a lot of spirobenzofuranoid dibenzocyclooctadiene compounds have been found in *K. heteroclita*. Tetrahydrofura compounds have been found in *K. longipedunculata*. 18 (13→12)-abeo-lanostane and nortriterpenoid compounds have been found only in *K. coccinea* (Liu et al., 2014). The different chemical constituents can influence the curative effect and security. The chemometrics analysis can make up for the shortage of molecular identification and has successfully been applied to identify the three *Kadsura* crude drug.

In this study, the DNA sequence analyzes, the recheck of morphology and chemical characteristics applied to identify the three *Kadsura* crude drug. The identification of medicinal materials between *K. longipedunculata* and *K. heteroclita*

remained unresolved by the existing molecular fragments. The chemical characterization shows that the chemometric of chemical composition owned higher resolution to discriminate three crude drugs of the *Kadsura* and helpful to differentiate the source of samples and judge the consistency of three *Kadsura* species which make up for the shortage of molecular identification. This paper conducts a comprehensive analysis on three *Kadsura* crude drugs and provides a new research route for the confused herbs by molecular phylogeny, morphology and chemical composition.

AUTHOR CONTRIBUTIONS

JL involved field survey, performed operation of the whole experiments, and wrote the manuscript. XZ and XW assisted with JL in the experiments. YQ and HL responsible for provided the technical guidance and designed the experiments. BZ and PX improved the manuscript.

FUNDING

The authors are grateful for the financial support provided by the National Natural Sciences Foundation of China (Nos. 81373913 and 81703650) and CAMS Initiative for Innovative Medicine (CAMS-I2M-1-010).

ACKNOWLEDGMENTS

We thank the reviewers for carefully reviewing our manuscript and making many valuable suggestions.

REFERENCES

Academiae Sinicae Edita (2004). *Flora Republicae Popularis Sinicae*. Beijing: Science Press.

Bandelt, H.-J., Forster, P., and Röhl, A. (1999). Median-joining networks for inferring intraspecific phylogenies. *Mol. Boil. Evol.* 16, 37–48. doi: 10.1093/oxfordjournals.molbev.a026036

CBOL Plant Working Group (2009). A DNA barcode for land plants. *Proc. Natl. Acad. Sci. U.S.A.* 106, 12794–12797. doi: 10.1073/pnas.0905845106

Chen, D. F., Xu, G. J., Yang, X. W., Hattori, M., Tezuka, Y., Kikuchi, T., et al. (1992). Dibenzocyclooctadiene lignans from *Kadsura heteroclita*. *Phytochemistry* 31, 629–632. doi: 10.1016/0031-9422(92)90049-V

Chen, M., Jia, Z. W., and Chen, D. F. (2006). Heteroclitin H, a new lignan from *Kadsura heteroclita*. *J. Asian Natl. Prod. Res.* 8, 643–648. doi: 10.1080/10286020500209053

Chen, P., Zhengou, W., and Peiping, X. (1999). *History and Development of Traditional Chinese Medicine*. Beijing: Science Press.

Chen, S. L., Yao, H., Han, J. P., Liu, C., Song, J. Y., Shi, L. C., et al. (2010). Validation of the ITS2 Region as a novel dna barcode for identifying medicinal plant species. *PLoS One* 5:e8613. doi: 10.1371/journal.pone.0008613

Chen, Y. G., Wang, P., Lin, Z. W., Sun, H. D., Qin, G. W., and Xie, Y. Y. (1998). Dibenzocyclooctadiene lignans from *Kadsura angustifolia*. *Phytochemistry* 48, 1059–1062. doi: 10.1016/S0031-9422(97)00996-5

Chinese Pharmacopeia Commission (2015). *Pharmacopoeia of the People's Republicof China Version (2015)*. Beijing: Chinese Medical Science Press.

Cubero-Leon, E., Peñalver, R., and Maquet, A. (2014). Review on metabolomics for food authentication. *Food Res. Int.* 60, 95–107. doi: 10.1016/j.foodres.2013.11.041

de Boer, H. J., Ichim, M. C., and Newmaster, S. G. (2015). DNA barcoding and pharmacovigilance of herbal medicines. *Drug Safety* 38, 611–620. doi: 10.1007/s40264-015-0306-8

Deng, W., Wang, Y., Liu, Z., Cheng, H., and Xue, Y. (2014). HemI: a toolkit for illustrating heatmaps. *PLoS One* 9:e111988. doi: 10.1371/journal.pone.0111988

Flora of China Edita (2013). *Flora of China*. Beijing: Science Press, 39–41.

FuJian Food and Drug Administration (2006). *Chinese Materia Medica Standards of FuJian Province*. Fujian: HaiFeng Press.

Gao, X. M., Pu, J. X., Xiao, W. L., Huang, S. X., Lou, L. G., and Sun, H. D. (2008). Kadcoccilactones K-R, triterpenoids from *Kadsura coccinea*. *Tetrahedron* 64, 11673–11679. doi: 10.1016/j.tet.2008.10.011

Gao, X. M., Pu, J. X., Zhao, Y., Yang, L. B., and Sun, H. D. (2012). Lignans from *Kadsura angustifolia* and *Kadsura coccinea*. *J. Asian Natl. Prod. Res.* 14, 129–134. doi: 10.1080/10286020.2011.637922

Guangdong Food and Drug Administration (2004). *Chinese Materia Medica Standards of Guang Dong Province*. Guangzhou: Guangdong Science and Technology Press.

GuangXi Zhuang Autonomous Region Health Department (1992). *Chinese Materia Medica Standards of Guang Xi Province*. Nanning: Guangxi Science and Technology Press.

Guo, Y. J., Guo, H. J., Liu, J. S., Li, X. W., and Qi, Y. D. (2015). Advances in studies on chemical constituents in *Kadsura longipedunculata* and their pharmacological activities. *Mod. Chin. Med.* 17, 1350–1358.

Hall, T. A. (1999). BioEdit: a user-friendly biological sequence alignment editor and analysis program for Windows 95/98/NT. *Nucl. Acids Symp. Ser.* 41, 95–98.

Han, G. Q., Dai, P., Xue, R., Arison, B. H., Lankin, D. C., and Hwang, S. B. (1992). Dibenzocyclooctadiene lignans with platelet-activating factor (PAF) antagonist activity from *Kadsura heteroclita*. *J. Chin. Pharm. Sci.* 1, 20–27.

Kress, W. J., Wurdack, K. J., Zimmer, E. A., Weigt, L. A., and Janzen, D. H. (2005). Use of DNA barcodes to identify flowering plants. *Proc. Natl. Acad. Sci.* 102, 8369–8374. doi: 10.1073/pnas.0503123102

Kuo, Y. H., Li, S. Y., Wu, M. D., Huang, R. L., Yang, K. L., and Chen, C. F. (1999). A new anti-HBeAg lignan, kadsumarin A, from *Kadsura matsudai* and *Schizandra arisanensis*. *Chem. Pharm. Bull.* 47, 1047–1048. doi: 10.1248/cpb.47.1047

Li, L. N., Xue, H., and Tan, R. (1985). Dibenzocyclooctadiene lignans from roots and stems of *Kadsura coccinea*. *Planta Med.* 51, 297–300. doi: 10.1055/s-2007-969495

Li, Y., Wang, Y., Tai, W., Yang, L., Chen, Y., Chen, C., et al. (2015). Challenges and solutions of pharmacokinetics for efficacy and safety of traditional Chinese medicine. *Curr. Drug Metab.* 16, 756–776. doi: 10.2174/1389200216091512011114223

Liu, H. T., Qi, Y. D., Xu, L. J., Peng, Y., Zhang, B. G., and Xiao, P. G. (2012). Ethnopharmacological investigation of Schisandraceae plants in China. *China J. Chin. Mater. Med.* 37, 1353–1359.

Liu, H. T., Xu, L. J., Peng, Y., Li, R. T., and Xiao, P. G. (2009). Chemical study on ethyl acetate soluble portion of *Kadsura oblongifolia*. *China J. Chin. Mater. Med.* 34, 864–866.

Liu, J. S., Huang, M. F., and Zhou, H. X. (1991). Kadsulignan C and D, two novel lignans from *Kadsura longipedunculata*. *Can. J. Chem.* 69, 1403–1407. doi: 10.1139/v91-207

Liu, J. S., and Li, L. (1995). Kadsulignans L-N, three dibenzocyclooctadiene lignans from *Kadsura coccinea*. *Phytochemistry* 38, 241–245. doi: 10.1016/0031-9422(94)00557-A

Liu, J. S., Qi, Y. D., Lai, H. W., Zhang, J., Jia, X. G., Liu, H., et al. (2014). Genus *Kadsura*, a good source with considerable characteristic chemical constituents and potential bioactivities. *Phytomedicine* 21, 1092–1097. doi: 10.1016/j.phymed.2014.01.015

Liu, J. X., and Pan, Y. P. (1991). Isolation and structures of schisantherin J and schisanlactone F. *Yaoxue Xuebao* 49, 308–312.

Liu, Z., Wang, D., Li, D., and Zhang, S. (2017). Quality evaluation of Juniperus rigida sieb. et zucc. based on phenolic profiles, bioactivity, and hplc fingerprint combined with chemometrics. *Front. Pharmacol.* 8:198. doi: 10.3389/fphar.2017.00198

Ma, W. H., Ma, X. L., Lu, Y., and Chen, D. F. (2009). Lignans and triterpenoids from the stems of *Kadsura induta*. *Helv. Chim. Acta* 92, 709–715. doi: 10.1002/hlca.200800363

Masssart, D. L., Vandeginste, B. G. M., Deming, S. N., Michotte, Y., and Kaufman, L. (1998). *Data Handling in Science and Technology. Chemometrics: A Textbook*. Amsterdam: Elsevier.

Saunders, R. M. (1998). Monograph of *Kadsura* (Schisandraceae). *Syst. Bot. Monogr.* 1:106. doi: 10.2307/25096646

Shen, Y. C., Lin, Y. C., Cheng, Y. B., Chiang, M. Y., Liou, S. S., and Khalil, A. T. (2009). Dibenzocyclooctadiene lignans from *Kadsura philippinensis*. *Phytochemistry* 70, 114–120. doi: 10.1016/j.phytochem.2008.11.005

Song, H. H., Kim, D. Y., Woo, S., Lee, H. K., and Oh, S. R. (2013). An approach for simultaneous determination for geographical origins of Korean Panax ginseng by UPLC-QTOF/MS coupled with OPLS-DA models. *J. Gins. Res.* 37:341. doi: 10.5142/jgr.2013.37.341

Sun, R., Song, H. C., Wang, C. R., Shen, K. Z., Xu, Y. B., Gao, Y. X., et al. (2011). Compounds from *Kadsura angustifolia* with anti-HIV activity. *Bioorg. Med. Chem. Lett.* 21, 961–965. doi: 10.1016/j.bmcl.2010.12.055

Thompson, J. D., Gibson, T. J., Plewniak, F., Jeanmougin, F., and Higgins, D. G. (1997). The Clustal_X windows interface: flexible strategies for multiple sequence alignment aided by quality analysis tools. *Nucleic Acids Res.* 25, 4876–4882. doi: 10.1093/nar/25.24.4876

Wolfe, K. H., Li, W. H., and Sharp, P. M. (1987). Rates of nucleotide substitution vary greatly among plant mitochondrial, chloroplast, and nuclear DNAs. *Proc. Natl. Acad. Sci.* 84, 9054–9058. doi: 10.1073/pnas.84.24.9054

Wu, Z. Y., Raven, P. H., and Hong, D. Y. (2008). *Flora of China*, Vol. 7. Beijing: Science Press.

Xia, J. G., Mandal, R. I, Sinelnikov, V., Broadhurst, D., and Wishart, D. S. (2012). MetaboAnalyst 2.0-a comprehensive server for metabonomic data analysis. *Nucleic Acids Res.* 40, 127–133. doi: 10.1093/nar/gks374

Yang, J. H., Zhang, H. Y., Wen, J., Du, X., Chen, J. H., Zhang, H. B., et al. (2011). Dibenzocyclooctadiene lignans with antineurodegenerative potential from *Kadsura ananosma*. *J. Nat. Prod.* 74, 1028–1035. doi: 10.1021/np1009288

Yao, Y., Chen, H., Xie, L., and Rao, X. (2013). Assessing the temperature influence on the soluble solids content of watermelon juice as measured by visible and near-infrared spectroscopy and chemometrics. *J. Food Eng.* 119, 22–27. doi: 10.1016/j.jfoodeng.2013.04.033

Zhang, J., Chen, M., Dong, X., Lin, R., Fan, J., and Chen, Z. (2015). Evaluation of four commonly used DNA barcoding loci for Chinese medicinal plants of the family schisandraceae. *PLoS One* 10:e0125574. doi: 10.1371/journal.pone.0125574

2

Screening and Identification of Cardioprotective Compounds from Wenxin Keli by Activity Index Approach and *in vivo* Zebrafish Model

Hao Liu[1], Xuechun Chen[1], Xiaoping Zhao[2]*, Buchang Zhao[3], Ke Qian[3], Yang Shi[3], Mirko Baruscotti[4]* and Yi Wang[1]*

[1] Pharmaceutical Informatics Institute, College of Pharmaceutical Sciences, Zhejiang University, Hangzhou, China, [2] School of Basic Medical Sciences, Zhejiang Chinese Medical University, Hangzhou, China, [3] Shandong Danhong Pharmaceutical Co., Ltd., Heze, China, [4] Department of Bioscienze, The PaceLab, University of Milano, Milan, Italy

*Correspondence:
Xiaoping Zhao
zhaoxiaoping@zcmu.edu.cn
Mirko Baruscotti
mirko.baruscotti@unimi.it
Yi Wang
mysky@zju.edu.cn

Wenxin Keli (WXKL) is a widely used Chinese botanical drug for the treatment of arrhythmia, which is consisted of four herbs and amber. In the present study, we analyzed the chemical composition of WXKL using liquid chromatography coupled with high-resolution mass spectrometry (LC-HRMS) to tentatively identify 71 compounds. Through typical separate procession, the total extract of WXKL was divided into fractions for further bioassays. Cardiomyocytes and zebrafish larvae were applied for assessment. *In vivo* arrhythmia model in Cmlc2-GFP transgenic zebrafish was induced by terfenadine, which exhibited obvious reduction of heart rate and occurrence of atrioventricular block. Dynamic beating of heart was recorded by fluorescent microscope and sensitive camera to automatically recognize the rhythm of heartbeat in zebrafish larvae. By integrating the chemical information of WXKL and corresponding bioactivities of these fractions, activity index (AI) of each identified compound was calculated to screen potential active compounds. The results showed that dozens of compounds including ginsenoside Rg_1, ginsenoside Re, notoginsenoside R_1, lobetyolin, and lobetyolinin were contributed to cardioprotective effects of WXKL. The anti-arrhythmic activities of five compounds were further validated in larvae model and mature zebrafish by measuring electrocardiogram (ECG). Our findings provide a successful example for rapid discovery of bioactive compounds from traditional Chinese medicine (TCM) by activity index based approach coupled with *in vivo* zebrafish model.

Keywords: Wenxin Keli, arrhythmia, zebrafish, cardioprotection, drug screen

INTRODUCTION

Natural products have played important roles in healthcare system throughout history and will continue to be served as huge and invaluable resource for the discovery of drug candidates. Traditional Chinese Medicine (TCM), widely used in Eastern Asian countries, has been regarded as an important part of natural products for the therapy of various diseases (Wang et al., 2012). The discovery of bioactive constituents from TCM is the key step in the modernization of TCM.

As a consequence, developing high throughput methods with satisfied sensitivity for identifying active compounds from complex mixtures of TCM is in great demand. In past two decades, many efforts have been made for rapidly screening of compounds from TCM. Artemisinin (qinghaosu) with antimalarial effect is a successful and impressive example as the gift from TCM (Tu, 2011).

Arrhythmia occurs with abnormal beating of heart myocardium, generally represent disorder of ion channels or cardiomyopathy, can be classified with disorders of impulse formation or conduction. Arrhythmia has intricate pathogenesis, in general, most cardiovascular diseases such as heart failure always accompany with arrhythmia. Some types of arrhythmias are capable of triggering cardiac arrest and sudden death. Unfortunately, most of the antiarrhythmic drugs lack specificity and have numerous adverse effects (Page and Roden, 2005). TCMs have multitargets and synergy effect that benefit with those complex diseases (Li et al., 2011). Wenxin Keli (WXKL) is one of the widely used Chinese patent medicine for arrhythmia and heart failure, and is the first Chinese-developed anti-arrhythmic medicine approved by the China Food and Drug Administration (CFDA) and approved by Chinese Pharmacopeia (ChP), and consists of *Codonopsis pilosula, Polygonatum sibiricum, Radix Notoginseng, Nardostachys jatamansi, Succinum*. Researches in decades have proved that WXKL can suppress and prevent cardiac arrhythmias, including atrial and ventricular arrhythmias (Xing et al., 2013; He et al., 2016; Wang et al., 2016; Li et al., 2017), and inhibit multiple ion channels (Chen et al., 2013; Yang et al., 2017), especially the atrial-selective inhibition of sodium-channel current (Burashnikov et al., 2012), and effect on late Na current (Xue et al., 2013).

Arrhythmia is difficult to model *in vitro*, multiple elements may contribute to the final arrhythmia including genetic predisposition, extrinsic injury, environmental exposures, and stochastic processes. Cell-based model unable to fully reveal the pathological process of arrhythmia. On the other hand, using animal model for screening is costly. Zebrafish (*Danio rerio*) has been a model for biomedical research for decades and is ideal for phenotype-based screen in various ways. The generation time of adult fish is about 3 months and it is easy to maintain a great number of zebrafish with low cost and needn't much space. The embryogenesis can be finished in 24 h post-fertilization (hpf) and each pair of fish can produce more than hundred eggs and the mating is not depended on season. More attractively, their embryos are transparent and most organs including the heart, liver, intestine, and kidney develop in 96 hpf that can be clearly visualized (Barros et al., 2008). The larvae can be manipulated in well-plate and live with a little fluid and is permeable to small molecules (Zhang et al., 2003; Kari et al., 2007). These traits make it possible to establish an easy and high-throughput model to assay the effects of drug candidates on internal organs in the live organism. Zebrafish are easy to genetic manipulation to simulate human disease (Asnani and Peterson, 2014). As a developmental and genetic model, zebrafish has been used for anti-cancer compounds discovery, chemicals toxicity assessment, and so on. Zebrafish heart is highly comparable with human heart in structures, functions, signal pathways, and ion channels

(Hu et al., 2000) and is particularly suitable for the study of the cardiovascular system. Here, we used terfenadine, an antihistamine drug but also a potent hERG blocker and QT prolonger (Dhillon et al., 2013), and was reported that had pro-arrhythmic effects (Chaudhari et al., 2013), to induce the heart disturbance of zebrafish.

In the present study, we simultaneously used cell-based and zebrafish-based model to assess the cardioprotective and anti-arrhythmia effect of WXKL and the separated fractions, and combined HRMS and chemometric analysis to identify bioactive compounds from WXKL. H9c2 cell damaged by H_2O_2 were conducted to evaluate the protective activity of fractions. *In vivo* arrhythmic model based on Cmlc2-GFP transgenic (Tg) zebrafish was applied and the heart rate and rhythm of larvae were measured to evaluate pharmacological effects. The cell viability and heart rate recovery of zebrafish were transformed as the bioactivity coefficient and correlated with the compounds constitute in fractions from WXKL to calculate active index of every compounds. The entire process is illustrated in **Figure 1**. With both *in vitro* and *in vivo* assessment and active index calculation, several compounds including ginsenoside Rg$_1$, ginsenoside Re, notoginsenoside R$_1$, lobetyolin, lobetyolinin were selected to validate the activity on larvae and mature fish.

MATERIALS AND METHODS
Materials and Reagents
Wenxin Keli was obtained from Shanxi Buchang Pharmaceutical Co., Ltd (Shanxi, China). Ginsenoside Rg$_1$, Ginsenoside Re, Notoginsenoside R$_1$ were purchased from Winherb Medical Tech. Co., Ltd (Shanghai, China). Lobetyolin was obtained from Push Bio-Tech (Chengdu, China). Extract of codonopsis glycosides was obtained from Dasfbio (Nanjing, China).

HPLC-grade acetonitrile and methanol were purchased from Merck (Darmstadt, Germany). Formic acid (HPLC grade) was purchased from Roe Scientific (Newark, DE, USA). Ethanol was purchased from Zhejiang Changqing Chemical (Hangzhou, China). Deionized water was prepared with an Elga PURELAB flex system (ELGA LabWater, UK).

High-glucose Dulbecco's modified Eagle's medium, fetal bovine serum, trypsin-EDTA and antibiotics (100 U/ml penicillin G and 100 g/mL streptomycin) were obtained from Gibico BRL (Grand Island, NY, USA). Tert-Butyl hydroperoxide solution, Thiazolyl Blue Tereazolium Bromide, Terfenadine, DMSO, N-Phenylthiourea (PTU), and Tricaine were acquired from Sigma–Aldrich (St. Louis, MO, USA).

Apparatus
Tecan infinite M1000 system (Tecan, Zurich, Switzerland). AB TripleTOF 5600^{plus} System (AB SCIEX, Framingham, USA), coupled to a Waters ACQUITY UPLC^{TM} system (Waters, MA, USA). Finnigan LCQ DecaXP^{plus} mass spectrometer equipped with an ESI source (Thermo, MA, USA) coupled to Agilent 1100 liquid chromatography (Agilent, Waldbronn, Germany). Agilent 1200 preparative performance liquid chromatography (Agilent, Waldbronn, Germany). Leica DMI 3000B Fluorescence Inversion Microscope System (Leica Microsystems Inc., USA), Andor Zyla

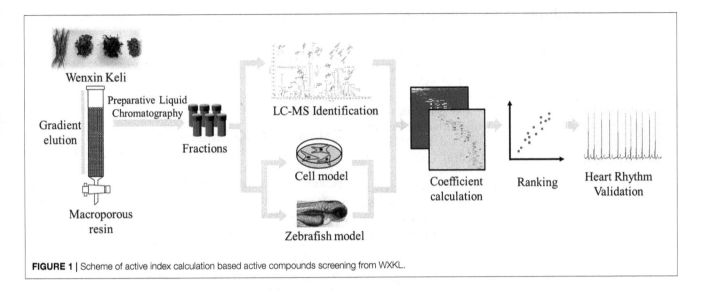

FIGURE 1 | Scheme of active index calculation based active compounds screening from WXKL.

5.5 sCMOS Cameras (Oxford Instruments plc, Tubney Woods, Abingdon, UK). IX-100F Zebrafish system (iWorx Systems, Inc., USA).

Characterization of Major Compounds of WXKL by LC–HRMS

Chemical composition of WXKL was characterized by AB TripleTOF 5600^{plus} System coupled to a Waters Acquity UPLC system. The MS conditions: scan range m/z 100–2,000. Negative ion mode: source voltage was−4.5 kV, and the source temperature was 550°C. Positive ion mode: source voltage was +5.5 kV, and the source temperature was 600°C. The pressure of Gas 1 (Air) and Gas 2 (Air) were set to 50 psi. The pressure of Curtain Gas (N_2) was set to 35 psi. Maximum allowed error was set to ±5 ppm. Declustering potential (DP), 100 V; collision energy (CE), 10 V. For MS/MS acquisition mode, the parameters were almost the same except that the collision energy (CE) was set at 50 ± 20 V, ion release delay (IRD) at 67, ion release width (IRW) at 25. The acquisition parameters for Finnigan LCQ DecaXP^{plus} mass spectrometer were as follows: nebulizing gas, high purity nitrogen (N_2); collusion gas, high-purity helium (He); ion spray voltage:−3 kV; capillary temperature: 350°C; capillary voltage:−15 V; mass range: m/z 100–1,500. Chromatographic separation was carried out on an Agilent Zorbax SB-C18 analytical column (4.6 × 250 mm I.D., 5 μm; Agilent Technologies, USA). The mobile phase consisted of water (A) and acetonitrile (B) both containing 0.05% v/v formic acid. A gradient program was used as follows: 0–5 min, 10% B; 5–15 min, 10–25% B; 15–35 min, 25–35% B; 35–40 min, 35–40% B; 40–45 min, 40–70% B; 45–55 min, 70–95% B; 55–65 min: 95% B. The flow rate was 0.5 mL/min, the column temperature was 30°C, and the injection volume was 20 μL.

Cell Culture and Anti-Oxidation Assays

H9c2 cell were obtained from Cell Bank of the Chinese Academy of Science (Shanghai, China) and cultured in high glucose Dulbecco's modified Eagle's medium supplemented containing 10% fetal bovine serum (FBS) and antibiotics (100 units/mL penicillin and 100 μg/mL streptomycin). The cultures were maintained at 37°C in a humidified atmosphere of 5% CO_2. The anti-oxidation activity of each fraction was determined by tetrazolium based colorimetric assay (MTT assay). Briefly, cells (5×10^4 cell/mL) were seeded to 96-well plates for 24 h and then treated with fractions of WXKL for another 24 h prior to 150 μM H_2O_2 exposure in fresh medium for 3 h, After that, 100 μL 0.5 mg/mL MTT in fresh medium replaced the former medium for 4 h at 37°C. Then, the medium was replaced by 100 μL DMSO and vibrated for 10 min. The cell viabilities of tested fractions were determined by measuring the optimal densities (ODs) of untreated cells (control), the cells exposed to H_2O_2 (model), and the cells pre-incubated with components (tested). The activities of the components were calculated using the following formula: Survival rate% = OD of tested/OD of control. Protection rate% = (OD of model – OD of tested)/(OD of model – OD of control).

Zebrafish Husbandry and Management

Heterozygotes and homozygote transgenic Cmlc2-GFP zebrafish expressing green fluorescent protein (GFP) exclusively in myocardium were provided by Zebrafish Resource Center, Zhejiang University School of Medicine (Hangzhou, China) and maintained according to established standard procedures. Two parent zebrafish were placed separately in a mating box equipped with a separator to protect the eggs from being eaten. Spawning was induced in the morning and embryos from each box were collected and rinsed with system fish water (containing 0.3% Instant Ocean Salt in deionized water with final pH 6.9–7.2, conductivity 450–550 μs/cm, and hardness of about 90 mg/L NaHCO$_3$). The embryos were maintained in the Petri dish with system fish water and transferred to the incubator and incubated at 28°C. This study was granted by the Institutional Animal Care and Use Committee of the Laboratory Animal Center, Zhejiang University. We followed the relevant guidelines from the Laboratory Animal Center of Zhejiang University.

Zebrafish Arrhythmia Model and Drug Incubation

In 24 hpf, larvae with fluorescence were picked under fluorescent microscope and membranes of these larvae were ruptured artificially. Larvae were distributed into a 24-well plate and 8–10 larvae in each well with system fish water added with 0.2 mM N-Phenylthiourea (PTU) and 6 nM methylene blue for treatment. Set groups by wells, including Control, Model, and Treat. Terfenadine was stocked in DMSO at 100 mM, fractions of WXKL was stocked in DMSO at 100 mg/mL and fish water was used to dilute the stock to appropriate concentration. The model group was only given terfenadine, and the treat groups were given terfenadine and corresponding fractions. In 48 hpf incubating, the previous medium was discarded, and added fractions and terfenadine working solution, according to the groups, and filled to 2 mL with fish water medium in each well. The final concentrations of terfenadine was 6 μM. The fractions were diluted to appropriate concentration, mostly 50 μg/mL and some were 25, 12.5, 6.25 μg/mL, depending on the toxicity refer to cell assay.

Heartbeat Recording

In 72 hpf, the beating of zebrafish heart was recorded under florescence with Leica DMI 3000B Fluorescence Inversion Microscope System (Leica). The readout speed of the sCMOS camera was set at 10 frames or 20 frames per second with 4 × 4 pixel binning. L5 filter cube (excitation wave length of 480 nm and emission wave length of 527 nm). One hundred continuous dynamic images were captured by Zyla 5.5 sCMOS Cameras (Andor), subsequently were recognized by Matlab. The area of heart in each picture was measured. The area change with time was supposed to exhibit the heart rhythm. The heartbeats were also recorded manually for accuracy. We calculated the heartbeat of ventricle uniformly.

Calculation of the Activity Indexes

The recovery rate (R_i) of the components were calculated using the following formula:

$$R_i = \frac{B_i - B_M}{B_C - B_M} \times 100\%$$

R_i: normalized heart rate recovery rate of fraction i; B_i: beats of larvae treated by fraction i; B_M: beats of larvae treated by terfenadine; B_C: beats of larvae treated in control group.

The peak area of each compound was normalized according to the following formula:

$$A_j = \frac{A_{i,j}}{\sum_{i=1}^{m} A_{i,j}}$$

A_j: normalized values of peak area of constituent j in fraction i; $A_{i,j}$: peak area of compound j in fraction i; m: the numbers of fractions obtained from whole extract.

The activity indexes of compounds were given by the following formula:

$$AI_j = \sum (R_i \times A_j)$$

AI_j: activity index of compound j.

Zebrafish ECG Measurement

The ECG of zebrafish was measured by IX-100F Zebrafish system (iWorx Systems, Inc., USA). Zebrafish was anesthetic at first and positioned on its back on a fish-bed. Use a paper to gently remove excess water and ensure that the fins are not crossing the belly of the fish. Place the fish-bed with the fish, head to the right, in the chamber and position it under Ag/AgCl surface electrodes. The two electrodes were placed axially along the center-line of the fish's belly and the forward electrode should be placed close to the gills. ECG was recorded by LabScribe v3 software (iWorx System Inc., USA).

Statistical Analysis

The data are expressed as mean ± standard deviation (SD). Parameter comparisons between groups were made with one-way ANOVA analysis of variance. GraphPad prism 7 software (GraphPad Software, USA) was used to carry out statistical analysis. $P < 0.05$ was considered statistically significant.

RESULTS AND DISCUSSION

The Chemical Composition of Wenxin Keli Extract

The main compounds of WXKL include sugar, glycosides, lignans, polyynes, saponins, iridoid glycosides, detailed information is listed in **Table 1**. The negative ion model base peak LC-MS chromatograms of WXKL was showed as **Figure 2**. We collected 71 compounds information of MS/MS and identified 53 compounds primarily, including saponins, phenylpropanoids, polyacetylene, triterpenoid, and others. Twenty-seven compounds of them belong to *Notoginseng*, including notoginsenoside R_1, ginsenoside Rg_1, ginsenoside Re, ginsenoside Ra_3, ginsenoside Rb_1, notoginsenoside R_2, ginsenoside Rc, ginsenoside Rd and so on. Sixteen compounds belong to *Codonopsis*, including tangshenoside V, lobetyolinin, lobetyolin, atractylenolide III, gentisic acid β-D-glucoside, syringin, hexyl 6-O-β-D-glucopyranosyl-β-D-glucopyranoside, hexyl 2-O-β-D-glucopyranosyl-beta-D-glucopyranoside and others. Besides, 5 were identified from *Polygonatum*, and 2 were from *Nard* (**Table 1**).

Evaluating Cardioprotective Effect of Components by Zebrafish Arrhythmia Model

We first performed standard isolation by preparative chromatography to obtain fractions, which were analyzed by Finnigan LCQ DecaXP^plus mass spectrometer. The mass spectrums of every fractions were shown in **Supplementary Material**.

TABLE 1 | Chromatographic and mass spectral data of the constituents of WXKL.

Peak No.	t_R (min)	Identification	Detected (m/z)	Molecular formula	Error (ppm)	MS/MS (m/z)	Source
1	4.427	Raffinose	503.1598	$C_{18}H_{32}O_{16}$	−3.9	383.1174 221.0651 179.0548	
2	4.58	Sucrose or lactose	341.1089	$C_{12}H_{22}O_{11}$	−1.9	179.0555 $[M-H-C_6H_{10}O_5]^-$ 161.0459 $[M-H-C_6H_{12}O_6]^-$ 119.0349 $[M-H-C_6H_{10}O_5-2CH_2O]^-$ 101.0247 $[M-H-C_6H_{10}O_5-2CH_2O-H_2O]^-$	
3	6.533	Difructose anhydride III	323.0976	$C_{12}H_{20}O_{10}$	−2.4	99.0459	
4	8.104	Unknown	326.124	$C_{15}H_{21}NO_7$	−1.6	164.0708 $[M-H-Glc]^-$	
5	9.508	Vanillic acid 4-O-neohesperidoside	475.1446	$C_{20}H_{28}O_{13}$	−2.3	167.0345 $[M-H-Glc-Rha]^-$ 152.011 $[M-H-2C_6H_{11}O_5]^-$ 108.0218 $[M-H-2C_6H_{11}O_5-CO_2]^-$	HJ
6	10.07	Gentisic acid β-D-glucoside	315.0718	$C_{13}H_{16}O_9$	−1.1	153.0182 $[M-H-Glc]^-$ 152.0110 $[M-H-Glc-H]^-$ 109.0289 $[M-H-Glc-CO_2]^-$ 108.0217 $[M-H-Glc-H-CO_2]^-$	DS
7	10.35	Unknown	375.1287	$C_{16}H_{24}O_{10}$	−2.6	213.0757 $[M-H-Glc]^-$ 169.0860 $[M-H-Glc-CO_2]^-$ 151.0752 $[M-H-Glc-CO_2-H_2O]^-$ 125.0607 $[M-H-Glc-C_3H_4O_3]^-$	
8	13.103	Neochlorogenic acid	353.0876	$C_{16}H_{18}O_9$	−0.6	191.0560 $[M-H-C_9H_6O_3]^-$ 179.0344 $[M-H-C_7H_{10}O_5]^-$ 173.0456 $[M-H-C_9H_8O_4]^-$ 135.0453 $[M-H-C_8H_{10}O_7]^-$ 107.0503 $[M-H-C_{10}H_{14}O_7]^-$	DS
9	14.29	Syringin	371.1339	$C_{17}H_{24}O_9$	−2.3	417.1396 $[M-H+FA]^-$	DS
10	15.697	Codonopilate A Or Codonopilate B	718.2728	$C_{49}H_{82}O_3$	None	598.2277 335.1248 303.1002	DS
11	15.917	Chlorogenic acid	353.0877	$C_{16}H_{18}O_9$	−0.3	191.0557 $[M-H-C_9H_6O_3]^-$ 179.0352 $[M-H-C_7H_{10}O_5]^-$ 173.0449 $[M-H-C_9H_8O_4]^-$ 135.0446 $[M-H-C_8H_{10}O_7]^-$	DS
12	16.263	Cryptochlorogenic acid	353.0873	$C_{16}H_{18}O_9$	−1.4	191.0560 $[M-H-C_9H_6O_3]^-$ 179.0344 $[M-H-C_7H_{10}O_5]^-$ 173.0456 $[M-H-C_9H_8O_4]^-$ 135.0453 $[M-H-C_8H_{10}O_7]^-$ 107.0503 $[M-H-C_{10}H_{14}O_7]^-$	DS
13	17.038	Unknown	779.2739	$C_{37}H_{48}O_{18}$	−3.7	437.1571 $[M-H-Glc-C_6H_{12}O_6]^-$	HJ
14	17.529	Vina-ginsenoside R_{15}	815.2829	$C_{33}H_{52}O_{23}$	0.3	861.3002 $[M-H+FA]^-$ 653.4300 $[M-H-Glc]^-$ 491.3754 $[M-H-2Glc]^-$	SQ
15	17.562	Unknown	617.2197	$C_{31}H_{38}O_{13}$	−6.9	663.2250 $[M-H+FA]^-$ 437.1574 $[M-H-C_6H_{12}O_6]^-$ 365.1357 293.1143	
16	17.874	Unknown	455.1662	$C_{32}H_{24}O_3$	2	293.1151 $[M-H-Glc]^-$	

(Continued)

TABLE 1 | Continued

Peak No.	t_R (min)	Identification	Detected (m/z)	Molecular formula	Error (ppm)	MS/MS (m/z)	Source
17	19.878	Hexyl 6-O-β-D-glucopyranosyl-β-D-glucopyranoside	425.2017	$C_{18}H_{34}O_{11}$	−2.7	471.2076 [M-H+FA]$^-$ 179.0560 [M-H-$C_{12}H_{22}O_5$]$^-$ 143.0327 [M-H-$C_6H_{14}O$-$C_6H_{12}O_6$]$^-$ 101.0243 [M-H-$C_{12}H_{20}O_{10}$]$^-$	DS
18	20.04	Deoxyloganic Acid	359.1342	$C_{16}H_{24}O_9$	−1.5	197.081 [M-H-Glc]$^-$ 153.0917 [M-H-Glc-CO_2]$^-$ 135.0811 [M-H-Glc-CO_2-H_2O]$^-$	DS or HJ
19	20.132	Hexyl 2-O-β-D-glucopyranosyl-β-D-glucopyranoside	425.2017	$C_{18}H_{34}O_{11}$	−2.7	263.1492 [M-H-$C_6H_{10}O_5$]$^-$ 179.0560 [M-H-$C_{12}H_{22}O_5$]$^-$ 143.0327 [M-H-$C_6H_{14}O$-$C_6H_{12}O_6$]$^-$ 101.0243 [M-H-$C_{12}H_{20}O_{10}$]$^-$	
20	20.678	Tangshenoside V	469.1348	$C_{21}H_{26}O_{12}$	−0.7	325.0923 [M-H-$C_6H_8O_4$]$^-$ 265.0717 [M-H-$C_8H_{12}O_6$]$^-$ 235.0608 [M-H-$C_9H_{14}O_7$]$^-$ 205.05 [M-H-$C_{10}H_{16}O_8$]$^-$ 163.0396 [M-H-$C_{12}H_{18}O_9$]$^-$ 145.0289 [M-H-$C_{12}H_{18}O_9$-H_2O]$^-$ 99.0465 [M-H-$C_{15}H_{18}O_8$-CO_2]$^-$	DS
21	21.697	Unknown	313.1649	$C_{16}H_{26}O_6$	−2.4	359.1688 [M-H+FA]$^-$	
22	22.033	Lobetyolinin	557.2232	$C_{26}H_{38}O_{13}$	−1.4	603.2292 [M-H+FA]- 323.0984 [M-H-$C_{14}H_{18}O_3$]$^-$ 233.1166 [M-H-$C_{12}H_{20}O_{10}$]$^-$ 221.0661 [M-H-$C_{18}H_{24}O_6$]$^-$ 179.0554 [M-H-$C_{20}H_{26}O_7$]$^-$ 161.045 [M-H-$C_{20}H_{28}O_8$]$^-$ 119.0347 [M-H-$C_{18}H_{30}O_{12}$]$^-$	DS
23	22.621	20-(β-D-glucopyranosyloxy)-ginsenoside Rf or Vina-ginsenoside R_4	961.5399	$C_{48}H_{82}O_{19}$	2.2	1007.5456 [M-H+FA]$^-$ 799.493[M-H-Glc]$^-$ 637.4365[M-H-2Glc]$^-$	SQ
24	23.362	Notoginsenoside R_1	931.5281	$C_{47}H_{80}O_{18}$	1	977.534 [M-H+FA]$^-$ 799.4936 [M-H-Xyl]$^-$ 769.4832 [M-H-Glc]$^-$ 637.4373 [M-H-Xyl-Glc]$^-$ 475.3832 [M-H-Xyl-2Glc]$^-$	SQ
25	24.286	Isoheptanol 2(S)-O-β-D-xylopyranosyl-(1→6)-O-β-D-glucopyranoside Or isoheptanol 2(S)-O-β-D-apiofuranosyl-(1→6)-O-β-D-glucopyranoside Or n-hexanol O-rutinoside	409.2071	$C_{18}H_{34}O_{10}$	−2	276.0881 [M-H-133]$^-$ 217.0494 [M-H-192]$^-$	HJ
26	24.923	Ginsenoside Re	945.5443	$C_{48}H_{82}O_{18}$	1.5	991.5504 [M-H+FA]$^-$ 783.4995 [M-H-Glc]$^-$ 637.4377 [M-H-Glc-Rha]$^-$	SQ
27	25.073	Ginsenoside Rg_1	799.4859	$C_{42}H_{72}O_{14}$	1.2	845.4913 [M-H+FA]$^-$ 637.4392 [M-H-Glc]$^-$ 475.3822 [M-H-2Glc]$^-$ 391.2879 [M-H-2Glc-C_6H_{12}]$^-$	SQ

(Continued)

TABLE 1 | Continued

Peak No.	t_R (min)	Identification	Detected (m/z)	Molecular formula	Error (ppm)	MS/MS (m/z)	Source
28	25.963	Lobetyolin	395.1705	$C_{20}H_{28}O_8$	−1.6	441.1765 [M-H+FA]$^-$ 233.1180 [M-H-Glc]$^-$ 215.1060 [M-H-Glc-H$_2$O]$^-$ 185.0968 [M-H-Glc-H$_2$O-CH$_2$O]$^-$ 159.0813 [M-H-Glc-H$_2$O-C$_3$H$_4$O]$^-$ 143.0711 [M-H-Glc-C$_7$H$_6$]$^-$ 125.0603 [M-H-Glc-C$_7$H$_6$-H$_2$O]$^-$	DS
29	27.235	2,2,6-trimethylcyclohexanone	187.0982	$C_9H_{16}O_4$	3.3		GS
30	28.512	Unknown	445.0772	$C_{21}H_{18}O_{11}$	−1	269.0448 [M-H-C$_6$H$_8$O$_6$]$^-$	DS or HJ
31	28.796	Notoginsenoside G	959.5233	$C_{48}H_{80}O_{19}$	1.2	1005.5306 [M-H+FA]$^-$	SQ
32	30.678	14-hydroxy-lactarolide A	297.1338	$C_{15}H_{22}O_6$	−1.9	343.1383 [M-H+FA]$^-$ 235.1724 [M-H-62]$^-$ 191.1431 [M-H-106(62+46)]$^-$	
33	31.183	Vina-ginsenoside R$_2$	827.4801	$C_{43}H_{72}O_{15}$	0.3	781.4769 [M-H-HCOOH]$^-$	SQ
34	33.446	Madecassic acid Or terminolic acid	503.3373	$C_{30}H_{48}O_6$	−1	459.3116 [M-H-CO$_2$]$^-$	
35	33.772	Unknown	419.1448	$C_{32}H_{20}O$	1.6		
36	34.161	Unknown	401.135	$C_{32}H_{18}$	3.6		
37	35.266	Notoginsenoside Fa	1239.6392	$C_{59}H_{100}O_{27}$	1	1285.645 [M-H+FA]$^-$ 1107.603 [M-H- C$_5$H$_8$O$_4$]$^-$ 945.551 [M-H- C$_5$H$_8$O$_4$-Glc]$^-$ 783.4893 [M-H- C$_5$H$_8$O$_4$-2Glc]$^-$ 621.4405 [M-H- C$_5$H$_8$O$_4$-3Glc]$^-$	SQ
38	35.949	Unknown	276.0879	$C_{14}H_{15}NO_5$	0.6		
39	36.816	Ginsenoside Ra$_3$	1239.6398	$C_{59}H_{100}O_{27}$	1.5	1285.6455 [M-H+FA]$^-$ 1107.603 [M-H- C$_5$H$_8$O$_4$]$^-$ 945.551 [M-H- C$_5$H$_8$O$_4$-Glc]$^-$ 783.4893 [M-H- C$_5$H$_8$O$_4$-2Glc]$^-$ 621.4405 [M-H- C$_5$H$_8$O$_4$-3Glc]$^-$	SQ
40	37.686	Chikusetsusaponin L$_5$ Or Chikusetsusaponin LM$_2$	901.517	$C_{46}H_{78}O_{17}$	0.4	947.5234 [M-H+FA]$^-$ 769.4828 [M-H-132]$^-$	SQ
41	38.845	Notoginsenoside R$_4$	1239.6381	$C_{59}H_{100}O_{27}$	0.1	1285.645 [M-H+FA]$^-$ 1107.603 [M-H- C$_5$H$_8$O$_4$]$^-$ 945.551 [M-H- C$_5$H$_8$O$_4$Glc]$^-$ 783.4893 [M-H- C$_5$H$_8$O$_4$-2Glc]$^-$ 621.4405 [M-H- C$_5$H$_8$O$_4$-3Glc]$^-$	SQ
42	39.161	Ginsenoside Rb$_1$	1107.5963	$C_{54}H_{92}O_{23}$	0.6	1153.6012 [M-H+FA]$^-$ 1061.5274 [M-H-46]$^-$ 945.554 [M-H-Glc]$^-$	SQ
43	39.855	Notoginsenoside R$_2$	769.4742	$C_{41}H_{70}O_{13}$	−0.2	815.4801 [M-H+FA]$^-$ 637.4367 [M-H-Xyl]$^-$ 619.4250 [M-H-Xyl-H$_2$O]$^-$ 475.3813 [M-H-Xyl-Glc]$^-$ 391.2869 [M-H-Xyl-Glc-C$_6$H$_{12}$]$^-$	SQ
44	39.923	Polygonatoside D or isomer	899.465	$C_{45}H_{72}O_{18}$	0.5	753.2310 [M-H-Rha]$^-$ 737.4188 [M-H-Glc]$^-$ 429.2190 [M-H-2Glc-Rha]$^-$	HJ

(Continued)

TABLE 1 | Continued

Peak No.	t_R (min)	Identification	Detected (m/z)	Molecular formula	Error (ppm)	MS/MS (m/z)	Source
45	41.725	S-ginsenoside Rg$_2$	783.4894	$C_{42}H_{72}O_{13}$	−0.8	829.4958 [M-H+FA]$^-$ 637.4348 [M-H-Rha]$^-$ 475.3809 [M-H-Rha-Glc]$^-$	SQ
46	42.073	Ginsenoside Rc	1077.585	$C_{53}H_{90}O_{22}$	−0.1	1123.5909 [M-H+FA]$^-$ 945.5531 [M-H- $C_5H_8O_4$]$^-$ 783.4964 [M-H- $C_5H_8O_4$-Glc]$^-$ 621.4409 [M-H- $C_5H_8O_4$-2Glc]$^-$ 459.3871 [M-H- $C_5H_8O_4$-3Glc]$^-$	SQ
47	42.147	R-ginsenoside Rg$_2$	783.4896	$C_{42}H_{72}O_{13}$	−0.5		SQ
48	42.422	Ginsenoside Rb$_2$	1077.585	$C_{53}H_{90}O_{22}$	−0.1	1123.5909 [M-H+FA]$^-$	SQ
49	42.533	(20R)-Ginsenoside Rh$_1$	637.4309	$C_{36}H_{62}O_9$	−1.9	683.4371 [M-H+FA]$^-$ 475.3793 [M-H-Glc]$^-$	SQ
50	43.06	Ginsenoside Rb$_3$	1077.585	$C_{53}H_{90}O_{22}$	−0.1	1123.5909 [M-H+FA]$^-$	SQ
51	43.469	Ginsenoside Rh$_1$	637.4308	$C_{36}H_{62}O_9$	−2.1	683.4374 [M-H+FA]$^-$ 475.3793 [M-H-Glc]$^-$	SQ
52	43.835	Unknown	489.3205	$C_{29}H_{46}O_6$	−3.4	535.3265 [M-H+FA]$^-$	
53	44.41	5,6,9-trihydroxy-octadec-7-enoic acid	329.2332	$C_{18}H_{34}O_5$	−0.4	229.1443 211.1338	DS
54	44.788	Ginsenoside Rd	945.5423	$C_{48}H_{82}O_{18}$	−0.6	991.5476 [M-H+FA]$^-$ 783.4963 [M-H-Glc]$^-$ 621.4396 [M-H-2Glc]$^-$	SQ
55	45.359	Ginsenoside F$_1$	637.4308	$C_{36}H_{62}O_9$	−2.1	683.4374 [M-H+FA]$^-$ 475.3793 [M-H-Glc]$^-$	SQ
56	46.429	Unknown	677.2456	$C_{33}H_{42}O_{15}$	0.7		
57	46.468	Unknown	501.3214	$C_{30}H_{46}O_6$	−1.5	547.3264 [M-H+FA]$^-$	
58	47.455	Notoginsenside T$_5$	751.4631	$C_{41}H_{68}O_{12}$	−0.9	797.4692 [M-H+FA]$^-$ 619.4254 [M-H- $C_5H_8O_4$]$^-$	DS
59	47.995	Aractylenolide III	247.1343	$C_{15}H_{20}O_3$	1.3		DS
60	48.41	Unknown	487.3042	$C_{29}H_{44}O_6$	−4.7	533.3104 [M-H+FA]$^-$ 441.3025 [M-H-46]$^-$	
61	48.933	20(S)-Ginsenoside Rg$_3$	783.4897	$C_{42}H_{72}O_{13}$	−0.4	829.4962 [M-H+FA]$^-$ 621.4415 [M-H-Glc]$^-$ 459.3859 [M-H-2Glc]$^-$	SQ
62	48.975	Ginsenoside Rh$_4$ Or Ginsenoside Rk$_3$	619.4192	$C_{36}H_{60}O_8$	−3.8	665.4272 [M-H+FA]$^-$	SQ
63	49.098	20(R)-Ginsenoside Rg$_3$	783.4895	$C_{42}H_{72}O_{13}$	−0.7	829.4962 [M-H+FA]$^-$ 621.4415 [M-H-Glc]$^-$ 459.3856 [M-H-2Glc]$^-$	SQ
64	49.71	3-(4′-hydroxy-benzyl)-5,7-dihydroxy-6,8-dimethyl-chroman-4-one	313.1078	$C_{18}H_{18}O_5$	−1.1	207.0649 [M-H-C_7H_6O]$^-$ 205.0502 [M-H-C_7H_8O]$^-$ 179.0700 [M-H-$C_9H_{10}O$]$^-$ 165.0549 [M-H-$C_9H_8O_2$]$^-$	HJ
65	50.172	Unknown	485.326	$C_{30}H_{46}O_5$	−2.6	531.3322 [M-H+FA]$^-$ 441.3002 [M-H-CO_2]$^-$	
66	50.573	Lobetyol	247.1342	$C_{14}H_{18}O$	0.9	247.1342 [M-H+FA]$^-$	DS
67	50.819	Nardosinone	249.1497	$C_{15}H_{22}O_3$	0.3	295.1550 [M-H+FA]$^-$	GS
68	52.662	Unknown	457.2949	$C_{28}H_{42}O_5$	−2.3	295.2452 [M-H-Glc]$^-$	

(Continued)

TABLE 1 | Continued

Peak No.	t_R (min)	Identification	Detected (m/z)	Molecular formula	Error (ppm)	MS/MS (m/z)	Source
69	52.921	Ginsenoside Rk$_1$ Or Ginsenoside Rg$_5$	765.4785	$C_{42}H_{70}O_{12}$	−1.2	811.4851 [M-H+FA]$^-$ 603.4289 [M-H-Glc]$^-$ 279.1597 [M-H-3Glc]$^-$	SQ
70	53.449	Unknown	455.2793	$C_{28}H_{40}O_5$	−2.2	501.2858 [M-H+FA]$^-$ 411.2912 [M-H-CO$_2$]$^-$	
71	55.169	Unknown	499.3056	$C_{30}H_{44}O_6$	−1.8	545.3107 [M-H+FA]$^-$ 455.3182 [M-H-CO$_2$]$^-$ 411.3280 [M-H-2CO$_2$]$^-$	

DS, Codonopsis pilosula; HJ, Polygonatum sibiricum; SQ, Radix Notoginseng, GS, Nardostachys jatamansi.

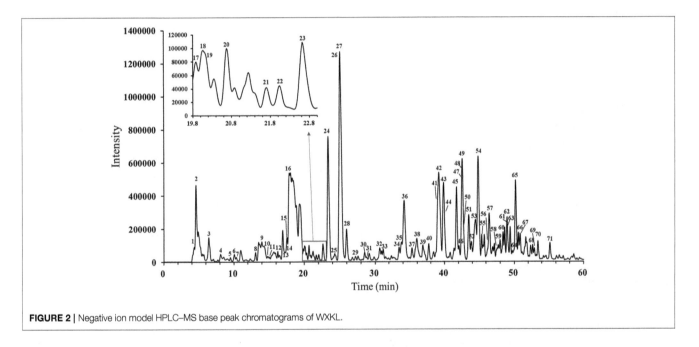

FIGURE 2 | Negative ion model HPLC–MS base peak chromatograms of WXKL.

Oxidative stress plays a key role in the pathogenesis of various diseases (Furukawa et al., 2004). These fractions were then evaluated the protective activity on H9c2 cell damaged by H$_2$O$_2$. The toxicity of all fractions were tested at first, and the safe concentration of most fraction were 50 μg/mL, and some were 25/12.5/6.25 μg/mL to insure no toxicity. The cell viability with these fractions treated were shown in **Supplementary Material**.

Zebrafish (*D. rerio*) has been an ideal model for drug screening (Goldsmith, 2004). There have been many applications of zebrafish as a high-throughput screening model and cardiotoxicity risk assessment of drug candidates (Wen et al., 2012; Zhu et al., 2014). Here we used Cmlc2-GFP Tg zebrafish as the base. This transgenic line expressing GFP exclusively in myocardium driven by promoter cmlc2 (cardiac myosin light chain 2 gene) (Huang et al., 2003). Terfenadine has been reported can induce QT prolongation in zebrafish and guinea pig (Milan et al., 2006; Lu et al., 2012; Chaudhari et al., 2013), which is

associated with ventricular tachyarrhythmia (Gowda et al., 2004). Terfenadine causes QT prolongation in adult zebrafish, also demonstrate in zebrafish embryos (Langheinrich et al., 2003).

As shown in **Figure 3**, terfenadine had less effect on the structure of the heart (**Figure 3A**) but influenced the rhythm of beat obviously (**Figure 3B**). The rhythm of heartbeat was exhibited through the area change of heart analyzed by Matlab. It's obvious that the control groups performed fast and regular rhythm (about 180 beats/min), and in the model groups, the heart rate were down to 80–100 beats/min with irregular heartbeats after incubated with terfenadine for 24 h, and some showed typically atrioventricular block (Peal et al., 2011), while co-incubated with WXKL stabilized the rhythm (**Figure 3B, Supplementary Videos**). And WXKL and its fractions performed varying affection on heart rate. Fraction 1 and Fraction 2 and former part of Fraction 3 showed beneficial effect on heart rate, while the remaining parts of Fraction 3 lowered the rate even more (**Figure 3C**).

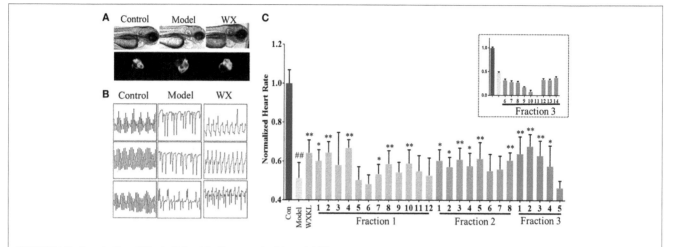

FIGURE 3 | Cardioprotection of Wenxin Keli and fractions on zebrafish model. **(A)** Represent images of heart structures in zebrafish under bright-field and fluorescence. **(B)** Represent images of heartbeat rhythm of different groups exhibited by Matlab. **(C)** Normalized heart rate of zebrafish larvae influenced by WXKL fractions. $n \geq 8$. $^{\#\#}P < 0.01$ vs. control, $^{*}P < 0.05$, $^{**}P < 0.01$ vs. model.

Screening Active Compounds by Activity Indexes Calculation and Ranking

Activity index (AI) of each compound was calculated according to mathematical formulae proposed in our previous study. It was assumed that the compounds with positive activity index might be active and has contribution to the activity of whole formula to some extent (Wang et al., 2014). The relative intensities of the identified compounds in each fraction were visually presented in a heatmap (**Figure 4A**). After multiply corresponding bioactivity coefficient (i.e., heart rate recovery rate) of each fraction, the heatmap was converted into a bio-active map, and the red and gray color represent good or bad effect, respectively. The calculated scores were exhibited as histogram on the right (**Figure 4B**). The detailed scores were listed in **Supplementary Material**. We plot compounds with the effect on cardiomyocytes and the heart rate of zebrafish (**Figure 4C**), the compounds in upper right region represented a better activity.

Validation of Active Compounds

According to the scores, Ginsenoside Rg_1, Ginsenoside Re, Notoginsenoside R_1, Lobetyolin, Lobetyolinin were selected to validate activity, considering the available. Lobetyolinin was prepared and enriched by ourselves from commercial codonopsis glycosides. Their toxicity was confirmed before. We increased the dosage of terfenadine and shortened the incubation time as an acute injury model to improve significance when validating the active of pure compounds by reason of the pure compounds were not strong enough to exhibit activity in original method. After pre-treated with compounds ($50\,\mu M$) for $24\,h$, the larvae were treated with $15\,\mu M$ terfenadine for $2\,h$ and recorded heartbeat under fluorescent. As the consequence, the heart rate of larvae was recovered in varying degree (**Figure 5A**). Ginsenoside Rg_1 and lobetyolinin exhibited better activities. Meanwhile, ECG of adult zebrafish treated with compound was measured. The heart rate of normal zebrafish was around 100 beats/min, and after treated with $25\,\mu M$ terfenadine for $1\,h$, the heart rate was

down and occurred irregular rhythm (**Figure 5B**). Lobetyolinin pre-treated for $6\,h$ recovered the heart rate and represent electrocardiograms were showed as **Figure 5C**.

DISCUSSION

A few researches described the chemical components of WXKL. Wang et al. established a database for the chemical components of the five herbs in WXKL for active compounds predication (Wang et al., 2017), however, all the compounds were acquired from database refer to the herb not the real composition of the patent drug, and the chemical components probably change during the manufactory process. We analyzed the extract of WXKL directly with LC-HRMS at beginning, but the analytic method we established still has limitation. Actually, the compounds in Fraction 2 weren't separated clearly and seemed have low mass spectrum response, which make this portion of fractions have similar composition. Compounds identified from *Nard* and *Succinum* were rare, maybe for the reason that the main constitutes of *Nard* and *Succinum* are volatile oil, which are more appropriate analyzed by gas chromatography–mass spectrometry (GC–MS). According to report, the extracts of *Nard* significantly blocked I_{Na} and I_{Ito} of rat ventricular myocytes (Liu et al., 2009). The active compounds we predicted especially on the top are minor composition were difficult to get standard substance for bioactive assays except ginsenoside Re, ginsenoside Rg_1 and notoginsenoside R_1, which limited the further validation. We attempted to isolate substances such as lobetyolinin from extracts of *C. pilosula*. It has reported that ginsenoside Re has negative effect on cardiac contractility and autorhythmicity (Peng et al., 2012), ginsenoside Rg_1 prolonged ventricular refractoriness and repolarization (Wu et al., 1995), notoginsenoside R_1 has protective effects on cardiovascular system (Li et al., 2014). Related activity of lobetyolin has few reports.

Drug-induced model is a common approach, verapamil and terfenadine were applied to develop a zebrafish heart failure

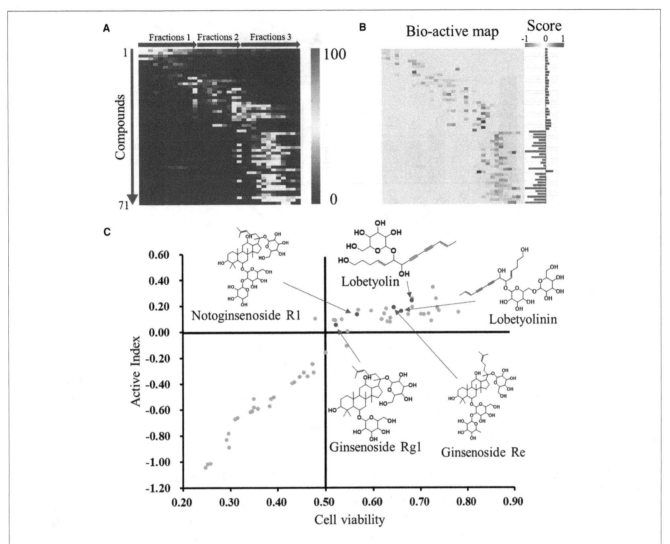

FIGURE 4 | Identification of active compounds by coefficient ranking. **(A)** Heatmap for relative content of identified compounds in each WXKL fractions. **(B)** Bio-active map was converted from content map and corresponding bioactivity coefficient in each fraction, and active indexes of identified compounds were calculated and showed on the right. **(C)** Compounds were plot by cell protection and bio-active scores and mass spectrum of several compounds on top. X axis means the contribution of compounds to the cardiomyocytes protection. Y axis means the AI of compounds.

model (Zhu et al., 2018). QT prolonging is a typical characteristic of arrhythmia which also can be induced by cisapride and astemizole besides terfenadine (Langheinrich et al., 2003). It has to be considered that drug treated by oral may cause unstable effect, so design rational approaches of drug treatment is necessary. Chaudhari et al. performed parenteral administration of terfenadine with different doses and recorded ECG to assess drug-induced QTc prolongation in zebrafish. Those with the doses above 1 mg/kg were observed some proarrhythmic effects such as Ventricular Premature Contractions, Ventricular Tachycardia, Atrio-Ventricular (AV) Block, and Torsade de pointes (TdP) (Chaudhari et al., 2013). However, the cardiotoxic of terfenadine is possible not associated with QT prolongation and the occurrence of TdPs, but with marked widening of the QRS complex and other cardiac arrhythmias (Hondeghem et al., 2011). It's reported that terfenadine caused non-TdP like VT/VF

by slowing of conduction via blockade of I_{Na} (Lu et al., 2012). In addition, transgenic zebrafish lines are also feasible to avoid the unstable results of drug induce method. Several mutants were identified that exhibited arrhythmias (Milan and Macrae, 2008) like the bradycardic line *slo mo*, with variable degrees of sinoatrial or atrioventricular heart block (Baker et al., 1997). Besides, some mutants exhibited recessive lethal phenotypes included mutants such as *tremblor* (Langenbacher et al., 2005), *island beat* (Rottbauer et al., 2001), and *reggae* (Hassel et al., 2008). The Tg line that express fluorescent proteins (e.g., Cmlc2-GFP) was beneficial for optical measurement from the other perspective.

ECG (electrocardiogram) abnormalities is the critical characteristic of arrhythmia. Several ECG measurement equipments for zebrafish have been developed, and mostly of them consist of electrode or micropipette and electrical filter (Milan et al., 2006; Chaudhari et al., 2013; Dhillon et al.,

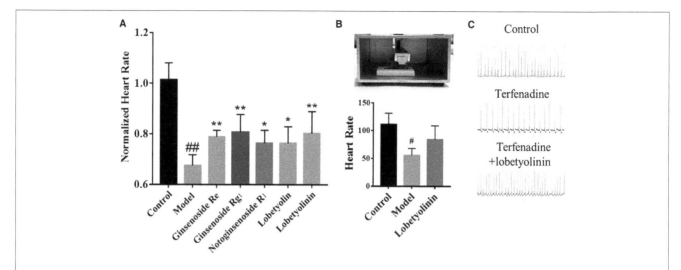

FIGURE 5 | (A) Normalized heart rate of zebrafish larvae treated with compounds. $n = 7$. $^{\#}P < 0.05$ vs. control, $^{\#\#}P < 0.01$ vs. control, $^{*}P < 0.05$, $^{**}P < 0.01$ vs. model. **(B)** The schematic of ECG measurement, and the result of different group. $n = 3$. **(C)** Represent electrocardiograms of adult zebrafish treated in different groups.

2013). Detection of 3 dpf larva is also possible (Chi et al., 2008). However, the invasive injury and anesthesia could cause damage to the individual. As for high throughput screening, a fast and stable method of ECG measurement is required, but existing devices seem not compatibility. Computerized recognition of ECGs has become a well-established practice, assisting to classify long-term ECG recordings, which suggests new approaches like Machine Learning are able to recognize and classify the rhythm signal. For instance, automatic classification of single-lead ECG signals with Deep learning (also known as unsupervised feature learning or representation learning) was established (Singh et al., 2018). A new semi-supervised approach based on deep learning and active learning for classification of electrocardiogram signals is proposed (Sayantan et al., 2018). Though several algorithms have focused on automatically classifying heartbeats in ECGs, the scalability failure to handle large intra-class variations wherein the robustness of many existing ECG classification techniques remains limited. We have acquired plenty of dynamic images of different conditions of heartbeat and attempt to establish the relationship between waveform and define characteristic to classify the phenotype. Rhythm classify method based on image processing will be a non-invasive measurement of heart regulation.

In conclusion, we identified 71 compounds from extract of WXKL by LC-HRMS, and firstly utilized a transgenic zebrafish cmlc2-GFP induced by terfenadine as an animal model for screening active compounds from WXKL. After recording heartbeat that affected by fractions under a fluorescent microscope, a convenient image process was applied to exhibit the rhythm of heartbeat. Subsequently, we integrated chemometric analysis with bio-activity *in vivo* model of corresponding fractions and calculated active index of identified compounds. Ginsenoside Rg$_1$, ginsenoside Re, notoginsenoside R$_1$, lobetyolin, and lobetyolinin were selected to validate activity.

Measurement of ECG of adult zebrafish also performed as a complement. Our results suggest that integrate bio-assay and substantial analysis to perform active index calculation improve the efficiency of active compounds discovering from TCM, and this approach is possible to be applied for the research of complex diseases.

AUTHOR CONTRIBUTIONS

HL and XC designed and performed the experimental work. BZ, KQ, and YS provided the WXKL patent drug and related herb and extract. MB guided the theory of cardiac electrophysiology and pharmacology. All authors proofread the paper and provided feedback.

FUNDING

This study was supported by the National Key Scientific and Technological Project of China (grant 2017ZX09301012), and National Natural Science Foundation of China (No. 81774151, No. 81822047), the Fundamental Research Funds for the Central Universities (2016FZA7016).

SUPPLEMENTARY MATERIAL

Supplementary Table 1 | Bioactive-coefficient ranking of identified compounds.

Supplementary Figure 1 | LC-MS chromatograms of fractions of WXKL. Some fractions were not enough for analysis so were not showed here.

Supplementary Figure 2 | Anti-oxidation activity of WXKL fractions. **(A)** Protection rate of all fractions of WXKL, $n = 3$. **(B)** Dose-response of selected fractions that has protective activity.

Supplementary Figure 3 | Dose effect of Terfenadine on heart rate of zebrafish. **P < 0.01 vs. control. n = 8.

Video 1 | Side view of heart of zebrafish larva in normal group.

Video 2 | Vertical view of heart of zebrafish larva in normal group.

Video 3 | Side view of heart of zebrafish larva in terfenadine group.

Video 4 | Vertical view of heart of zebrafish larva in terfenadine group.

Video 5 | Side view of heart of zebrafish larva in WXKL group.

Video 6 | Vertical view of heart of zebrafish larva in WXKL group.

REFERENCES

Asnani, A., and Peterson, R. T. (2014). The zebrafish as a tool to identify novel therapies for human cardiovascular disease. *Dis. Model. Mech.* 7, 763–767. doi: 10.1242/dmm.016170

Baker, K., Warren, K. S., Yellen, G., and Fishman, M. C. (1997). Defective "pacemaker" current (Ih) in a zebrafish mutant with a slow heart rate. *Proc. Natl. Acad. Sci. U.S.A.* 94, 4554–4559. doi: 10.1073/pnas.94.9.4554

Barros, T. P., Alderton, W. K., Reynolds, H. M., Roach, A. G., and Berghmans, S. (2008). Zebrafish: an emerging technology for in vivo pharmacological assessment to identify potential safety liabilities in early drug discovery. *Br. J. Pharmacol.* 154, 1400–1413. doi: 10.1038/bjp.2008.249

Burashnikov, A., Petroski, A., Hu, D., Barajas-Martinez, H., and Antzelevitch, C. (2012). Atrial-selective inhibition of sodium-channel current by Wenxin Keli is effective in suppressing atrial fibrillation. *Heart Rhythm* 9, 125–131. doi: 10.1016/j.hrthm.2011.08.027

Chaudhari, G. H., Chennubhotla, K. S., Chatti, K., and Kulkarni, P. (2013). Optimization of the adult zebrafish ECG method for assessment of drug-induced QTc prolongation. *J. Pharmacol. Toxicol. Methods* 67, 115–120. doi: 10.1016/j.vascn.2013.01.007

Chen, Y., Li, Y., Guo, L., Chen, W., Zhao, M., Gao, Y., et al. (2013). Effects of wenxin keli on the action potential and L-type calcium current in rats with transverse aortic constriction-induced heart failure. *Evid. Based Complement. Alternat. Med.* 2013:572078. doi: 10.1155/2013/572078

Chi, N. C., Shaw, R. M., Jungblut, B., Huisken, J., Ferrer, T., Arnaout, R., et al. (2008). Genetic and physiologic dissection of the vertebrate cardiac conduction system. *PLoS Biol.* 6:e109. doi: 10.1371/journal.pbio.0060109

Dhillon, S. S., Doro, E., Magyary, I., Egginton, S., Sik, A., and Muller, F. (2013). Optimisation of embryonic and larval ECG measurement in zebrafish for quantifying the effect of QT prolonging drugs. *PLoS ONE* 8:e60552. doi: 10.1371/journal.pone.0060552

Furukawa, S., Fujita, T., Shimabukuro, M., Iwaki, M., Yamada, Y., Nakajima, Y., et al. (2004). Increased oxidative stress in obesity and its impact on metabolic syndrome. *J. Clin. Invest.* 114, 1752–1761. doi: 10.1172/J.C.I.21625

Goldsmith, P. (2004). Zebrafish as a pharmacological tool: the how, why and when. *Curr. Opin. Pharmacol.* 4, 504–512. doi: 10.1016/j.coph.2004.04.005

Gowda, R. M., Khan, I. A., Wilbur, S. L., Vasavada, B. C., and Sacchi, T. J. (2004). Torsade de pointes: the clinical considerations. *Int. J. Cardiol.* 96, 1–6. doi: 10.1016/j.ijcard.2003.04.055

Hassel, D., Scholz, E. P., Trano, N., Friedrich, O., Just, S., Meder, B., et al. (2008). Deficient zebrafish ether-a-go-go-related gene channel gating causes short-QT syndrome in zebrafish reggae mutants. *Circulation* 117, 866–875. doi: 10.1161/CIRCULATIONAHA.107.752220

He, M., Lv, Z., Yang, Z. W., Huang, J. L., and Liu, F. (2016). Efficacy and safety of Chinese herbal medicine Wenxin Keli for ventricular premature be ats: a systematic review. *Complement. Ther. Med.* 29, 181–189. doi: 10.1016/j.ctim.2016.10.007

Hondeghem, L. M., Dujardin, K., Hoffmann, P., Dumotier, B., and De Clerck, F. (2011). Drug-induced QTC prolongation dangerously underestimates proarrhythmic potential: lessons from terfenadine. *J. Cardiovasc. Pharmacol.* 57, 589–597. doi: 10.1097/FJC.0b013e3182135e91

Hu, N., Sedmera, D., Yost, H. J., and Clark, E. B. (2000). Structure and function of the developing zebrafish heart. *Anat. Rec.* 260, 148–157. doi: 10.1002/1097-0185(20001001)260:2<148::AID-AR50>3.0.CO;2-X

Huang, C. J., Tu, C. T., Hsiao, C. D., Hsieh, F. J., and Tsai, H. J. (2003). Germ-line transmission of a myocardium-specific GFP transgene reveals critical regulatory elements in the cardiac myosin light chain 2 promoter of zebrafish. *Dev. Dyn.* 228, 30–40. doi: 10.1002/dvdy.10356

Kari, G., Rodeck, U., and Dicker, A. P. (2007). Zebrafish: an emerging model system for human disease and drug discovery. *Clin. Pharmacol. Ther.* 82, 70–80. doi: 10.1038/sj.clpt.6100223

Langenbacher, A. D., Dong, Y., Shu, X., Choi, J., Nicoll, D. A., Goldhaber, J. I., et al. (2005). Mutation in sodium-calcium exchanger 1 (NCX1) causes cardiac fibrillation in zebrafish. *Proc. Natl. Acad. Sci. U.S.A.* 102, 17699–17704. doi: 10.1073/pnas.0502679102

Langheinrich, U., Vacun, G., and Wagner, T. (2003). Zebrafish embryos express an orthologue of HERG and are sensitive toward a range of QT-prolonging drugs inducing severe arrhythmia. *Toxicol. Appl. Pharmacol.* 193, 370–382. doi: 10.1016/j.taap.2003.07.012

Li, C., Li, Q., Liu, Y. Y., Wang, M. X., Pan, C. S., Yan, L., et al. (2014). Protective effects of Notoginsenoside R1 on intestinal ischemia-reperfusion injury in rats. *Am. J. Physiol. Gastrointest. Liver Physiol.* 306, G111–G122. doi: 10.1152/ajpgi.00123.2013

Li, M., Qiu, R., Tian, G., Zhang, X., Li, C., Chen, S., et al. (2017). Wenxin Keli for ventricular premature complexes with heart failure: a systematic review and meta-analysis of randomized clinical trials. *Complement. Ther. Med.* 33, 85–93. doi: 10.1016/j.ctim.2017.06.006

Li, S., Zhang, B., and Zhang, N. (2011). Network target for screening synergistic drug combinations with application to traditional Chinese medicine. *BMC Syst. Biol.* 5(Suppl. 1):S10. doi: 10.1186/1752-0509-5-S1-S10

Liu, Y., Guo, J., Zhang, P., Li, J., and Li, C. (2009). The effects of nardostachys chinensis batal extract on the sodium current and transient outward potassium current of rat ventricular myocytes. *Chinese J. Card. Pacing Electrophysiol.* 23, 533–535. doi: 10.13333/j.cnki.cjcpe.2009.06.002

Lu, H. R., Hermans, A. N., and Gallacher, D. J. (2012). Does terfenadine-induced ventricular tachycardia/fibrillation directly relate to its QT prolongation and Torsades de Pointes? *Br. J. Pharmacol.* 166, 1490–1502. doi: 10.1111/j.1476-5381.2012.01880.x

Milan, D. J., Jones, I. L., Ellinor, P. T., and Macrae, C. A. (2006). In vivo recording of adult zebrafish electrocardiogram and assessment of drug-induced QT prolongation. *Am. J. Physiol. Heart Circ. Physiol.* 291, H269–H273. doi: 10.1152/ajpheart.00960.2005

Milan, D. J., and Macrae, C. A. (2008). Zebrafish genetic models for arrhythmia. *Prog. Biophys. Mol. Biol.* 98, 301–308. doi: 10.1016/j.pbiomolbio.2009.01.011

Page, R. L., and Roden, D. M. (2005). Drug therapy for atrial fibrillation: where do we go from here? *Nat. Rev. Drug Discov.* 4, 899–910. doi: 10.1038/nrd1876

Peal, D. S., Mills, R. W., Lynch, S. N., Mosley, J. M., Lim, E., Ellinor, P. T., et al. (2011). Novel chemical suppressors of long QT syndrome identified by an *in vivo* functional screen. *Circulation* 123, 23–30. doi: 10.1161/CIRCULATIONAHA.110.003731

Peng, L., Sun, S., Xie, L. H., Wicks, S. M., and Xie, J. T. (2012). Ginsenoside Re: pharmacological effects on cardiovascular system. *Cardiovasc. Ther.* 30, e183–188. doi: 10.1111/j.1755-5922.2011.00271.x

Rottbauer, W., Baker, K., Wo, Z. G., Mohideen, M. A., Cantiello, H. F., and Fishman, M. C. (2001). Growth and function of the embryonic heart depend upon the cardiac-specific L-type calcium channel alpha1 subunit. *Dev. Cell* 1, 265–275. doi: 10.1016/S1534-5807(01)00023-5

Sayantan, G., Kien, P. T., and Kadambari, K. V. (2018). Classification of ECG beats using deep belief network and active learning. *Med. Biol. Eng. Comput.* 56, 1887–1898. doi: 10.1007/s11517-018-1815-2

Singh, R. S., Saini, B. S., and Sunkaria, R. K. (2018). Detection of coronary artery disease by reduced features and extreme learning machine. *Clujul Med* 91, 166–175. doi: 10.15386/cjmed-882

Tu, Y. (2011). The discovery of artemisinin (qinghaosu) and gifts from Chinese medicine. *Nat. Med.* 17, 1217–1220. doi: 10.1038/nm.2471

Wang, S., Chen, P., Jiang, W., Wu, L., Chen, L., Fan, X., et al. (2014). Identification of the effective constituents for anti-inflammatory activity of Ju-Zhi-Jiang-Tang, an ancient traditional Chinese medicine formula. *J. Chromatogr. A* 1348, 105–124. doi: 10.1016/j.chroma.2014.04.084

Wang, T., Lu, M., Du, Q., Yao, X., Zhang, P., Chen, X., et al. (2017). An integrated anti-arrhythmic target network of a Chinese medicine compound, Wenxin Keli, revealed by combined machine learning and molecular pathway analysis. *Mol. Biosyst.* 13, 1018–1030. doi: 10.1039/C7MB00003K

Wang, X., Wang, Y., Feng, X., Lu, Y., Zhang, Y., Wang, W., et al. (2016). Systematic review and meta-analysis of randomized controlled trials on Wenxin keli. *Drug Des. Devel. Ther.* 10, 3725–3736. doi: 10.2147/DDDT.S112333

Wang, Y., Fan, X., Qu, H., Gao, X., and Cheng, Y. (2012). Strategies and techniques for multi-component drug design from medicinal herbs and traditional Chinese medicine. *Curr. Top. Med. Chem.* 12, 1356–1362. doi: 10.2174/156802612801319034

Wen, D., Liu, A., Chen, F., Yang, J., and Dai, R. (2012). Validation of visualized transgenic zebrafish as a high throughput model to assay bradycardia related cardio toxicity risk candidates. *J. Appl. Toxicol.* 32, 834–842. doi: 10.1002/jat.2755

Wu, W., Zhang, X. M., Liu, P. M., Li, J. M., and Wang, J. F. (1995). Effects of Panax notoginseng saponin Rg1 on cardiac electrophysiological properties and ventricular fibrillation threshold in dogs. *Zhongguo Yao Li Xue Bao* 16, 459–463.

Xing, Y., Gao, Y., Chen, J., Zhu, H., Wu, A., Yang, Q., et al. (2013). Wenxin-Keli regulates the calcium/calmodulin-dependent protein kinase II signal transduction pathway and inhibits cardiac arrhythmia in rats with myocardial infarction. *Evid. Based Complement. Alternat. Med.* 2013:464508. doi: 10.1155/2013/464508

Xue, X., Guo, D., Sun, H., Wang, D., Li, J., Liu, T., et al. (2013). Wenxin Keli suppresses ventricular triggered arrhythmias via selective inhibition of late sodium current. *Pacing Clin. Electrophysiol.* 36, 732–740. doi: 10.1111/pace.12109

Yang, X., Chen, Y., Li, Y., Ren, X., Xing, Y., and Shang, H. (2017). Effects of Wenxin Keli on cardiac hypertrophy and arrhythmia via regulation of the calcium/calmodulin dependent kinase II signaling pathway. *Biomed Res. Int.* 2017:1569235. doi: 10.1155/2017/1569235

Zhang, C., Willett, C., and Fremgen, T. (2003). Zebrafish: an animal model for toxicological studies. *Curr. Protoc. Toxicol.* Chapter 1, Unit 1.7. doi: 10.1002/0471140856.tx0107s17

Zhu, J. J., Xu, Y. Q., He, J. H., Yu, H. P., Huang, C. J., Gao, J. M., et al. (2014). Human cardiotoxic drugs delivered by soaking and microinjection induce cardiovascular toxicity in zebrafish. *J. Appl. Toxicol.* 34, 139–148. doi: 10.1002/jat.2843

Zhu, X. Y., Wu, S. Q., Guo, S. Y., Yang, H., Xia, B., Li, P., et al. (2018). A zebrafish heart failure model for assessing therapeutic agents. *Zebrafish* 15, 243–253. doi: 10.1089/zeb.2017.1546

3

Detection of Seasonal Variation in *Aloe* Polysaccharides Using Carbohydrate Detecting Microarrays

Louise Isager Ahl[1]*, Narjes Al-Husseini[1], Sara Al-Helle[1], Dan Staerk[2], Olwen M. Grace[3], William G. T. Willats[4], Jozef Mravec[5], Bodil Jørgensen[5] and Nina Rønsted[1]*

[1] Natural History Museum of Denmark, University of Copenhagen, Copenhagen, Denmark, [2] Department of Drug Design and Pharmacology, University of Copenhagen, Copenhagen, Denmark, [3] Comparative Plant and Fungal Biology, Royal Botanic Gardens Kew, Richmond, United Kingdom, [4] School of Natural and Environmental Sciences, Newcastle University, Newcastle upon Tyne, United Kingdom, [5] Department of Plant and Environmental Sciences, University of Copenhagen, Frederiksberg, Denmark

*Correspondence:
Louise Isager Ahl
louise.ahl@snm.ku.dk
Nina Rønsted
nronsted@snm.ku.dk

Aloe vera gel is a globally popular natural product used for the treatment of skin conditions. Its useful properties are attributed to the presence of bioactive polysaccharides. Nearly 25% of the 600 species in the genus *Aloe* are used locally in traditional medicine, indicating that the bioactive components in *Aloe vera* may be common across the genus *Aloe*. The complexity of the polysaccharides has hindered development of relevant assays for authentication of *Aloe* products. Carbohydrate detecting microarrays have recently been suggested as a method for profiling *Aloe* polysaccharide composition. The aim of this study was to use carbohydrate detecting microarrays to investigate the seasonal variation in the polysaccharide composition of two medicinal and two non-medicinal *Aloe* species over the course of a year. Microscopy was used to explore where in the cells the bioactive polysaccharides are present and predict their functional role in the cell wall structure. The carbohydrate detecting microarrays analyses showed distinctive differences in the polysaccharide composition between the different species and carbohydrate detecting microarrays therefore has potential as a complementary screening method directly targeting the presence and composition of relevant polysaccharides. The results also show changes in the polysaccharide composition over the year within the investigated species, which may be of importance for commercial growing in optimizing harvest times to obtain higher yield of relevant polysaccharides.

Keywords: *Aloe*, authentication, carbohydrate detecting microarrays, plant cell walls, polysaccharides, seasonal variation, succulent tissue

INTRODUCTION

The succulent *Aloe vera* L. leaf tissue is a natural product used globally in a wide range of household commodities (Grace et al., 2015). By the end of 2016, *Aloe vera* leaf tissue had reached a revenue of US\$ 1.6 billion and it is estimated that the revenue will exceed US\$ 3.3 billion by 2026 (Future Market Insights, 2016). The succulent inner leaf tissue, the gel, is a polysaccharide rich matrix containing high amounts of mannan (polymannose), which enables the tissue to hold larger amounts of water (Reynolds and Dweck, 1999; Ni et al., 2004; Grace et al., 2015). The genus *Aloe*, to which *Aloe vera* belongs, contains more than 500 different species out of which at least 25% are used medicinally mainly by indigenous communities in the areas where they occur naturally (Grace, 2011).

From the *Aloe* leaves, two different medicinal products can be derived – the excudate and the gel. The often yellow and bitter exudate comes from aloitic cells (specialized cells in relation to the vascular bundles, that excrete af mixture of compounds used for medicinal purposes (Reynolds, 2004) in the outer leaf mesophyll, and contains a range of compounds used as purgative (Grace et al., 2009). The colorless polysaccharide-rich gel from the inner leaf is used topically for treatment of wounds, minor burns, and skin irritation or internally for a range of different applications (Grindlay and Reynolds, 1986; Reynolds and Dweck, 1999; Hamman, 2008; Grace et al., 2009). Due to the complexity of the polysaccharides, the composition and bioactivity of *Aloe* gel is not well understood, and there is a lack of useful methods for analysis and authentication (Bozzi et al., 2007; Grace and Rønsted, 2017).

The plant cell wall is an insoluble entity composed almost entirely of complex polysaccharides arranged in an intricate matrix (Cosgrove, 2005; Albersheim, 2011). The main non-cellulosic polysaccharides in *Aloe* inner leaf mesophyll are hemicelluloses and pectins. Hemicelluloses cover a range of different polysaccharides with xyloglucans usually being the principal ones (Albersheim, 2011; Pedersen et al., 2012). Another hemicellulose mannan, and in particular an acetylated form of it, have been of particular interest in relation to *Aloe* research as it is considered the most likely bioactive component in the gels (Reynolds and Dweck, 1999; Talmadge et al., 2004; Simões et al., 2012). Plant cell wall polysaccharides are traditionally investigated indirectly using monosaccharide analyses (Albersheim, 2011; Grace et al., 2013), but by the complete break-down of the plant cell wall, information is inevitably lost about the tertiary structure and chemical construction of the polymers, why development of methods targeting polysaccharides or at least oligosaccharides have been highly sought after (Fangel et al., 2012; Krešimir et al., 2017).

The ability to analyze and distinguish between polysaccharide compositions in different plant tissues, between different batches, and between species are especially important in plants containing bioactive polysaccharides used for medicinal purposes like the acetylated mannan of *Aloe vera* (Femenia et al., 1999; Ahl et al., 2018; Minjares-Fuentes et al., 2018). Mannan is not only a common plant cell wall polysaccharide, but it is also often found in tissues related to water storage (Stancato et al., 2001). The acetylated mannan (polymannose) from *Aloe vera* has been linked to induced tissue repair in humans (Reynolds and Dweck, 1999; Xing et al., 2014; Thunyakitpisal et al., 2017), whereas a de-acetylation of mannan have been shown to result in a loss of bioactivity (Chokboribal et al., 2015).

Polysaccharide and phenolic compound contents are expected to vary with age of the plant, between batches,

and with season and rainfall or water availability (Hu et al., 2003; Beppu et al., 2006; Cristiano et al., 2016). Harvesting and subsequent processing including drying of *Aloe* gel can also influence the content and composition of bioactive compounds including causing de-acetylation of mannan polymers (Minjares-Fuentes et al., 2016; Sriariyakul et al., 2016).

The efficacy and safety of herbal products can be compromised through accidental adulteration, misidentification and deliberate contamination, which can lead to lack of the desired effect at best, or severe side effects due to the presence of toxic compounds in worst case scenarios (Ernst, 2004; van Breemen and Farnsworth, 2008; Gilbert, 2011; Saslis-Lagoudakis et al., 2015). To ensure the efficacy and safety of herbal products, their qualitative and quantitative composition are regulated by international and national monographs such as the European Pharmacopeia by the European Directorate for the Quality of Medicines and Healthcare (EDQM, 2016), which presents a series of monographs for herbal products, including recommended tests for identification and quality of the plant species included in these products.

Two bulk *Aloe* herbal products are included in the European Pharmacopeia (EDQM, 2016), namely *Aloe barbadensis* (a synonym of the accepted name, *Aloe vera* L.), and *Aloe capensis* (a synonym of the accepted name, *Aloe ferox* Mill.), but both are based on the detection of hydroxyanthracene derivatives in the juice (exudate). A World Health Organization [WHO] (1999) monograph is available on *Aloe vera* gel recommending a chromatographic assay (t'Hart et al., 1989; World Health Organization [WHO], 1999), but no quantitative requirements of content has been proposed.

Considering the global use and appraisal of *Aloe vera* gel and its acclaimed beneficial effects, there is an urgent need for establishing reliable, and relevant authentication methods. In addition to ensuring the safety and efficacy of *Aloe* herbal products, an authentication method can also be used to assist in control of illegal harvesting and trade. All *Aloe* species except *Aloe vera* are prohibited from trade under the Convention on International Trade in Endangered Species as described in appendix II (CITES, 2017).

Due to the complexity of the polysaccharides, no efficient standard method exists for neither qualitative nor quantitative authentication of polysaccharide composition in *Aloe* herbal products (Grace et al., 2013; Minjares-Fuentes et al., 2018). Full structural identification of polysaccharides can currently only be achieved through a complex combination of spectroscopic techniques (Simões et al., 2012; Shi et al., 2018). However, a number of indirect methods exist, such as ^{1}H-NMR spectroscopy, which can be used to verify the presence of specific structural groups, such as the acetyl groups of the acetylated mannan (Bozzi et al., 2007; Campestrini et al., 2013).

Structure–activity relationships suggest that monosaccharide composition and branching patterns play an important role in the bioactivity of plant polysaccharides (Paulsen and Barsett, 2005). As a proxy, the constituent monosaccharides have therefore been suggested as a tool for authenticating *Aloe*-based products (O'Brian et al., 2011; Minjares-Fuentes et al., 2018). Several analytical techniques are in use including colorimetric and spectrophotometric fingerprinting methods, and chromatographic methods, which can efficiently separate, identify, and quantify the monosaccharides (t'Hart et al., 1989; Eberendu et al., 2005; Nazeam et al., 2017; Zhang et al., 2018). However, little is known about the relationship between polysaccharide composition and therapeutic value of the leaf mesophyll in *Aloe,* and it is recommended that future authentication focus on developing methods targeting the polysaccharides (Grace et al., 2013).

Carbohydrate detecting microarrays (Moller et al., 2007) have been proposed as a possible method for qualitative comparison of polysaccharide composition between *Aloe* species and in *Aloe* herbal products (Ahl et al., 2018). Carbohydrate detecting microarrays is a high-throughput method allowing for the simultaneous investigation of numerous samples at the same time. However, carbohydrate microarrays are limited by what antibodies are available and the effectiveness of extractions and immobilization. The most optimal use of the method in relation to authentication is as a complementary screening tool prior to analyses like ^{1}H-NMR spectrometry analysis for more in-depth knowledge of the present *Aloe* compounds (Campestrini et al., 2013; Minjares-Fuentes et al., 2018). For the purpose of obtaining quantitative data, GC-MS profiling of monosaccharides is also still a useful method (Grace et al., 2013).

The aim of the present study was to use carbohydrate detecting microarrays to investigate the seasonal variation in the polysaccharide composition of two medicinal and two non-medicinal aloes over the course of a year. Microarray profiling was complemented by microscopy to understand where in the cells the bioactive polysaccharides are present.

MATERIALS AND METHODS

Plant Material

Four species were chosen for this study to represent medicinal and or non-medicinal usage, but also based on their growth form, geographical distribution, and leaf size (**Table 1**). *Aloe vera* is a short-stemmed species growing in large clumps, and is probably native to the Arabian Peninsula (Grace et al., 2015). *Aloe arborescens* is a widespread species in the southern part of the African continent. The two medicinal aloes are very different in terms of habit, growth form and distribution, with *A. arborescens* growing up to 3 m in height compared to *A. vera* being a maximum of 1 m tall. Both non-medicinal species selected for this study are native to Madagascar, with *A. decaryi* being a narrow endemic growing in a pendulous or sprawling habit in thickets near sea level. *Aloe vaombe,* on the other hand is a widespread tree growing up to 5 m tall at altitudes of 50–1200 m (Carter et al., 2011).

Plant material was sampled from the living collections of the Botanical Garden, Natural History Museum of Denmark,

University of Copenhagen, Denmark, and vouchers are deposited in Herbarium C (**Table 1**).

Plants of the four species were mature (+20 years old) when sampled and were grown under glass in conditions mimicking the daylight changes and water availability of the region they come from (**Table 1**). Samples were collected in triplicates for each species once a month from June 26th, 2017 to June 25th, 2018. Seasonality are expressed as northern hemisphere spring (March–May), summer (June–August), autumn (September–November), and winter (December–February) for the greenhouse-grown material, although the natural habitat of most aloes is in the southern hemisphere (**Table 1**). Two different types of fresh samples were taken at each collection point. To reduce the risk of contamination with phenolic compounds, which can bind and lead to masking of epitopes in the carbohydrate detecting microarrays, only the inner leaf mesophyll was carefully collected for carbohydrate detecting microarray analysis. Sections including epidermis were collected for microscopy investigations.

Ph. Eur. reference material for *Aloe vera* (product number 103504) and *A. capensis* (product number 203304) was obtained from Alfred Galke, Bad Grund, Germany, and was used as a standard (EDQM, 2016).

Microarray Profiling of Polysaccharides

Polysaccharide data was obtained by following the protocol described by Ahl et al. (2018), which in turn was modified from that of Moller et al. (2007) to accommodate the unique properties of the *Aloe* tissue (**Figure 1**). The succulent inner leaf mesophyll was collected in three biological replicates from the four selected *Aloe* species each month for a full year. The tissue was carefully excised from mature leaves, and immediately placed in labeled Falcon tubes (Corning, New York, United States) before they were snap frozen in liquid nitrogen. The collected samples were kept at –20°C for 24 h before they were freeze dried, weighed, and milled prior to extractions. Samples of approximately 5 mg were weighed to 1 decimal accuracy from each biological replicate and placed in Corning 8-strip cluster tubes (Merck Life Science, Darmstadt, Germany). Samples were homogenized in a Tissuelyser II (Gentec Biosciences, Columbia) using glass beads prior to extractions.

Extractions were carried out in three-step sequential series and for each sample, the extractant volume was adjusted to accommodate the exact weight of each sample reaching a ratio of 10 mg sample to 300 µL extraction solvent. The extraction series is based on the work by Moller et al. (2007) and adjusted according to Ahl et al. (2018). The glass beads used for homogenization were kept in the tube to enhance the extraction of polysaccharides during the sequential steps. The following solvents were used: dH_2O – targeting primarily soluble unbound or loosely bound polysaccharides including mannans, 50 mM CDTA (*trans*-1,2-diaminocyclohexane-*N,N,N′,N′*-tetraacetic acid monohydrate, pH 7.5, Merck Life Science, Darmstadt, Germany) – targeting primarily pectins and some hemicelluloses, and finally 4 mM NaOH – targeting

TABLE 1 | Biogeographical, morphological, and usage of the selected Aloe species found in the wild.

		Plant name			
		Aloe decaryi Guillaumine	Aloe vaombe Decorse & Poiss	Aloe vera L. Burm.f.	Aloe arborescens Miller
In situ	Region (s)	Madagascan	Madagascan	Only in cultivation	Southern African Zambezian
	Country	Madagascar	Madagascar	Only in cultivation	South Africa (L, M, KN, EC, WC) Swaziland Malawi MozambiqueZimbabwe
	Distribution	Limited – island	Widespread – island	Naturalised	Widespread
	Ecological adaptations	Thick coastal scrub	Dry thorn-bush	NA	Rocky slopes, sometimes dense bush
	Altitude min (m)	Sea level	50	NA	Sea level
	Altitude max (m)	Sea level	1200	NA	2800
	Type	Pendulous/sprawling	Tree	Stemless - large clumps, few-branched	Tree
	Fresh sap	NA	Deep purple	Yellow	NA
	Dry sap	NA	Deep purple	Yellow	NA
	Lenght (cm) leaves min	15	80	40	50
	Lenght (cm) leaves max	19	100	60	60
	Whith (cm) leaves min	0.8	15	6	5
	Whith (cm) leaves min	1.2	20	7	7
	Leaf color	Uniformly dull green	Dull green	Grey-green with brownish tinge	Dull green to grey-green
	Teeth	Present	Present	Present	Present
	Flower color	Rose-red to scarlet	Bright crimson	Yellow	Scarlet
	Usage	non-medicinal	non-medicinal	medicinal	medicinal
	Year scientifically identified	1941	1912	1768	1768
Greenhouse	Voucher details	Ahl P1977-5375	Ahl S1985-0546	Ahl P1991-5289	Ahl 1997-0785
	Spring watering	1–2 times per week	1–2 times per week	1–2 times per week	1–2 times per week
	Summer watering	2–3 times per week	2–3 times per week	2–3 times per week	2–3 times per week
	Fall watering	1–2 times per week	1–2 times per week	1–2 times per week	1–2 times per week
	Winter watering	1–2 times per week	1–2 times per week	Every 3rd week	Every 3rd week
	Extra light in winter	Yes	Yes	No	No
	Temperature (°C)	18–22	18–22	13–17	13–17
	Fertilizer	NPK standard	NPK standard	NPK standard	NPK standard

The cultivated species were grown in two different greenhouses depending on their natural habitat. Aloe arborescens and Aloe vera did not get additional light during the winter months, but Aloe vaombe and Aloe decaryi did, as they grow mainly in the winter months. Watering was generally done according to the directions above, but if a time period had been particularly sunny watering was increased and if the period had been more cloudy watering was decreased. Temperature were adjusted to be within the listed ranges. Vouchers are deposited in Herbarium C, National History Museum of Denmark, University of Copenhagen, Denmark.

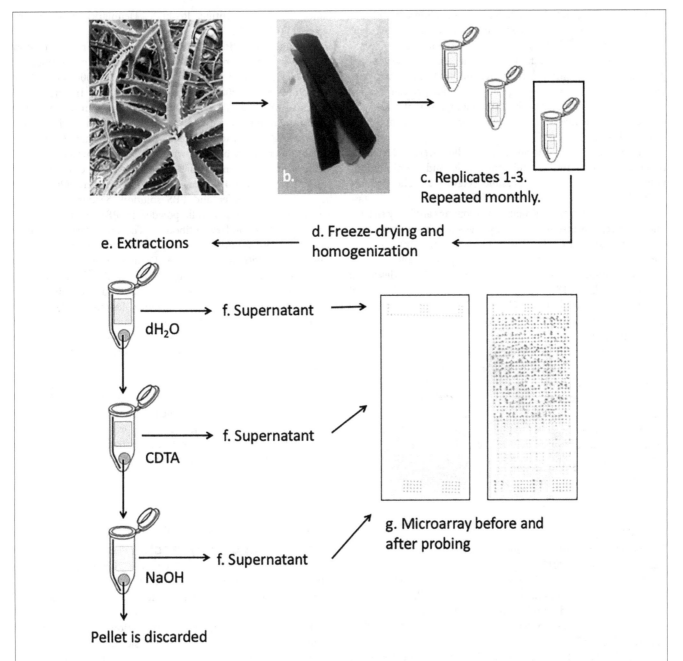

FIGURE 1 | Schematic presentation of the CoMPP method illustrated with *Aloe arborescens*. Species are sampled in triplicates and prepared for extractions. The supernatant from each sequential extraction step is printed separately in technical replicates on nitrocellulose membranes. The printed microarrays are then probed with a selection of molecular probes.

primarily hemicelluloses. For all three extraction steps samples were shaken in a Tissuelyzer at 27 s^{-1} for 2 min before the speed was reduced to 6 s^{-1} for 2 h. All extractions were carried out at room temperature. After the extractions, samples were centrifuged at 4000 RPM (Thermo Fisher Scientific, Waltham, MA, United States) for 10 min before the supernatant was carefully removed and transferred to a labeled 0.5 mL Eppendorf tube (Eppendorf, Hamburg, Germany). Extractions were carried out on the pellet, and

extracts were kept at 4°C during the subsequent extractions to minimize degradation.

Once extractions were done for all samples, fourfold dilution series were made for each sample in a 384-well microtiter plate (Merck Life Science, Darmstadt, Germany). Dilutions were made using Arrayjet buffer (55.2% glycerol, 44% water, 0.8% Triton X-100). The 384-well microplates with the diluted extracts were centrifuged at 3000 RPM (Thermo-Fisher Scientific, Waltham, MA, United States) for 10 min before they were printed on a 0.45 μm nitrocellulose membrane (Whatman, Maidstone, United Kingdom) using an Arrayjet Sprint (Arrayjet, Edinburgh, United Kingdom) piezoelectric robotic printer. For each sample, the dilution series was printed in four technical replicates on each microarray, to yield a total of 48 spots per plant specimen per harvest (16 spots per extraction step). The three biological replicates were extracted and printed on three separate days using the approach described above.

Fifteen primary monoclonal antibodies were selected to cover as many types of different pectic and hemicellulotic polysaccharide epitopes as possible (**Figure 2**). The primary antibodies were paired with either alkaline phosphatase conjugated anti-rat or anti-mouse as secondary antibody (Merck Life Science, Darmstadt, Germany) depending on the origin of the primary antibody. The printed arrays from all three identical extraction rounds were developed, quantified and analyzed simultaneously following the procedures described by Ahl et al. (2018). The final tally of arrays developed for this study accounts to 47 arrays: 1 for each antibody and extraction round, plus two for negative controls of the secondary antibodies.

For the data analysis averages were calculated using both the dilution series for each sample and the array triplicates (total of 48 data points per sample). The full data set was visualized in a heatmap format with all antibodies and their binding shown in the **Figure 2**. The highest mean value of the entire dataset was assigned the value of 100%, and the remainder of the data were adjusted accordingly and normalized with a 5% cut off (represented with a zero – "0"). All data analyses were carried out in Microsoft Excel for Mac, version 16.16.4 (181110), 2018.

Microscopy

The microscopy work was done on samples from the summer collection in August 2017.

Sections from all four *Aloe* species were also stained with 1% Toluidine blue for 10 min, washed twice in distilled water and mounted on glass slides under a coverslip. Images were taken on Olympus BX41 microscope with a mounted Olympus ColorView I camera (**Figure 3**).

Tissue pieces of approximately 3 mm in diameter were excised from the sampled material and fixed for 30 min in 4% formaldehyde prepared from paraformaldehyde in phosphate-buffered saline (PBS). Sections were washed twice in PBS, before they were dehydrated in a series of methanol:water solutions until reaching a final concentration of 100% methanol. The methanol was then substituted with a methanol:LR White resin mixture (1:1) for 8– 10 h. Sections were then transferred to a pure LR resin overnight. The specimens were organized in gelatine capsules filled with pure LR resin. The final polymerization was performed overnight in a 60°C oven. 1 μm-thick sections were made from each species using a Leica EM-UC7 ultramicrotome (Leica, Roskilde, Denmark) and glass knives, and subsequently adhered on Superfrost

Slides (Thermo Scientific, Roskilde, Denmark) in a drop of water at 60°C.

Immunolocalization of different polysaccharides in resin sections was performed following the procedure described by Mravec et al. (2017) using the antibodies BS-400-4 and LM21 (Pettolino et al., 2001; Marcus et al., 2010). In short, leaf sections were placed on individual glass microscope slides, and a hydrophobic circle was drawn around each section with a PAP pen (Merck Life Science, Darmstadt, Germany). Sections were then blocked with a 5% milk powder and PBS solution for 15 min, before probing with the monoclonal antibodies (**Figures 4**, **5**) for 1 h. Antibodies were diluted 1:10 in a 5% milk powder and PBS solution. Sections were then washed twice with 5% milk powder in PBS solution, before probing with secondary antibodies. The secondary antibodies used were either anti-rat or anti-mouse conjugated to Alexa Fluor 555 (Invitrogen, Roskilde, Denmark) at 1:300 dilution in 3% bovine serum albumin (BSA) in PBS. Leaf sections were then washed three times in PBS, and counterstained with Calcofluor White (Merck Life Science, Darmstadt, Germany) at 0.1 mg/ml concentration for 10 min. Finally, the leaf sections were washed one last time before being mounted in CitiFluor, an antifading reagent (Agar Scientific, Essex, United Kingdom).

The fluorescently labeled samples were scanned using a Leica SP5 confocal laser scanning microscope equipped with UV diode (405 nm), Ar (488 nm), and HeNe (543 nm) lasers at either 20X or 63X water objectives. Pictures were processed with GIMP2 software for color enhancement and contrast. Control samples were treated equally for comparison.

RESULTS

Aloe Inner Leaf Mesophyll Structure and Localization of Polysaccharides

Distinctive morphological differences between the four different *Aloe* leaves investigated for this study were observed (**Figure 3**). The amount of inner leaf mesophyll varied from a thin layer in *A. vaombe* to a thicker many-celled layer in *A. vera*. The micrographic observation of toluidine blue stained resin sections showed the basic anatomical structure is conserved between the *Aloe* species. Below epidermis, is the outer mesophyll made of app. 15 layers of round or slightly elongated parenchymatic cells with size of 40– 100 μm in diameter followed by the inner mesophyll of enlarged water storage cells reaching 300 μm in diameter. These observations showed that the overall thickness of the *Aloe* leaves is largely determined by the thickness of the inner mesophyll.

Two mannan-specific antibodies (BS-400-4 and LM21) were used to investigate the localization of mannans in the mesophyll layers. The exact specificity of the mannan-binding antibody BS-400-4 is $(1\rightarrow4)$-β-mannan/galacto-$(1\rightarrow4)$-β-mannan (Pettolino et al., 2001). The probed micrographs (**Figures 4**, **5**) show that that the majority of mannan is found in the cytosol inside the cells, and in very different amounts depending on

		All extractions combined																
		Pectins							Hemicelluloses								2°Ab control	
		Homogalacturonan					RGI		Mannan				XG	Glucan		Xylan	Negative	
Species	Season	JIM5	JIM7	LM18	LM19	LM20	LM5	LM6	LM21	LM22	BS-400-4	CCRC-170	LM25	BS-400-2	BS-400-3	LM23	Neg. R	Neg. M
Aloe arborescens	Fall	0	5	17	21	0	5	0	24	0	79	56	24	0	0	0	0	0
Aloe arborescens	Spring	0	7	16	19	0	5	0	22	0	72	51	22	0	0	0	0	0
Aloe arborescens	Summer	6	9	21	26	7	11	0	29	0	85	62	27	0	0	0	0	0
Aloe arborescens	Winter	0	7	18	22	0	6	0	24	0	76	54	24	0	0	0	0	0
Aloe decaryi	Fall	0	6	11	16	0	0	0	35	0	83	48	20	0	0	0	0	0
Aloe decaryi	Spring	0	0	10	14	0	0	0	33	0	83	48	20	0	0	0	0	0
Aloe decaryi	Summer	0	0	12	16	0	0	0	43	0	90	54	22	0	0	0	0	0
Aloe decaryi	Winter	0	0	10	14	0	0	0	35	0	86	48	19	0	0	0	0	0
Aloe vaombe	Fall	6	9	18	21	8	0	0	45	0	91	58	28	0	0	0	0	0
Aloe vaombe	Spring	0	0	17	20	0	7	0	40	0	90	53	26	0	0	0	0	0
Aloe vaombe	Summer	8	12	21	26	11	6	0	47	0	93	58	29	0	0	0	0	0
Aloe vaombe	Winter	0	5	15	20	0	5	0	40	0	91	57	26	0	0	0	0	0
Aloe Vera	Fall	0	16	0	7	15	0	0	28	0	74	39	18	0	0	0	0	0
Aloe Vera	Spring	0	14	0	7	13	0	0	25	0	69	40	15	0	0	0	0	0
Aloe Vera	Summer	0	17	0	6	18	0	0	37	0	84	45	16	0	0	0	0	0
Aloe Vera	Winter	0	13	0	8	11	0	0	32	0	78	42	17	0	0	0	0	0
Aloe Ferox	Standard	0	0	7	7	0	0	0	11	0	36	23	0	0	0	0	0	0
Aloe vera	Standard	0	0	14	15	0	8	9	49	0	100	63	24	0	0	0	0	0

Polymer	Code	Epitope	Origin	Reference
Pectin	JIM5	Homogalactauronan with a low DE	Rat	VandenBosch et al. (1989); Willats et al. (2000); Clausen et al. (2003)
	JIM7	Homogalactauronan with a high DE	Rat	VandenBosch et al. (1989); Willats et al. (2000); Clausen et al. (2003)
	LM18	Partially methylesterified homogalactauronan	Rat	Verhertbruggen et al. (2009)
	LM19	Partially methylesterified homogalactauronan	Rat	Verhertbruggen et al. (2009)
	LM20	Partially methylesterified homogalactauronan	Rat	Verhertbruggen et al. (2009)
	LM5	(1→4)-β-D-galactan	Rat	Jones et al. 1997
	LM6	(1→5)-α-L-arabinan	Rat	Willats et al. (1998); Lee et al. (2005); Verhertbruggen et al. (2009)
Mannan	BS-400-4	(1→4)-β-D-mannan	Mouse	Pettolino et al. (2001)
	LM21	(1→4)-β-D-mannan/galactomannan/glucomannan	Rat	Marcus et al. (2010)
	LM22	(1→4)-β-D-mannan/galactomannan/glucomannan	Rat	Marcus et al. (2010)
	CCRC-170	Acetylated mannan	Mouse	Pattathil et al. (2012); Zhang et al. (2014)
Xyloglucan	LM25	Xyloglucan	Rat	Pedersen et al. (2012)
Xylan	LM23	(1→4)-β-D-xylan	Rat	Manabe et al. (2011); Pedersen et al. (2012); Torode et al. (2015)
Glucan	BS-400-2	(1→3)-β-D-glucan	Mouse	Meikle et al. (1991)
	BS-400-3	(1→3)(1→4)-β-D-glucan	Mouse	Meikle et al. (1994)

FIGURE 2 | All extractions are summarized per season. The Ph. Eur. Material extractions (standards) are also summarized for each species. All tested antibodies are included. Included antibodies and their target epitope as well as the origin of the antibody and where their bindings have been described is listed below the heatmap. DE, degree of esterification; RGI, rhamno-galacturonan; KG, kyloglycan; Neg. R, anti-rat; Neg. M, anti-mouse. The highest mean value of the entire dataset was assigned the value of 100%, and the remainder of the data were adjusted accordingly and normalized with a 5% cut off (represented with a zero – "0").

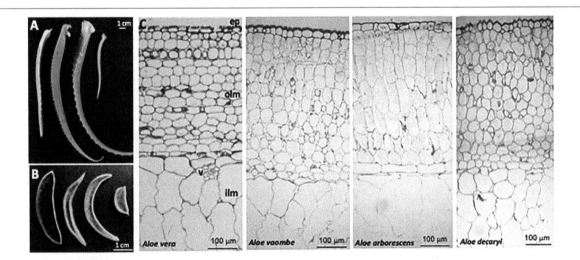

FIGURE 3 | Anatomy of four *Aloe* species, **(A)** Leaves and **(B)** cross-sections from left to right of *Aloe vera*, *A. vaombe*, *A. arborescens* and *A. decaryi*. **(C)** Cross-sections from left to right of *Aloe vera*, *A. voombe*, *A. arborescens* and *A. decaryi* stained with Toluidine blue. Marked are ep, epidermis; olm, outer leaf mesophyll; v, vasculature; ilm, inner leaf mesophyll.

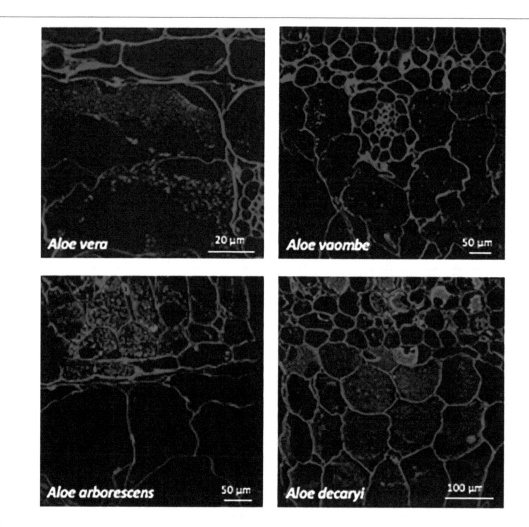

FIGURE 4 | Immunolabeling using the mannan specific monoclonal antibody BS-400-4 (red channel). Overlay with CalcofluorWhite (blue channel) counterstain to visualize cell walls.

the species. In *A. vaombe* the mannan seems to be almost entirely embedded in the wall. The mannan polymers do not seem to form a continuous entity, but rather appear as granules. In *A. decaryi* the mannan granules fill up almost the entire inside of the cells, whereas there were distinct vacuoles in the gatherings of mannan polymers in *A. vera* and *A. arborescens*. Additionally, in *A. arborescens* it seems like mannan is primarily present in the outer mesophyll and only present in thin bands around the edges in the inner mesophyll. The mannan-specific antibody LM21 binds β-(1→4)-manno-oligosaccharides from DP2 to DP5, but it also displays a wider recognition including mannan, glucomannan and galactomannan polysaccharides (Marcus et al., 2010). Based on the histological micrographs (**Figure 5**) from the four *Aloe* species there appear to be very little mannan present in the mesophyll when LM21 is used to detect it. Again, in *A. vaombe*, the mannan seems to be almost embedded in the wall, whereas the distribution resembles the binding pattern of BS-400-4 more in the remaining three species although in a lower concentration. In *A. vera*, *A. arborescens*, and *A. decaryi* the mannan recognized

by LM21 also seems to be granulated rather than a dense sheet (**Figure 4**).

Polysaccharide Profile Variation Between Species

Binding studies of 15 primary monoclonal antibodies representing different pectic and hemicellulotic polysaccharide epitopes show differences between the four *Aloe* species in polysaccharide compositions of their inner leaf mesophyll (**Figures 2, 6**). As expected, the sequential extraction series resulted in the extraction of a mixture of polysaccharides. **Figure 2** presents a summary of the pooled serial extractions for each species and each antibody, in order to investigate if the total amounts of polysaccharides change over the course of a year, whereas detailed results for each of the three extraction solvents (H_2O, CDTA, and NaOH) are shown in the **Supplementary Material**. In **Figure 6**, species-specific heatmaps including only the antibodies that recognized epitopes in the material are depicted

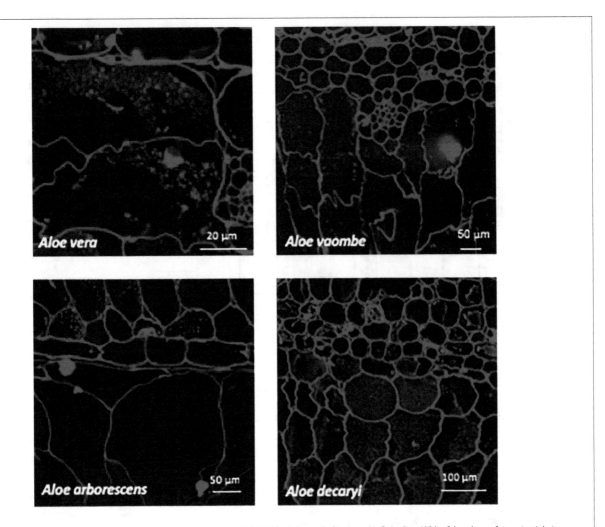

FIGURE 5 | Immunolabeling using the mannan specific monoclonal antibody LM21 (red channel). Overlay with Calcofluor White (blue channel) counterstain to visualize cell walls.

along with graphs showing the changes in mannan epitopes over time.

For all species mannan and xyloglycan epitopes were detected, although in various amounts. *A. vaombe* contained the highest amounts of mannan in the water extractions as detected by all three mannan-specific antibodies (LM21, BS-400-4, and CCRC-170) seen in **Figure 6** (Pettolino et al., 2001; Marcus et al., 2010; Pattathil et al., 2012; Zhang et al., 2014). For all species, the CCRC-170, binding acetylated mannan, the signal completely disappears in the spring and summer samples during the NaOH extraction, but re-appear in lower concentrations during the fall and winter.

The most distinct changes between species are found in the pectin profiles and this has also been observed in other studies (Ahl et al., 2018). In relation to specific antibodies, only *A. vaombe* and *A. arborescens* show binding from JIM5, targeting low methylated homogalacturonan – the backbone of the pectin polymer (Vandenbosch et al., 1989; Willats et al., 2000; Clausen et al., 2003). High-methylated homogalacturonan (JIM7), expressed by the binding of JIM7, is primarily released

from the matrix in the CDTA extraction, but only in very low amounts from *A. decaryi*. Slightly more is released from *A. arborescens* and *A. vaombe*. The highest amounts of JIM7 is released from *A. vera* reaching almost double the amount when all seasons and extractions are combined (**Figure 2**; Vandenbosch et al., 1989; Willats et al., 2000; Clausen et al., 2003). Three different antibodies are detecting partially methylated homogalacturonan – LM18, LM19, and LM20 (Verhertbruggen et al., 2009). Despite being described as binding to the same type of epitope there are clear differences in the binding patterns of the three antibodies. There is binding for LM18 and LM19 in all selected species, but LM20 does not show any binding to *A. decaryi* and also has a very low binding to *A. vaombe* and *A. arborescens*, but then binds strongly to *A. vera* in the same pattern as JIM7 did. In terms of LM18 and LM19, *A. vera* is the species with the lowest binding with amounts hardly above the background cut-off. The three remaining species all express strong binding to both LM18 and LM19 with noticeable differences between the seasons. For all three species relative amounts of the polysaccharides are

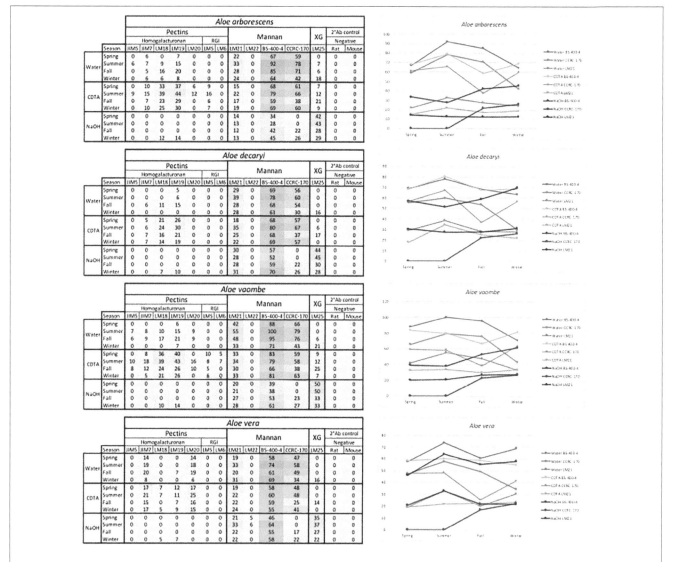

FIGURE 6 | Species specific heatmaps and graphs showing the changes in mannan over time in the three sequential extractions. RGI, rhamno-galacturonan; XG, xyloglycan; Meg. R, anti-rat; Neg. M, anti-mouse. The highest mean value of the entire dataset was assigned the value of 100%, and the remainder of the data were adjusted accordingly and normalized with a 5% cut off (represented with a zero – "0").

almost doubled in the spring and summer periods compared to fall and winter.

In this study two antibodies targeting galactan and arabinan epitopes on rhamno-galacturonan, a pectin side-chain, was included – LM5 and LM6 (Jones et al., 1997; Willats et al., 1998; Lee et al., 2005). LM6 only bound to *A. vaombe* in the CDTA extraction of the spring and summer periods, but very weakly. Similarly, LM5 only showed binding in the CDTA extractions of *A. vaombe* and *A. arborescens*. Again, the binding showed low amounts of galactan with the highest values found in the spring and summer periods. Whereas seasonal differences were clearly detectable in the different extraction steps (**Figure 6** and **Supplementary Material**), the combined heatmap (**Figure 2**) shows that even though changes do occur over a 12-month period they are much subtler when considering the pooled extracts. The summer amounts are still the highest for almost all antibodies

and all species. The differences between the species are still clearly visible even when extraction data is pooled (**Figure 2**).

DISCUSSION

Organization of Mannans in the Succulent Tissue of Aloes

The microscopy work was done to determine the placement of the polysaccharides within the succulent tissue and determine the differences and similarities between the four species – *A. arborescens*, *A. decaryi*, *A. vaombe*, and *A. vera*. The microscopy work has overall corroborated the carbohydrate detecting microarrays results both in terms of species differences and the localization of specific polymers recognized by the same set of antibodies as were used for the carbohydrate detecting microarrays. However, on the histological micrographs, *A. vaombe* appeared to contain a low amount of mannan based on the detection of LM21 and BS-400-4 and only in the cell wall, whereas the carbohydrate detecting microarrays analysis of the comparable summer samples showed *A. vaombe* to be the one investigated species containing the most of both epitopes. In the microscopy study the focus was on the bioactive polysaccharide mannan using the antibodies BS-400-4 and LM21. Both anti-mannan antibodies detected the polymers in all species, but in *A. arborescens*, the signal from both antibodies BS-400-4 and LM21 was more pronounced in the outer mesophyll cells than in the inner leaf mesophyll (**Figures 4**, **5**, respectively). This could indicate that the outer cell layers are more used for storage than the inner most cells are, assuming mannans function as storage polymers (Stancato et al., 2001). In *A. vaombe* the signals from the mannan recognizing antibodies were generally weaker, and the mannan appeared to be embedded in the cell wall with only very low amounts of the polysaccharide located in the cytosol. In terms of mannan amounts and distribution based on the histological micrographs, *A. vera* and *A. decaryi* seem to be containing the highest amounts of mannan, suggesting *A. decaryi* potentially could also be a source of medicinally relevant mannans. *A. arborescens* also contained larger amounts of mannan, but not throughout the mesophyll as did *A. vera* and *A. decaryi*. The extensive medicinal use of *A. arborescens* indicates that it is the quantity rather than the specific localization of the polysaccharides in the mesophyll that determines the medicinal quality of the mannan.

Structural Function of *Aloe* Polysaccharides in the Cell Wall

A very general description of a plant cell wall is based on a scaffold of linear cellulose strands bound together by an array of hemicelluloses embedded in a pectin matrix (Cosgrove, 2005; Albersheim, 2011). The main non-cellulosic polysaccharides detected by carbohydrate detecting microarrays in *Aloe* inner leaf mesophyll are pectins and two kinds of hemicelluloses – mannans and xyloglucan. Whereas the acetylated mannan is interesting from a medicinal point of view, from a plant cell wall perspective, the xyloglucan is likely to be the primary one binding the cellulose strands together as the mannan seems to be present in granulates more than as a flat sheet when looking at the histological micrographs. A large concentration of mannan was released in the water extraction also suggesting that these polymers are very loosely bound in the matrix, as tightly bound hemicelluloses would normally be expected to require NaOH for bulk release (Hansen et al., 2014). The release of xyloglucan in the NaOH extraction thus further supports the idea that this polysaccharide is more tightly bound in the cell wall participating in the general scaffold together with cellulose. Neither xylan nor glucans were detected in the carbohydrate detecting microarrays analyses (seen by the lack of detection by antibodies LM23, BS-400-2, and BS-400-3) and comparatively,

xyloglucan contains more side-chains than xylan, which could likely have an effect on the cell wall structure (Meikle et al., 1991; Manabe et al., 2011; Pedersen et al., 2012; Torode et al., 2015). However, negative detection of a polysaccharide is not evidence of its absence, as its presence could be under the level of detection for the method or not expressed in the studied material. The acetylation of the mannan might be an important factor in relation to the types of bindings formed between the mannan and the scaffold polysaccharides. The detected pectin epitope changes over the season and between the extractions supports this idea of a highly flexible matrix.

Composition and Variation of *Aloe* Polysaccharides

The expectation of finding highly acetylated mannans in at least the *Aloe vera* gel was supported in particular by the binding of CCRC-170, as this antibody has a known target epitope containing acetylations (Pattathil et al., 2012; Zhang et al., 2014). The antibody BS-400-4 bound most strongly to the *Aloe* extractions indicating that the tissue contains high amounts of loosely bound $(1{\to}4)$-β-D-mannan. We observed a complete lack of binding from the mannan-specific antibody LM22 compared to the binding seen for LM21. Both epitopes was shown to bind mannans by Marcus et al. (2010), although their study was focused on mannan derived oligosaccharides from *Amorphophallus cognac* K. Koch and *Seratonia siliqua* L., which may be structurally different from *Aloe* derived mannans. In particular LM22 has been reported to bind strongly to galactomannan, whereas LM21 binds to glucomannan and the lack of binding of LM21 may therefore suggest glucomannan is not present in *Aloe* (Marcus et al., 2010). The acetylation of mannan has been a concern with regards to the mannan recognizing antibodies as previous studies using the same set of antibodies failed to show any binding (Ahl et al., 2018). In the present study, however, the method has been optimized, especially in terms of sample wait-time, meaning the polysaccharides printed on the nitrocellulose were of a better quality. If samples sit for too long between extraction and printing, signals are likely to fade or even disappear, and a similar situation is expected if samples are frozen (personal observation).

Based on the carbohydrate detecting microarrays results, seasonal variation was detected in the quantity of polysaccharides. The monthly variation was subtle, but when data was pooled according to season, distinct differences were seen. The changes were primarily seen in the binding patterns of pectin and mannan-specific antibodies. Variation in cell wall composition is well-known and reflects the flexibility of the cell wall (Albersheim, 2011). When all data for each species was pooled per season as shown in **Figure 2** the changes were not as obvious as when the three extractions steps were compared separately. There was a clear trend, however, of the plants having the highest amounts of polysaccharides in June, July, and August. The optimal harvest time for obtaining higher yield of the sought-after polysaccharides might change from location to location. The ability to detect change in mannan content could therefore be of importance to the *Aloe* industry for planning of harvest time in plantations.

Potential of Carbohydrate Detecting Microarrays for Authentication of *Aloe* Products

Acetylated mannan from *Aloe vera* has been linked to induced tissue repair in humans for decades (Reynolds and Dweck, 1999; Xing et al., 2014; Thunyakitpisal et al., 2017), but traditionally more than 25% of the genus *Aloe species* (about 150 taxa) have been used to treat a range of conditions (Grace et al., 2009). The primary aim of this study was to investigate if carbohydrate detecting microarrays could be used as a complementary method to detect a seasonal variation in the polysaccharide composition of the selected aloes – two medicinally used and two non-medicinally used. Based on our results, each species had a distinct polysaccharide profile, yet the two medicinally used species (*A. vera* and *A. arborescens*) were more similar to each other than they were to the two non-medicinally used species in terms of both pectin and to some extent mannans. Although, it was possible to differentiate between the *Aloe* species based on carbohydrate detecting microarrays analyses of the investigated samples, the profiles are distinct enough to use carbohydrate detecting microarrays to discriminate unambiguously between individual species. Furthermore, the observed seasonal variation supports the stand that carbohydrate detecting microarrays should not be used as a stand-alone means of analysis to authenticate an *Aloe vera* product. Additional replicate samples would also be needed to explore potential within species variation. However, the similarities and differences between the polysaccharide compositions of the medicinally used species and the non-medicinally ones may potentially be useful to identify the group of medicinal aloes.

As carbohydrate detecting microarrays are primarily a qualitative method, they cannot be used for quantitative authentication of products, but could be suitable to detect if a product actually contains polysaccharides in a composition that could be related to *Aloe vera* or another medicinally used species. The most important antibodies to use for such a screen would be both the mannan-specific ones from which we saw signals in this study, but also pectin-specific antibodies, which showed more differentiation of species. In terms of feasibility for authentication of *Aloe* polysaccharides, carbohydrate detecting microarrays is a high-throughput method capable of simultaneously analyzing 10–20 different samples. Apart from the investment in a microarrayer, the running costs include non-specialist lab equipment, nitrocellulose for printing, and a few selected antibodies. For the analysis of fewer samples, a commercial services analysis of freeze-dried and milled samples could

possibly be set up with laboratories having the set up in house. One additional concern is the availability of relevant standardized reference material for comparison. Aloes are rich in phenolic compounds, which can bind and lead to masking of epitopes, and it is therefore important to only use inner leaf mesophyll for the carbohydrate detecting microarray analysis. The commercial plant material of *Aloe vera* and *A. ferox* obtained here as Ph. Eur. reference standard is whole above ground plant material, whereas the monographs specify either exudate or inner leaf mesophyll depending on intended use and the whole plant extracts included here also differed in polysaccharide composition and content (**Figure 2** and **Supplementary Material**). Consequently, there is a need for a more specific definition of what should be considered standard Ph. Eur. reference material.

CONCLUSION

The histological micrographs showed differences between species in terms of the amounts of mannan present in different parts of the aloe leaf tissue. The micrographs revealed that the polysaccharides serve as structural hemicellulose in the cell wall but can also function as a storage polysaccharide within the cytosol of *Aloe* species. In terms of Quality Control and Standardization of Plant Based Medicines – carbohydrate detecting microarrays were able to detect differences between species and seasonal variation in composition and abundance of polysaccharides and relevant antibodies are available to screen for the acetylated mannans hypothesized to be responsible for the acclaimed bioactivities of *Aloe* gel. Carbohydrate detecting microarrays therefore has potential as a complementary screening method directly targeting the presence and composition of relevant polysaccharides. The observed seasonal variation may be of importance for commercial growing to optimize harvest times. In addition to seasonal variation, we would expect potential variation of polysaccharides according to the age and origin of the plants, as well as the impact of the local growing conditions, and of storage conditions further down the production line. The carbohydrate detecting microarrays method could thus be used to provide relevant information about variation of the polysaccharides in individual plantations allowing optimization of yield.

AUTHOR CONTRIBUTIONS

LA designed the study together with NR and OG, conducted the probing with the antibodies, supervised NA-H and SA-H together with DS and NR, and wrote the manuscript together with NR. LA, NA-H, and SA-H collected and prepared the samples. NA-H and SA-H conducted the carbohydrate detecting microarrays extractions and printing under guidance of LA. LA and BJ conducted the data analysis. JM conducted the microscopy imaging and interpreted the results together with LA. All authors contributed to the discussions and to the final version of the manuscript.

FUNDING

This research was supported by grants from the Villum Foundation, Planet Project #9283 to WW, BJ, and NR and #17489 to JM.

ACKNOWLEDGMENTS

We thank gardener Martin Årseth-Hansen, Botanical Garden, Natural History Museum of Denmark, for growing the plant material, and Jeanett Hansen for help in the laboratory at PLEN, and Henriette L. Pedersen for discussion on carbohydrate detecting microarrays methods and results.

REFERENCES

Ahl, L. I., Grace, O. M., Pedersen, H. L., Willats, W. G. T., Jørgensen, B., and Rønsted, N. (2018). Analyses of *Aloe* polysaccharides using carbohydrate microarray profiling. *J. AOAC Int.* 101, 1711–1719. doi: 10.5740/jaoacint.18-0120

Albersheim, P. (2011). *Plant Cell Walls?: from Chemistry to Biology.* Taylor, MI: Garland Science.

Beppu, H., Shimpo, K., Chihara, T., Kaneko, T., Tamai, I., Yamaji, S., et al. (2006). Antidiabetic effects of dietary administration of *Aloe arborescens* Miller components on multiple low-dose streptozotocin-induced diabetes in mice: investigation on hypoglycemic action and systemic absorption dynamics of aloe components. *J. Ethnopharmacol.* 103, 468–477. doi: 10.1016/j.jep.2005.10.034

Bozzi, A., Perrin, C., Austin, S., and Arce Vera, F. (2007). Quality and authenticity of commercial *Aloe Vera* gel powders. *Food Chem.* 103, 22–30. doi: 10.1016/j.foodchem.2006.05.061

Campestrini, L. H., Silveira, J. L. M., Duarte, M. E. R., Koop, H. S., and Noseda, M. D. (2013). NMR and rheological study of *Aloe barbadensis* partially acetylated glucomannan. *Carbohydr. Polym.* 94, 511–519. doi: 10.1016/j.carbpol.2013.01.020

Carter, S., Lavranos, J. J., Newton, L. E., and Walker, C. C. (2011). *Aloes the Definitive Guide.* Richmond, VA: Royal Botanic Gardens Kew. doi: 10.1016/j.carbpol.2013.01.020

Chokboribal, J., Tachaboonyakiat, W., Sangvanich, P., Ruangpornvisuti, V., Jettanacheawchankit, S., and Thunyakitpisal, P. (2015). Deacetylation affects the physical properties and bioactivity of acemannan, an extracted polysaccharide from *Aloe vera. Carbohydr. Polym.* 133, 556–566. doi: 10.1016/j.carbpol.2015.07.039

CITES (2017). *CITES Appendices I, II, III. Convection,* 61. doi: 10.1016/j.carbpol.2015.07.039

Clausen, M. H., Willats, W. G. T., and Knox, J. P. (2003). Synthetic methyl hexagalacturonate hapten inhibitors of anti-homogalacturonan monoclonal antibodies LM7, JIM5 and JIM7. *Carbohydr. Res.* 338, 1797–1800. doi: 10.1016/S0008-6215(03)00272-6

Cosgrove, D. J. (2005). Growth of the plant cell wall. *Nat. Rev. Mol. Cell Biol.* 6, 850–861. doi: 10.1038/nrm1746

Cristiano, G., Murillo-Amador, B., and De Lucia, B. (2016). Propagation techniques and agronomic requirements for the cultivation of Barbados *Aloe (Aloe vera* (L.) Burm. F.) — a review. *Front. Plant Sci.* 7:1410. doi: 10.3389/fpls.2016.01410

Eberendu, A. R., Luta, G., Edwards, J. A., Mcanalley, B. H., Davis, B., Rodriguez, S., et al. (2005). Quantitative colorimetric analysis of *Aloe* polysaccharides as a measure of *Aloe vera* quality in commercial products. *J. AOAC Int.* 88, 684–691.

EDQM (2016). *European Pharmacopoeia (Ph. Eur.), 9th Edn.* (accessed December 11, 2018).

Ernst, E. (2004). Risks of herbal medicinal products. *Pharmacoepidemiol. Drug Saf.* 13, 767–771. doi: 10.1002/pds.1014

Fangel, J. U., Pedersen, H. L., Vidal-Melgosa, S., Ahl, L. I., Salmean, A. A., Egelund, J., et al. (2012). Carbohydrate microarrays in plant science. *Methods Mol. Biol.* 918, 351–362. doi: 10.1007/978-1-61779-995-2_19

Femenia, A., Sanchez, E. S., Simal, S., Rossell, C., Sánchez, E. S., Simal, S., et al. (1999). Compositional features of polysaccharides from *Aloe vera (Aloe barbadensis* Miller) plant tissues. *Carbohydr. Polym.* 39, 109–117. doi: 10.1016/S0144-8617(98)00163-5

Future Market Insights (2016). *Global Demand for Aloe vera Extracts to Reach 60,720 Tonnes in 2016; Emergence of Innovative, High-Quality and Cost-Effective Products Ramping up Adoption.* Pune: Future Market Insights. doi: 10.1016/s0144-8617(98)00163-5

Gilbert, N. (2011). Herbal medicine rule book: can Western guidelines govern Eastern herbal traditions? *Nature* 480, 598–599.

Grace, O. M. (2011). Current perspectives on the economic botany of the genus *Aloe* L. (Xanthorrhoeaceae). *S. Afr. J. Bot.* 77, 980–987. doi: 10.1016/J.Sajb.2011.07.002

Grace, O. M., Buerki, S., Symonds, M. R., Forest, F., van Wyk, A. E., Smith, G. F., et al. (2015). Evolutionary history and leaf succulence as explanations for medicinal use in aloes and the global popularity of *Aloe vera. BMC Evol. Biol.* 15:29. doi: 10.1186/s12862-015-0291-7

Grace, O. M., Dzajic, A., Jäger, A. K., Nyberg, N. T., Önder, A., and Rønsted, N. (2013). Monosaccharide analysis of succulent leaf tissue in *Aloe. Phytochemistry* 93, 79–87. doi: 10.1016/j.phytochem.2013.03.015

Grace, O. M., and Rønsted, N. (2017). "Comparative biology of aloes and related genera in the context of recent phylogenetic evidence", in *Diversity and Phylogeny of the Monocotyledons,* Memoirs of The New York Botanical Garden Vol. 118, eds L. M. Campbell, J. I. Davis, A. W. Meerow, R. F. C. Naczi, D. W. Stevenson, and W. W. Thomas (New York, NY: NYBG Press), 100–112. doi: 10.21135/893275341.006

Grace, O. M., Simmonds, M. S. J., Smith, G. F., and Van Wyk, A. E. (2009). Documented utility and biocultural value of *Aloe* L. (Asphodelaceae): a review. *Econ. Bot.* 63, 167–178. doi: 10.1007/s12231-009-9082-7

Grindlay, D., and Reynolds, T. (1986). The *Aloe vera* phenomenon: a review of the properties and modern uses of the leaf parenchyma gel. *J. Ethnopharmacol.* 16, 117–151. doi: 10.1016/0378-8741(86)90085-1

Hamman, J. H. (2008). Composition and applications of *Aloe vera* leaf gel. *Molecules* 13, 1599–1616. doi: 10.3390/Molecules13081599

Hansen, M. A. T., Ahl, L. I., Pedersen, H. L., Westereng, B., Willats, W. G. T., Jørgensen, H., et al. (2014). Extractability and digestibility of plant cell wall polysaccharides during hydrothermal and enzymatic degradation of wheat straw (*Triticum aestivum* L.). *Ind. Crops Prod.* 55, 63–69. doi: 10.1016/j.indcrop.2014.02.002

Hu, Y., Xu, J., and Hu, Q. (2003). Evaluation of antioxidant potential of *Aloe vera (Aloe barbadensis* Miller) extracts. *J. Agric. Food Chem.* 51, 7788–7791. doi: 10.1021/jf034255i

Jones, L., Seymour, G. B., and Knox, J. P. (1997). Localization of pectic galactan in tomato cell walls using a monoclonal antibody specific to (1-4)-[beta]-D-Galactan. *Plant Physiol.* 113, 1405–1412. doi: 10.1104/pp.113.4.1405

Krešimir, S., Fangel, J. U., Rydahl, M. G., Pedersen, H. L., Vidal-Melgosa, S., and Willats, W. G. T. (2017). "Carbohydrate microarray technology applied to high-throughput mapping of plant cell wall glycans using Comprehensive Microarray Polymer Profiling (CoMPP)," in *High-Throughput Glycomics and Glycoproteomics,* eds G. Lauc and M. Wuhrer (New York, NY: Springer Science+Business Media), 147–166. doi: 10.1007/978-1-4939-6493-2

Lee, K. J. D., Sakata, Y., Mau, S., Pettolino, F., Bacic, A., Quatrano, R. S., et al. (2005). Arabinogalactan proteins are required for apical cell extension in the moss *Physcomitrella patens. Plant Cell* 17, 3051–3065. doi: 10.1105/tpc.105.034413.for

Manabe, Y., Nafisi, M., Verhertbruggen, Y., Orfila, C., Gille, S., Rautengarten, C., et al. (2011). Loss-of-function mutation of reduced wall acetylation in *Arabidopsis* leads to reduced cell wall acetylation and increased resistance to *Botrytis cinerea*. *Plant Physiol*. 155, 1068–1078. doi: 10.1104/pp.110.168989

Marcus, S. E., Blake, A. W., Benians, T. A. S., Lee, K. J. D., Poyser, C., Donaldson, L., et al. (2010). Restricted access of proteins to mannan polysaccharides in intact plant cell walls. *Plant J*. 64, 191–203. doi: 10.1111/J.1365-313x.2010.04319.X

Meikle, P. J., Bonig, I., Hoogenraad, N. J., Clarke, A. E., and Stone, B. A. (1991). The location of (1-3)-beta-glucans in the walls of pollen tubes of *Nicotiana alata* using a (1-3)-beta-glucan-specific monoclonal antibody. *Planta* 185, 1–8. doi: 10.1007/BF00194507

Minjares-Fuentes, R., Femenia, A., Comas-Serra, F., Rosselló, C., Rodríguez-González, V. M., González-Laredo, R. F., et al. (2016). Effect of different drying procedures on physicochemical properties and flow behavior of *Aloe vera* (*Aloe barbadensis* Miller) gel. *LWT Food Sci. Technol*. 74, 378–386. doi: 10.1016/j.lwt.2016.07.060

Minjares-Fuentes, R., Femenia, A., and Rodriguez-Gonzalez, V. M. (2018). Compositional and structural features of the main bioactive polysaccharides present in the *Aloe vera* plant. *J. AOAC Int*. 101, 1711–1719. doi: 10.5740/jaoacint.18-0119

Moller, I., Sørensen, I., Bernal, A. J., Blaukopf, C., Lee, K., Øbro, J., et al. (2007). High-throughput mapping of cell-wall polymers within and between plants using novel microarrays. *Plant J*. 50, 1118–1128. doi: 10.1111/j.1365-313X.2007.03114.x

Mravec, J., Kračun, S. K., Rydahl, M. G., Westereng, B., Pontiggia, D., De Lorenzo, G., et al. (2017). An oligogalacturonide-derived molecular probe demonstrates the dynamics of calcium-mediated pectin complexation in cell walls of tip-growing structures. *Plant J*. 91, 534–546. doi: 10.1111/tpj.13574

Nazeam, J. A., Gad, H. A., El-Hefnawy, H. M., and Singab, A. N. B. (2017). Chromatographic separation and detection methods of *Aloe arborescens* Miller constituents: a systematic review. *J. Chromatogr. B Anal. Technol. Biomed. Life Sci*. 1058, 57–67. doi: 10.1016/j.jchromb.2017.04.044

Ni, Y., Turner, D., Yates, K. M., and Tizard, I. (2004). Isolation and characterization of structural components of *Aloe vera* L. leaf pulp. *Int. Immunopharmacol*. 4, 1745–1755. doi: 10.1016/J.Intimp.2004.07.006

O'Brian, C., Van Wyk, B.-E., and Van Heerden, F. R. (2011). Physical and chemical characteristics of *Aloe ferox* leaf gel. *S. Afr. J. Bot*. 77, 988–995. doi: 10.1016/j.sajb.2011.08.004

Pattathil, S., Avci, U., Miller, J. S., and Hahn, M. G. (2012). Immunological approaches to plant cell wall and biomass characterization: glycome profiling. *Methods Mol. Biol*. 908, 61–72. doi: 10.1007/978-1-61779-956-3

Paulsen, B. S., and Barsett, H. (2005). "Bioactive pectic polysaccharides," in *Polysaccharides 1: Structure, Characterization and Use*, ed. T. Heinze (Berlin: Springer), 69–101. doi: 10.1007/B136817

Pedersen, H. L., Fangel, J. U., McCleary, B., Ruzanski, C., Rydahl, M. G., Ralet, M.-C., et al. (2012). Versatile high resolution oligosaccharide microarrays for plant glycobiology and cell wall research. *J. Biol. Chem*. 287, 39429–39438. doi: 10.1074/jbc.M112.396598

Pettolino, F. A., Hoogenraad, N. J., Ferguson, C., Bacic, A., Johnson, E., and Stone, B. A. (2001). A (1-4)-beta-mannan-specific monoclonal antibody and its use in the immunocytochemical location of galactomannans. *Planta* 214, 235–242. doi: 10.1007/s004250100606

Reynolds, T. (2004). "*Aloe* chemistry," in *Aloes: the Genus Aloe*, ed. T. Reynolds (Boca Raton, FL: CRC Press), 39–74.

Reynolds, T., and Dweck, A. C. (1999). *Aloe vera* leaf gel: a review update. *J. Ethnopharmacol*. 68, 3–37. doi: 10.1016/S0378-8741(99)00085-9

Saslis-Lagoudakis, C. H., Iwanycki, N. E., Bruun-Lund, S., Petersen, G., Seberg, O., Jäger, A. K., et al. (2015). Identification of common horsetail (*Equisetum arvense* L.; Equisetaceae) using thin layer chromatography versus DNA barcoding. *Sci. Rep*. 5:11942. doi: 10.1038/srep11942

Shi, X. D., Yin, J. Y., Huang, X. J., Que, Z. Q., and Nie, S. P. (2018). Structural and conformational characterization of linear O-acetyl-glucomannan purified from gel of *Aloe barbadensis* Miller. *Int. J. Biol. Macromol*. 120, 2373–2380. doi: 10.1016/j.ijbiomac.2018.09.005

Simões, J., Nunes, F. M., Domingues, P., Coimbra, M. A., and Domingues, M. R. (2012). Mass spectrometry characterization of an *Aloe vera* mannan presenting immunostimulatory activity. *Carbohydr. Polym*. 90, 229–236. doi: 10.1016/j.carbpol.2012.05.029

Sriariyakul, W., Swasdisevi, T., Devahastin, S., and Soponronnarit, S. (2016). Drying of *Aloe vera* puree using hot air in combination with far-infrared radiation and high-voltage electric field: drying kinetics, energy consumption and product quality evaluation. *Food Bioprod. Process*. 100, 391–400. doi: 10.1016/j.fbp.2016.08.012

Stancato, G. C., Buckeridge, M. S., and Mazzafera, P. (2001). Effect of a drought period on the mobilisation of non-structural carbohydrates, photosynthetic efficiency and water status in an epiphytic orchid. *Plant Physiol. Biochem*. 39, 1009–1016. doi: 10.1016/S0981-9428(01)01321-3

Talmadge, J., Chavez, J., Jacobs, L., Munger, C., Chinnah, T., Chow, J. T., et al. (2004). Fractionation of *Aloe vera* L. inner gel, purification and molecular profiling of activity. *Int. Immunopharmacol*. 4, 1757–1773. doi: 10.1016/J.Intimp.2004.07.013

t'Hart, L., van den Berg, A., Kuis, L., van Dijk, H., and Labadie, R. (1989). An anti-complementary polysaccharide with immunological adjuvant activity from the leaf parenchyma gel of *Aloe vera*. *Planta Med*. 55, 509–512. doi: 10.1055/s-2006-962082

Thunyakitpisal, P., Ruangpornvisuti, V., Kengkwasing, P., Chokboribal, J., and Sangvanich, P. (2017). Acemannan increases NF-κB/DNA binding and IL-6/-8 expression by selectively binding Toll-like receptor-5 in human gingival fibroblasts. *Carbohydr. Polym*. 161, 149–157. doi: 10.1016/j.carbpol.2016.12.034

Torode, T. A., Marcus, S. E., Jam, M., Tonon, T., Blackburn, R. S., Hervé, C., et al. (2015). Monoclonal antibodies directed to fucoidan preparations from brown algae. *PLoS One* 10:e0118366. doi: 10.1371/journal.pone.0118366

van Breemen, R. B., and Farnsworth, N. R. (2008). Ensuring the safety of botanical dietary supplements. *Am. J. Clin. Nutr*. 87, 509–513.

Vandenbosch, K. A., Bradley, D. J., Knox, J. P., Perotto, S., Butcher, G. W., and Brewin, N. J. (1989). Common components of the infection thread matrix and the intercellular space identified by immunocytochemical analysis of pea nodules and uninfected roots. *Eur. Mol. Biol. Organ. J*. 8, 335–341. doi: 10.1002/j.1460-2075.1989.tb03382.x

Verhertbruggen, Y., Marcus, S. E., Haeger, A., Ordaz-Ortiz, J. J., and Knox, J. P. (2009). An extended set of monoclonal antibodies to pectic homogalacturonan. *Carbohydr. Res*. 344, 1858–1862. doi: 10.1016/j.carres.2008.11.010

Willats, W. G. T., Limberg, G., Buchholt, H. C., Van Alebeek, G. J., Benen, J., Christensen, T. M. I. E., et al. (2000). Analysis of pectic epitopes recognised by hybridoma and phage display monoclonal antibodies using defined oligosaccharides, polysaccharides, and enzymatic degradation. *Carbohydr. Res*. 327, 309–320. doi: 10.1016/S0008-6215(00)00039-2

Willats, W. G. T., Marcus, S. E., and Knox, J. P. (1998). Generation of a monoclonal antibody specific to (1-5)-beta-l-arabinan. *Carbohydr. Res*. 308, 149–152. doi: 10.1016/S0008-6215(98)00070-6

World Health Organization [WHO] (1999). WHO monographs on selected medicinal plants. *Essent. Med. Heal. Prod. Inf. Portal* 1, 183–194.

Xing, W., Guo, W., Zou, C. H., Fu, T. T., Li, X. Y., Zhu, M., et al. (2014). Acemannan accelerates cell proliferation and skin wound healing through AKT/mTOR signaling pathway. *J. Dermatol. Sci*. 79, 101–109. doi: 10.1016/j.jdermsci.2015.03.016

Zhang, X., Rogowski, A., Zhao, L., Hahn, M. G., Avci, U., Knox, J. P., et al. (2014). Understanding how the complex molecular architecture of mannan-degrading hydrolases contributes to plant cell wall degradation. *J. Biol. Chem*. 289, 2002–2012. doi: 10.1074/jbc.M113.527770

Zhang, Y., Bao, Z., Ye, X., and Xie, Z. (2018). Chemical investigation of major constituents in Aloe vera leaves and several commercial Aloe juice powders. *J. AOAC Int*. 101, 1741–1751. doi: 10.5740/jaoacint.18-0122

DNA Metabarcoding Authentication of Ayurvedic Herbal Products on the European Market Raises Concerns of Quality and Fidelity

*Gopalakrishnan Saroja Seethapathy[1,2], Ancuta-Cristina Raclariu-Manolica[1,3], Jarl Andreas Anmarkrud[1], Helle Wangensteen[2] and Hugo J. de Boer[1]**

[1] Natural History Museum, University of Oslo, Oslo, Norway, [2] Department of Pharmaceutical Chemistry, School of Pharmacy, University of Oslo, Oslo, Norway, [3] Stejarul Research Centre for Biological Sciences, National Institute of Research and Development for Biological Sciences, Piatra Neamt, Romania

Correspondence:
Hugo J. de Boer
hugo.deboer@nhm.uio.no

Ayurveda is one of the oldest systems of medicine in the world, but the growing commercial interest in Ayurveda based products has increased the incentive for adulteration and substitution within this herbal market. Fraudulent practices such as the use of undeclared fillers and use of other species of inferior quality is driven both by the increased as well as insufficient supply capacity of especially wild plant species. Developing novel strategies to exhaustively assess and monitor both the quality of raw materials and final marketed herbal products is a challenge in herbal pharmacovigilance. Seventy-nine Ayurvedic herbal products sold as tablets, capsules, powders, and extracts were randomly purchased via e-commerce and pharmacies across Europe, and DNA metabarcoding was used to assess the ability of this method to authenticate these products. Our analysis reveals that only two out of 12 single ingredient products contained only one species as labeled, eight out of 27 multiple ingredient products contained none of the species listed on the label, and the remaining 19 products contained 1 to 5 of the species listed on the label along with many other species not specified on the label. The fidelity for single ingredient products was 67%, the overall ingredient fidelity for multi ingredient products was 21%, and for all products 24%. The low level of fidelity raises concerns about the reliability of the products, and detection of threatened species raises further concerns about illegal plant trade. The study highlights the necessity for quality control of the marketed herbal products and shows that DNA metabarcoding is an effective analytical approach to authenticate complex multi ingredient herbal products. However, effort needs to be done to standardize the protocols for DNA metabarcoding before this approach can be implemented as routine analytical approaches for plant identification, and approved for use in regulated procedures.

Keywords: Ayurvedic herbal products, botanical authentication, DNA barcoding, herbal medicines, pharmacovigilance, quality control

INTRODUCTION

Ayurveda, or Ayurvedic medicine, is one of the oldest systems of traditional medicine (TM), with origins in India more than 3,000 years ago. Nowadays Ayurveda is popular and used worldwide in complementary and alternative healthcare and medical practices (CAM) (World Health Organization [WHO], 2013). Ayurvedic formulations are obtained using an average of 80% botanicals, 12% animals, and 8% minerals, and are used as raw materials and preparations such as extracts (Joshi et al., 2017). About 7,000 plant species are used for medicinal purposes in India, from which, about 1,200 species have been reported to be actively traded (Goraya and Ved, 2017). The total commercial demand for herbal material in India, in 2014 and 2015, was estimated to be in excess of 512,000 tons, with a market value of 1 billion USD (Goraya and Ved, 2017). India has more than 8,000 licensed manufacturing units for medicinal products and the increasing level of consumption of herbal products exceed the supply capacity for some plant species (Goraya and Ved, 2017). In order to ensure a level of uniformity of the therapeutic formula and the ingredients used, the Ayurvedic formulary and Ayurvedic Pharmacopeia of India was published by the Government of India as a legally binding document describing the quality, purity, and strength of selected drugs that are manufactured, distributed and sold by the licensed manufacturers in India (Joshi et al., 2017).

As many other TMs, Ayurvedic herbal medicines, require quality assurances for their wider usage and acceptability in CAM practicing countries (World Health Organization [WHO], 2013). The growing demand for Ayurveda encourages an industry for mass production of herbal products, leading to the use of large quantities of plant raw material, mainly harvested from the wild flora (Valiathan, 2006; Goraya and Ved, 2017; Joshi et al., 2017). Many of the Indian medicinal plant species are in short supply due to the lack of cultivation and several wild species are not available in sufficient quantities for commercial exploitation (Goraya and Ved, 2017). The intensive use of herbal products increases the incentive for adulteration and substitution in the medicinal plant trade (Newmaster et al., 2013). This awareness of content irregularities calls attention to the quality of the traded mass produced herbal products with direct impact on their efficacy and safety (Leonti and Casu, 2013). One of the pharmacognostic parameters to assure quality, safety and efficacy of a herbal medicine is the utilization of correctly identified medicinal plants used as raw material (Evans, 2009). Several new strategies and appropriate standard methods have been proposed to exhaustively assess and monitor both the quality of raw materials and marketed herbal products (Barnes, 2003; De Boer et al., 2015). Standard methods routinely used to assess herbal material, preparations and products rely on morphological characters, microscopy, and chemical fingerprinting [i.e., thin–layer chromatography', high–performance liquid chromatography (HPLC), and gas chromatography (GC)] (De Boer et al., 2015; Parveen et al., 2016). These methods are quick and cost-effective techniques for primary qualitative analysis of raw material and derived herbal products. Alternatively, the use of more advanced methods for identification and quantification of chemical marker compounds

is becoming popular [i.e., liquid chromatography (LC)–mass spectrometry (MS), GC-MS, and LC-nuclear magnetic resonance (NMR)], but requires valuable instrumentation (Jiang et al., 2010; Wang et al., 2017; Zhang et al., 2017; Raclariu et al., 2018a).

Various important issues influence the quality of Ayurvedic herbal products and they need to be carefully taken into consideration when determining the analytical method of choice for quality control. The herbal products are usually complex mixtures of plant material and/or extracts and excipients, and results of manifold processing steps. To apply only standard analytical methods may pose serious challenges to the accuracy of herbal product quality control. Furthermore, adulteration by the deliberate use or admixture of substitutes and undeclared plant fillers, fraudulent adulteration by using fillers of botanical origin or plant materials of inferior quality (Zhang et al., 2012), the addition of pharmaceuticals or other synthetic substances in order to reach an expected effect or a certain level of marker compounds (Calahan et al., 2016; Rocha et al., 2016) raises concerns about the quality and safety of the herbal products. Multiple plant species as source for botanical drug as allowed in different pharmacopeias, as well as the accidental substitutions, all raise concerns ranging from simple misleading labeling to potential serious adverse drug reactions (Ernst, 1998; Heubl, 2010; Gilbert, 2011) or poisoning due to toxic contaminants (Chan, 2003).

All the standard analytical approaches, including sensory and chemical inspection may have a good resolution in quality control by detecting the quality and quantity of specific lead or phytochemical marker compounds. However, they are generally not applicable in identifying target plant species within a complex herbal product, and show low ability to detect non-targeted plant ingredients in herbal products (De Boer et al., 2015). To overcome this limitation, DNA-based approaches have been proposed as useful analytical tools for the quality control of herbs and herbal products (Parveen et al., 2016). DNA barcoding is a cost-effective, species-level identification based upon the use of short and standardized gene regions, known as 'barcodes' (Hebert et al., 2003). Several reviews have corroborated the diverse applicability of DNA barcoding in the field of medicinal plant research (Techen et al., 2014; De Boer et al., 2015). Initially used as an identification tool, DNA barcoding is now applied in the industrial quality assurance context to authenticate a wide range of herbal products (De Boer et al., 2015; Parveen et al., 2016; Sgamma et al., 2017).

The combination of High-Throughput Sequencing (HTS) and DNA barcoding, known as DNA metabarcoding, enables simultaneous high-throughput multi-taxa identification by using the extracellular and/or total DNA extracted from complex samples containing DNA of different origins (Taberlet et al., 2012). Several studies have utilized this approach in identifying and authenticating medicinal plants and derived herbal products. For example, *Echinacea* species, *Hypericum perforatum*, and *Veronica officinalis* were detected in 89, 68 and 15%, respectively, of the investigated herbal products (Raclariu et al., 2017a,b, 2018b). Similarly, Ivanova et al. (2016) found that 15 tested herbal supplements contained non-listed, non-filler plant DNA, and Cheng et al. (2014) showed that the quality of 27 tested herbal preparations was highly affected by the presence of contaminants. Coghlan et al. (2012) revealed the species composition of 15 highly processed traditional Chinese medicines using DNA metabarcoding, and showed that the products contained species included on CITES appendices I and II. A number of studies in India have surveyed herbal raw drug markets and tested the authenticity of the herbal drugs using DNA barcoding. These studies reported that 24% of raw drug samples of *Phyllanthus amarus* Schumach. & Thonn. were substituted with other phenotypically similar *Phyllanthus* species (Srirama et al., 2010). Similar substitution were reported for other species, such as *Sida cordifolia* L. (76%) (Vassou et al., 2015), *Cinnamomum verum* J.Presl (70%) (Swetha et al., 2014), *Myristica fragrans* Houtt. (60%) (Swetha et al., 2017), *Senna auriculata* (L.) Roxb. (50%) (Seethapathy et al., 2015), *Senna tora* (L.) Roxb. (37%) (Seethapathy et al., 2015) and *Senna alexandrina* Mill. (8%) (Seethapathy et al., 2015). Furthermore, Vassou et al. (2016) reported that 21% of raw drugs in Indian herbal markets were unauthentic. Shanmughanandhan et al. (2016) found that 60% of 93 herbal products sold in the form of capsules and plant powders in local stores in India were adulterated. Studies that combined spectroscopic methods, such as NMR, with DNA barcoding or microscopy to authenticate herbal products, reported 80% adulteration in *Saraca asoca* (Urumarudappa et al., 2016), 80% in *Berberis aristata* (Srivastava and Rawat, 2013) and 22% in *Piper nigrum* (Parvathy et al., 2014). All these studies utilizing DNA barcoding and metabarcoding have highlighted the concerns over the quality and good labeling practices of herbal products (Coghlan et al., 2012; Ivanova et al., 2016; Raclariu et al., 2017a,b; Veldman et al., 2017).

The aim of this study was threefold. First, we aimed to test the composition and fidelity of Ayurvedic products marketed in Europe using DNA metabarcoding. Secondly, we aimed to analyze the presence of any red listed species listed on the product label and used as ingredients using DNA metabarcoding. Our final aim was to evaluate the ability of DNA metabarcoding to identify the presence of authentic species, any substitution and adulteration and/or presence of other off labeled plant species.

MATERIALS AND METHODS

Sample Collection

Seventy-nine Ayurvedic herbal products sold as tablets ($n = 30$), capsules ($n = 30$), powders ($n = 16$), and extracts ($n = 3$) were purchased via e-commerce ($n = 53$) and pharmacies ($n = 26$), from Norway ($n = 21$), Romania ($n = 26$), and Sweden ($n = 32$). Based on the label information, 26 were single plant ingredient products, 39 contained between two to ten plant ingredients, and 14 products contained between eleven to 27 plant ingredients (**Supplementary Table S1**). The products contained a total of 159 plant species belonging to 132 genera and 60 families (**Supplementary Table S2**). It was also confirmed that nrITS sequences of all the 159 plant species labeled in the analyzed herbal products were available within the NCBI/GenBank database (**Supplementary Table S2**). The accepted binomial

names and authors of the plants species used as ingredients were validated using The Plant List (2013). The Ayurvedic herbal products were imported into Norway for scientific analyses under Norwegian Medicines Agency license no. 16/04551–2. An overview of the products, including label information, but not the producer/importer name, lot number, expiration date or any other information that could lead to the identification of that specific product, can be found in **Supplementary Table S1**.

DNA Extraction, Amplicon Generation, and High Throughput Sequencing

The 79 Ayurvedic herbal products were processed depending on their pharmaceutical formulation, in addition to an extraction blank per DNA extraction round. A small amount of each herbal product, about 200 mg, was homogenized using 3–5 zirconium grinding beads in a Mini-Beadbeater-1 (Biospec Products Inc., Bartlesville, Oklahoma, United States). The total DNA from each product was extracted from homogenized contents using CTAB extraction (Doyle and Doyle, 1987). The final elution volume was 100 μl. Extracted DNA was quantified using a Qubit 2.0 Fluorometer and Qubit dsDNA HS Assay Kit (Invitrogen, Carlsbad, California, United States). All amplicon libraries, defined as PCR amplified products from a study sample, were prepared in three replicates. For each replicate two nuclear ribosomal target sequences were amplified, the internal transcribed spacers nrITS1 and nrITS2, respectively. The fusion primers included the annealing motif from the Sun et al. (1994) plant-specific primer pairs 17SE and 5.8I1, and 5.8I2 and 26SE. The forward primers included the Ion Torrent A adapter, a 10 bp multiplex identifier tag following the IonXpress setup for Ion Torrent (Thermo Fisher Scientific, Carlsbad, California, United States). The reverse primer included the truncated P1 (trP1) tags in addition to the annealing motif. Expected amplicon sizes were 300–350 bp.

Polymerase chain reactions were carried out using DNA extracted from the herbal products in final reaction volumes of 25 μl including 0.5 μl of template DNA solution (ranging from 0.5 to 2 ng/μl), 1X Q5 reaction buffer (New England Biolabs Inc., United Kingdom), 0.6 μM of each primer (Biolegio B.V., Netherlands), 200 nM dNTPs, 5 U Q5 High-Fidelity DNA Polymerase (New England Biolabs Inc., United Kingdom) and 1X Q5 High GC enhancer. The PCR cycling protocol consisted of initial denaturation at 98°C for 30 s, followed by 35 cycles of denaturation at 98°C for 10 s, annealing at 56°C for nrITS1 or 71°C for nrITS2 for 30 s, and elongation at 72°C for 30 s, followed by a final elongation step at 72°C for 2 min. Three PCR negative controls of the extraction blanks were included per amplification to control for external and cross sample contamination. After PCR, the amplicons were purified using Illustra Exostar (GE Healthcare, Chicago, Illinois, United States) in accordance with the manufacturer protocols. The molarity of each amplicon library was measured using a qPCR based assay (CFX96 Touch Real-Time PCR Detection System, Bio-Rad, Hercules, California, United States). The equimolar amounts of each amplicon library were merged and sequenced using an Ion Torrent Personal Genomic Machine (Thermo Fisher Scientific) as described by Raclariu et al. (2017a).

Bioinformatics Analysis

The sequencing read data were analyzed and demultiplexed into FASTQ files, per sample, using Torrent Suite version 5.0.4 (LT), and each of the replicates was analyzed individually. FASTQ read files were processed using the HTS-barcode-checker pipeline available as a Galaxy pipeline at the Naturalis Biodiversity Center[1] (Lammers et al., 2014). Using the HTS pipeline, nrITS1 and nrITS2 primer sequences were used to demultiplex the sequencing reads per sample and to filter out reads that did not match any of the primers. PRINSEQ was used to determine filtering and trimming values based on read lengths and Phred read quality. All reads with a mean Phred quality score of less than 26 were filtered out, as well as reads with a length of less than 200 bp. The remaining reads were trimmed to a maximum length of 380 bp. CD-HIT-EST was used to cluster reads into molecular operational taxonomic units (MOTUs) defined by a sequence similarity of >99% and a minimum number of ten reads. The consensus sequences of non-singleton MOTUs were queried using BLAST against a reference nucleotide sequence database, with a maximum e-value of 0.05, a minimum hit length of 100 bp and sequence identity of >97%. The number of reads per MOTU, as well as the BLAST results per MOTU, were compiled using custom scripts from the HTS Barcode Checker pipeline (Lammers et al., 2014). The reference sequence database consisted of a local copy of the NCBI/GenBank nucleotide database that is refreshed monthly. These parameters were applied to each of the replicates. A species was considered and validated as being present within the product only if this was detected in at least 2 out of the 3 replicates.

Presence and Abundance of Species Across Samples

To assess species diversity within each sample, and to obtain insights into the dominant species within the Ayurvedic herbal products, the read abundances were normalized by dividing the number of reads for a MOTU by the total number of reads per sample. As a result, the read counts are transformed into a proportion of reads found per species within each sample (**Supplementary Tables S3, S4**). Furthermore, MOTUs detected in at least two out of the three replicates, for each sample, were categorized into expected-detected (MOTUs corresponding to species listed on the product label versus species detected in the analysis), expected-not detected (MOTUs corresponding to species listed on the product label but not detected in the analysis), and not expected-detected (MOTUs corresponding to species non-listed on the product label but detected in the analysis) (**Supplementary Table S5**). The total occurrences of MOTUs per category of expected and detected were evaluated (**Supplementary Table S5**), and a matrix of

[1]http://145.136.240.164:8080/

correlation was generated using ClustVis (Metsalu and Vilo, 2015).

RESULTS

Fidelity of Ayurvedic Products

The genomic DNA extracts were highly variable in quantity and quality. Total DNA concentration for each of the 79 herbal products is provided in **Supplementary Table S6**. **Table 1** shows the average DNA yield for each of the investigated herbal product types. The result shows that three samples labeled as containing only standardized extracts yielded an average of 0.5 ng/µl DNA, whereas tablets, capsules and powders yielded an average of 5.8, 9.6, and 44.7 ng/µl DNA, respectively. Out of 79 products used in the study, 10 tablets were also labeled to contain extracts in addition to crude plant material (#6, #12, #13, #14, #17, #18, #20, #21, #38, and #74). PCR amplification for nrITS1 and nrITS2 regions were performed for all 79 samples, and amplicons were generated for all replicates for nrITS1 and nrITS2 (for samples and concentrations see **Supplementary Table S6**). The extraction blanks yielded no molecular operational taxonomic units (MOTUs) with nrITS1 and nrITS2 primers.

The sequencing success rate was 44% for ITS1 and 41% for ITS2 (**Supplementary Table S6**). Thirty-five products out of 79 (44%) yielded no MOTUs in any of the replicates either for nrITS1 or nrITS2 that fulfilled our quality criteria, and they were excluded from the results and the further discussion (#11, #20–22, #28, #29, #33, #35, #37–39, #41–51, #53, #54, #56, #57, #59, #62, 64, #65, #67, #71, #72, #76, and #78). These products consisted of 13 tablets, 11 capsules, and 11 powders (**Supplementary Table S6**). The products that yielded MOTUs were represented by 17 tablets, 19 capsules, 5 powders, and 3 extracts (**Supplementary Table S7**).

A total of 188 different plant species belonging to 154 genera and 65 families were identified from the retained MOTUs using BLAST. The separate analyses resulted in 131 plant species (110 genus and 53 families) for nrITS1, and 101 plant species (84 genus and 39 families) for nrITS2. The number of species detected per sample ranged from one to 42. After applying our quality selection criteria, where a species was considered and validated as being present within the product only if it was detected in at least 2 out of the 3 replicates, five additional products (#4, #15, #24, #25, and #26 includes 2 tablets and 3 extracts) that failed to yield the same MOTU in any of the replicates were discarded. The remaining 39 products resulted in a total of 97 plant species belonging to 40 families (62 species for nrITS1, and 60 species for nrITS2). The species detected for all the replicates for both ITS1 and ITS2, were merged for each sample for further analyses (**Figure 1** and **Supplementary Tables S3, S7**).

Figure 2 illustrates the fidelity of herbal products between various product forms, country, and method of acquisition. In ten out of twelve single ingredient products that were labeled as containing only one species, we detected multiple species (exceptions #5 and #52), from which six contained the species labeled on the product together with other species, whereas four products did not contained the species listed on the product

TABLE 1 | Genomic DNA yield and amplicon concentrations per herbal product type.

Product type	No. of herbal products	Average genomic DNA concentration (ng/µl) (SD)	Average amplicon concentration quantified by qPCR (ng/µl)						No. of products yielding DNA sequences	No. of products analyzed post filtering
			nrITS1			nrITS2				
			Replicate 1 (SD)	Replicate 2 (SD)	Replicate 3 (SD)	Replicate 1 (SD)	Replicate 2 (SD)	Replicate 3 (SD)		
Tablets	30	5.8 (6)	5.0 (7)	4.3 (4)	7.7 (15)	7.1 (10)	4.9 (4)	15.3 (18)	20	19
Capsules	30	9.6 (12)	6.2 (11)	6.0 (11)	5.1 (9)	5.8 (9)	4.2 (5)	8.3 (13)	16	15
Powders	16	44.7 (63)	19.2 (25)	3.4 (6)	2.4 (3)	9.4 (19)	4.0 (11)	8.3 (18)	5	5
Extracts	3	0.5 (0.5)	3.4 (0.4)	2.4 (2)	2.4 (2)	20.3 (13)	8.5 (4)	21 (19)	3	–

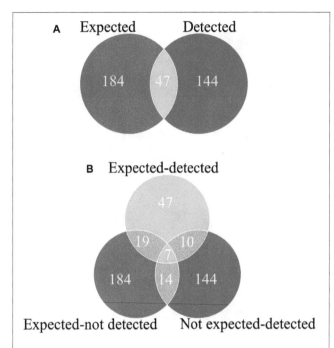

FIGURE 1 | Discrepancies between listed species and detected species using DNA metabarcoding in Ayurvedic herbal products. **(A)** Total number of occurrences of expected species as labeled in the herbal products and detected species using DNA metabarcoding. **(B)** Total number of detected species occurred among expected species as labeled in herbal products (expected-detected), the number of undetected species among the expected species as labeled (expected-not detected), and the number of detected unexpected species (not expected-detected) found in herbal products using DNA metabarcoding. The overlapping numbers are the same species detected in herbal products as expected, detected and unexpected detected.

label but contained several other non-listed species. Out of 27 successfully analyzed multiple ingredient products, 8 (29.6%) products contained none of the species listed on the label, and the remaining 19 products contained between one to five species listed on the label along with many other species not specified on the product label. The fidelity rate for single ingredient products was 67% (8 out of 12), and the overall ingredient fidelity (detected species from product label/total number of species on label) for multi ingredient products was 21% and for all products 24%. **Table 2** shows the top ten products with highest fidelity is also relatively high in the level of substitution, whereas **Table 3** shows the top ten products with highest adulteration and its fidelity.

Figure 3 depicts all 97 detected species based on the relative abundance of read numbers in 39 herbal products per type under the categories of expected-detected, expected-not detected, and not expected-detected.

Plant Ingredients in Herbal Products

A total of 159 plant species belonging to 132 genera and 60 families were specified on the labels of the 79 Ayurvedic herbal products used in this study. Assessing the source and availability of these plants, we found that 83 plants species are solely harvested from wild, and 31 of these are under various threat levels, including critically endangered and protected species, such

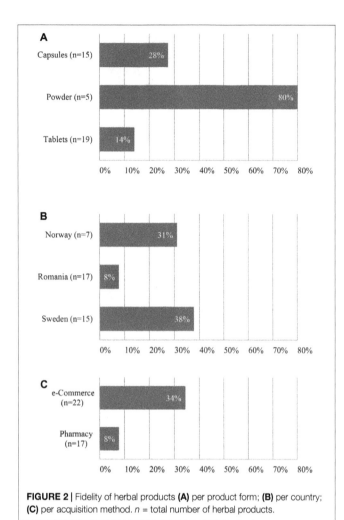

FIGURE 2 | Fidelity of herbal products **(A)** per product form; **(B)** per country; **(C)** per acquisition method. *n* = total number of herbal products.

i.e., *Celastrus paniculatus*, *Glycyrrhiza glabra*, *Gymnema sylvestre*, and *Saraca asoca*, whereas the remaining threatened species were not detected despite being included as labeled ingredients (**Figure 3** and **Supplementary Table S7**). The following species were found in over 20% of the products: *Withania somnifera* (L.) Dunal (39%), *Tribulus terrestris* L. (27%), *Convolvulus prostratus* Forssk. (23%), *Coriandrum sativum* L. (23%), *Ipomoea parasitica* (Kunth) G. Don (23%), *Ocimum basilicum* L. (23%) and *Senna alexandrina* Mill. (23%) (**Figure 3** and **Supplementary Table S3**). Seventeen are present in more than 10% of samples are listed in the **Supplementary Table S3**.

DISCUSSION

The British Pharmacopeia is one the first to publish a specific methods section on DNA barcoding, and in the 2016 version it included a new methods appendix on "Deoxyribonucleic acid (DNA) based identification techniques for herbal drugs" to create a framework for compliance of DNA barcoding with regulatory requirements (British Pharmacopeia Commission, 2016; Sgamma et al., 2017). However, DNA barcoding and metabarcoding are not yet widespread validated methods for use in the regulatory context of quality control. Several studies advocate its usefulness for herbal product authentication and pharmacovigilance either as a standard method or as a complementary method (Ivanova et al., 2016; Raclariu et al., 2017a,b, 2018a; Sgamma et al., 2017). In this study, DNA metabarcoding was used as an analytical approach in Ayurveda herbal product authentication.

A number of studies have shown that the quality of the extraction substrate influences amplification and sequencing success (Ivanova et al., 2016; Raclariu et al., 2017a, 2018b). In addition the presence of DNA in the extraction substrates is influenced by degradation during the harvesting, drying, storage, and industrial processing of plant material (Novak et al., 2007). The success rate in generating raw sequence reads from the herbal products, and the number of products from which MOTUs could be identified per product after applying strict trimming and filtering quality criteria, reduced the number of

as *Pterocarpus marsupium* Roxb., *Pterocarpus santalinus* L.f., *Santalum album* L., and *Saraca asoca* (Roxb.) Willd. (**Figure 4** and **Supplementary Table S2**; Ved and Goraya, 2007; Envis Frlht, 2017; Goraya and Ved, 2017). The DNA metabarcoding analysis confirms the presence of four of these threatened species,

TABLE 2 | Top ten products with the highest fidelity and their level of adulteration.

Herbal product code	Product type	No. species on label	Detected by DNA metabarcoding	Fidelity (Expected-detected, absolute)	Fidelity (Expected-detected, relative)	Adulteration (Detected-Not expected, absolute)	Adulteration (Detected-Not expected, relative)
34	Tablets	8	15	5	63%	10	67%
31	Tablets	10	7	5	50%	2	29%
36	Tablets	13	7	4	31%	3	43%
73	Tablets	14	14	3	21%	11	79%
74	Tablets	9	5	3	33%	2	40%
66	Capsules	6	5	3	50%	2	40%
7	Capsules	6	5	2	33%	3	60%
75	Tablets	3	3	2	67%	1	33%
69	Capsules	1	13	1	100%	12	92%
3	Tablets	4	9	1	25%	8	89%

TABLE 3 | Top ten products with the highest adulteration and their fidelity.

Herbal product code	Product type	No species on label	Detected by DNA metabarcoding	Fidelity (Expected-detected, absolute)	Fidelity (Expected-detected, relative)	Adulteration (Detected-Not expected, absolute)	Adulteration (Detected-Not expected, relative)
69	Capsules	1	13	1	100%	12	92%
32	Tablets	6	12	0	0%	12	100%
73	Tablets	14	14	3	21%	11	79%
34	Tablets	8	15	5	63%	10	67%
3	Tablets	4	9	1	25%	8	89%
68	Capsules	1	8	0	0%	8	100%
40	Capsules	4	8	1	25%	7	88%
27	Capsules	1	8	1	100%	7	88%
6	Tablets	9	7	1	11%	6	86%
23	Tablets	4	7	1	25%	6	86%

samples yielding DNA metabarcoding results from 79 to 39 samples. In this study, 44% of products did not yield MOTUs in any of the replicates either for nrITS1 or nrITS2. Also, in the herbal products labeled to contain only extracts, no plant DNA was detected. The undetected MOTUs in these products could be related to the methodological framework of DNA metabarcoding such as DNA extraction protocol, suitability of primer pair sequences, amplification protocols in PCR for the library preparation, sequencing platform, filtering, quality thresholds, and chimera removal, and clustering thresholds (De Boer et al., 2017; Sgamma et al., 2017; Raclariu et al., 2018b). In addition, extraction of crude herbal drugs either in pre-processing or manufacturing can reduce the availability of plant DNA from those species, especially if material is extracted in boiling water or alcohol, and evaporated or dried at high temperatures.

Considerable incongruences were observed between the detected species and those listed on the label of the products. Similarly, Raclariu et al. (2017b) demonstrated the ability of DNA metabarcoding in detecting *Hypericum* species in complex herbal formulations, and revealed the incongruence between constituent species and those listed on the label in all products. Also, De Boer et al. (2017) performed DNA metabarcoding analyses on 55 commercial products based on orchids (*salep*) purchased in Iran, Turkey, Greece, and Germany, and concluded that there are significant differences in labeled and detected species. They also highlighted the applicability of DNA metabarcoding in targeted efforts for conservation of endangered orchid species. In our study, we detected a total of 97 species in 39 products that passed our quality criteria, and most of the identified species are likely ingredients of Ayurvedic herbal products. Detection of certain species is improbable given their distribution or unlikely use, and these include *Achillea millefolium* L., *Anchusa italica* Retz., *Calluna vulgaris* (L.) Hull, *Damrongia cyanantha* Triboun, *Fraxinus albicans* Buckley and *Trigastrotheca molluginea* F.Muell. The identification of these plant species may be explained by *(i)* amplified PCR chimeras; *(ii)* false-positive BLAST identifications due to incomplete or error-prone reference

databases; or *(iii)* presence of pollen from wind pollinating species, and this confirms previously raised concerns about the hypersensitivity of DNA metabarcoding (De Boer et al., 2017).

Out of 97 species detected in the DNA metabarcoding analysis, 40 species are sourced from wild, 38 species are cultivated, and 15 species are sourced from both wild and cultivation. Similarly, among the 89 species which were not detected in the analysis, 62 species are mainly sourced from wild, including endangered species such as *Embelia ribes* Burm.f., *Pterocarpus marsupium* Roxb., *Pterocarpus santalinus* L.f., *Pueraria tuberosa* (Willd.) DC., and *Santalum album* L. Understanding, the discrepancies between the species detected using DNA metabarcoding and those listed on the label of the products require careful consideration. In DNA metabarcoding analyses, the level of similarity clustering thresholds (>97, >99, and 100%) have an impact on the number and size of assigned MOTUs (Raclariu et al., 2017a). In this study, we used a 99% clustering threshold similar to previously published studies (Raclariu et al., 2017a; Veldman et al., 2017). Furthermore, to limit the impact of sequencing errors, which are known to affect the Ion Torrent sequencing platform (Salipante et al., 2014) and which could lead to the formation of false MOTUs, we used only the clusters that contained a minimum of 10 reads. In addition, by using three replicates for each sample and marker, we reduced further noise by accepting MOTUs only if present in more than one replicate. Furthermore, the strict filtering and trimming thresholds for base calling, length and quality, and strict clustering criteria for MOTUs formation, increase confidence of the results. As reported by previous studies (Ivanova et al., 2016; Raclariu et al., 2017b), the results related to the authentication of herbal products using DNA metabarcoding need to focus primarily on checking the presence of the labeled ingredients and contaminants. The presence of non-listed species may be explained by various factors, including but not limited to the deliberate adulteration and unintentional substitution that may occur from the early stage of the supply chain of medicinal plants (i.e., cultivation, transport, and storage), to the manufacturing

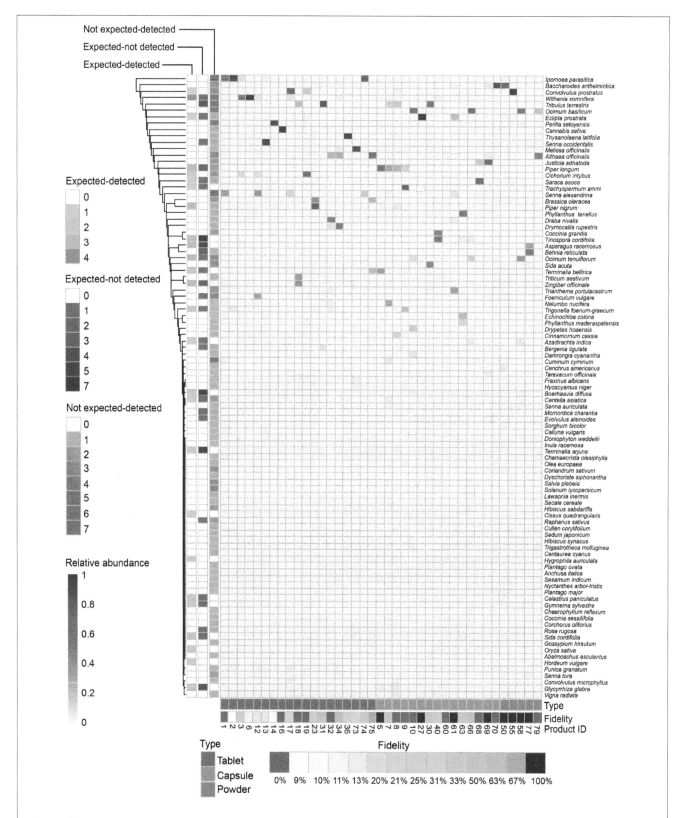

FIGURE 3 | Detection of species in Ayurvedic herbal products. Species (y-axis) are colored by relative abundance of normalized read numbers. Species are categorized in expected-detected and not expected-detected, based on the total number of occurrences, whereas the category expected-not detected is based on the number of times that the species is expected but not detected. Species are clustered by Euclidean distances. Ayurvedic samples (x-axis) are numbered with product code and grouped by product type.

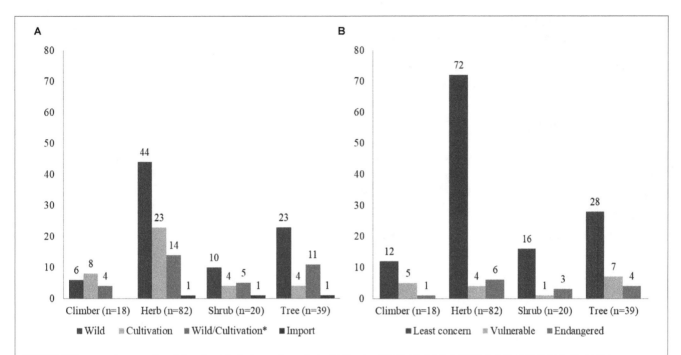

FIGURE 4 | Source and conservation status of species in Ayurvedic products. **(A)** Source of plants labeled as ingredients in the herbal products studied. **(B)** Conservation status of plants labeled as ingredients in the herbal products studied. *N* = total number of species. *Wild/Cultivation denotes that the plants species are sourced both from wild and cultivation.

process and the commercialization of the final products. DNA metabarcoding is a highly sensitive method and even traces of DNA, e.g., contamination from grains of pollinating species or plant dust in the manufacturing process, can be detected and identified.

The advantage of DNA metabarcoding is its ability to simultaneously identify total species diversity within complex multi-ingredient and processed mixtures. Importantly, DNA metabarcoding data is used for qualitative evaluation only, to determine presence of taxa, and not for quantitative assessment of relative species abundance based on read numbers, as many variables considerably impact the obtained sequence read results (Staats et al., 2016). In the context of the quality control of herbal products, DNA metabarcoding does not provide any quantitative nor qualitative information of the active metabolites in the raw plant material or the resulting preparation, and this narrows its applicability only to identification and authentication procedures. Thus, if product safety control relies on threshold levels of specific marker compounds, absence of toxins, allergens and admixed pharmaceuticals, then other methods may be more relevant than DNA-based composition analysis. On the other hand, if product fidelity, species substitution or adulteration is suspected then the latter method outperforms in terms of resolution.

The results of this study reveal that there is a need for a better quality control of herbal products. A novel analytical approach should eventually use a combination of innovative high throughput methods that complement the standard ones recommended today.

CONCLUSION

Assessment of Ayurvedic herbal medicines using DNA metabarcoding provides insight into species diversity in these products and highlights a marked incongruence between species listed as ingredients on the product labels and those detected from DNA present in the samples. Detection of not-listed and not-expected species first and foremost suggests irregularities in the manufacturing process. The presence of foreign plant material could be due accidental reasons, such as contamination from insufficiently cleaned bags, containers, mills, conveyors, and other equipment, or co-occurrence of weeds in cultivation, pollen from wind pollinated species or seeds from wind-dispersed species. However, foreign plant material could also result from fraud, i.e., substitution, adulteration and/or admixture of other species. Interpretation of incongruences should focus on the detected species in the products, and less on the failure to detect species as there are many steps in manufacturing processes that could lead to degradation or loss of DNA beyond detectable limits, e.g., alcoholic extraction, decoction and drying of material at high temperatures. Our study showed that the investigated herbal products contained species not listed on the product labels, and this reveals a clear need for improved quality control. A novel analytical approach should eventually use a combination of advanced chemical methods and innovative high throughput sequencing to complement the standard ones recommended today. The findings of our study show that DNA metabarocoding is a promising tool for quality evaluation of herbal products and pharmacovigilance, and a good candidate for an effective use as a regulatory tool to authenticate complex herbal products. However, standardization of protocols is necessary before DNA metabarcoding can be implemented as a routine analytical approach and approved by competent authorities for use in a regulatory framework.

AUTHOR CONTRIBUTIONS

GS, ACRM, HW, and HdB conceived the experiment. GS collected the material and carried out the molecular lab work and analysis together with ACRM. JA carried out high-throughput sequencing together with GS. GS wrote the manuscript together with HdB. All authors contributed to and approved the final version of the manuscript.

FUNDING

GS was supported through the University of Oslo by the Quota Scheme of the Norwegian Centre for International Cooperation in Higher Education.

ACKNOWLEDGMENTS

The authors acknowledge the help received in the DNA laboratory and genetic analyses from Audun Schrøder-Nielsen and Birgitte Lisbeth Graae Thorbek. Data storage was provided by UNINETT Sigma2 (project no. NS9080K) – the Norwegian national infrastructure for high performance computing and data storage.

REFERENCES

Barnes, J. (2003). Pharmacovigilance of herbal medicines. *Drug Saf.* 26, 829–851. doi: 10.2165/00002018-200326120-00001

British Pharmacopeia Commission (2016). *British Pharmacopoeia 2016. Deoxyribonucleic acid (DNA) Based Identification Techniques for Herbal Drugs. Appendix XI V.* London: TSO.

Calahan, J., Howard, D., Almalki, A. J., Gupta, M. P., and Calderón, A. I. (2016). Chemical adulterants in herbal medicinal products: a review. *Planta Med.* 82, 505–515. doi: 10.1055/s-0042-103495

Chan, K. (2003). Some aspects of toxic contaminants in herbal medicines. *Chemosphere* 52, 1361–1371. doi: 10.1016/S0045-6535(03)00471-5

Cheng, X., Su, X., Chen, X., Zhao, H., Bo, C., Xu, J., et al. (2014). Biological ingredient analysis of traditional Chinese medicine preparation based on high-throughput sequencing: the story for Liuwei Dihuang Wan. *Sci. Rep.* 4:5147. doi: 10.1038/srep05147

Coghlan, M. L., Haile, J., Houston, J., Murray, D. C., White, N. E., Moolhuijzen, P., et al. (2012). Deep sequencing of plant and animal DNA contained within Traditional Chinese Medicines reveals legality issues and health safety concerns. *PLoS Genet.* 8:e1002657. doi: 10.1371/journal.pgen.1002657

De Boer, H. J., Ghorbani, A., Manzanilla, V., Raclariu, A.-C., Kreziou, A., Ounjai, S., et al. (2017). DNA metabarcoding of orchid-derived products reveals widespread illegal orchid trade. *Proc. R. Soc. Lond. B Biol. Sci.* 284:20171182. doi: 10.1098/rspb.2017.1182

De Boer, H. J., Ichim, M. C., and Newmaster, S. G. (2015). DNA barcoding and pharmacovigilance of herbal medicines. *Drug Saf.* 38, 611–620. doi: 10.1007/s40264-015-0306-8

Doyle, J., and Doyle, J. (1987). A rapid DNA isolation procedure for small quantities of fresh leaf tissue. *Phytochem. Bull* 19, 11–15.

Envis Frlht (2017). *"ENVIS Resource Partner on Medicinal Plants".* Available at: http://envis.frlht.org/ [accessed July 27, 2017].

Ernst, E. (1998). Harmless herbs? A review of the recent literature. *Am. J. Med. Sci.* 104, 170–178. doi: 10.1016/S0002-9343(97)00397-5

Evans, W. C. (2009). *Trease and Evans' Pharmacognosy E-Book.* Amsterdam: Elsevier Health Sciences.

Gilbert, N. (2011). Regulations: herbal medicine rule book. *Nature* 480, S98–S99. doi: 10.1038/480S98a

Goraya, G. S., and Ved, D. K. (2017). *Medicinal Plants in India: An Assessment of their Demand and Supply.* Dehradun: Ministry of AYUSH.

Hebert, P., Cywinska, A., Ball, S., and Ewaard, J. (2003). Biological identifications through DNA barcodes. *Proc. R. Soc. Lond. B Biol. Sci.* 270, 313–321. doi: 10.1098/rspb.2002.2218

Heubl, G. (2010). New aspects of DNA-based authentication of Chinese medicinal plants by molecular biological techniques. *Planta Med.* 76, 1963–1974. doi: 10.1055/s-0030-1250519

Ivanova, N. V., Kuzmina, M. L., Braukmann, T. W. A., Borisenko, A. V., and Zakharov, E. V. (2016). Authentication of herbal supplements using next-generation sequencing. *PLoS One* 11:e0156426. doi: 10.1371/journal.pone.0156426

Jiang, Y., David, B., Tu, P., and Barbin, Y. (2010). Recent analytical approaches in quality control of traditional Chinese medicines—a review. *Anal. Chim. Acta* 657, 9–18. doi: 10.1016/j.aca.2009.10.024

Joshi, V. K., Joshi, A., and Dhiman, K. S. (2017). The Ayurvedic Pharmacopoeia of India, development and perspectives. *J. Ethnopharmacol.* 197, 32–38. doi: 10.1016/j.jep.2016.07.030

Lammers, Y., Peelen, T., Vos, R. A., and Gravendeel, B. (2014). The HTS barcode checker pipeline, a tool for automated detection of illegally traded species from high-throughput sequencing data. *BMC Bioinformatics* 15:44. doi: 10.1186/1471-2105-15-44

Leonti, M., and Casu, L. (2013). Traditional medicines and globalization: current and future perspectives in ethnopharmacology. *Front. Pharmacol.* 4:92. doi: 10.3389/fphar.2013.00092

Metsalu, T., and Vilo, J. (2015). ClustVis: a web tool for visualizing clustering of multivariate data using principal component analysis and heatmap. *Nucleic Acids Res.* 43, W566–W570. doi: 10.1093/nar/gkv468

Newmaster, S. G., Grguric, M., Shanmughanandhan, D., Ramalingam, S., and Ragupathy, S. (2013). DNA barcoding detects contamination and substitution in North American herbal products. *BMC Med.* 11:222. doi: 10.1186/1741-7015-11-222

Novak, J., Grausgruber-Gröger, S., and Lukas, B. (2007). DNA-based authentication of plant extracts. *Food Res. Int.* 40, 388–392. doi: 10.1016/j.foodres.2006.10.015

Parvathy, V. A., Swetha, V. P., Sheeja, T. E., Leela, N. K., Chempakam, B., and Sasikumar, B. (2014). DNA barcoding to detect chilli adulteration in traded black pepper powder. *Food Biotechnol.* 28, 25–40. doi: 10.1080/08905436.2013.870078

Parveen, I., Gafner, S., Techen, N., Murch, S. J., and Khan, I. A. (2016). DNA barcoding for the identification of botanicals in herbal medicine and dietary supplements: strengths and limitations. *Planta Med.* 82, 1225–1235. doi: 10.1055/s-0042-111208

Raclariu, A. C., Mocan, A., Popa, M. O., Vlase, L., Ichim, M. C., Crisan, G., et al. (2017a). Veronica officinalis product authentication using DNA metabarcoding and HPLC-MS reveals widespread adulteration with Veronica chamaedrys. *Front. Pharmacol.* 8:378. doi: 10.3389/fphar.2017.00378

Raclariu, A. C., Paltinean, R., Vlase, L., Labarre, A., Manzanilla, V., Ichim, M. C., et al. (2017b). Comparative authentication of Hypericum perforatum herbal products using DNA metabarcoding, TLC and HPLC-MS. *Sci. Rep.* 7:1291. doi: 10.1038/s41598-017-01389-w

Raclariu, A. C., Heinrich, M., Ichim, M. C., and De Boer, H. (2018a). Benefits and limitations of DNA barcoding and metabarcoding in herbal product authentication. *Phytochem. Anal.* 29, 123–128. doi: 10.1002/pca.2732

Raclariu, A. C., Tebrencu, C. E., Ichim, M. C., Ciuperca, O. T., Brysting, A. K., and De Boer, H. J. (2018b). What's in the box? Authentication of Echinacea herbal products using DNA metabarcoding and HPTLC. *Phytomedicine* 44, 32–38. doi: 10.1016/j.phymed.2018.03.058

Rocha, T., Amaral, J. S., and Oliveira, M. B. P. P. (2016). Adulteration of dietary supplements by the illegal addition of synthetic drugs: a review. *Compr. Rev. Food Sci. Food Saf.* 15, 43–62. doi: 10.1111/1541-4337.12173

Salipante, S., Kawashima, T., Rosenthal, C., Hoogestraat, D., Cummings, L., Sengupta, D., et al. (2014). Performance comparison of illumina and ion torrent next-generation sequencing platforms for 16S rRNA-based bacterial community profiling. *Appl. Environ. Microbiol.* 80, 7583–7591. doi: 10.1128/AEM.02206-14

Seethapathy, G. S., Ganesh, D., Santhosh Kumar, J. U., Senthilkumar, U., Newmaster, S. G., Ragupathy, S., et al. (2015). Assessing product adulteration in natural health products for laxative yielding plants, Cassia, Senna, and Chamaecrista, in Southern India using DNA barcoding. *Int. J. Legal Med.* 129, 693–700. doi: 10.1007/s00414-014-1120-z

Sgamma, T., Lockie-Williams, C., Kreuzer, M., Williams, S., Scheyhing, U., Koch, E., et al. (2017). DNA barcoding for industrial quality assurance. *Planta Med.* 83, 1117–1129. doi: 10.1055/s-0043-113448

Shanmughanandhan, D., Ragupathy, S., Newmaster, S. G., Mohanasundaram, S., and Sathishkumar, R. (2016). Estimating herbal product authentication and adulteration in India using a vouchered, DNA-based biological reference material library. *Drug Saf.* 39, 1211–1227. doi: 10.1007/s40264-016-0459-0

Srirama, R., Senthilkumar, U., Sreejayan, N., Ravikanth, G., Gurumurthy, B. R., Shivanna, M. B., et al. (2010). Assessing species admixtures in raw drug trade of Phyllanthus, a hepato-protective plant using molecular tools. *J. Ethnopharmacol.* 130, 208–215. doi: 10.1016/j.jep.2010.04.042

Srivastava, S., and Rawat, A. K. (2013). Quality evaluation of ayurvedic crude drug daruharidra, its allied species, and commercial samples from herbal drug markets of India. *Evid. Based Complement. Alternat. Med.* 2013:472973. doi: 10.1155/2013/472973

Staats, M., Arulandhu, A. J., Gravendeel, B., Holst-Jensen, A., Scholtens, I., Peelen, T., et al. (2016). Advances in DNA metabarcoding for food and wildlife forensic species identification. *Anal. Bioanal. Chem.* 408, 4615–4630. doi: 10.1007/s00216-016-9595-8

Sun, Y., Skinner, D. Z., Liang, G. H., and Hulbert, S. H. (1994). Phylogenetic analysis of sorghum and related taxa using internal transcribed spacers of nuclear ribosomal DNA. *Theor. Appl. Genet.* 89, 26–32. doi: 10.1007/BF00226978

Swetha, V. P., Parvathy, V. A., Sheeja, T. E., and Sasikumar, B. (2014). DNA barcoding for discriminating the economically important *Cinnamomum verum* from its adulterants. *Food Biotechnol.* 28, 183–194. doi: 10.1080/08905436.2014.931239

Swetha, V. P., Parvathy, V. A., Sheeja, T. E., and Sasikumar, B. (2017). Authentication of *Myristica fragrans* Houtt. using DNA barcoding. *Food Control* 73, 1010–1015. doi: 10.1016/j.foodcont.2016.10.004

Taberlet, P., Coissac, E., Pompanon, F., Brochmann, C., and Willerslev, E. (2012). Towards next generation biodiversity assessment using DNA metabarcoding. *Mol. Ecol.* 21, 2045–2050. doi: 10.1111/j.1365-294X.2012.05470.x

Techen, N., Parveen, I., Pan, Z., and Khan, I. A. (2014). DNA barcoding of medicinal plant material for identification. *Curr. Opin. Biotechnol.* 25, 103–110. doi: 10.1016/j.copbio.2013.09.010

The Plant List (2013). *Version 1.1.* Available at: http://www.theplantlist.org/ [accessed July 25, 2018].

Urumarudappa, S. K., Gogna, N., Newmaster, S. G., Venkatarangaiah, K., Subramanyam, R., Saroja, S. G., et al. (2016). DNA barcoding and NMR spectroscopy-based assessment of species adulteration in the raw herbal trade of *Saraca asoca* (Roxb.) Willd, an important medicinal plant. *Int. J. Legal Med.* 130, 1457–1470. doi: 10.1007/s00414-016-1436-y

Valiathan, M. S. (2006). Ayurveda: putting the house in order. *Curr. Sci.* 90, 5–6.

Vassou, S. L., Kusuma, G., and Parani, M. (2015). DNA barcoding for species identification from dried and powdered plant parts: a case study with authentication of the raw drug market samples of *Sida cordifolia. Gene* 559, 86–93. doi: 10.1016/j.gene.2015.01.025

Vassou, S. L., Nithaniyal, S., Raju, B., and Parani, M. (2016). Creation of reference DNA barcode library and authentication of medicinal plant raw drugs used in Ayurvedic medicine. *BMC Complement. Altern. Med.* 16:186. doi: 10.1186/s12906-016-1086-0

Ved, D. K., and Goraya, G. S. (2007). *Demand and Supply of Medicinal Plants in India.* New Delhi: NMPB.

Veldman, S., Gravendeel, B., Otieno, J. N., Lammers, Y., Duijm, E., Nieman, A., et al. (2017). High-throughput sequencing of African chikanda cake highlights conservation challenges in orchids. *Biodivers. Conserv.* 26, 2029–2046. doi: 10.1007/s10531-017-1343-7

Wang, L., Liu, L. F., Wang, J. Y., Shi, Z. Q., Chang, W. Q., Chen, M. L., et al. (2017). A strategy to identify and quantify closely related adulterant herbal materials by mass spectrometry-based partial least squares regression. *Anal. Chim. Acta* 977, 28–35. doi: 10.1016/j.aca.2017.04.023

World Health Organization [WHO] (2013). *WHO traditional medicine strategy: 2014-2023.* Available at: http://www.who.int/medicines/publications/traditional/trm_strategy14_23/en/ [accessed July 27, 2017].

Zhang, A., Sun, H., Yan, G., and Wang, X. (2017). Recent developments and emerging trends of mass spectrometry for herbal ingredients analysis. *Trends Analyt. Chem.* 94, 70–76. doi: 10.1016/j.trac.2017.07.007

Zhang, J., Wider, B., Shang, H., Li, X., and Ernst, E. (2012). Quality of herbal medicines: challenges and solutions. *Complement. Ther. Med.* 20, 100–106. doi: 10.1016/j.ctim.2011.09.004

5

Simultaneous Extraction and Determination of Compounds with Different Polarities from Platycladi Cacumen by AQ C$_{18}$-Based Vortex-Homogenized Matrix Solid-Phase Dispersion with Ionic Liquid

Mingya Ding[1,2], Jin Li[1,2†], Shuhan Zou[1,2], Ge Tang[3], Xiumei Gao[1,2] and Yan-xu Chang[1,2†]*

[1] Tianjin State Key Laboratory of Modern Chinese Medicine, Tianjin University of Traditional Chinese Medicine, Tianjin, China,
[2] Tianjin Key Laboratory of Phytochemistry and Pharmaceutical Analysis, Tianjin University of Traditional Chinese Medicine, Tianjin, China, [3] Department of Nephrology, The First Teaching Hospital, Tianjin University of Traditional Chinese Medicine, Tianjin, China

Correspondence:
Yan-xu Chang
Tcmcyx@126.com;
tcmcyx@tjutcm.edu.cn

†*These authors have contributed equally to this work*

This study presented a rapid, simple and environmentally friendly method of employing AQ C$_{18}$-based vortex-homogenized matrix solid-phase dispersion with ionic liquid (AQ C$_{18}$-IL-VHMSPD) for the extraction of compounds with different polarities from Platycladi Cacumen (PC) samples by ultra high-performance liquid chromatography with PDA detection. AQ C$_{18}$ (aqua C$_{18}$) and ionic liquid ([Bmim]BF$_4$) were used as the adsorbent and green elution reagent in vortex-homogenized MSPD procedure. The AQ C$_{18}$-IL-VHMSPD conditions were optimized by studying several experimental parameters including the type of ionic liquid, the type of adsorbent, ratio of sample to adsorbent, the concentration and volume of ionic liquid, grinding time and vortex time. The recoveries of the target compounds were in the range of 96.9–104% with relative standard deviation values no more than 2.8%. The limits of detection and limits of quantitation were in the range of 0.2–1.2 and 1.0–5.4 ng mL^{-1}, respectively. Compared with the traditional ultrasonic-assisted extraction, the developed AQ C$_{18}$-IL-VHMSPD method required less sample, reagent and time. It was concluded that the AQ C$_{18}$-IL-VHMSPD method was a powerful method for the extraction and quantification of the high polarity and low polarity compounds in traditional Chinese medicines samples.

Keywords: AQ C$_{18}$, ionic liquid, Platycladi Cacumen, UHPLC, vortex-homogenized matrix solid-phase dispersion

INTRODUCTION

Platycladi Cacumen (PC), namely Cebaiye, derived from the dry twigs and leaves of *Platycladus orientalis* (L.) Franco, is one of the most commonly used traditional Chinese medicines (TCMs). It has been applied in many TCM formulations for thousands of years. It was recorded that the PC could cool the blood to stanch bleeding, dispel pathogenic wind, remove dampness and resolve phlegm (Chinese Pharmacopoeia Commission, 2015). Recently, it was confirmed that PC has antimicrobial, anti-tumor, anti-inflammatory, anti-oxidant activities and neuroprotective effect (Hassanzadeh et al., 2001; Emami et al., 2011; Zaugg et al., 2011; Fan et al., 2012; Zhang et al., 2013). Flavonoids are regarded as the material basis for the efficacy. The main flavonoid glycosides consists of myricitrin, isoquercitrin, and quercitrin. In addition, there is a large amount of biflavonoids in PC. Among these biflavonoids, hinokiflavone, and amentoflavone are the representative ones (Lu et al., 2006). These five flavonoids with different polarities have been reported to exert a therapeutic effect on diseases in previous literatures (Ma and Wu, 2013). Thus, the complete extraction and precise analysis of the five compounds (**Figure 1**) with different polarities are particularly crucial for quality control and pharmacological investigations of herbal PC.

The conventional methods for the extraction of PC included the ultrasonic-assisted extraction (UAE) with HPLC-UV or UPLC-DAD (Zhuang et al., 2017, 2018), the microwave-based extraction with ultraviolet–visible detection, and heat reflux extraction with UPLC-DAD (Chen et al., 2007; Shan et al., 2018). However, these methods normally require a great deal of organic reagent, which arouse the environment pollution. Besides, the longer extraction time was another shortage. Matrix solid-phase dispersion (MSPD) is a comprehensive sample preparation method in which sample homogenization, disruption, extraction, fractionation and purification were simultaneously performed in one step and a shorter extraction time and less organic solvent were required (Barker et al., 1989; García-López et al., 2008). At present, many MSPD methods have been successfully applied for various samples (Liu et al., 2008; Vela-Soria et al., 2014). Recently, a vortex-homogenized MSPD (VHMSPD) technique not only retained the superiority of the traditional MSPD method but also overcame the shortage of the loss of analytes in complex procedures (Du et al., 2018a,b). However, no information about VHMSPD was available for the analysis of Platycladi Cacumen in the literature.

The adsorbent used in the MSPD procedure acts a pivotal part in improving the extraction efficiency of target analytes (Cao et al., 2016). Most applications of MSPD have utilized the silica gel matrix material and absorptive matrix materials. PSA, NH₂, CN, COOH, C₈, C₁₈ (end capped), C₁₈-N (no end capped) and AQ C₁₈ were silica gel matrix material. Florisil was absorptive matrix materials. Compared with C₁₈, more silanol groups linking to the surface of C₁₈-N, which could provide the additional polar interactions. A certain proportion of polar functional groups were added to the surface of non-polar materials of AQ C₁₈, which not only has the higher adsorption capacity on low polarity target compounds, but also greatly increases the adsorption capacity of high polarity target compounds. Thus, AQ C₁₈ could be used to extract high polarity and low polarity target compounds from traditional Chinese medicines. To our knowledge, no reference on the use of AQ C₁₈ as an adsorbent for the extraction of TCMs by VHMSPD has been reported.

Ionic liquids (ILs) are characterized by diverse combinations of organic or inorganic anions and organic cations. Recently, they have been widely used as green elution reagent for

microextraction due to the advantages of high thermal stability, negligible vapor pressure and good solubility for inorganic and organic compounds (Han et al., 2012). It was reported that ILs could interact with analytes by various mechanisms such as π-π, electrostatic force, hydrogen bonding, ion-dipole, inclusion complex etc. (Qiu et al., 2012). Thus, the green ILs were applied for extracting analytes using VHMSPD method in the TCMs.

In this study, an AQ C₁₈-based vortex-homogenized matrix solid phase dispersion with ionic liquids (AQ C18-IL-VHMSPD) technique with UHPLC-PDA was first established for simultaneous determination of compounds with different polarities from Platycladi Cacumen including three high polarity flavonoid glycosides (myricitrin, isoquercitrin and quercitrin) and two low polarity bioflavonoids (hinokiflavone and amentoflavone). The combination of AQ C₁₈ and ionic liquid was applied to extract natural compounds in the vortex-homogenized matrix solid phase dispersion procedure. Some parameters such as type of adsorbent, sample/adsorbent ratio, and type and concentration of eluent were optimized to obtain a good extraction efficiency in detail. Furthermore, the five compounds were extracted by using the conventional ultrasonic-assisted extraction to evaluate the feasibility of the developed AQ C₁₈-IL-VHMSPD method.

MATERIALS AND METHODS

Chemicals and Reagents

Reference standards of myricitrin, isoquercitrin, quercitrin, amentoflavone and hinokiflavone were purchased from Chengdu Desite Bio-Technology Co., Ltd., (Chengdu, China). PSA (40–60 μm, 60 A), NH₂ (40–60 μm, 60 A), CN (50 μm, 60 A), COOH (50 μm, 60 A), Florisil (60–100 μm, 80 A), C₈ (50 μm, 60 A), C₁₈ (50 μm, 60 A), C₁₈-N (50 μm, 60 A) and AQ C₁₈ (50 μm, 60 A) were supplied from Agela Technologies. 1-butyl-3-methylimidazolium tetrafluoroborate ([Bmim]BF₄), 1-hexyl-3-methylimidazolium tetrafluoroborate ([Hmim]BF₄), 1-octyl-3-methylimidazolium tetrafluoroborate ([Omim]BF₄), 1-butyl-3-methylimidazolium hexafluorophosphate ([Bmim]PF₆) and 1-octyl-3-methylimidazolium hexafluorophosphate ([Omim]PF₆) were purchased from Shanghai Chengjie Chemical Co., Ltd., HPLC-grade acetonitrile and methanol were purchased from Dikma Technologies Inc., United States. HPLC-grade formic acid was purchased from Tedia Company, Inc. (Tedia, Fairfield, OH, United States). Deionized water was purified from a Milli-Q academic ultra-pure water system (Millipore, Milford, MA, United States). Other chemical reagents were of analytical grade. All the solutions were filtered through a 0.22 μm filter membrane before UPLC analysis.

Plant Material

A total of 8 batches of Platycladi Cacumen and its processed products were collected from different regions of China and authenticated by Dr. Yan-xu Chang (Tianjin University of Traditional Chinese Medicine). All samples were pulverized

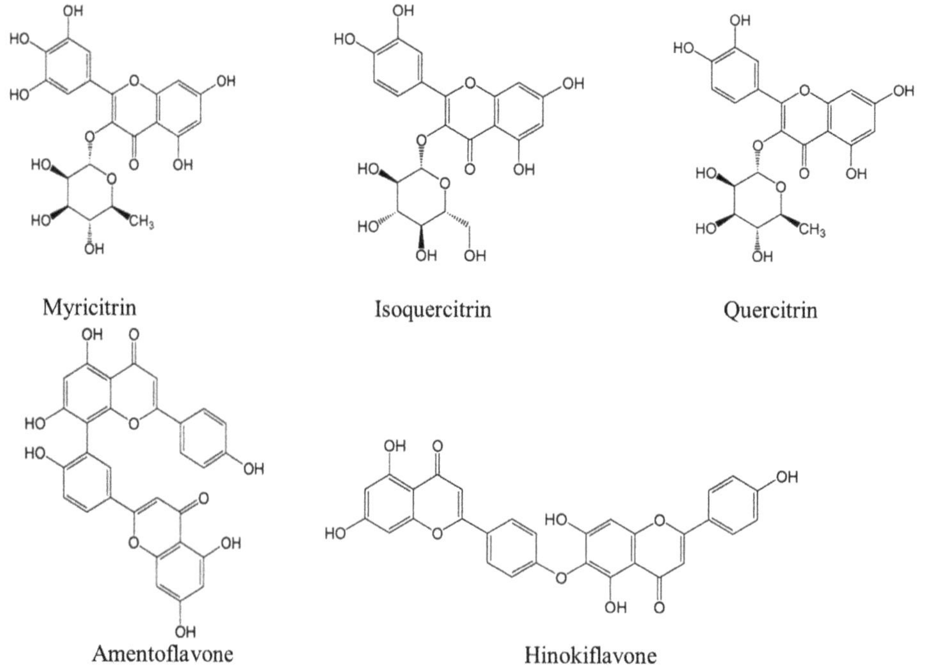

FIGURE 1 | The chemical structures of five compounds assayed in Platycladi Cacumen sample.

using a pulverizer (Zhongcheng Pharmaceutical Machinery) after being dried at 60°C for 24 h, then passed through a 100-mesh sieve.

Preparation of Standard Solutions

The standard stock solutions of myricitrin, isoquercitrin, quercitrin, hinokiflavone and amentoflavone were separately prepared in methanol. Myricitrin and quercitrin were 2 mg mL^{-1}. Isoquercitrin, hinokiflavone and amentoflavone were 1 mg mL^{-1}. The appropriate amount solution of all standards was diluted with methanol to obtain eight different appropriate concentrations for calibration curves. The concentrations of myricitrin, isoquercitrin, quercitrin, hinokiflavone and amentoflavone were in the range of 0.4–100, 0.08–20, 0.8–200, 0.2–50, and 0.2–50 μg mL^{-1}, respectively. The related standard solutions were stored at 4°C.

Ultra High-Performance Liquid Chromatography With PDA Detection (UHPLC-PDA) Analysis

The chromatographic analysis was performed on a Waters ACQUITY UPLC System (Waters Co., Milford, MA, United States) that consisted of a photodiode array (PDA). The workstation controlled by Empower 2 software was employed to collect and analyze data. The separation was performed on an ACQUITY UPLC BEH C$_{18}$ column (2.1 mm × 100 mm, 1.7 μm, Waters) at the flow rate of 0.3 mL min^{-1}. The mobile phase consisted of water with 0.1% formic acid (eluent A) and acetonitrile (eluent B) using

a gradient elution: 0–2 min, 5–37% B; 2–9 min, 37–67% B; 9–10 min, 67–85% B; 10–13 min, 85–95% B; 13–15 min, 95–5% B, then post run 6 min. The column temperature was maintained at 30°C and the injection volume was 1 μL. The detection wavelength was set at 340 nm. Under the above chromatographic conditions, the chromatographic peaks of analytes included samples and standard solutions were separated excellently (**Figure 2**).

AQ C$_{18}$-Based Vortex-Homogenized Matrix Solid-Phase Dispersion With Ionic Liquid Procedure

An aliquot of 25 mg of the previously crushed sample and 50 mg adsorbents (AQ C$_{18}$) were put into an agate mortar gradually. The mixture was grinded with a pestle for 3 min. Once completely dispersed, the mixture was transferred into a 4 mL polypropylene tube. 1.5 mL elution reagent ([Bmim]BF$_4$) was added and then thoroughly shaken by vortex for 45 s. Subsequently, the tubes were placed into a centrifuge at 14000 rpm for 10 min. The supernatant liquor was collected and 1 uL was injected into the UHPLC for analysis. The schematic diagram of AQ C$_{18}$-IL-VHMSPD method was exhibited in **Figure 3**.

Ultrasonic Extraction

According to the Chinese Pharmacopoeia 2015, the dried PC samples (0.500 g) were precisely weighed and introduced into a 100 mL Erlenmeyer flask, then mixed with 20 mL methanol. Finally the mixture was extracted ultrasonically (40 kHz, 96% power) for 30 min and the weight loss of the solution was

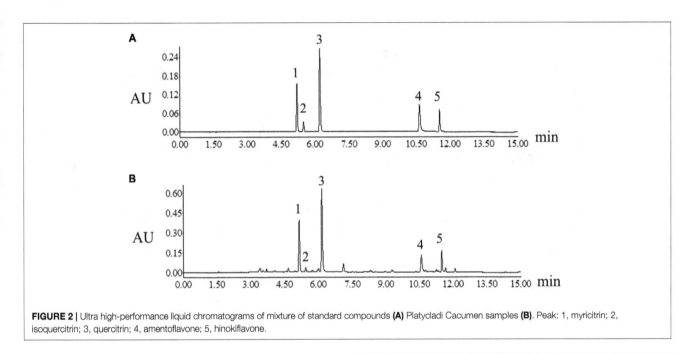

FIGURE 2 | Ultra high-performance liquid chromatograms of mixture of standard compounds **(A)** Platycladi Cacumen samples **(B)**. Peak: 1, myricitrin; 2, isoquercitrin; 3, quercitrin; 4, amentoflavone; 5, hinokiflavone.

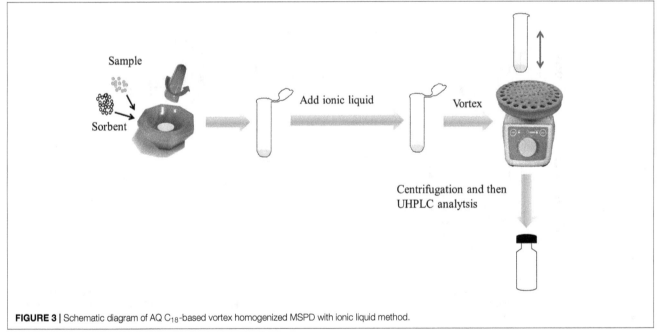

FIGURE 3 | Schematic diagram of AQ C_{18}-based vortex homogenized MSPD with ionic liquid method.

complemented with methanol. All the extract solution was filtrated through a 0.22 μm filter membrane and 1 μL filter liquor was injected into the UPLC-PDA for further analysis.

Optimization of AQ C_{18}-IL-VHMSPD Parameters

To obtain a good extraction efficiency of the target compounds, several experimental parameters including the type of adsorbent, ratio of sample to adsorbent, type and concentration of the eluting solvent, and grinding time were investigated. Each test was repeated in triplicate.

Several adsorbents were investigated including PSA, NH_2, CN, COOH, Florisil, C_8, C_{18}, C_{18}-N and AQ C_{18}. An aliquot of 25 mg PC samples and 50 mg adsorbents were transferred into an agate mortar, then grinded for 3 min. The eluent was 1.5 mL 90 mM ILs and 3 min was chosen as vortex time. Different types of ILs such as [Bmim]BF_4, [Hmim]BF_4, [Omim]BF_4, [Bmim]PF_6 and [Omim]PF_6 were optimized. Then, four levels of concentration of [Bmim]BF_4 (50, 70, 90, and 110 mM) and volumes of IL (0.5–2 mL) were considered to be optimized. The ratio of sample to adsorbent (1:0, 1:1, 1:2, and 1:3) was considered to investigate while the other conditions remained unchanged. In addition, the vortex time (15, 30, 45,

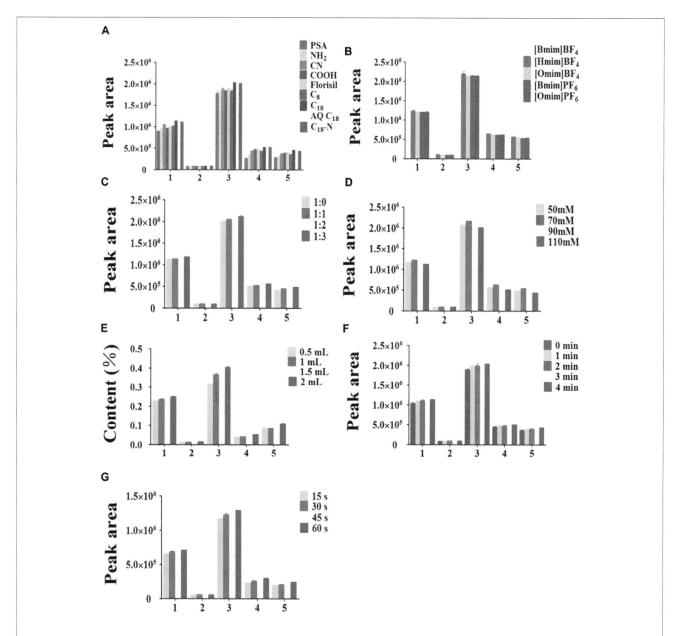

FIGURE 4 | Effects of parameters on extraction efficiency of five peak: (1) myricitrin, (2) isoquercitrin, (3) quercitrin, (4) hinokiflavone, (5) amentoflavone, **(A)** type of the adsorbent, **(B)** type of the ionic liquid, **(C)** ratio of sample to adsorbent, **(D)** ionic liquid concentration, **(E)** ionic liquid volume, **(F)** grinding time, **(G)** vortex time. The errors bars represent RSD (n = 3).

and 60 s) and grinding time (0, 1, 2, 3, and 4 min) were also tested.

RESULTS AND DISCUSSION

Optimization of the AQ C$_{18}$-IL-VHMSPD Method

Type of Adsorbent

In the development of the MSPD procedure, it is crucial to employ a suitable dispersing adsorbent. The adsorbent is not only used as a disruption and dispersion agent that

destroys the structure of samples for the extraction of the target compounds, but also as a purificant that removes the interfering substance of matrix. In the present study, nine types of adsorbent were evaluated. As **Figure 4A** shows, the analytes has the strongly retention when PSA, NH$_2$, CN, COOH, Florisil and C$_8$ were used as adsorbent. The reason was that the analytes bonded with the adsorbent too tightly to be eluted effectively. C$_{18}$-N and C$_{18}$ produced the equivalent extraction efficiency, but not dramatically better than AQ C$_{18}$. One probable explanation was that the abundant Si-O-Si and Si-OH groups formed hydrogen bonds between adsorbent and analytes. Additionally, the interaction force may be supplied by the silica, including hydrogen bonding and electrostatic interaction. Therefore, AQ C_{18} was chosen as the optimal adsorbent for the subsequent extraction procedure.

Type of Ionic Liquid

An appropriate type of elution solvent is a significant parameter to obtain good extraction efficiency for target analytes. The elution solvent should have a similar polarity as target analytes, which is easy to disrupt the interaction between the target analytes and the adsorbent (García-Mayor et al., 2012). [Bmim]BF$_4$, [Hmim]BF$_4$, [Omim]BF$_4$, [Bmim]PF$_6$ and [Omim]PF$_6$ are five common ionic liquids. To select the most appropriate one, these five ILs were evaluated based on the extraction efficiency of the target analytes in the MSPD procedure. As shown in **Figure 4B**, the elution efficiency of ILs was affected by the alkyl chain length of cation and the types of anion. It was quite obvious that the peak areas of the five target compounds were significantly increased from [Omim]BF$_4$ to [Bmim]BF$_4$. The mechanism of this phenomenon is that the hydrogen bonding interaction was weakening between the target analytes and imidazolium rings when alkyl chain length was increased with the same anion BF$_4^-$. Although [Bmim]BF$_4$ and [Bmim]PF$_6$ had the same cation, the highest peak areas of all analytes were observed with the BF$_4^-$ anion. The possible reason is that the combination of anion BF$_4^-$ and analytes generated the stronger electrostatic interaction. Overall, [Bmim]BF$_4$ was chosen as the optimum elution solvent for the next experiment.

Ratio of Sample to Adsorbent

The mass ratio of adsorbent to sample is a significant parameter affecting the extraction yield of the target analytes from the samples (Rodrigues et al., 2010; Xu et al., 2016). An appropriate ratio of sample to adsorbent not only guarantees that the sample is completely homogenized and dispersed in the adsorbent, but also decreases the loss of sample in the blending procedure. It can be seen in **Figure 4C** that the peak areas of the five target compounds were distinctly increased when the sample/adsorbent ratio increased from 1:0 to 1:2. The possible reason was that the larger the amount of adsorbent, the stronger the molecular interaction produced, such as hydrogen bonding and electrostatic force between analytes and adsorbents. However, further increment of the sample/adsorbent ratio led to a slightly decrease of the extraction efficiency. The reason may be that the excessive adsorbent generated such a strong interaction between the five compounds and AQ C_{18} that eluent could not completely eluted. Thus, sample/sorbent ratio of 1:2 was selected.

Concentration and Volume of Ionic Liquid

The concentration and volume of [Bmim]BF$_4$ are also crucial parameters affecting the extraction yield of the target analytes in the elution process. The results (**Figure 4D**) showed that the peak areas of target compounds were gradually increased from 50 to 90 mM. A possible reason was that the π-π, electrostatic

and hydrogen-bond interactions between the [Bmim]BF$_4$ and target analytes were stronger than the interaction of the analytes and adsorbent, while the extraction efficiency was slightly decreased following the increment of the concentration of [Bmim]BF$_4$. This phenomenon could be ascribed to the intensive viscosity, which gave rise to poor capacity to transfer the target analytes from adsorbent into eluent. Thus, 90 mM [Bmim]BF$_4$ seemed to be the optimum concentration for further experiments.

To attain the highest extraction efficiency with the minimum volumes of ILs, 0.5 mL to 2 mL volume of 90 mM [Bmim]BF$_4$ were investigated. **Figure 4E** demonstrates that the contents of the five compounds were increased from 0.5 to 1.5 mL. The reason could be that the stronger interaction was generated between analytes and eluant along with the increase of the volume of eluant. Nevertheless, the peak areas of the five compounds remained unchanged when the volume kept increasing. *T*-test was introduced to evaluate the differences between two groups by Microsoft excel (version 2010). The results showed that there was no significant difference between 1.5 and 2 mL of 90 mM [Bmim]BF$_4$. Consequently, 1.5 mL of [Bmim]BF$_4$ was used in the following MSPD extraction procedure.

Grinding Time

The grinding time is a vital parameter of great concern in the VH-MSPD method. In order to evaluate the effect of different grinding times, five time intervals at 0, 1, 2, 3, and 4 min were tested. As the results show in **Figure 4F**, the peak areas of the 5 target analytes were increased with increasing grinding time from 1 to 3 min. It was likely that the longer grinding time caused a stronger interaction force between AQ C_{18} and analytes, facilitating the transfer of the target analytes from samples into the adsorbent. However, the extraction efficiency employing 3 min-grinding was approximately equal to that of 4 min-grinding. Thus, the grinding time for 3 min was chosen for further experiments.

Vortex Time

Previous studies have proven that vortex time is an important factor influencing the extraction efficiency. As shown in **Figure 4G**, the peak areas of the five target compounds were significantly increased as the vortex time increased from 15 to 30 s. However, increasing the vortex time to 60 s resulted in a slightly decline of the peak areas. Thus, 45 s was chosen as the optimal vortex time. Eventually, the optimized AQ C_{18}-IL-VHMSPD conditions were determined to be 25 mg PC sample, 50 mg AQ C_{18}, grinding time of 3 min, 1.5 mL 90 mM [Bmim]BF4 as the elution solvent and 45 s vortex time.

Method Validation
Selectivity and Linearity

The calibration curves (*n* = 8) of 5 analytes were obtained by performing the peak areas as Y-axis, versus the concentration in μg mL^{-1} as X-axis, which ranged from 0.08 to 200 μg mL^{-1}.

TABLE 1 | Linearity, limits of detection (LOD), limit of quantification (LOQ), and repeatability of the proposed method ($n = 6$).

Compounds	Regressive equation	Linear range (μg/mL)	R^2	LOD (μg/mL)	LOQ (μg/mL)	Repeatability RSD (%)
Myricitrin	$y = 18697x + 4126.3$	0.4–100	1	0.0003	0.001	1.9
Isoquercitrin	$y = 20257x + 593.13$	0.08–20	0.9999	0.0002	0.0054	0.9
Quercitrin	$y = 18819x + 9536.7$	0.8–200	0.9999	0.0002	0.001	1.3
Amentoflavone	$y = 40153x - 1750.5$	0.2–50	0.9997	0.0012	0.004	3.7
Hinokiflavone	$y = 59804x + 2041.5$	0.2–50	0.9999	0.0008	0.002	1.9

TABLE 2 | The results of precision and stability.

Compounds	Concentration (μg/mL)	Intra-day		Inter-day		Stability	
		RSD (%)	Accuracy (%)	RSD (%)	Accuracy (%)	RSD (%)	Remain (%)
Myricitrin	1	1.4	96.9	1.7	96.2	1.4	98.2
	5	0.5	99.9	1.5	99.4	1.2	98.9
	25	1.4	101	2.1	101	0.9	101
Isoquercitrin	0.2	1.3	97.8	2.0	96.4	1.2	95.8
	1	0.9	98.5	0.9	98.2	1.4	97.6
	5	1.5	103	2.1	103	1.0	103
Quercitrin	2	1.3	97.4	1.7	97.4	1.3	95.4
	10	0.6	95.5	1.3	98.4	1.1	97.0
	50	1.5	95.2	2.2	96.4	0.9	96.4
Amentoflavone	0.4	0.8	113	2.7	115	2.6	115
	2	0.9	104	0.6	104	1.6	103
	10	3.3	104	3.1	104	1.8	104
Hinokiflavone	0.4	0.4	97.3	0.2	97.5	1.5	97.6
	2	0.4	100	0.5	101	0.8	100
	10	0.7	97.4	1.0	97.4	0.4	97.4

TABLE 3 | The results of recovery test ($n = 6$).

Compounds	Original (μg)	Spiked (μg)	Detected (μg)	Average recovery (%)	RSD (%)
Myricitrin	60.85	25	85.5	98.4	2.5
Isoquercitrin	4.34	2.5	6.8	96.9	2.8
Quercitrin	107.84	50	159.6	104	1.6
Amentoflavone	11.38	5	16.5	102	0.6
Hinokiflavone	6.30	1.25	7.5	98.4	1.9

The correlation coefficients (R^2) of each analyte were higher than 0.9997 (**Table 1**).

Limits of Detection and Quantification

Limits of detection (LOD) and limit of quantification (LOQ) were employed to assess the sensitivity of the developed method. They were estimated as the concentrations of the analytes when the signal-to-noise (S/N) ratio reached 3 and 10 individually. The LODs of the five compounds ranged from 0.0002 to 0.0012 μg mL^{-1}, while the LOQs ranged from 0.001 to 0.0054 μg mL^{-1} (**Table 1**).

Reproducibility

The repeatability was evaluated by six parallel AQ C$_{18}$-IL-VHMSPD extracts of a PC sample. As summarized in **Table 1**, the values of relative standard deviations (RSDs) were all less than 3.7%. It was confirmed from the results that the developed method had good reproducibility during experiment.

Precision, Stability and Recovery

Instrumental precision was expressed as intra-day and inter-day precision by determining the relative standard deviations (RSDs) at three levels of concentrations in six replicates of each compounds. Intra-day precision and inter-day precision were tested in a single day and within continuous 3 days, respectively. The validation results are presented in **Table 2**, the accuracies were within the range of 95.2–104.2% (RSD $\leq$ 3.3%) and 96.2–114.6% (RSD $\leq$ 3.1%) for intra-day precision and inter-day precision, respectively.

The stability was investigated by analyzing the accuracies of three levels of concentrations of five compounds at room temperature condition over 24 h. The accuracies of five compounds were in a range of 95.8–114.8%, while with the RSDs

TABLE 4 | Contents of the five flavonoids of Platycladi Cacumen samples from 8 batches (*n* = 6).

No.	Production region	Content (mg/g)				
		Myricitrin	Isoquercitrin	Quercitrin	Amentoflavone	Hinokiflavone
1[a]	Shandong	2.05 ± 0.01	0.16 ± 0.00	3.76 ± 0.03	0.44 ± 0.01	0.25 ± 0.01
1*	Shandong	2.02 ± 0.00	0.16 ± 0.00	3.73 ± 0.01	0.46 ± 0.01	0.24 ± 0.01
2[a]	Anhui	2.03 ± 0.04	0.16 ± 0.00	3.83 ± 0.03	0.46 ± 0.01	0.25 ± 0.00
2*	Anhui	1.99 ± 0.02	0.16 ± 0.00	3.82 ± 0.01	0.46 ± 0.00	0.26 ± 0.01
3[a]	Unknown	2.10 ± 0.04	0.16 ± 0.00	4.13 ± 0.04	0.46 ± 0.00	0.24 ± 0.00
4[a]	Unknown	1.64 ± 0.03	0.11 ± 0.00	3.41 ± 0.05	0.48 ± 0.01	0.26 ± 0.01
5[a]	Unknown	1.89 ± 0.02	0.15 ± 0.00	3.83 ± 0.01	0.40 ± 0.01	0.20 ± 0.00
6[a]	Unknown	2.01 ± 0.05	0.16 ± 0.00	3.76 ± 0.10	0.40 ± 0.01	0.20 ± 0.01
7[b]	Anhui	0.17 ± 0.01	0.01 ± 0.00	0.25 ± 0.03	0.06 ± 0.01	0.04 ± 0.00
8[b]	Unknown	0.06 ± 0.00	0.00 ± 0.00	0.03 ± 0.00	0.02 ± 0.00	0.02 ± 0.00

[a]Crude Platycladi Cacumen samples; [b]processed Platycladi Cacumen samples; *the certain Platycladi Cacumen sample was extracted by the authoritative extract method (Pharmacopoeia of China 2015).

TABLE 5 | Comparison of the AQ C_{18}-IL-VHMSPD method with other methods in the determination of compounds in Platycladi Cacumen sample.

No.	Extracted compounds	Sample amounts (mg)	Type of solvent	Solvent volume (mL)	Extraction method	Extraction time (min)	Detection method	Detection time (min)	Reference
1	Myricitrin, isoquercitrin, quercitrin, myricetin, afzelin, quercetin, kaempferol, amentoflavone, hinokiflavone	500	75% ethanol	10	UAE[a]	60	UPLC-DAD	24	Zhuang et al., 2018
2	Myricitrin; quercitrin; amentoflavone; hinokiflavone	25	Deep eutectic solvents	1	UAE[a]	30	HPLC-UV	28	Zhuang et al., 2017
3	Myricitrin, isoquercitrin, quercitrin, afzelin, cupressuflavone, amentoflavone hinokiflavone	1000	Ethanol–water (75:25)	50	Reflux	28	UPLC-DAD	30	Shan et al., 2018
4	Myricitrin, isoquercitrin, quercitrin, amentoflavone hinokiflavone	25	Ionic liquid	1.5	AQ C_{18}-IL-VHMSPD	0.75	UPLC-PDA	15	This work

were both no more than 2.6%, showing that the analytes were stable from 0 to 24 h at room temperature.

To verify the accuracy of the proposed method, recovery tests were performed by analyzing the spiked sample in triplicate. Unspiked samples and spiked samples were simultaneously extracted using the optimum AQ C_{18}-IL-VHMSPD procedures. The results are listed in **Table 3**. The mean recoveries of 5 compounds were all in the range of 96.9–103.6% and the RSDs were all less than 2.8%, which demonstrated that the proposed AQ C_{18}-IL-VHMSPD method was reliable and effective.

Application

All of the above analysis results demonstrated that the proposed method had applicable value. Thus, the developed AQ C_{18}-IL-VHMSPD method was employed to analyze the target compounds with different polarities using the last-optimized conditions in six batches of crude Platycladi Cacumen and two batches of carbonized Platycladi Cacumen obtained from various producing areas. The contents of myricitrin, isoquercitrin, quercitrin, amentoflavone and hinokiflavone in crude PC were in the range of 1.64–2.10, 0.11–0.16, 3.41–4.13, 0.40–0.48, and

0.20–0.26 mg g^{-1}, individually (**Table 4**). Furthermore, the contents of myricitrin, isoquercitrin, quercitrin, amentoflavone and hinokiflavone in carbonized PC were in the range of 0.06–0.17, 0.00–0.01, 0.03–0.25, 0.02–0.06, and 0.02–0.04 mg g^{-1}, respectively. The results clearly revealed that the contents of the five target compounds were remarkably decreased after processing.

In order to compare the proposed AQ C_{18}-IL-VHMSPD method with conventional ultrasonic-assisted extraction from Pharmacopoeia of China 2015, the contents of the five target compounds from the same batches of PC were determined by these two methods. It was found that there was no significantly difference between the contents of the five components by two methods. The results indicated that the developed AQ C_{18}-IL-VHMSPD method had the almost same effectiveness as the method of Pharmacopoeia of China 2015 for extracting PC.

Comparison With Other Methods

To evaluate the performance of the proposed AQ C_{18}-IL-VHMSPD method, several methods including ultrasonic assisted extraction and reflux extraction were introduced to compare the sample amount, extraction solvent, solvent volume, extraction time and detection time. As summarized in **Table 5**, it is obviously observed that the developed AQ C_{18}-IL-VHMSPD method has the lower extraction time and detection time in contrast with other methods. Except for the method 2 in **Table 5** (deep eutectic solvents based ultrasonic assisted extraction) and the AQ C_{18}-IL-VHMSPD method, other methods all employed a large volume of organic solvent. Moreover, the proposed method required less extraction time and detection time than deep eutectic solvents based ultrasonic assisted extraction method. Overall, these results indicated that the AQ C_{18}-IL-VHMSPD method was a rapid, simple and environmentally friendly method for the extraction of the high polarity and low polarity compounds in PC samples.

CONCLUSION

An environmentally friendly sample pretreatment method, AQ C_{18}-based vortex-homogenized matrix solid-phase dispersion with ionic liquid was successfully developed to extract and quantify the target analytes with different polarity from Platycladi Cacumen by UHPLC-PDA. AQ C_{18} was employed as the

adsorbent to improve the adsorption capacity of compounds of different polarity. The use of green ionic liquids reduced the environment pollution. Compared with other extraction methods (UAE and reflux extraction), the present method is rapid, time-saving and efficient. This proposed method could be used for determination of compounds with different polarity from other traditional Chinese medicines.

AUTHOR CONTRIBUTIONS

Y-xC, GT, XG, and JL designed the experiments. MD and SZ performed the experiments. MD wrote the manuscript.

FUNDING

This research was supported National Natural Science Foundation of China (81374050 and 81703702) and Special Program of Talents Development for Excellent Youth Scholars in Tianjin of China.

REFERENCES

Barker, S. A., Long, A. R., and Short, C. R. (1989). Isolation of drug residues from tissues by solid phase dispersion. *J. Chromatogr. A* 475, 353–361. doi: 10.1016/S0021-9673(01)89689-8

Cao, J., Peng, L. Q., and Xu, J. J. (2016). Microcrystalline cellulose based matrix solid phase dispersion microextration for isomeric triterpenoid acids in loquat leaves by ultrahigh-performance liquid chromatography and quadrupole time-of-flight mass spectrometry. *J. Chromatogr. A* 1472, 16–26. doi: 10.1016/j.chroma.2016.10.034

Chen, L. G., Ding, L., Yu, A. M., Yang, R. L., Wang, X. P., Li, J. T., et al. (2007). Continuous determination of total flavonoids in *Platycladus orientalis* (L.) Franco by dynamic microwave-assisted extraction coupled with on-line derivatization and ultraviolet-visible detection. *Anal. Chim. Acta* 596, 164–170. doi: 10.1016/j.aca.2007.05.063

Chinese Pharmacopoeia Commission (2015). *Pharmacopoeia of the People's Republic of China*, Vol. 1. Beijing: China Medical Science and Technology Press.

Du, K. Z., Li, J., Bai, Y., An, M. R., Gao, X. M., and Chang, Y. X. (2018a). A green ionic liquid-based vortex-forced MSPD method for the simultaneous determination of 5-HMF and iridoid glycosides from *Fructus corni* by ultra-high performance liquid chromatography. *Food Chem.* 244, 190–196. doi: 10.1016/j.foodchem.2017.10.057

Du, K. Z., Li, J., Tian, F., and Chang, Y. X. (2018b). Non-ionic detergent triton X-114 based vortex-synchronized matrix solid-phase dispersion method for the simultaneous determination of six compounds with various polarities from *Forsythiae Fructus* by ultra high-performance liquid chromatography. *J. Pharm. Biomed. Anal.* 150, 59–66. doi: 10.1016/j.jpba.2017.12.003

Emami, S. A., Asgary, S., Ardekani, M. R. S., Naderi, G. A., Kasher, T., Aslani, S., et al. (2011). Antioxidant activity in some in vitro oxidative systems of the essential oils from the fruit and the leaves of *Platycladus orientalis*. *J. Essent. Oil Res.* 23, 83–90. doi: 10.1016/j.jep.2011.05.019

Fan, S. Y., Zeng, H. W., Pei, Y. H., Li, L., Ye, J., Pan, Y. X., et al. (2012). The anti-inflammatory activities of an extract and compounds isolated from *Platycladus orientalis* (Linnaeus) Franco in vitro and ex vivo. *J. Ethnopharmacol.* 141, 647–652. doi: 10.1016/j.jep.2011.05.019

García-López, M., Canosa, P., and Rodríguez, I. (2008). Trends and recent applications of matrix solid-phase dispersion. *Anal. Bioanal. Chem.* 391, 963–974. doi: 10.1007/s00216-008-1898-y

García-Mayor, M. A., Gallego-Picó, A., Garcinuño, R. M., Fernández-Hernando, P., and Durand-Alegría, J. S. (2012). Matrix solid-phase dispersion method for

the determination of macrolide antibiotics in sheep's milk. *Food Chem.* 134, 553–558. doi: 10.1016/j.foodchem.2012.02.120

Han, D. D., Tang, B. K., Lee, Y. R., and Row, K. H. (2012). Application of ionic liquid in liquid phase microextraction technology. *J. Sep. Sci.* 35, 2949–2961. doi: 10.1002/jssc.201200486

Hassanzadeh, M. K., Rahimizadeh, M., Fazly Bazzaz, B. S., Emami, S. A., and Assili, J. (2001). Chemical and antimicrobial studies of *Platyclaus orientalis* essential oils. *Pharm. Biol.* 39, 388–390. doi: 10.1076/phbi.39.5.388.5894

Liu, H. C., Li, Q. W., Li, S. P., Zou, Y. H., and Gu, A. Y. (2008). The rapid determination of artemisinin by post-column derivatization high-performance liquid chromatography using matrix solid-phase dispersion method. *J. Chromatogra. Sci.* 46, 122–126. doi: 10.1093/chromsci/46.2.122

Lu, Y. H., Liu, Z. Y., Wang, Z. T., and Wei, D. Z. (2006). Quality evaluation of *Platycladus orientalis* (L.) Franco through simultaneous determination of four bioactive flavonoids by high-performance liquid chromatography. *J. Pharm. Biomed. Anal.* 41, 1186–1190. doi: 10.1016/j.jpba.2006.02.054

Ma, R., and Wu, S. B. (2013). Research progress about pharmacological effect mechanism of flavonoids in traditional Chinese medicine. *Chin. Pharmacovigil. J.* 10, 286–290. doi: 10.3969/j.issn.1672-8629.2013.05.008

Qiu, H. D., Mallik, A. K., Takafuji, M., Liu, X., Jiang, S. X., and Ihara, H. (2012). A new imidazolium-embedded C18 stationary phase with enhanced performance in reversed phase liquid chromatography. *Anal. Chim. Acta* 738, 95–101. doi: 10.1016/j.aca.2012.06.018

Rodrigues, S. A., Caldas, S. S., and Primel, E. G. (2010). A simple; efficient and environmentally friendly method for the extraction of pesticides from onion by matrix solid-phase dispersion with liquid chromatography-tandem mass spectrometric detection. *Anal. Chim. Acta* 678, 82–89. doi: 10.1016/j.aca.2010.08.026

Shan, M. Q., Li, S. F. Y., Yu, S., Qian, Y., Guo, S. C., Zhang, L., et al. (2018). Chemical fingerprint and quantitative analysis for the quality evaluation of *Platycladi cacumen* by ultra-performance liquid chromatography coupled with hierarchical cluster analysis. *J. Chromatogr. Sci.* 56, 41–48. doi: 10.1093/chromsci/bmx079

Vela-Soria, F., Rodríguez, I., Ballesteros, O., Zafra-Gómez, A., Ballesteros, L., Cela, R., et al. (2014). Simplified matrix solid phase dispersion procedure for the determination of parabens and benzophenone-ultraviolet filters in human placental tissue samples. *J. Chromatogr. A* 1371, 39–47. doi: 10.1016/j.chroma.2014.10.063

Xu, J. J., Cao, J., Peng, L. Q., Cao, W., Zhu, Q. Y., and Zhang, Q. Y. (2016). Characterization and determination of isomers in plants using trace matrix solid phase dispersion via ultrahigh performance liquid chromatography coupled with an ultraviolet detector and quadrupole time-of-flight tandem mass spectrometry. *J. Chromatogr. A* 1436, 64–72. doi: 10.1016/j.chroma.2016.01.046

Zaugg, J., Khom, S., Eigenmann, D., Baburin, I., Hamburger, M., and Hering, S. (2011). Identification and characterization of GABA(A) receptor modulatory diterpenes from *Biota orientalis* that decrease locomotor activity in mice. *J. Nat. Prod.* 74, 1764–1772. doi: 10.1021/np200317p

Zhang, J. F., Sun, G. L., Zhang, B., Sun, Z. G., and Li, Y. (2013). Study progress of oriental arborvitae pharmacological effects. *Lishizhen Med. Mater. Med. Res.* 24, 2231–2233. doi: 10.3969/j.issn.1008-0805.2013.09.087

Zhuang, B., Bi, Z. M., Wang, Z. Y., Duan, L., Lai, C. J. S., and Liu, E. H. (2018). Chemical profiling and quantitation of bioactive compounds in *Platycladi cacumen* by UPLC-Q-TOF-MS/MS and UPLC-DAD. *J. Pharm. Biomed. Anal.* 154, 207–215. doi: 10.1016/j.jpba.2018.03.005

Zhuang, B., Dou, L. L., Li, P., and Liu, E. H. (2017). Deep eutectic solvents as green media for extraction of flavonoid glycosides and aglycones from *Platycladi cacumen*. *J. Pharm. Biomed. Anal.* 134, 214–219. doi: 10.1016/j.jpba.2016.11.049

6

Chemical Analysis and Multi-Component Determination in Chinese Medicine Preparation Bupi Yishen Formula Using Ultra-High Performance Liquid Chromatography with Linear Ion Trap-Orbitrap Mass Spectrometry and Triple-Quadrupole Tandem Mass Spectrometry

Jing Zhang[†], Wen Xu[†], Peng Wang, Juan Huang, Jun-qi Bai, Zhi-hai Huang*, Xu-sheng Liu* and Xiao-hui Qiu*

Guangdong Provincial Key Laboratory of Clinical Research on Traditional Chinese Medicine Syndrome, The Second Clinical Medical College of Guangzhou University of Chinese Medicine, Guangdong Provincial Hospital of Traditional Chinese Medicine, Guangzhou, China

*Correspondence:
Zhi-hai Huang
zhhuang7308@163.com
Xu-sheng Liu
liuxu801@126.com
Xiao-hui Qiu
qiuxiaohui@gzucm.edu.cn

[†]*These authors have contributed equally to this work.*

Bupi Yishen Formula (BYF), a Chinese medicine preparation, has been clinically applied for the recovery of chronic kidney disease and for delaying its progress. Nevertheless, the chemical components in BYF have yet to be fully clarified. Ultra-high performance liquid chromatography with linear ion trap-Orbitrap mass spectrometry (UHPLC-LTQ-Orbitrap-MS^n) and triple-quadrupole tandem mass spectrometry (UHPLC-TQ-MS/MS) methods were developed for qualitative chemical profiling and multi-components quantitative analysis in BYF. The chromatographic separation was performed on a Phenomenex Kinetex C_{18} column (2.1 × 100 mm i.d., 1.7 μm) using gradient elution of water (A) and acetonitrile (B) both containing 0.1% formic acid. Eighty-six compounds, including flavones, saponins, phenolic acids, and other compounds were authenticated or temporarily deduced according to their retention behaviors, mass mensuration, and characteristic fragment ions with those elucidated reference substances or literatures. Among the herbal medicinal materials of the formula, Astragali Radix, Codonopsis Radix, Salviae Miltiorrhizae Radix Rhizoma, and Polygoni Multiflori Radix Praeparata contributed to the bulk of the dissolved metabolites of the formula extraction. In addition, seven analytes were simultaneously determined by UHPLC-TQ-MS/MS, which was validated and has managed to determine major components in BYF. The study indicated that the established qualitative and quantitative methods would be potent and dependable analytical tools for characterizing multi-constituent in complex prescriptions decoction and provided a basis for the evaluation of bioactive components in BYF.

Keywords: Chinese medicine preparation, chemical analysis, multi-component determination, linear ion trap-orbitrap, quality control

INTRODUCTION

Chinese herbal medicine is the main form of clinical prevention and treatment of Traditional Chinese Medicine (TCM), the composition of which is composed of many different ingredients, and the organic combination of these different ingredients is different from adding individual ingredients simply. The material basis of Chinese herbal medicine is to coordinate and interact with each other so as to achieve the integrate function. Different from western medicine research, studies on Chinese herbal compound emphasize the integrity of the complex prescription, which should not split off from intrinsic characteristics of TCM and pursuit monomer compound (Wang et al., 2005). The material base of single herb or prescription is active substance groups. These groups of active substances are compatibly combined according to certain requirements, which act on multiple targets and thus has pleiotropic effects by multiple pathways (Xiong et al., 2015). Therefore, it is imperative to use modern advanced techniques to intrinsically explain the material basis of Chinese herbal medicine and to elaborate the connotation of compatibility and its curative effect.

Bupi Yishen Formula (BYF) is a non-herbal combination preparation of TCM which possesses the basic characterization of formula compatibility of TCM. BYF is prepared from the extract mixture of nine herbs, namely Astragali Radix, Codonopsis Radix, Atractylodis Macrocephalae Rhizoma, Poria, Dioscoreae Rhizoma, Polygoni Multiflori Radix Praeparata, Cuscutae Semen, Coicis Semen, and Salviae Miltiorrhizae Radix Rhizoma (Liu et al., 2012). The clinical application of BYF is treating and delaying the progression of chronic kidney disease, including postponing chronic renal failure symptoms, defering early and mid-renal dysfunction, delaying entering the dialysis time, and protection of residual renal function (Mao et al., 2015). Modern pharmacological studies revealed that the decoction could effectively delay glomerular filtration rate (GFR) of patients on the fourth stage of chronic kidney disease. Unambiguously, detecting and identifying the major components in BYF is a prerequisite and the hinge to disclose the active constituents and how they produce the effectiveness.

In recent years, reports on global characterizations of complicated ingredients in TCM prescriptions continues to grow steadily due to the recently rapid development of multifarious hyphenated and hybrid mass spectrometry (MS). Analytical methods have exhibited good performance in analysis of unknown targets from TCM prescriptions, containing LC-ESI/MS (Dou et al., 2009; Shaw et al., 2012), LC-TOF/MS (Sun et al., 2013), LC/MS-IT-TOF, etc. (Hao et al., 2008; Liu et al., 2016).

Ultra-high performance liquid chromatography (UHPLC) has been utilized in many bioanalytical fields in recent years due to its rapid analysis and excellent separation (Simons et al., 2009; Ha et al., 2013). Equipped with a relatively short column with a low flow rate, UHPLC usually cost a remarkably shorter analysis time to achieve the same separation efficiency as HPLC. The hybrid LTQ-Orbitrap analytical platform, being composed of an ion trap coupled with an Orbitrap mass analyzer, enables two scan types obtained at the same time. The Orbitrap provides relatively higher mass accuracy (<3 ppm) and mass resolution than a number of other mass spectrometers, which is available for determining exact molecular formulas (Dunn et al., 2008; Tchoumtchoua et al., 2013). Moreover, multi-stage MS^n mass spectra can be detected using ion trap by data-dependent scan and also minimize total analysis time, owing to its trigger for fragment spectra of target ions, and avoiding duplication by dynamic exclusion settings (Qiu et al., 2013). Thus, the LTQ-Orbitrap platform provides elemental compositions as well as multiple-stage mass data, which allow fast, sensitive, and reliable detecting, thus facilitating the identification of unknown compounds. Constituents of BYF could be structurally classified based on similar carbon skeletons, which should share a similar fragmentation pathway of each type and hence generate common characteristic product ions. Thus, mass spectra analysis for structural identifications could be facilitated by proposed strategies. In our previous study, the combination of UHPLC and LTQ-Orbitrap-MS^n has been successfully used in analyzing multiple components in single herbal extracts (Xu et al., 2014; Wang et al., 2015; Zhang et al., 2015). In this study, we attempt to exploit it to detect and identify the TCM prescription, which contain hundreds of different chemical constituents.

The present work attempted to establish an expeditious UHPLC-LTQ-Orbitrap-MS^n applicable approach for rapid separation and reliable identification of major constituents in BYF extract. Several strategies were used during the process, such as diagnostic fragment ions screening and fragment monitoring. In the decoction, eighty-six components altogether were identified or tentatively identified according to retention time and MS spectra data. Besides, a quantitative analysis approach has been constructed by Ultra-high performance liquid chromatography with triple quadrupole mass spectrometry (UHPLC-TQ-MS/MS). Seven representative compounds of relatively high contents unequivocally identified, were selected as marker components to evaluate the quality of BYF. The UHPLC-LTQ-Orbitrap MS^n, and UHPLC-TQ-MS/MS platforms were proved as potent tools for both rapid qualitative and quantitative detection and analysis of complicated constituents from natural resources and the study facilitated the comprehensive quality control of BYF.

EXPERIMENTAL

Chemicals, Reagents, and Materials

Chemical references including calycosin-7-O-β-D-glucopyranoside, calycosin, formononetin, astragulin, salvianolic acid B, (E)-2,3,5,4'-Tetrahydroxystilbene-2-O-glucopyranoside ((E)-THSG) Astragaloside I, Astragaloside II, Astragaloside III, Astragaloside IV, soyasaponin I, lobetyolin, emodin were bought from Must (Chengdu, China). Rosmarinic acid, lithospermic acid, formononetin-7-O-glucopyranoside were from Yuanye (Shanghai, China). Salvianolic acid A was purchased from Feiyu (Jiangsu, China). Isomucronulatol-7-O-glucoside, 9, 10-di-methoxypterocarpan-3-O-β-D-glucopyranoside were isolated from *Astragalus membranaceus* and provided by Prof. Zhu Dayuan from Shanghai Institute of Materia Medica. (S)-THSG, emodin-8-O-β-D-glucoside and physcion-8-O-β-D-glucoside were isolated from *Polygonum multiflorum* in our lab. The purity of each standard was determined by HPLC (≥95%) and their structures were confirmed by MS, ^{1}H-NMR, and ^{13}C-NMR. All references were deliquated with methanol for at a concentration of 50.0 μg/mL.

HPLC-grade Acetonitrile, methanol, and formic acid were from Sigma Aldrich (MO, USA). Ultra-pure water was prepared by a Milli-Q water system (Millipore, MA, USA). Other reagents and chemicals were of analytical grade.

Astragali Radix (No. 11050419, Neimenggu), Codonopsis Radix (No. 110653271, Gansu), Atractylodis Macrocephalae Rhizoma (No. 110600711, zhejiang), Poria (No. 110506341, Hunan), Dioscoreae Rhizoma (No. 121001014, Henan), Polygoni Multiflori Radix Praeparata (No. 110400831, Henan), Cuscutae Semen (No. 110502581, Shandong), Coicis Semen (No. 110600371, Guizhou), and Salviae Miltiorrhizae Radix Rhizoma (No. 110601741, Anhui) were from Kangmei(Guangdong, China). They were authenticated by Dr. Huang Zhihai and the specimens were preserved in Guangdong Provincial Hospital of TCM. Two batches of BYF concentrated granule was produced in the pilot-scale by Peili Pharmaceutical Co., Ltd. (NanNing, China).

Preparation of Calibration Standard Solutions

Standard of seven compounds was accurately weighed and dissolved in methanol separately to prepare the stock solution of each. A mixed stock solution was obtained, containing seven stock solutions, giving a concentration of 15.30 μg/mL for calycosin-7-O-Glc, 6.45 μg/mL for calycosin, 644.80 μg/mL for (*E*)-THSG, 6.03 μg/mL for astragulin, 15.60 μg/mL for rosmarinic acid, 8.10 μg/mL for salvianolic acid A, 0.812 μg/mL for salvianolic acid B, respectively. Daidzein (50.0 μg/mL) was also prepared with methanol to obtain the internal standard (IS) stock solution. To construct calibration curves, the mixed stock solution was continuously diluted for series concentrations at 1/2, 1/4, 1/8, 1/16, 1/32, 1/64, and 1/128 of the original one. In a 2 mL volumetric flask, 0.2 mL of each concentration solution above, as well as 100 μL IS solutions were added, and all concentrations were finally diluted to 2 mL with 18% aqueous methanol. The acquired solutions were conserved at 4°C in refrigerator until use. All the solutions were filtered through 0.22 μm membranes before analysis.

Sample Preparation

(i) Extraction of crude drugs: A total 125 g dry pieces of nine medicinal materials were mixed by prescription ratio and extracted with boiling water (1:10) for three times (45,30, and 30 min, respectively), filtered through gauze. Then three filtrates were combined and vacuum evaporated to recover the solvent at 56°C, and then BYF extract could be obtained. Extract was transferred into 250 mL volumetric flask, then adjusted to desired level with 10% methanol solution (final crude drug concentration was 0.5 g/mL). Solid-phase extraction (SPE) with C-18 column (ProElut, 200 mg, 3 mL column volume) was used for the pretreatment procedure, which had been conditioned with

methanol (2 mL) and water (2 mL). After 1.0 mL of BYF extract was loaded, the column was washed by 10% methanol (2 mL), and eluted with 1.0 mL 100% methanol slowly. The dry pieces of each herb were disposed through the same procedure, thus individual decoction was obtained. All the sample solutions were passed through 0.22 μm membranes prior to analysis.

(ii) Pretreatment of decoction for quantitative study: The lyophilized powder of BYF decoction was produced by freeze-drying. 11.20 g lyophilized powder was acquired from 100 mL of BYF decoction. Five hundred and sixty milligrams of BYF was filtered, a 0.1 mL portion of which was added with 10 μL of the IS solution, and then was diluted with methanol to 5 mL. The sample solutions were passed through 0.22 μm membranes.

(iii) Pretreatment of BYF concentrated granule: Concentrated granule (2.0 g) was accurately weighed and precisely dissolved in 100 mL of 80% aqueous methanol, and then refluxed for 1 h. The extract was cooled down to room temperature, weighed and made up a deficiency by 80% methanol, which was then treated in the same way as (ii).

UHPLC-LTQ-Orbitrap-MS^n Conditions

Chromatographic separation was conducted by a Thermo Accela UHPLC system (San Joes, USA) comprising an autosampler, a quaternary pump, a diode-array detector (DAD), and a column compartment settled to room temperature. A Phenomenex Kinetex C_{18} column (2.1 × 100 mm i.d., 1.7 μm) was utilized for sample separating. The mobile phase was mixture of water (A) and acetonitrile (B), both containing 0.1% formic acid. The elution gradient was set as follows: 0–12 min (10–25% B), 12–25 min (25–32% B), 15–42 min (32–56% B), 42–51 min (56–95% B). The injection volume of samples was 2 μL with a flow rate of mobile phase at 200 μL/min.

For qualitative experiments, a Thermo Fisher Scientific LTQ-Orbitrap XL hybrid mass spectrometer (Bremen, Germany) was hyphenated to the LC instrument via an electron spray ionization (ESI) interface. The samples were determined in negative mode. The ESI parameters were set (spray voltage was −3.5 KV; capillary temperature was 325°C; tube lens voltage was −76 V; Sheath gas and auxiliary gases were 45 and 6 units, respectively). The Orbitrap mass analyzer was set up the full scan mass range at m/z 120–1,200 of 30,000 resolution in centroided-type mass mode. In data-dependent MS^n acquisition, the most intense ions were always selected for online MS^2-MS^3 analysis by FT and MS^4-MS^5 analysis by LTQ, and dynamic exclusion detection was also conducted during the process for repetition prevention. Dynamic exclusion parameters was set as follows: Repeat count, 2; Repeat duration, 0.35 min; Exclusion duration, 1.0 min; Exclusion mass width, 3 amu. The collision energy for collision-induced dissociation (CID) was set as 30 % of maximum.

The number and types of expected atoms were fixed as follows for possible elemental composition of components: carbons ≤50, hydrogens ≤80, oxygens ≤30, nitrogens ≤2. The accuracy error threshold was set at 3 ppm. The software of Thermo Fisher Scientific Xcalibur 2.1 was applied for data analysis.

UHPLC-TQ-MS/MS Analysis

An Accela™ UPLC system and a Thermo Scientific TSQ Quantum Ultra triple-quadrupole spectrometer (San Jose, USA) fitted with an ESI probe were employed for quantitative analysis. The separation column, column temperature, and the mobile phase were identical with those of qualitative conditions, with a gradient elution of 18–39% B at 0–5 min, 39–65% B at 5–7 min, 65–95% B at 7–9 min at 10–12 min with a flow rate at 250 μL/min. The injection volume was set at 5 μL.

Multiple reaction monitoring (MRM) was used for MS data acquisition and the conditions were designed as below: capillary temperature was 400°C; capillary voltage was 2.5 kV for negative mode and 3.0 kV for positive mode; sheath gas (N_2) was pressure 40 psi; auxiliary gas was 8 psi; the dwell time was 100 ms. The detection parameters of target compounds were summarized in **Table 1**. Peak areas of each analyte and IS acquired in MRM mode were employed for calibration curve establishing. Data were collected and analyzed by Thermo Xcalibur 2.1.0 Software.

Validation of Quantitative Method

The linear calibration curves were established by the analyte/IS ratio of each analyte (peak area ratio between each analyte and IS). Diluted standard solutions were successively analyzed until a signal-to-noise ratio (S/N) 3:1 and 10:1 were reached, respectively, to measure the limit of detection (LOD) and limit of quantification (LOQ) of each target compound. The intra-day precision was evaluated by detecting six times during 1 day, while the inter-day precision was assessed for 3 days in a row. Repeatability was obtained by six independent sample solutions using identical procedure in section Sample Preparation and variations were displayed by the relative standard deviation (RSD). One sample solution was tested at room temperature at different times within 24 h for stability evaluation. The recovery test was validated by adding known amounts of mixed reference solution to sample solutions at three concentration levels.

RESULTS AND DISCUSSION

Optimization of Extraction Procedure and Analysis Conditions

Variable factors during extraction procedures of BYF granule, including extraction solvent (water, 50, 80, and 100% methanol),

method (reflux and sonication), solvent volume (30, 60, and 100 mL), and time (15, 30, 45, and 60 min) were optimized so as to extract the compounds efficiently. The optimized method was finally determined to extract the BYF granule with 100 ml of 80% methanol by refluxed for 1 h.

The UHPLC conditions were optimized, containing type of column, column temperature, mobile phase system, and flow rate. The Phenomenex Kinetex C_{18} column was selected based upon our previous multi-constituents analysis. Besides, different kinds of mobile phases were tested (acetonitrile and methanol with added modifiers, including formic acid, acetic acid, and ammonium acetate). A combination of acetonitrile and water both containing 0.1% (v/v) formic acid was found not only compatible to MS analysis, but also suitable for compounds separation for qualitative analysis. Comparing the TIC of the negative and positive modes, signal response was found more sensitive to the majority of components in negative mode, thus the MS^n data were detected in negative mode. The total ion chromatogram of BYF was acquired for structure confirmation (shown in **Figure 1**).

Characterization of Constituents in BYF Extract

BYF extract was analyzed using the optimized UHPLC-LTQ-Orbitrap-MS^n method. To elucidate the chemical components, known compounds were identified by comparing with the data of reference standards. Based on the MS^n analysis of the authentic compounds, the characteristic fragmentation behaviors of each type with the same carbon skeleton were conducted, and thus applied the obtained rules to structure characterization of their derivatives. For other unknown compounds, the structures were tentatively identified according to MS^n spectra and previous data in literatures. Eighty-six compounds in all were identified or tentatively identified (**Table 2**), including 15 flavones, 10 saponins, 12 phenolic acids, and other compounds. Nine herbs made markedly different chemical contributions to BYF. Specifically, the major constituents in BYF extract came from Astragali Radix (25 compounds), Codonopsis Radix (18 compounds), Salviae Miltiorrhizae (11 compounds), Cuscutae Semen (16 compounds), and Polygoni Multiflori Radix Praeparata (6 compounds).

TABLE 1 | Chromatographic retention time, MRM parameters, and collision energy for the seven investigated compounds.

Analytes	t_R (min)	Ionization mode	Precursor ion (m/z)	Product ion (m/z)	Collision energy (eV)
Calycosin-7-O-Glc	2.33	ESI(+)	447.13	285.10	27
(E)-THSG	2.65	ESI(−)	405.02	243.04	21
Astragulin	3.18	ESI(−)	447.02	255.04	35
Rosmarinic acid	3.71	ESI(−)	359.99	161.03	20
Salvianolic acid A	4.73	ESI(−)	492.99	295.03	18
Salvianolic acid B	4.21	ESI(−)	717.00	321.03	33
Calycosin	4.88	ESI(−)	283.36	268.04	24
IS daidzein	4.47	ESI(+)	254.90	199.01	23

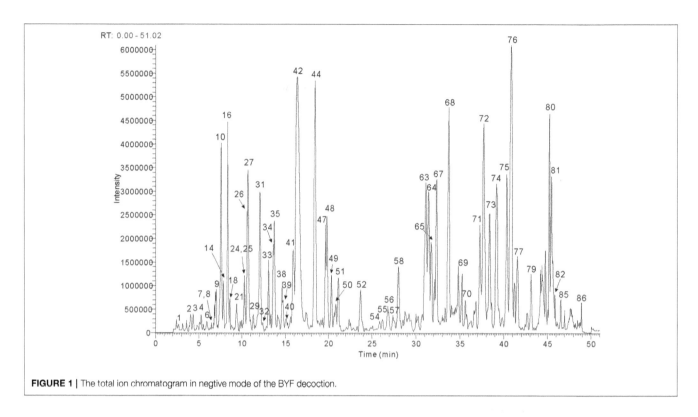

FIGURE 1 | The total ion chromatogram in negtive mode of the BYF decoction.

Compounds From Astragali Radix

Isoflavones and saponins, the major bioactive compounds in Astragali Radix, have various effects such as tonic, immunostimulant, cardioprotective diuretic, and hepatoprotective properties (Xu et al., 2006; Auyeung et al., 2009). In our work, 20 compounds from RA were totally characterized in BYF, including 12 isoflavones and 8 saponins. By comparing with information of reference standards, calycosin-7-O-β-D-glycoside, ononin, calycosin, formononetin, isomucronulatol-7-O-β-D-glucoside, 9,10-diMP-3-O-glucoside, 9,10-di-methoxypterocarpan-3-O-β-D-glucopyranoside, Astragaloside I, Astragaloside II, Astragaloside III, Astragaloside IV, and soyasaponin I were identified. Based on the MS^n analysis of these authentic compounds, the characteristic fragmentation behaviors of isoflavones and saponins were proposed in our previous study (Zhang et al., 2015), which were applied for the structure elucidation of their derivatives.

The MS^2 spectra of Compound 39 and Compound 55 exhibited characteristic product ions [M-C$_2$H$_2$O]$^-$ (m/z 475.1 and 429.1) and [M-glu-C$_2$H$_2$O]$^-$ (m/z 283.1 and 267.1), and their characteristic product ions yielded from the aglycone ion coincided with those of calycosin and formononetin. Based on the cleavage rules of loss of acetyl (42 Da) and acetylglucosyl (204 Da) groups, the two compounds were deduced as acetyl-glucoside of calycosin and formononetin.

Astragalosides from BYF decoction were mainly constituted by cycloastragenol aglycone, while aglycone ions or ions originated from the neutral loss of different glycosyl moiety in their MS^2 spectra. Take Compound 69 as an example, the [M-H]$^-$ ion was m/z 783.450 20 (C$_{41}$H$_{67}$O$_{14}^-$), which easily lose the

sugar units in its MS^2 spectra and gained typical product ions at m/z 651, 621, 489 from the loss of one xylose ([M-132]$^-$), one glucose ([M-164 (glu)]$^-$), one xylose and glucose ([M-132 (xyl)-164 (glu)]$^-$), respectively. In addition, one soyasaponin (Compound 78) of lower content from Astragali Radix was found in BYF decoction.

Compounds From Codonopsis Radix

The identified compounds of Codonopsis Radix in BYF can be classified into four main classes, namely, phenylpropanoid glycosides, acetylene glycosides, hexyl (hexenol) glycosides (Lin et al., 2013). In (-)ESI-MS spectra of BYF decoction, apart from phenylpropanoid glycosides (including compounds 8, 12, 23, 37, and 40) existing in [M-H]$^-$ ion forms, others displayed as both [M+HCOO]$^-$ and [M-H]$^-$ ions.

By comparing the retention time values and mass data with those of the references, Compound 8 and 30 were unambiguously identified as tangshenoside I and lobetyolin, which are the representative compounds of phenylpropanoid glycosides and acetylene glycosides in Radix Codonopsis. Their MS^n spectra and proposed fragmentation pathways were summarized in **Figures 2A–C, 3, 4**, respectively. The [M-H]$^-$ ion and the typical ions in the MS^2 spectra of Compound 19 (C$_{26}$H$_{37}$O$_{13}^-$), namely, m/z 557.2 [M-H]$^-$, 467.2 [M-C$_7$H$_6$]$^-$, 341.1 [M-C$_{14}$H$_{17}$O$_2$]$^-$, were all 162 Da less compared to those of Compound 30, demonstrating that they have identical site cleavage. Compound 19 was therefore characterized as lobetyolinin by comparison with the literature (Kanji et al., 2003).

Compounds 37 and 40 were identified as diastereomers by the same deprotonated ions at m/z 823.265 8 (C$_{38}$H$_{47}$O$_{20}^-$) and the

TABLE 2 | Compounds detected and identified in BYF decoction.

No.	t_R/min	$[M-H]^-$ (Mass error, ppm)	Characteristic fragment ions	Molecular formula	Compounds	Resources
1	2.67	353.086 82 (−0.44)	MS^2 [353]: 191.1, 179.0	$C_{16}H_{18}O_9$	3-Caffeoyl-quinic acid	Cs
2	4.01	353.086 76 (−0.49)	MS^2 [353]: 191.1, 179.0	$C_{16}H_{18}O_9$	5-Caffeoyl-quinic acid	Cs
			MS^2 [191]: 173.0, 127.0			
3	4.35	353.086 98 (−0.28)	MS^2 [353]: 191.1, 179.0, 173.0	$C_{16}H_{18}O_9$	4-Caffeoyl-quinic acid	Cs
			MS^2 [191]: 173.0, 127.0			
4	5.30	469.191 35^a (−0.22)	MS^2 [469]: 423.2	$C_{18}H_{32}O_{11}$	(S)-3-Hexenyl-β-D-sophoriside	Cr
		423.185 76 (−0.32)	MS^3 [423]: 261.1, 221.1, 179.1, 161.1			
5	5.48	350.196 08^b (−0.12)	MS^3 [350]: 250.1, 205.1, 161.1	$C_{19}H_{28}NO_5^+$	Codonopyrrolidium A^c	Cr
6	5.84	469.191 25^a (−0.32)	MS^2 [469]: 423.2	$C_{18}H_{32}O_{11}$	(E)-2-Hexenyl-β-D-sophoriside	Cr
		423.185 91 (−0.60)	MS^3 [423]: 261.1, 221.1, 179.1, 161.0			
7	6.44	405.118 07 (0.06)	MS^2 [405]: 243.1	$C_{20}H_{22}O_9$	(Z)-THSG	Pm
			MS^2[243]: 225.1, 215.1, 201.0, 173.0, 149.0, 137.0			
8	6.52	677.228 09 (−0.65)	MS^2[677]: 497.2, 453.2, 261.1,	$C_{29}H_{42}O_{18}$	Tangshenoside I	Cr
			MS^3[261]: 99.1, 161.1			
9	6.96	471.207 40^a (0.18)	MS^2[471]: 425.2	$C_{18}H_{34}O_{11}$	Hexyl β-sophoroside	Cr
		425.201 57 (−0.17)	MS^3[425]: 263.1, 161.0			
10	7.50	491.118 65^a (0.25)	MS^2[417]: 283.1	$C_{22}H_{22}O_{10}$	Calycosin-7-O-β-D-glup	Ar
			MS^3[283]: 268.0			
			MS^4[268]: 240.0, 224.0, 211.0, 184.0			
11	7.45	595.129 33 (−0.03)	MS^2[595]: 463.1, 301.0, 300.0	$C_{26}H_{28}O_{16}$	Quercetin 3-O-(2-O-apisyl)-galactoside	Cs
			MS^3[300]: 271.0, 255.0			
			MS^4[271]: 243.0, 227.01, 199.0			
12	7.70	469.133 51 (−0.54)	MS^2 [469]: 325.1, 265.1, 235.1	$C_{21}H_{26}O_{12}$	Tangshenoside IV isomer	Cr
			MS^3 [325]: 265.1, 235.1			
13	7.74	441.196 66^a (0.01)	MS^2 [395]: 263.1, 161.0	$C_{17}H_{32}O_{10}$	Hexyl-(pen)-glup	Cr
		395.191 10 (−0.21)				
14	7.79	633.180 91 (−0.49)	MS^2 [633]: 471.1, 307.1	$C_{30}H_{34}O_{15}$	Unknown	Cs
			MS^3[307]: 247.1, 205, 187, 163.1, 145.0			
15	7.97	521.128 72^a (0.25)	MS^2[521]: 475.1, 359.1, 313.1, 298.1, 207.0	$C_{23}H_{24}O_{11}$	Odoratin-glup	Ar
			MS^3[313]: 298.0, 283.0, 270.0			
16	8.32	405.118 47 (−0.09)	MS^2 [405]: 243.1	$C_{20}H_{22}O_9$	(E)-THSG	Pm
			MS^2[243]: 225.1, 215.1, 201.0, 173.0, 149.0, 137.0			
17	8.40	309.154 85^a (0.46)	MS^2 [309]: 263.1	$C_{12}H_{24}O_6$	Hexyl β-D-glup	Cr
			MS^3 [263]: 161.1			
18	8.54	463.087 52 (0.42)	MS^2[595]: 463.1, 301.0, 300.0	$C_{21}H_{20}O_{12}$	Quercetin 3-O-galactoside (hyperoside)	Cs
			MS^3[301]: 271.0, 255.0, 179.0, 151.0			
19	8.88	603.227 84^a (−0.51)	MS2 [603]: 557.2, 467.2, 341.1, 323.1	$C_{26}H_{38}O_{13}$	Lobetyolinin	Cr
20	9.10	557.128 11 (−0.86)	MS^2[557]: 405.1, 313.1, 243.1	$C_{27}H_{25}O_{13}$	2,3,5,4'-Tetrahydroxystilbene-2-(galloyl)-O-glc	Pm
			MS^3[313]: 169.0, 295.0			
21	9.32	261.133 79 (0.53)	MS^2[261]: 187.1, 125.1	$C_{12}H_{22}O_6$	Hexenyl-β-D-glup	Cr
22	9.40	565.191 10^a (−1.01)	MS^2[519]: 357.1	$C_{26}H_{32}O_{11}$	Unknown	
		519.185 85 (−0.79)	MS^2[357]: 151.0, 136.0			

(Continued)

TABLE 2 | Continued

No.	t_R/min	[M–H]⁻ (Mass error, ppm)	Characteristic fragment ions	Molecular formula	Compounds	Resources
23	9.72	469.133 82 (−0.23)	MS²[469]: 407.1, 367.1, 325.1 MS³[325]: 163.0, 119.1	$C_{21}H_{26}O_{12}$	Tangshenoside V	Cr
24	10.21	417.081 63[M-H]⁻ (0.01)	MS²[417]: 373.1, 175.0 MS²[307]: 175.0	$C_{20}H_{17}O_{10}$	Salvianolic acid D	Sm
25	10.30	537.102 29 (−1.9)	MS²[537]: 493.1, 339.0, 295.1 MS³[339]: 321.0, 295.1, 185.0	$C_{27}H_{22}O_{12}$	Salvianolic acid H or I	Sm
26	10.60	187.097 35 (0.89)	MS²[187]: 125.1, 97.1	$C_9H_{16}O_4$	Azelaic acid	Co / Cr
27	10.69	447.092 41 (−0.33)	MS²[447]: 327.0, 285.0, 284.0 MS³[284]: 255.0, 227.0	$C_{21}H_{20}O_{11}$	Astragulin	Cs
28	10.83	507.113 01ᵃ (−0.31)	MS²[507]: 461.1, 299.1 MS³[299]: 284.0 MS⁴[284]: 256.0, 227.0, 212.0	$C_{22}H_{22}O_{11}$	Pratensein-7-O-Glu	Ar
29	11.30	477.102 60 (−1.5)	MS²[477]: 314.0 MS³[314]: 285.0, 271.0, 243.0	$C_{22}H_{22}O_{12}$	Unknown	/
30	11.86	441.175 29ᵃ (−0.23) 395.169 65 (−0.40)	MS² [441]: 395.1, 305.1, 215.1, 185.1, 179.1	$C_{20}H_{28}O_8$	Lobetyolin	Cr
31	12.03	359.076 51 (0.36)	MS² [359]: 223.0, 197.1, 179.0, 161.0	$C_{18}H_6O_8$	Rosmarimic acid	Sm
32	12.33	537.102 48 (−0.27)	MS²[537]: 493.1, 339.0, 295.1 MS²[493]: 321.0, 295.1	$C_{27}H_{22}O_{12}$	Salvianolic acid H or I	Sm
33	13.03	723.499 08ᵃ (0.78) 677.493 90 (1.08)	MS²[677]: 451.3 MS²[677]: 433.4, 225.1	$C_{48}H_{68}O_5$	Unknown	Cr/Am/Dr/ Ar
34	13.56	537.102 97 (0.22)	MS²[537]: 493.1 MS³[493]: 295.1 MS⁴[295]: 277.1, 159.0, 109.0	$C_{27}H_{22}O_{12}$	Lithospermic acid	Sm
35	13.69	475.123 66ᵃ (0.17)	MS²[475]: 429.1, 267.1, MS³[267]: 252.0, 22.9, 208.1	$C_{22}H_{22}O_9$	Formononetin-7-O-Glc	Ar
36	14.43	505.133 64ᵃ (−0.42)	MS²[475]: 297.1, MS³[297]: 282.1, MS⁴[282]: 267.1, 254.1, 239.1	$C_{23}H_{24}O_{10}$	6,4′-Dimethoxyisoflavone-7-O-Glc	Ar
37	14.48	823.265 87 (0.35)	MS² [823]: 497.2, 453.2, 261.1	$C_{38}H_{48}O_{20}$	6‴-Trans-p-coumaroyl-tangshenoside I	Cr
38	14.60	471.128 48 (−1.4)	MS² [471]: 307.1 MS³[307]: 247.1, 187.0, 163.1, 145.0	$C_{24}H_{24}O_{10}$	Unknown	Cs
39	14.74	533.128 66ᵃ (−1.6)	MS²[533]: 487.1, 445.1, 283.1 MS³[283]: 268.0 MS⁴[268]: 240.0, 224.0, 211.0	$C_{24}H_{24}O_{11}$	Calycosin-7-O-glc-6″-O-acetate	Ar
40	15.13	823.265 81 (0.34)	MS² [823]: 497.2, 453.2, 261.1	$C_{38}H_{48}O_{20}$	6‴-Cis-p-coumaroyl-tangshenoside I	Cr
41	15.92	269.092 59 (−0.03)	MS²[269]: 225.1 MS³[225]: 207.1, 183.1, 166.1, 156.1	$C_{15}H_{14}O_3N_2$	Cuscutamine	Cs
42	16.38	717.144 65 (-0.36)	MS²[717]: 519.1, 321.0 MS³[519]: 339.0, 321.0 MS⁴[321]: 293.0, 279.1, 277.1 MS⁵[279]: 251.1	$C_{36}H_{30}O_{16}$	Salvianolic acid B	Sm
43	16.43	507.150 36ᵃ (0.66)	MS²[507]: 461.1, 299.1, 284.1	$C_{23}H_{26}O_{10}$	9,10-Di-methoxypterocarpan-3-O-β-D-glucopyranoside	Ar

(Continued)

TABLE 2 | Continued

No.	t_R/min	[M–H]$^-$ (Mass error, ppm)	Characteristic fragment ions	Molecular formula	Compounds	Resources
			MS^3[299]: 284.1, 269.0, 241.0			
44	18.40	283.060 73 (0.63)	MS^2[283]: 268.0, 240.0, 224.0, 211.0	$C_{16}H_{12}O_5$	Calycosin	Ar
45	18.54	509.165 44^a (0.08)	MS^2[509]: 463.1, 445.1, 346.1, 301.1, 286.0	$C_{23}H_{28}O_{10}$	Isomucronulatol-7-O-β-D-glucopyranoside	Ar
			MS^3[301]: 286.1, 135.0, 109.0			
46	19.37	523.123 23 (–0.27)	MS^2[523]: 491.1, 343.1, 325.1, 293.0	–	–	–
47	19.63	493.113 16 (–0.6)	MS^2[493]: 295.1	$C_{26}H_{22}O_{10}$	Salvianolic acid A	Sm
			MS^3[295]: 277.1, 267, 185, 159.0, 109.0			
48	19.81	717.143 92 (–1.09)	MS^2[717]: 519.1	$C_{36}H_{30}O_{16}$	Salvianolic acid E	Sm
			MS^3[519]: 339.0, 321,.0			
			MS^4[321]: 279.1, 251.1			
49	20.34	551.118 35 (–1.0)	MS^2[551]: 519.1	$C_{28}H_{24}O_{12}$	Monomethyl lithospermater	Sm
			MS^3[519]: 353.1, 321.0			
50	20.81	431.097 08(–0.19)	MS^2[431]: 269.0	$C_{21}H_{20}O_{10}$	Emodin-8-O-glc	Pm
			MS^3[269]: 225.0, 241.0			
			MS^4[225]: 181.0, 210.0			
51	21.14	493.112 70 (–0.22)	MS^2[493]: 295.1	$C_{26}H_{22}O_{10}$	Isomer of Salvianolic acid A	Sm
			MS^3[295]: 277.1, 267.1, 185.1	$C_{36}H_{30}O_{15}$		
52	23.68	491.097 23 (–0.04)	MS^2[491]: 293.0, 311.1	$C_{26}H_{20}O_{10}$	Salvianolic acid C	Sm
			MS^3[293]: 276.0, 265.0, 249.1			
53	24.23	577.154 30 (–0.88)	–	$C_{27}H_{30}O_{14}$	Unknown	
54	25.32	297.076 02 (0.27)	MS^2[297]: 282.1, 267.1, 254.1, 239.1	$C_{17}H_{14}O_5$	7-Hydroxy-6,4'-dimethoxyisoflavone	Ar
55	26.18	517.133 67^a (–0.38)	MS^2[517]: 429.1, 267.1	$C_{24}H_{24}O_{10}$	Formononetin-7-O-β-D-glycoside-6''-O-acetate	Ar
			MS^3[267]: 252.0			
			MS^4[252]: 223.1, 208.1			
56	26.85	285.039 64 (–0.27)	MS^2[285]: 257.0, 229.1, 213.1, 169.1, 199.1, 151.0	$C_{15}H_{10}O_6$	Kaempferol or luteolin	Cs
57	27.86	299.055 33 (0.32)	MS^2[299]: 284.1, 271.1, 255.1, 240.1, 227.0	$C_{16}H_{12}O_6$	Rhamnocitrin	Ar
58	28.03	327.217 10 (0.50)	MS^2[327]: 291.2, 229.1, 211.1, 171.1	$C_{18}H_{32}O_5$	9,12,13-Trihydroxy-octadec-10,15-dienoic acid	Sm / Cr
			MS^3[229]: 211.1			
59	28.28	549.159 85^a (–0.42)	MS^2[549]: 485.1, 459.1, 415.1, 299.1	$C_{25}H_{28}O_{11}$	9,10-Di-methoxypterocarpan-3-O-β-D-glucopyranoside-acetate	Ar
			MS^3[299]: 284.1, 269.0, 241.0			
60	29.56	991.509 34^a (–1.50)	MS^2[991]: 783.5, 765.5, 489.4	$C_{47}H_{78}O_{19}$	Astragaloside VI or VII	Ar
61	29.99	671.138 73 (–0.80)	MS^2[671]: 473.1	$C_{35}H_{29}O_{14}$	Unknown	-
			MS^3[473]: 339.1, 321.0			
62	30.51	491.118 59^a (0.19)	MS^2[445]: 283.1	$C_{22}H_{22}O_{10}$	Physcion-8-O-glc	Pm
		445.112 92 (–0.01)	MS^2[283]: 268.0, 240.0			
			MS^2[240]: 212.0, 184.1			
63	31.13	267.065 92 (0.7)	MS^2[267]: 252.0	$C_{16}H_{12}O_4$	Formononetin	Ar
			MS^3[252]: 223.0, 208.0, 132.0			
64	31.42	329.232 70 (0.45)	MS^2[329]: 311.2, 293.2, 229.1, 211.1	$C_{18}H_{34}O_5$	9,12,13-Trihydroxy-octadec-10-enoic acid	Cr
			MS^3[171]: 153.0, 127.1, 125.1			

(Continued)

TABLE 2 | Continued

No.	t_R/min	[M–H]⁻ (Mass error, ppm)	Characteristic fragment ions	Molecular formula	Compounds	Resources
65	31.72	329.232 64 (−0.16)	MS² [329]: 311.2, 293.2, 229.1, 211.1 MS³ [229]: 211.1, 209.1	$C_{18}H_{34}O_5$	5,6,9-Trihydroxy-octadec-7-enoic acid	Cr / Co
66	33.03	991.508 61[a] (−2.22)	MS²[991]: 783.5, 765.5, 621.4, 489.4	$C_{47}H_{78}O_{19}$	Astragaloside V	Ar
67	32.35	843.421 45 (−0.57)	MS²[843]: 797.4, 779.4, 633.5	$C_{38}H_{68}O_{20}$	Cuscutic acid C/Isomer	Cs
68	33.70	843.421 08 (−0.94)	MS²[843]: 797.4, 779.4, 633.5	$C_{38}H_{68}O_{20}$	Cuscutic acid C/Isomer	Cs
69	35.23	829.456 18[a] (−1.83) 783.450 20 (−2.33)	MS²[783]: 651.4, 621.4, 489.4	$C_{41}H_{68}O_{14}$	Astragaloside IV	Ar
70	35.62	829.455 26[a] (−2.75) 783.450 26 (−2.27)	MS²[783]: 621.4, 489.4	$C_{41}H_{68}O_{14}$	Astragaloside III	Ar
71	37.26	885.431 03 (−2.10)	MS²[885]: 839.4, 821.4, 633.3	$C_{40}H_{70}O_{21}$	Unknown	Cs
72	37.70	885.431 27 (−1.31)	MS²[885]: 839.4, 821.4, 633.3	$C_{40}H_{70}O_{21}$	Unknown	Cs
73	38.35	885.431 09 (−1.49)	MS²[885]: 839.4, 821.4, 633.3	$C_{40}H_{70}O_{21}$	Unknown	Cs
74	39.13	885.431 27 (−1.31)	MS²[885]: 839.4, 821.4, 635.3	$C_{40}H_{70}O_{21}$	Unknown	Cs
75	40.30	871.467 29[a] (−1.29) 825.460 75 (−2.35)	MS²[825]: 783.5, 765.4, 489.4	$C_{43}H_{70}O_{15}$	Astragaloside II	Ar
76	40.78	885.431 40 (−1.18)	MS²[885]: 839.4, 821.4, 633.5	$C_{40}H_{70}O_{21}$	Acely-cuscutic acid C	Cs
77	41.54	681.367 55 (−1.6)	–	$C_{32}H_{58}O_{15}$	Unknown	
78	42.40	987.513 61[a] (−2.31) 941.508 18 (−2.26)	MS²[941]: 923.5, 795.5, 615.4, 457.4, 437.4	$C_{48}H_{78}O_{18}$	Soyasaponin I	Ar
79	43.14	871.466 67[a] (−1.91) 825.460 57 (−2.52)	MS²[871]:783.5, 765.5, 717.4, 633.4, 603.4, 489.4	$C_{43}H_{70}O_{15}$	Isoastragaloside II	Ar
80	45.19	913.477 66[a] (-1.48) 867.471 07 (−2.59)	MS²[867]: 825.5, 807.5, 765.5, 747.5, 729.5, 717.4, 705.5, 699.4, 633.4, 567.4, 489.4	$C_{45}H_{72}O_{16}$	Astragaloside I	Ar
81	45.45	295.227 36 (0.59)	MS²[295]: 277.2, 195.1, 171.1 MS³[277]: 233.2	$C_{18}H_{32}O_3$	Coronaric acid	Co
82	45.49	913.476 5[a] (−2.58)	MS³[867]: 825.5, 807.5, 765.5, 747.5, 729.5, 717.4, 705.4, 699.4, 633.4, 567.4, 489.4	$C_{45}H_{72}O_{16}$	Isoastragaloside I	Ar
83	45.80	269.045 04 (0.59)	MS²[269]: 225.0 MS³[225]: 181.0, 210.0	$C_{15}H_{10}O_5$	Emodin	Pm
84	45.86	915.493 23[a] (−1.56)	–	$C_{45}H_{72}O_{16}$	Dioscin	Dr
85	46.55	955.487 79 (−1.92)	MS²[955]: 891.5, 763.5, 701.4, 613.4, 523.4	$C_{47}H_{74}O_{17}$	Acetylastragaloside I	Ar
86	48.91	339.231 75 (−0.3)	MS²[339]: 163.1	$C_{23}H_{32}O_2$	Unknown	–

[a][M+HCOO⁻]⁻; [b][M+H]⁺; [c]only detected in positive mode.

Cs, Cuscutae Semen; Cr, Codonopsis Radix; Pm, Polygoni Multiflori Radix Praeparata; Ar, Astragali Radix; Sm, Salviae Miltiorrhizae Radix Rhizoma; Co, Coicis Semen; Am, Atractylodis Macrocephalae Rhizoma; Dr, Dioscoreae Rhizoma; P, Poria; pen, pentoside; glup, glucopyranoside.

same productions at m/z 497.2, m/z 453.2, and m/z 261.1, and they could be differentiated by their elution order. Their log P calculated by Discovery Studio were 0.47 and 0.59. As cis-isomers with lower polarity could by eluted relatively later than trans-isomers, compounds 37 and 40 were identified as 6‴-trans- and 6‴-cis-p-coumaroyl-tangshenoside I.

Compounds 9, 13, and 17 exhibited the [M+HCOO⁻]⁻ precursor ion at m/z 471.207 40, 441.196 66, and 309.154 85, and their MS² and MS³ spectra all yielded ions at m/z

263.1 ($C_{12}H_{23}O_6^-$) and 161.1 ($C_6H_9O_5^-$) as the base peak, respectively. It is inferred that Compounds 9 and 13 were, respectively, substituted by an additional glucopyranoside and pentoside compared to Compound 17. Compounds 9, 13, and 17 were tentatively characterized as hexyl β-sophoroside, hexyl-(pen)-glucopyranoside, and hexyl β-D-glucopyranoside.

Isomers (Compounds 4 and 6) were obtained by the EIC of m/z 423. Both of Them displayed [M-H]⁻ ion at m/z 423.185 76 ($C_{18}H_{31}O_{11}^-$) and their MS² spectra all exhibited

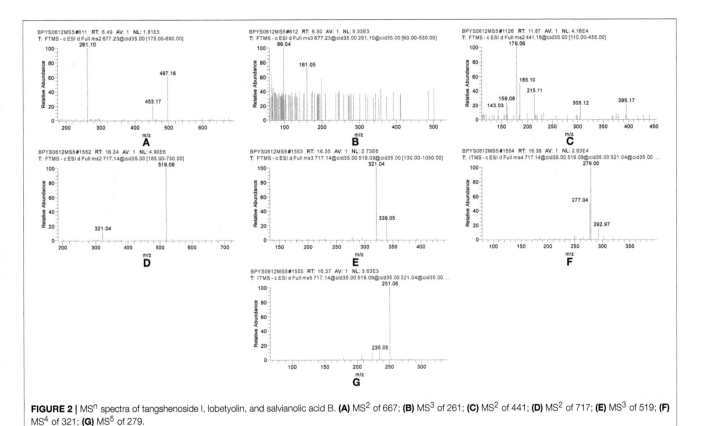

FIGURE 2 | MS^n spectra of tangshenoside I, lobetyolin, and salvianolic acid B. **(A)** MS^2 of 667; **(B)** MS^3 of 261; **(C)** MS^2 of 441; **(D)** MS^2 of 717; **(E)** MS^3 of 519; **(F)** MS^4 of 321; **(G)** MS^5 of 279.

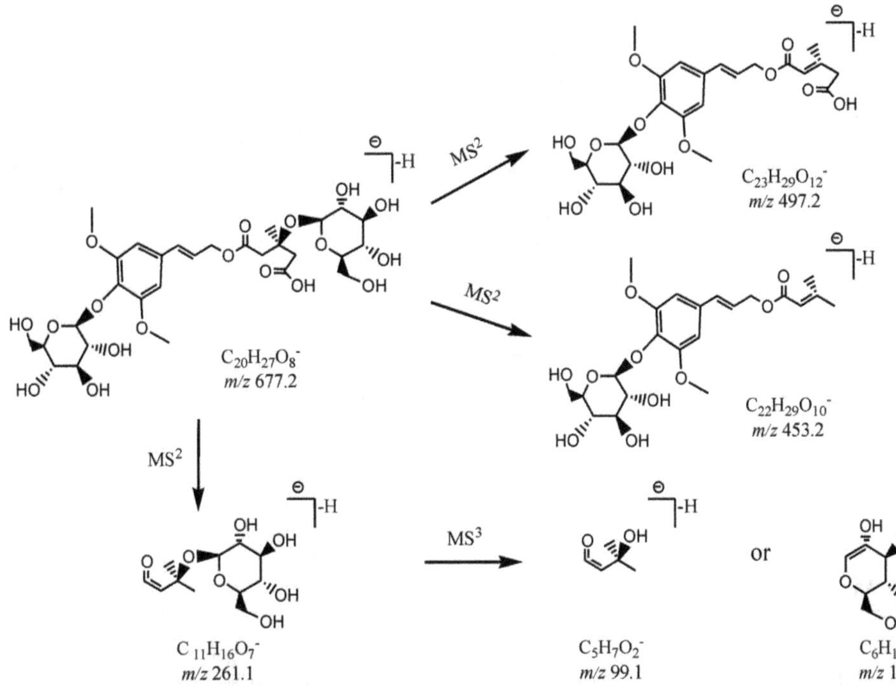

FIGURE 3 | The proposed MS^n fragmentation pathways of tangshenoside I.

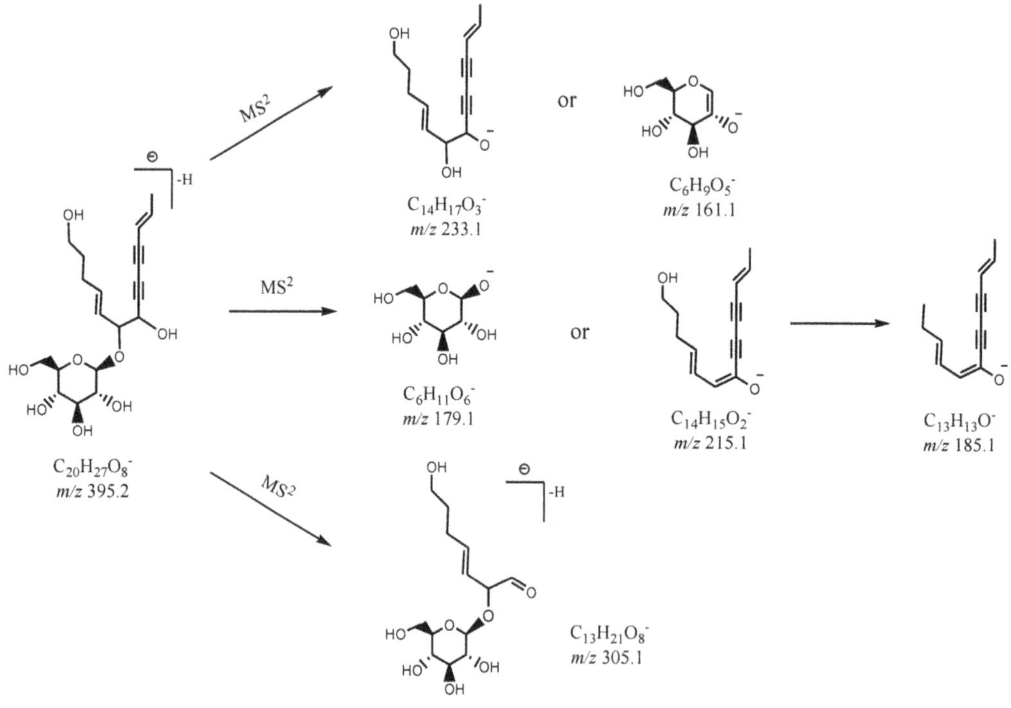

FIGURE 4 | The proposed MS^n fragmentation pathways of lobetyolin.

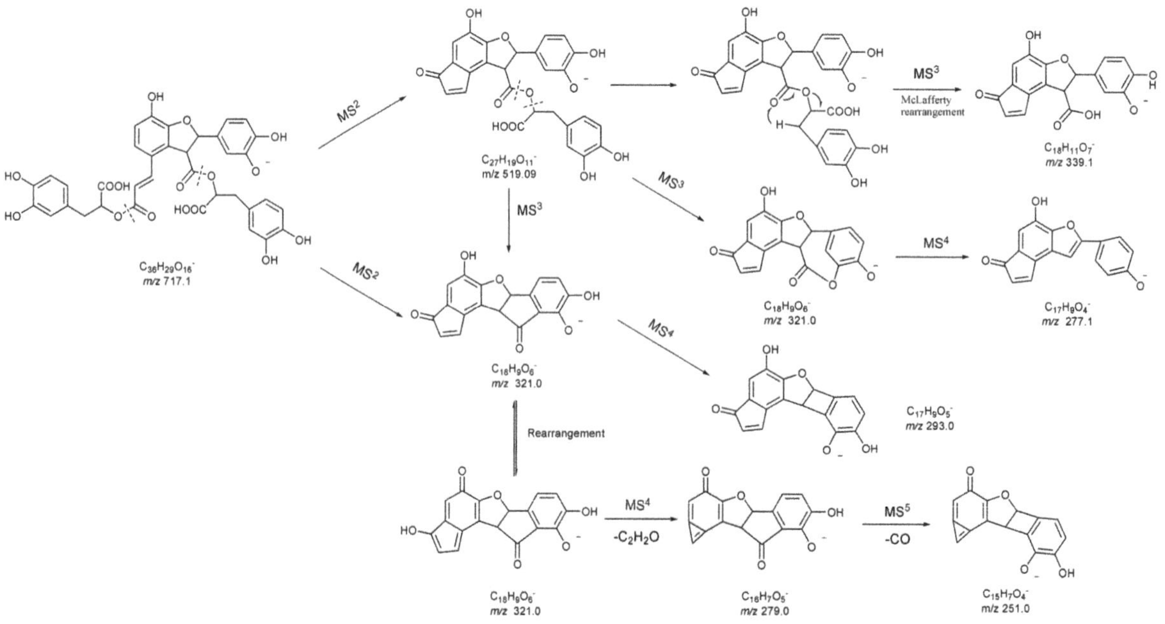

FIGURE 5 | The proposed MS^n fragmentation pathways of salvianolic acid B.

ion at m/z 261.1 $[M-H-C_6H_{10}O_5]^-$ and 161.1 $(C_6H_9O_5^-)$. Based on the fragmentation information and related literature (Tsai and Lin, 2010), they were primarily identified as (S)-3-hexenyl-β-D-sophoriside and (E)-2-hexenyl-β-D-sophoriside.

Their log P calculated by Discovery Studio were −1.9 and −2.0 and cis-isomers was eluted relatively later, therefore, compounds 4 and 6 were assigned as (S)-3-hexenyl-β-D-sophoriside and (E)-2-hexenyl-β-D-sophoriside.

TABLE 3 | Regression equations, linearity ranges, correlation coefficients, LOD, and LOQ data of the seven analytes.

Analytes	Regression equations	Linear range (ng/mL)	R^2	LOD[a] (ng/mL)	LOQ[b] (ng/mL)
Calycosin-7-O-Glc	$Y = 0.00591514X + 0.00256763$	11.48~765.0	0.9999	0.03	0.08
(E)-THSG	$Y = 0.000746494X - 0.0040087$	48.36~3,224.0	1.0000	0.02	0.04
Astragulin	$Y = 0.000933611X - 0.00599332$	4.523~301.5	0.9996	0.02	0.75
Rosmarinic acid	$Y = 0.000437025X - 0.00906707$	11.70~780.0	0.9994	0.98	3.91
Salvianolic acid A	$Y = 0.000390993X - 0.0022037$	6.075~405.0	0.9995	0.51	2.53
Salvianolic acid B	$Y = 0.000286894X + 0.004386$	609.0~40,600.0	0.9999	1.27	5.08
Calycosin	$Y = 0.00265233X + 0.00139572$	5.038~322.4	0.9995	0.04	0.15

[a]LOD, limit of detection.
[b]LOQ, limit of quantification.

TABLE 4 | Precision, repeatability, and stability of the seven investigated compounds.

Analytes	Precision (RSD %)				Repeatability (RSD%; $n = 6$)	Stability (RSD%; $n = 6$)
	Standard solution		BYF extract			
	Intra-day ($n = 6$)	Inter-day ($n = 3$)	Intra-day ($n = 6$)	Inter-day ($n = 3$)		
Calycosin-7-O-Glc	2.99	2.02	0.84	2.16	1.06	1.95
(E)-THSG	1.48	0.64	0.77	2.03	0.45	0.36
Astragulin	2.27	2.80	0.53	3.72	1.18	2.38
Rosmarinic acid	1.07	2.74	0.73	2.90	1.24	1.11
Salvianolic acid A	0.97	2.15	2.32	4.51	3.00	1.70
Salvianolic acid B	0.24	2.74	1.02	2.83	0.74	1.42
Calycosin	2.09	3.04	0.77	3.04	0.78	3.38

Compounds From Salviae Miltiorrhizae Radix Rhizoma

Salviae Miltiorrhizae Radix Rhizoma was mainly composed of hydrophilic salvianolic acids and lipophilic diterpenoid quinines (Wu et al., 2007). This research adopted the water extraction method so that the major ingredients of Salviae Miltiorrhizae Radix Rhizoma in the BYF are primarily salvianolic acids. This type of compounds has high molecular weight and a lot of homologs, which display similar ESI-MS^n behaviors for their differentiations.

Compound 42 displayed the [M-H]$^-$ ions at m/z 717.144 65 with the elemental composition of $C_{36}H_{30}O_{16}$. Its MS^2 spectrum gave diagnostic fragment ions at m/z 519.1 and 321.0, caused by the loss of one and two molecular unit of Danshensu, respectively. In the MS^3 spectrum, two distinctive ions at m/z 339.1 and 321.0, resulted from neutral loss of one danshensu and the McLafferty rearrangement, respectively, were observed. The CID of ion m/z 321.0 could further produced MS^4 and MS^5 spectra. Its MS^n spectra, as well as fragmentation pattern were shown in **Figures 2D–G, 5**. As its retention time and fragmentation ions were identical with those of the reference compound, Compound 42 was identified as salvianolic acid B.

As for the fragmentation pathway of Salvianolic acids, with Danshensu as their parent nucleus, their loss of H_2O and CO, as well as successive losses of Danshensu, occurred based on their MS spectra. Based on molecular weight and multi-stage information provided by MS^n, combining with literatures (Hu et al., 2005; Liu et al., 2007; Zhu et al., 2010), 11 phenolic acids in the prescription were identified accurately.

TABLE 5 | Recovery of the analytes.

Analytes	Initial (mg)	Added (mg)	Detected (mg)	Recovery (%)	RSD (%)
Calycosin-7-O-Glc	36.452	36.117	73.102	100.69	2.36
	45.465	45.147	90.417	100.76	
	54.716	54.176	110.166	103.44	
(E)-THSG	130.131	129.649	257.833	98.50	4.02
	161.804	161.901	328.248	102.80	
	194.186	194.367	386.662	99.03	
Astragulin	12.832	12.884	25.643	99.43	3.96
	16.183	16.100	32.122	99.00	
	19.397	19.316	37.913	95.86	
Rosmarinic acid	35.905	35.932	71.485	99.02	1.24
	45.219	44.928	89.772	99.16	
	53.911	53.924	107.457	99.30	
Salvianolic acid A	13.590	13.694	27.325	100.75	1.12
	17.258	17.107	34.256	100.74	
	20.036	20.542	40.565	101.07	
Salvianolic acid B	930.601	928.765	1,869.590	101.10	2.11
	1,162.726	1,160.186	2,309.808	98.87	
	1,395.901	1,393.148	2,806.526	101.25	
Calycosin	15.531	15.505	31.663	104.04	2.58
	19.362	19.374	39.527	104.08	
	23.197	23.243	46.378	99.73	

Compounds From Other Component Herbs

Phenolic constituents, including stilbenes and anthraquinones, were regarded as the main active components in Polygoni Multiflori Radix Praeparata (Chen et al., 2012). Most of these stilbenes previously reported were mainly 2,3,5,4′-tetrahydroxy substituted type (Liu et al., 2011). Compounds 7, 16, 50, 62, and 82 were indubitably distinguished as (E)-THSG, (S)-THSG, emodin-8-O-β-D-glucoside, physcion-8-O-β-D-glucoside, and emodin, by comparing their t_R-values and mass information with those of the standards. The MS and MS^2 spectra of Compounds 7, 16, and 20 showed characteristic ions at m/z 405.118 29 and 243.065 55, representing the corresponding elemental composition of $C_{20}H_{21}O_9^-$ and $C_{14}H_{11}O_4^-$, which was consistent with our previous studies (Qiu et al., 2013). Fragmentation behaviors of anthraquinones were also accordance with previous results.

The components in Cuscutae Semen are mainly phenolic acids and flavonoids. For example, The MS^2 and MS^3 spectra of Compounds 1, 2, and 3 were in accordance with those of 3-CQA (caffeoyl-quinic acid), 5-CQA, and 4-CQA available from the literature (Zhang et al., 2007). Although the fragmentation data of 5-CQA and 4-CQA were the same, retention time of 5-CQA was shorter in reversed-phase chromatography. Elution orders of the three isomers were consistent with the reported.

Compounds 67 and 68 both exhibited [M-H]⁻ ion at m/z 843.421 75 ($C_{38}H_{67}O_{20}^-$) and their MS^2 spectra all identical ions, they were tentatively identified as cuscutic acid C and its isomers. Five isomers of acely-Cuscutic acid C (Compounds 71, 72, 73, 74, and 76) were presented by ion extraction at m/z 885 from TIC. They showed identical precursor ion and MS^2 spectrum, while substituted position of their acetyl group was remained to be further studied.

Validation of Quantitative Method

Seven compounds, unequivocally identified with relatively high content in both the decoction and the granule, were selected as marker components to evaluate the quality of BYF. As the extraction process that we applied was through traditional method, which is extracted by water, the major components of high content were mainly water-soluble and highly polar compounds. These compounds have been observed at the early 25 min of the UHPLC-LTQ-Orbitrap-MS spectra. Meanwhile, those less polar compounds of much lower content emerged between 25 and 50 min, However, the relatively high peak area of such compounds in mass spectra has no direct relationship to their actual content in samples. Seven compounds for quantitative analysis were mainly phenolic and flavonoid compounds. Thus daidzein, a flavonoid, was chosen as the IS due

TABLE 6 | Contents (μg/g, $n = 3$) of the seven investigated compounds in the samples of BYF extract powder and BYF granule.

Analytes	Contents of BYF extract powder			Contents of BYF granule	
	1	2	3	1	2
Calycosin-7-O-Glc	244.124	246.061	251.827	122.741	137.846
(E)-THSG	382.673	466.849	438.201	270.693	305.022
Astragulin	52.899	61.430	57.947	27.192	39.693
Rosmarinic acid	10.447	29.943	23.690	63.700	103.399
Salvianolic acid A	11.303	18.126	19.853	97.021	108.978
Salvianolic acid B	5,395.621	5,769.462	5,507.373	2,059.143	2,671.567
Calycosin	38.498	43.058	40.046	16.167	11.441

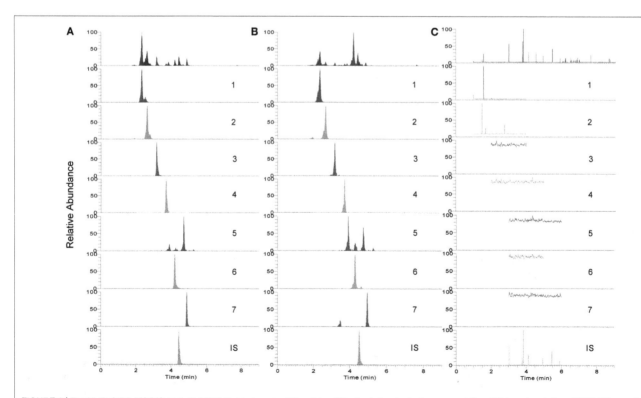

FIGURE 6 | The UHPLC-TQ-MS/MS analysis MRM chromatogram of 7 analytes. **(A)** mixed standard references solution; **(B)** sample solution of BYF; **(C)** negative samples; **1**, Calycosin-7-O-Glc; **2**, (E)-THSG; **3**, astragulin; **4**, rosmarinic acid; **5**, salvianolic acid A; **6**, salvianolic acid B; **7**, Calycosin; **IS**, Daidzein.

to its structural and polar similarity with the analytes, and no daidzein exist nor be detected in BYF.

Nice linearity with coefficients of determination ($R^2 > 0.9994$) were gained for the seven compounds. LOD and LOQ tests were carried out and listed in **Table 3**. The intra- or inter-day variations (RSD) were within the range of 0.24–2.99, 0.64–3.04, and 0.53–2.32%, 2.16–3.72% for mixed standard solution and sample solution, respectively (**Table 4**). Analytes in the sample solution were found stable for 24 h with a RSD <3.38%. Recoveries of the fourteen compounds ranged from 95.86 to 104.04% with RSD from 1.12 to 4.02% (shown in **Table 5**). As a result, the developed UHPLC-TQ-MS/MS method was considered as a sensitive, repeatable and accurate tool for the quantitative analysis of main compounds in BYF.

Application to Analysis of BYF Samples

The established UHPLC-TQ-MS/MS method was subsequently applied for quantitative analysis of both BYF decoction and its preparations. Two different batches of BYF extract powder and three different batches of BYF granule were detected using the developed method. MRM chromatograms of seven main compounds in BYF were displayed in **Figure 6**. The contents of the investigated compounds were determined and the outcomes were shown in **Table 6**.

As shown in **Table 6**, salvianolic acid B was found as the most abundant compound, and compared with BYF decoction, the contents of most investigated compounds are relative low in concentrated granule. This difference might result from manufacturing procedures, namely, concentration, mixing, granulation, and drying processes. Meanwhile, the contents of rosmarinic acid and salvianolic acid A were much higher in concentrated granule than in BYF decoction. The variability could be explained because salvianolic acid B could be degradated and oxidized in the manufacturing procedures thus transform to other phenolic acids, such as rosmarinic acid, salvianolic acid A, lithospermic acid, etc. (Zheng and Qu, 2012).

CONCLUSION

In this paper, chemical constituents of BYF were systematically investigated by UHPLC-LTQ-Orbitrap-MS^n and UHPLC-TQ-MS/MS methods, which provided comprehensively both qualitative and quantitative information for analysis of major components in BYF. Eighty-six compounds including flavones, saponins, phenolic acids, and other compounds were identified. The quantitative method was proved to have nice linearity, good accuracy, sensitivity, and repeatability. Although the bioactive components have not be determined, the present method will be helpful for providing the chemical basis for the further pharmacokinetic studies and effective quality evaluation of BYF, which would be of great importance for its safety use and mechanisms of action.

AUTHOR CONTRIBUTIONS

JZ and WX performed the experiments, analyzed the data, and wrote the paper. XL, ZH, and XQ conceived and designed the experiment, contributed reagent, materials, analysis tools, and revised the manuscript. PW, JH, and JB provided constructive suggestions for this research. All authors gave approval to the final version.

FUNDING

This work was supported by the Science and Technology Planning Project of Guangdong Province, China (2016A020226045, 2017A030313709, 2014A020221101, 2016A020226037, 2017B030314166), Pearl River S&T Nova Program of Guangzhou, China (201806010048), Special Subject of TCM Science and Technology Research of Guangdong Provincial Hospital of TCM, China (YN2016QJ07, YN2016QJ01) and Construction Project of TCM Hospital Preparation by Special Fund of Strong Province Construction in TCM, Guangdong, China (No. 6).

REFERENCES

Auyeung, K. K., Cho, C. H., and Ko, J. K. (2009). A novel anticancer effect of *Astragalus saponins*: transcriptional activation of NSAID-activated gene. *Int. J. Cancer.* 125, 1082–1091. doi: 10.1002/ijc.24397

Chen, Q., Zhang, S. Z., Ying, H. Z., Dai, X. Y., Li, X. X., Yu, C. H., et al. (2012). Chemical characterization and immunostimulatory effects of a polysaccharide from Polygoni Multiflori Radix Praeparata, in cyclophosphamide-induced anemic mice. *Carbohyd. Polym.* 88, 1476–1482. doi: 10.1016/j.carbpol.2012.02.055

Dou, S. S., Liu, L., Jiang, P., Zhang, W. D., and Liu, R. H. (2009). LC-DAD and LC-ESI-MS chromatographic fingerprinting and quantitative analysis for evaluation of the quality of Huang-Lian-Jie-Du-Tang. *Chromatographia* 69, 659–664. doi: 10.1365/s10337-008-0945-3

Dunn, W. B., Broadhurst, D., Brown, M., Baker, P. N., Redmand, C. W., Kenny, L. C., et al. (2008). Metabolic profiling of serum using Ultra Performance Liquid Chromatography and the LTQ-Orbitrap mass spectrometry system. *J. Chromatogr. B* 871, 288–298. doi: 10.1016/j.jchromb.2008.03.021

Ha, J., Shim, Y. S., Seo, D., Kim, K., Ito, M., and Nakagawa, H. (2013). Determination of 22 ginsenosides in ginseng products using ultra-high-performance liquid chromatography. *J. Chromatogr. Sci.* 51, 355–360. doi: 10.1093/chromsci/bms148

Hao, H. P., Cui, N., Wang, G. J., Xiang, B. R., Liang, Y., Xu, X. Y., et al. (2008). Global detection and identification of nontarget components from herbal preparations by liquid chromatography hybrid ion trap time-of-flight mass spectrometry and a strategy. *Anal. Chem.* 80, 8187–8194. doi: 10.1021/ac801356s

Hu, P., Liang, Q. L., Luo, G. A., Zhao, Z. Z., and Jiang, Z. H. (2005). Multi-component HPLC fingerprinting of radix *Salviae miltiorrhizae* and its LC-MS-MS identification. *Chem. Pharm. Bull.* 53, 677–683. doi: 10.1248/cpb.53.677

Kanji, I., Maiko, O., Li, Y., Toshihiro, F., Kunihide, M., and Norie, T. (2003). Polyacetylene glycosides from *Pratia nummularia* cultures. *Phytochemistry* 62, 643–646. doi: 10.1016/S0031-9422(02)00669-6

Lin, L. C., Tsai, T. H., and Kuo, C. L. (2013). Chemical constituents comparison of *Codonopsis tangshen, Codonopsis pilosula* var. modesta and *Codonopsis pilosula*. *Nat. Prod. Res.* 27:1812. doi: 10.1080/14786419.2013.778849

Liu, A. H., Lin, Y. H., Yang, M., Guo, H., Guan, S. H., Sun, J. H., et al. (2007). Development of the fingerprints for the quality of the roots of

Salvia miltiorrhiza and its related preparations by HPLC-DAD and LC-MS[n]. *J. Chromatogr. B. Analyt. Technol. Biomed. Life Sci.* 846, 32–41. doi: 10.1016/j.jchromb.2006.08.002

Liu, C. H., Ju, A. C., Zhou, D. Z., Li, D., Kou, J. P., Yu, B. Y., et al. (2016). Simultaneous qualitative and quantitative analysis of multiple chemical constituents in YiQiFuMai injection by ultra-fast liquid chromatography coupled with ion trap time-of-flight mass spectrometry. *Molecules* 21:640. doi: 10.3390/molecules21050640

Liu, X. S., Mao, W., Yang, N. Z., Zhou, C., Li, C., Zhang, L., et al. (2012). *Traditional Chinese Medicine Preparation for Treating Chronic Kidney Disease and its Preparation Method.* P.R.China, Patent No 201210029862.8. Beijing: State Intellectual Property Office of the P.R.C.

Liu, Z., Liu, Y. Y., Wang, C., Guo, N., Song, Z. Q., Wang, C., et al. (2011). Comparative analyses of chromatographic fingerprints of the roots of *Polygonum multiflorum* Thunb. and their processed products using RRLC/DAD/ESI-MSn. *Planta Med.* 77, 1855–1860. doi: 10.1055/s-0030-1271200

Mao, W., Zhang, L., Zou, C., Li, C., Wu, Y. F., Su, G. B., et al. (2015). Rationale and design of the Helping Ease Renal failure with Bupi Yishen compared with the Angiotensin II Antagonist Losartan (HERBAAL) trial: a randomized controlled trial in non-diabetes stage 4 chronic kidney disease. *BMC Complement. Altern. Med.* 15:316. doi: 10.1186/s12906-015-0830-1

Qiu, X. H., Zhang, J., Huang, Z. H., Zhu, D. Y., and Xu, W. (2013). Profiling of phenolic constituents in *Polygonum multiflorum* Thunb. by combination of ultra-high-pressure liquid chromatography with linear ion trap-Orbitrap mass spectrometry. *J. Chromatogr. A* 1292, 121–131. doi: 10.1016/j.chroma.2012.11.051

Shaw, L. H., Lin, L. C., and Tsai, T. H. (2012). HPLC-MS/MS analysis of a traditional Chinese medical formulation of Bu-Yang-Huan-Wu-Tang and its pharmacokinetics after oral administration to rats (pharmacokinetics of herbal formulation). *PLoS ONE* 7:e43848. doi: 10.1371/journal.pone.0043848

Simons, R., Vincken, J. P., Bakx, E. J., Verbruggen, M. A., and Gruppen, H. (2009). A rapid screening method for prenylated flavonoids with ultra-high-performance liquid chromatography/electrospray ionisation mass spectrometry in licorice root extracts. *Rapid Commun. Mass Spectrom.* 23, 3083–3093. doi: 10.1002/rcm.4215

Sun, L., Wei, H., Zhang, F., Gao, S. H., Zeng, Q. H., Lu, W. Q., et al. (2013). Qualitative analysis and quality control of traditional chinese medicine preparation tanreqing injection by LC-TOF/MS and HPLC-DAD-ELSD. *Anal. Methods* 5, 6431–6440. doi: 10.1039/C3AY40681D

Tchoumtchoua, J., Njamen, D., Mbanya, J. C., Skaltsounis, A., and Halabalaki, M. (2013). Structure-oriented UHPLC-LTQ Orbitrap-based approach as a dereplication strategy for the identification of isoflavonoids from *Amphimas pterocarpoides* crude extract. *J.Mass Spectrom.* 48, 561–575. doi: 10.1002/jms.3167

Tsai, T. H., and Lin, L. C. (2010). Phenolic glycosides and pyrrolidine alkaloids from *Codonopsis tangshen*. *Chem. Pharm. Bull.* 40, 1546–1550. doi: 10.1248/cpb.56.1546

Wang, J., Wang, Y. Y., and Yang, G. (2005). Methods and modes about the theory of traditional Chinese prescription composition. *China J. Chin. Mater. Med.* 30, 6–8. doi: 10.3321/j.issn:1001-5302.2005.01.002

Wang, T. H., Zhang, J., Qiu, X. H., Bai, J. Q., Gao, Y. H., and Xu, W. (2015). Application of ultra-high-performance liquid chromatography coupled with LTQ-orbitrap mass spectrometry for the qualitative and quantitative analysis of *Polygonum multiflorum* thumb. and its processed products. *Molecules* 21:E40. doi: 10.3390/molecules21010040

Wu, J. L., Yee, L. P., Jiang, Z. H., and Cai, Z. (2007). One single LC-MS/MS analysis for both phenolic components and tanshinones in Radix *Salviae miltiorrhizae* and its medicinal products. *Talanta* 73, 656–661. doi: 10.1016/j.talanta.2007.04.038

Xiong, X., Wang, P., Li, X., and Zhang, Y. (2015). Shenqi pill, a traditional Chinese herbal formula, for the treatment of hypertension: a systematic review. *Complement. Ther. Med.* 23, 484–493. doi: 10.1016/j.ctim.2015.04.008

Xu, F., Zhang, Y., Xiao, S., Lu, X., Yang, D., and Yang, X., et al. (2006). Absorption and metabolism of astragali radix decoction: *in silico, in vitro,* and a case study *in vivo. Drug Metab. Dispos.* 34, 913–924. doi: 10.1124/dmd.105.008300

Xu, W., Zhang, J., Zhu, D. Y., Huang, J., Huang, Z. H., Bai, J. Q., et al. (2014). Rapid separation and characterization of diterpenoid alkaloids in processed roots of *Aconitum carmichaeli* using ultra high performance liquid chromatography coupled with hybrid linear ion trap-Orbitrap tandem mass spectrometry. *J. Sep. Sci.* 37, 2864–2873. doi: 10.1002/jssc.201400365

Zhang, J., Xu, X. J., Xu, W., Huang, J., Zhu, D. Y., and Qiu, X. H. (2015). Rapid characterization and identification of flavonoids in Radix Astragali by ultra-high-pressure liquid chromatography coupled with linear ion trap-orbitrap mass spectrometry. *J. Chromatogr. Sci.* 53, 945–952. doi: 10.1093/chromsci/bmu155

Zhang, Y., Shi, P., Qu, H., and Cheng, Y. (2007). Characterization of phenolic compounds in *Erigeron breviscapus* by liquid chromatography coupled to electrospray ionization mass spectrometry. *Rapid Commun. Mass Spectrom.* 21, 2971–2984. doi: 10.1002/rcm.3166

Zheng, X. T., and Qu, H. B. (2012). Characterisation of the degradation of salvianolic acid B using an on-line spectroscopic analysis system and multivariate curve resolution. *Phytochem. Anal.* 23, 103–109. doi: 10.1002/pca.1330

Zhu, Z., Zhang, H., Zhao, L., Dong, X., Li, X., Chai, Y. F., et al. (2010). Rapid separation and identification of phenolic and diterpenoid constituents from Radix *Salvia miltiorrhizae* by high-performance liquid chromatography diode-array detection, electrospray ionization time-of-flight mass spectrometry and electrospray. *Rapid Commun. Mass Spectrom.* 21, 1855–1865. doi: 10.1002/rcm.3023

7

Selection of Reference Genes for Expression Analysis in Chinese Medicinal Herb *Huperzia serrata*

Mengquan Yang[1,2†], Shiwen Wu[1†], Wenjing You[1,2†], Amit Jaisi[1] and Youli Xiao[1,2,3]*

[1] CAS Key Laboratory of Synthetic Biology, CAS Center for Excellence in Molecular Plant Sciences, Institute of Plant Physiology and Ecology, Shanghai Institutes for Biological Sciences, Chinese Academy of Sciences, Shanghai, China, [2] University of Chinese Academy of Sciences, Beijing, China, [3] CAS-JIC Centre of Excellence in Plant and Microbial Sciences, Shanghai, China

*Correspondence:
Youli Xiao
ylxiao@sibs.ac.cn
[†] *These authors have contributed equally to this work*

Huperzine A (HupA) is a powerful and selective inhibitor of acetylcholinesterase. It has attracted widespread attention endangering the ultimate plant sources of Lycopodiaceae family. In this study, we used *Huperzia serrata*, extensively used in Traditional Chinese medicine (TCM), a slow growing vascular plant as the model plant of the *Lycopodiaceae* family to develop and validate the reference genes. We aim to use gene expression platform to understand the gene expression of different tissues and developmental stages of this medicinal herb. Eight candidate reference genes were selected based on RNA-seq data and evaluated with qRT-PCR. The expression of *L/ODC* and cytochrome P450s genes known for their involvement in lycopodium alkaloid biosynthesis, were also studied to validate the selected reference genes. The most stable genes were *TBP*, *GAPDH*, and their combination (*TBP + GAPDH*). We report for the first time the reference gene of *H. serrata's* different tissues which would provide important insights into understanding their biological functions comparing other *Lycopodiaceae* plants and facilitate a good biopharming approach.

Keywords: *Huperzia serrata*, lycopodium alkaloids, reference gene, real-time quantitative PCR, gene expression

INTRODUCTION

The *Lycopodiaceae* family comprises three main genera, namely, *Huperzia*, *Phlegmariurus*, and monotypic *Phylloglossum*. The morphological variability between *Phlegmariurus* and *Huperzia* has presented a taxonomic challenge. Interestingly, they possess similar chemical diversity, especially lycopodium alkaloids, such as huperzine A (HupA), a highly potent, selective, and reversible inhibitor of AchE (Zhao and Tang, 2002), hence, a lead candidate for Alzheimer's disease. HupA was initially isolated from the traditional Chinese medicine Qian Ceng Ta (*Huperzia serrata*). *H. serrata* is an economically important traditional Chinese herb that is used extensively for treatment of contusions, strains, swellings, schizophrenia, myasthenia gavis, and organophosphate poisoning since the Tang Dynasty (Ma et al., 2007; Xu et al., 2017). In the United States, *H. serrata* is marketed as a memory-enhancing dietary supplement (Ma and Gang, 2004). However, the wide clinical investigation and application of HupA are hampered by its poor supply from natural resource or uneconomical synthesis route (Benca, 2014). Moreover, extensive harvest for HupA has endangered *H. serrata* and other species in the Lycopodiaceae family. Synthetic biology approach offers an alternative potential source of HupA, but the inadequate understanding of its biosynthetic pathway restricts its production by metabolic engineering.

Current understanding of the biosynthesis of HupA and other lycopodium alkaloids originates from lysine and/or ornithine from feeding experiments and the pathway was initially proposed lysine/ornithine decarboxylase (*L/ODC*) as the first enzyme (Ma and Gang, 2004). Bunsupa and coauthors reported that *L/ODC* can catalyze the first step in the biosynthesis pathway of lysine-derived alkaloids, quinolizidine, and lycopodium alkaloids (**Figure 1**; Bunsupa et al., 2012, 2016). Furthermore, we cloned six *HsL/ODC* genes from *H. serrata* by degenerate method and characterized the function of one *HsL/ODC in vitro* and *in vivo* (Xu et al., 2017). A comprehensive relative quantitative metabolomic analysis of these alkaloids in different tissues of *H. serrata* was also performed by our group (Wu et al., 2018). However, the genes involved in skeleton formation and modification remain unclear (**Figure 1**, blue color; Yang et al., 2017).

Gene expression patterns in different plant tissues and growth developmental stages provide important insights into understanding their biological functions (Bustin, 2000; Vandesompele et al., 2002; Kozera and Rapacz, 2013). Transcriptome analysis and data mining have helped identify differentially expressed genes and measure the relative levels of their transcripts. Quantitative real-time PCR (qRT-PCR) provides a rapid, efficient, accurate, and reproducible method to present the mRNA transcription level in different samples or tissues and to validate data obtained from other methods (Vandesompele et al., 2002; Kozera and Rapacz, 2013; Zhang et al., 2017). The selection and validation of reference genes are the first steps in any qRT-PCR gene expression studies. The most commonly used genes for normalization of gene expression in different plant species include housekeeping genes, glyceraldehyde-3-phosphate dehydrogenase (*GAPDH*), β-*actin*, *tubulin*, and *18S* (Radonic et al., 2004; Niu et al., 2015; Martins et al., 2017). However, the transcript expression level of such genes is not always stable, especially in samples of different developmental stages and tissues and those subjected to stresses, leading to erroneous results (Radonic et al., 2004; Petriccione et al., 2015; Pombo et al., 2017). Hence, screening and validating reference genes for normalization of the gene expression levels are pivotal.

In this study, *actin*, *tubulin*, *18S*, *TBP*, *GAPDH*, *HSP90*, *MUB*, and *SAM* were selected as candidate reference genes based on global RNA-seq data. Their expression stabilities in the roots, stems, leaves, and sporangia of *H. serrata* in different developmental stages (2-, 3-, 4-, and 5-year old) were evaluated using geNorm, NormFinder, BestKeeper programs, comparative ΔCq method, and comprehensive stability rankings obtained from RefFinder. The expression of targeted genes, namely, *L/ODC* and cytochrome P450s, which are potentially involved in HupA biosynthesis, were used to validate the selected reference genes. This study is the first report to evaluate the expression stability of the reference genes in *H. serrata*. Results will be particularly useful in the selection of structural genes involved in HupA biosynthesis and research of Lycopodiaceae plants.

MATERIALS AND METHODS

Plant Materials

Plants of different growth periods (2-, 3-, 4-, and 5-year old) were collected from Xiangxi, Hunan, China in January 2017, identified as *H. serrata* (Thunb.) Trevis[1], and deposited at the Chinese herbarium with Barcode ID: 00019690[2]. The plants were carefully rinsed in running tap water, and soil was removed by hand. Root, stem, leaf, and sporangia were kept in collection tubes immediately after being separated from the plant, immersed in liquid nitrogen, and stored at −80°C until further use.

RNA Isolation and cDNA Synthesis

Total RNA was extracted from four different tissues of *H. serrata*, namely, root, stem, leaf, and sporangia with TIANGEN RNAprep Pure Plant Kit [Tiangen Biotech (Beijing) Co., Ltd.] according to the kit instructions. DNase I was used to digest contaminated DNA. The purified total RNA was quantified using Nanodrop (Agilent 2100, Agilent Technologies, United States) and 1% agarose gel. cDNA was synthesized as previously reported (Yang et al., 2017).

Reference Gene Selection and Primer Design

Eight reference genes (*actin*, *tubulin*, *18S*, *TBP*, *GAPDH*, *HSP90*, *MUB*, and *SAM*) were selected as potential candidates. All homologous in *H. serrata* were gathered by BLAST-search against the global RNA-seq data (Yang et al., 2017), and the candidate reference genes were selected with similar fragments per kilobase per million (FPKM) values determined in the four tissues (**Figure 2**). The primers of the candidate reference genes were designed, as listed in **Table 1**. The primer specificities were verified by the presence of a single DNA band with the expected size in 1.0% agarose gel electrophoresis and the presence of a single peak in qRT-PCR melting curve assays (**Figure 4**).

qRT-PCR Analysis

qRT-PCR amplification was performed as previously reported (Yang et al., 2017). Expression levels were recorded as cycle quantification (Cq). The PCR efficiency of each primer pair ($E = 10^{-1/\text{slope}} - 1$) was determined through slope of the amplification curve in the exponential phase, obtained by four fold series dilution of cDNA (Rutledge and Stewart, 2008).

Gene Expression Stability Analysis

The expression stability of the eight candidate reference genes across all tissues was evaluated with four algorithms, namely, geNorm (Vandesompele et al., 2002), NormFinder (Andersen et al., 2004), BestKeeper (Pfaffl et al., 2004), and ΔCq method. RefFinder (Xie et al., 2012), a web-based user-friendly comprehensive tool, was employed to generate the comprehensive ranking.

---

[1]http://www.theplantlist.org/tpl1.1/record/tro-26621719
[2]http://www.cvh.ac.cn/en/spm/HUST/00019690

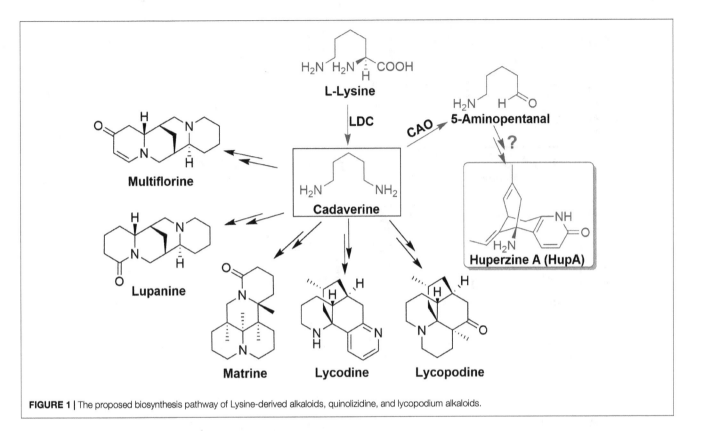

FIGURE 1 | The proposed biosynthesis pathway of Lysine-derived alkaloids, quinolizidine, and lycopodium alkaloids.

Validation of Identified Reference Genes

Previous studies have shown that *L/ODC* is the first key structure gene for precursor formation of HupA (Bunsupa et al., 2012, 2016; Xu et al., 2017). The homologues of the reported *L/ODC* (Unigene94988, Unigene94617) and four cytochrome P450 genes (CL9415.8, CL1143.2, Unigene1166, and Unigene25121) which were proposed to participate in the modification of HupA skeleton were also used to confirm the reliability of the selected reference genes by using the most two stable versus the least two stable genes.

RESULTS

RNA-Seq-Assisted Selection of Candidate Reference Genes and Primer Design

The eight reference genes (*actin, tubulin, 18S, TBP, GAPDH, HSP90, MUB,* and *SAM*) with similar FPKMs in four tissues were gathered, and primers were designed (**Table 1**, **Figure 3**, and **Supplementary Table S1**).

Expression Levels and Variations of Candidate Reference Genes

The PCR product of candidate reference genes were verified by electrophoresis in 1.0 % agarose gel showed only a single band. The presence of a single peak in qRT-PCR melting curve analysis for each of the eight sets of primers indicated high specificity

(**Figure 4**). qRT-PCR was performed to determine the expression levels of each candidate reference genes, and the Cq values showed differential transcript levels in the samples examined with low Cq values, which suggested transcript abundance. The mean Cq value of the eight candidate reference genes ranged from 13.57 to 31.72 (**Figure 5** and **Supplementary Table S1**). In all sample set, the mean Cq values showed a minimum of 15.35 and a maximum of 25.23 for the highest and lowest expression levels for *18S* and *TBP*, respectively. The coefficient of variation (CV) of the Cq values was also calculated to evaluate the expression levels of candidate reference genes of the four tissues, where low values represent low variability or maximum stability. The CV values of the eight reference genes among all samples ranged from 6.91 to 14.60%. *TBP* was the least variable reference gene with a CV of 6.91% among the eight candidate reference genes studied, and *HSP90* was the most variable with a CV of 14.60%. The stability ranking of all candidate reference genes on the basis of CV values is as follows: (most stable to least stable): *HSP90* < *MUB* < *SAM* < *18S* < *GAPDH* < *Actin* < *TBP* (**Figure 5**).

Stability of the Reference Gene

Expression stabilities of the eight candidate reference genes were determined using ΔCq, geNorm, NormFinder, and BestKeeper, and their overall stabilities were ranked by RefFinder across all the tissue samples.

ΔCq Analysis

The eight candidate reference genes from the most to least stable expression, as calculated by the ΔCq method, are listed

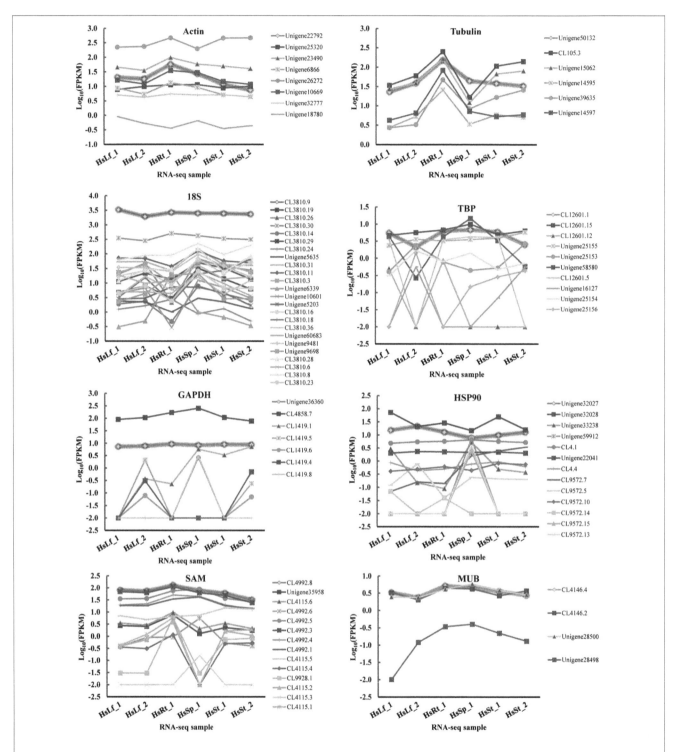

FIGURE 2 | FPKMs of candidate reference genes' homologs in six RNA-seq samples. The highlight lines indicate the selected candidate reference genes used in this study. Leaf: HsLf_1, HsLf_2; Root: HsRt_1; Sporangia: HsSp_1; Stem: HsSt_1, HsSt_2.

in **Table 2**. *GAPDH* and *TBP* were the most stable reference genes in the root and leaf. *Actin* and *TBP* were the most stable genes for the stem and sporangia, respectively. In sum, *TBP*, *Actin*, and *GAPDH* were the top three ideal reference genes.

geNorm Analysis

The stabilities of the eight candidate reference genes of *H. serrata* calculated using geNorm were ranked in the different tissues according to their M values, as shown in **Figure 6**. The lowest M value indicates the most stable reference gene, and the highest M

TABLE 1 | Primer sequences and amplification characters for the 8 candidate reference genes.

Gene	Gene ID	Definition	Primer sequence (5′ → 3′)		R^2	E
Actin	Unigene22792	β-Actin	Actin-F	GCTGTGGTTGTGAAGGAGTATC	0.9989	0.99
			Actin-R	GCTGTGCTGTCTCTGTATGC		
Tubulin	Unigene50132	Tubulin	Tubulin-F	AGTCTAGCGTCTGCGATATTG	0.9981	0.97
			Tubulin-R	CCATCTCATCCATACCTTCTCC		
18S	CL3810.9	18S ribosomal RNA	18S-F	CAACCATAAACGATGCCGAC	0.9935	1.01
			18S-R	CAGCCTTGCGACCATACTCCC		
TBP	CL12601.1	TATA binding protein	TBP-F	CACTGGCTGACTTCCTTCC	0.9987	0.93
			TBP-R	GGCAACTGTTATGTGATTCTCG		
GAPDH	Unigene36360	Glyceraldehyde 3-phosphate Dehydrogenase	GAPDH-F	GCCTGCTTCACCACCTTC	0.9960	0.95
			GAPDH-R	GCCTTCCGTGTTCCTACC		
HSP90	Unigene32027	Heat shock protein 90	HSP90-F	CTCACTCGCTCCCATTCC	0.9997	0.92
			HSP90-R	CGCCATCCTCAATCTCTACC		
MUB	CL4146.4	membrane-anchored ubiquitin-fold protein	MUB-F	CATCAGAAGGAAGCCATTGTG	0.9983	1.00
			MUB-R	CAGAAGAGCCAGCGTTCG		
SAM	CL4992.8	S-Adenosylmethionine decarboxylase	SAM-F	ATGTATTGTAGAATGAGCCTTACC	0.9977	0.95
			SAM-R	CAGCCAAAGAGATGACTAACG		

value indicates the least stable one. Using the criteria of M < 0.5, TBP and GAPDH were stable reference genes in the four tissues of root, stem, leaf, and sporangia. When the stabilities from all the samples were combined, TBP and GAPDH were also determined to be the most stable reference genes. By contrast, HSP90 and MUB were two common unstable reference genes in all tissues and developmental stages.

The pairwise variation (V_n/V_{n+1}) between two sequential normalization factors NF_n and NF_{n+1} was calculated by the geNorm algorithm to determine the optimal number of reference genes for accurate normalization. A cutoff value of 0.15 is the recommended threshold, which indicates that an additional reference gene will inconsiderably contribute to the normalization. The V3/4 values in the root and stem were less than 0.15 (**Figure 7**), which suggested that the top two reference genes were sufficient for accurate normalization. For the leaf, V5/6 was 0.126, which indicated that the top five reference genes (TBP, GAPDH, 18S, SAM, and actin) were needed for accurate normalization. For the sporangia, V3/4 was 0.148, which showed that three reference genes (actin, SAM, and TBP) were required.

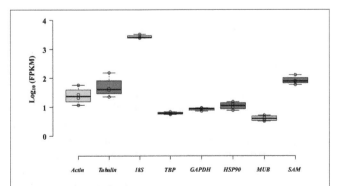

FIGURE 3 | Distribution of eight selected genes by using FPKMs determined in four tissues.

The value V2/3 for total was 0.129, which indicated that the most stable genes, TBP and GAPDH, could be used as the reference genes for the normalization of gene expression in H. serrata.

NormFinder Analysis

As shown in **Table 3**, TBP and GAPDH were the most stable genes (lowest stability value) in the root, leaf, and total subsets calculated using NormFinder. For the stem and sporangia samples, actin and TBP were the most stable reference genes. When all samples were taken to determine the stability of reference genes, the two most stable genes were TBP and GAPDH. SAM and actin also had low stability values, which indicated that the two reference genes were also suitable for qRT-PCR normalization, although not the most stable candidates.

BestKeeper Analysis

BestKeeper determined the stabilities of the candidate reference genes on the basis of their standard deviation (SD). Genes with SD > 1 were considered unacceptable reference genes. The genes are listed from most to least stability in **Table 4**. Actin was the most stable gene in the root and total subsets, GAPDH was the most stable genes in the stem and leaf subsets, and 18S was the most stable gene in the sporangia. Only MUB and HSP90 were unstable genes.

RefFinder Analysis

The rankings of the four algorithms were integrated by RefFinder to acquire reliable results for the expression stabilities of the eight candidate reference genes of H. serrata, and the results are shown in **Table 5**. The expression of GAPDH was ranked as the most stable in the root and leaf, and the expression of actin was ranked as the most stable in the stem and sporangia. The expression of TBP was ranked the most stable in total. By contrast, MUB and HSP90 were two least stable reference genes almost in all tissues calculated by all five programs. Overall, the best reference genes

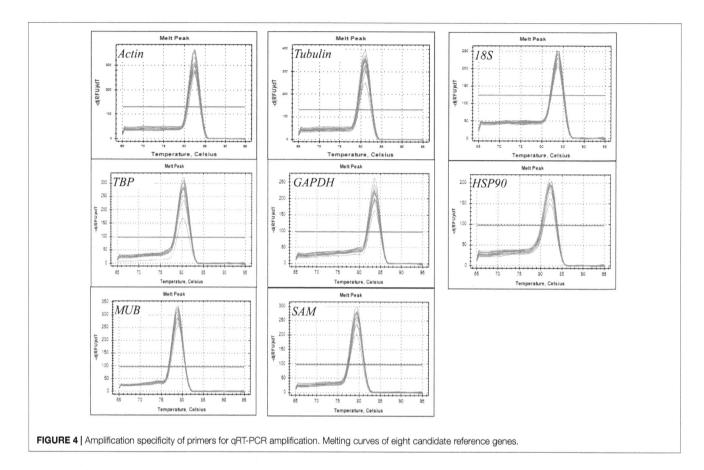

FIGURE 4 | Amplification specificity of primers for qRT-PCR amplification. Melting curves of eight candidate reference genes.

for accurate transcript normalization in all of the samples were *actin*, *GAPDH*, and *TBP*, which had the lowest geometric mean of the ranking values.

Validation of the Identified Reference Genes

The expression levels of HupA biosynthesis-related genes, *L/ODC* (Unigene94617, Unigene94988), and cytochrome P450s (CL94158.8, CL11443.2, Unigene1166, and Unigene25121) were

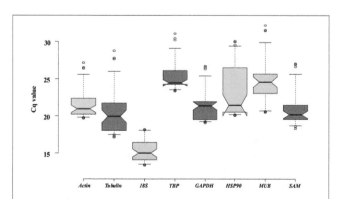

FIGURE 5 | Expression levels of eight candidate reference genes across all experimental samples. Distribution of Cq values of candidate reference genes in all samples. Boxplots show the 25 and 75th percentiles, mean, and outliers.

investigated using different reference genes in different tissues at different developmental stages to validate the selected candidate reference genes. Each of the two most stable reference genes (*TBP* and *GAPDH*), its combination (*TBP* + *GAPDH*), and the two least stable reference genes (*HSP90* and *MUB*) were used as internal controls. When using *TBP* alone, *GAPDH* alone, *MUB* alone, and the combination of *TBP* + *GAPDH* for normalization, the expression patterns were similar in all six validated genes. However, when the least stable gene *HSP90* was used for normalization, the expression patterns showed some differences (**Figure 8**). Thus, RNA Seq-assisted selection of candidate reference genes was helpful.

DISCUSSION

Standardization and quality assessment of traditional herbal formulations is of paramount importance in order to modernize. However, still major bottlenecks faced by the herbal industry is the unavailability of rigid quality control profiles, primarily because of the complexity and incomplete knowledge of the active medicinal compounds. *H. serrata*, a vulnerable group of slow-growing plant, extensively harvested by the traditional medicinal practitioners. It contains many active compounds, especially HupA whose contents differed significantly among the organs, varieties, age, and production areas of the herbal medicines (Ma et al., 2006). Hence, to address such variation

TABLE 2 | Expression stability of candidate reference genes as calculated by ΔCq.

Rank	Root		Stem		Leaf		Sporangia		Total*	
	Gene	Stability	Gene	Stability	Gene	Stability	Gene	Stability	Gene	Stability
1	GAPDH	1.34	Actin	1.01	GAPDH	1.14	Actin	1.34	TBP	1.03
2	TBP	1.37	TBP	1.03	TBP	1.15	TBP	1.39	Actin	1.06
3	SAM	1.39	GAPDH	1.04	SAM	1.33	SAM	1.42	GAPDH	1.07
4	Tubulin	1.48	Tubulin	1.18	18S	1.35	GAPDH	1.51	SAM	1.13
5	Actin	1.51	18S	1.26	Actin	1.38	Tubulin	1.66	18S	1.18
6	18S	1.81	SAM	1.27	Tubulin	1.38	18S	2.74	Tubulin	1.22
7	MUB	2.68	MUB	2.37	MUB	2.57	HSP90	2.92	MUB	2.63
8	HSP90	4.43	HSP90	3.08	HSP90	3.52	MUB	3.13	HSP90	3.44

* Total: Pooled samples from all treatments.

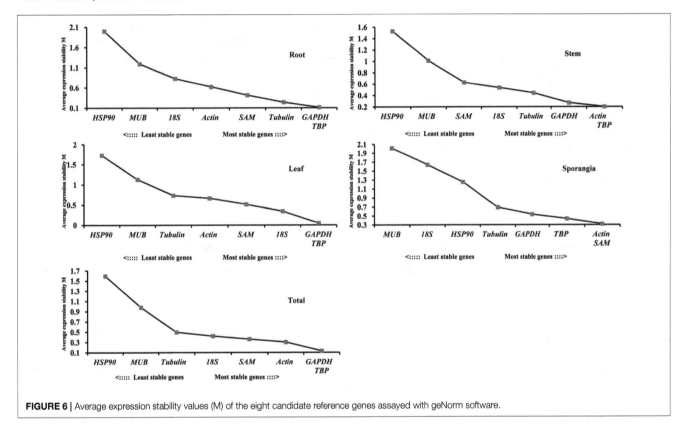

FIGURE 6 | Average expression stability values (M) of the eight candidate reference genes assayed with geNorm software.

in quality of medicinal material, studies has been directed towards understanding the molecular regulatory mechanisms of secondary metabolism through transcriptomics or functional genomics approaches.

Most of the modern plant research is often underpinned by the genetic approach creating transgenic lines to test the gene functions *in planta*. Inability to genetically transform any lycophytes species such as *H. serrata* has been challenging, and as such our understanding of Huperzia development lags significantly behind almost all other land plant lineages despite its traditional medicinal application. Recently, our group published the global RNA-seq of four different tissues which assisted us for the gene mining regards to the HupA biosynthesi (Yang et al., 2017). Elucidating the biosynthetic pathway is a prerequisite

to heterologous production of targeted metabolites limiting the overexploitation of the natural habitat. To our knowledge no suitable reference gene for this plant is available. It is important to select a suitable reference gene to study the different expression patterns in different varieties and different tissues in medicinal plants. Here, we report the use of eight genes (*actin, tubulin, 18S, TBP, GAPDH, HSP90, MUB,* and *SAM*), to select and validate the suitable reference genes for the qRT-PCR normalization in different tissues and developmental growth stages.

qRT-PCR is one of the most commonly used technologies for transcript expression analysis owing to its sensitivity and reproducibility (Derveaux et al., 2010). Coexpression analysis is a useful method to screen the candidate structure genes involved in specialized metabolite biosynthesis (Saito et al.,

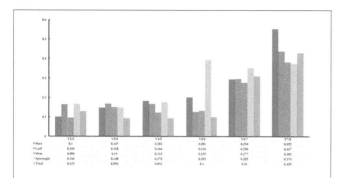

FIGURE 7 | Pairwise variation (V) of candidate reference genes, as calculated by geNorm software. Vn/Vn+1 values were used to determine the optimal number of reference genes.

2008). Normalization with stable reference genes is critical for obtaining accurate results from qRT-PCR data. Differential and coexpression analyses of the structural genes derived from qRT-PCR have been successful to screen UDP-dependent glucuronosyltransferase, which can catalyze continuous two-step glucuronosylation of glycyrrhetinic acid to yield (Xu et al., 2016). Hence, differential analysis coupled with coexpression analysis will be a useful method to screen the specific genes in the plants without genome information.

For *H. serrata*, the global RNA-seq data from four different tissues have been published, which can be directly used for differential and coexpression analyses. However, the suitable reference gene for this plant is still not selected, which may result in different expression patterns in different tissues or treatments. Here, eight reported reference genes (*actin, tubulin, 18S, TBP, GAPDH, HSP90, MUB,* and *SAM*) were selected and validated to discover the suitable reference genes for the qRT-PCR normalization in different tissues.

In the current study, four housekeeping genes (*GAPDH, actin, tubulin,* and *18S*) and other four genes (*TBP, SAM, HSP90,* and *MUB*) were used as query genes for the blast against the RNA-seq data (Yang et al., 2017) to find the homologous genes (Stanton et al., 2017). Genes with similar expression levels in four different tissues were selected as candidates as previously reported (Tan et al., 2015). In this study, the traditional reference genes, *GAPDH, actin, tubulin,* and *18S,* had good performances in CV values in qRT-PCR Cq values (CV < 10%), in line with the previous reports (Shivhare and Lata, 2016; Martins et al., 2017). The four most extensively used programs (ΔCq, geNorm, NormFinder, and BestKeeper) were used in this study for analyzing the stabilities of candidate reference genes to avoid selection of coregulated genes. The four programs showed a few differences in results; *TBP* and *GAPDH* were the most two stable reference genes, *MUB* and *HSP90* were the least stable reference genes, and others

TABLE 3 | Stability analysis of candidate reference genes, as assayed with NormFinder software.

Rank	Root		Stem		Leaf		Sporangia		Total*	
	Gene	Stability	Gene	Stability	Gene	Stability	Gene	Stability	Gene	Stability
1	TBP	0.005	Actin	0.006	TBP	0.001	Actin	0.006	TBP	0.005
2	GAPDH	0.005	TBP	0.006	GAPDH	0.001	TBP	0.006	GAPDH	0.005
3	SAM	0.008	GAPDH	0.007	SAM	0.020	SAM	0.007	SAM	0.007
4	Tubulin	0.014	Tubulin	0.024	Actin	0.023	GAPDH	0.028	Actin	0.007
5	Actin	0.025	SAM	0.027	18S	0.026	Tubulin	0.032	18S	0.014
6	18S	0.073	18S	0.049	Tubulin	0.034	18S	0.098	Tubulin	0.015
7	MUB	0.107	MUB	0.101	MUB	0.108	HSP90	0.106	MUB	0.107
8	HSP90	0.175	HSP90	0.132	HSP90	0.145	MUB	0.113	HSP90	0.139

* Total: Pooled samples from all treatments.

TABLE 4 | Stability analysis of candidate reference genes, as assayed with BestKeeper software.

Rank	Root			Stem			Leaf			Sporangia			Total*		
	Gene	SD	CV	Gene	SD	CV	Gene	SD	CV	Gene	SD	CV	Gene	SD	CV
1	Actin	0.49	2.40	GAPDH	0.23	1.18	GAPDH	0.32	1.47	18S	0.67	3.94	SAM	0.39	1.85
2	SAM	0.58	2.99	SAM	0.30	1.51	TBP	0.34	1.41	SAM	1.42	5.90	18S	0.40	2.58
3	18S	0.94	5.95	TBP	0.36	1.49	18S	0.36	2.58	Actin	1.53	6.46	Actin	0.51	2.39
4	GAPDH	0.96	4.67	Actin	0.43	2.12	SAM	0.43	2.13	GAPDH	1.67	7.14	TBP	0.65	2.56
5	TBP	1.01	3.96	18S	0.65	4.51	Tubulin	0.65	3.26	TBP	1.69	6.20	GAPDH	0.70	3.28
6	Tubulin	1.22	6.33	Tubulin	0.68	3.77	Actin	0.74	3.47	Tubulin	2.13	8.95	Tubulin	0.86	4.22
7	MUB	1.25	5.12	MUB	1.41	6.02	MUB	1.53	6.37	MUB	2.50	9.35	MUB	1.61	6.54
8	HSP90	3.36	14.52	HSP90	2.11	9.65	HSP90	2.41	10.71	HSP90	2.57	9.91	HSP90	2.34	10.02

* Total: Pooled samples from all treatments.

TABLE 5 | Expression stability of candidate reference genes, as assayed with RefFinder software.

Method	1	2	3	4	5	6	7	8
Ranking Order in Root (Better–Good–Average)								
Delta CT	GAPDH	TBP	SAM	Tubulin	Actin	18S	MUB	HSP90
BestKeeper	Actin	SAM	18S	GAPDH	TBP	Tubulin	MUB	HSP90
NormFinder	GAPDH	TBP	Tubulin	SAM	Actin	18S	MUB	HSP90
geNorm	TBP | GAPDH		Tubulin	SAM	Actin	18S	MUB	HSP90
Recommended comprehensive ranking	GAPDH	TBP	SAM	Actin	Tubulin	18S	MUB	HSP90
Ranking Order in Stem (Better–Good–Average)								
Delta CT	Actin	TBP	GAPDH	Tubulin	18S	SAM	MUB	HSP90
BestKeeper	GAPDH	SAM	TBP	Actin	18S	Tubulin	MUB	HSP90
NormFinder	Actin	TBP	GAPDH	Tubulin	SAM	18S	MUB	HSP90
geNorm	Actin | TBP		GAPDH	Tubulin	18S	SAM	MUB	HSP90
Recommended comprehensive ranking	Actin	TBP	GAPDH	SAM	Tubulin	18S	MUB	HSP90
Ranking Order in Leaf (Better–Good–Average)								
Delta CT	GAPDH	TBP	SAM	18S	Actin	Tubulin	MUB	HSP90
BestKeeper	GAPDH	TBP	18S	SAM	Tubulin	Actin	MUB	HSP90
NormFinder	GAPDH	TBP	18S	SAM	Actin	Tubulin	MUB	HSP90
geNorm	TBP | GAPDH		18S	SAM	Actin	Tubulin	MUB	HSP90
Recommended comprehensive ranking	GAPDH	TBP	18S	SAM	Actin	Tubulin	MUB	HSP90
Ranking Order in Sporangia (Better–Good–Average)								
Delta CT	Actin	TBP	SAM	GAPDH	Tubulin	18S	HSP90	MUB
BestKeeper	18S	SAM	Actin	GAPDH	TBP	Tubulin	MUB	HSP90
NormFinder	SAM	Actin	TBP	GAPDH	Tubulin	18S	HSP90	MUB
geNorm	Actin | SAM		TBP	GAPDH	Tubulin	HSP90	18S	MUB
Recommended comprehensive ranking	Actin	SAM	TBP	18S	GAPDH	Tubulin	HSP90	MUB
Ranking Order in Total (Better–Good–Average)								
Delta CT	TBP	Actin	GAPDH	SAM	18S	Tubulin	MUB	HSP90
BestKeeper	SAM	18S	Actin	TBP	GAPDH	Tubulin	MUB	HSP90
NormFinder	GAPDH	TBP	18S	Actin	SAM	Tubulin	MUB	HSP90
geNorm	TBP | GAPDH		Actin	SAM	18S	Tubulin	MUB	HSP90
Recommended comprehensive ranking	TBP	GAPDH	Actin	SAM	18S	Tubulin	MUB	HSP90

were midstable candidates with different rankings calculated by different programs.

Although *TBP* was the most stable candidate for all samples in our study, its expression level was very low, which was also observed in equine milk somatic cells and in *Aedes aegypti* (Cieslak et al., 2015; Dzaki et al., 2017). This low level was due to that the Cq values in qRT-PCR assays varied from 21.34 to 31.05 in all experiments with the five dilution cDNAs, which indicated that the *TBP* is a new plant species-dependent reference gene, hence suggesting a proper validation in each case. While, *GAPDH* exhibited good performance on qRT-PCR normalization in different tissues of plants of different developmental stages, as calculated by most of the programs. Hence, *GAPDH* alone is suitable for qRT-PCR normalization as a reference gene under different tissues. The few differences in reference genes showed in different programs were also in agreement with earlier studies (Jain et al., 2006; Cruz et al., 2009; Jain, 2009; Qi et al., 2016). The different rankings of the reference genes showed in different programs were also observed in *chrysanthemum* (Gu et al., 2011; Wang et al., 2015); thus, all these programs must be combined to evaluate the candidates for each species.

We further performed RT-qPCR experiments to investigate the expression levels of *L/ODC* genes, which were previously characterized in *H. serrata*, *Lycopodium clavatum*, and Leguminosae (Bunsupa et al., 2012; Bunsupa et al., 2016; Xu et al., 2017) by using the two most stable reference genes (*TBP* and *GAPDH*) and the two least stable reference genes (*MUB* and *HSP90*), to evaluate the eight selected reference genes. According to the pairwise analysis by geNorm software, two reference genes were sufficient for the normalization; thus, the combination of *TBP* and *GAPDH* was also used to calculate the expression level of targeted genes. Regardless of which reference gene was used, the expression patterns of

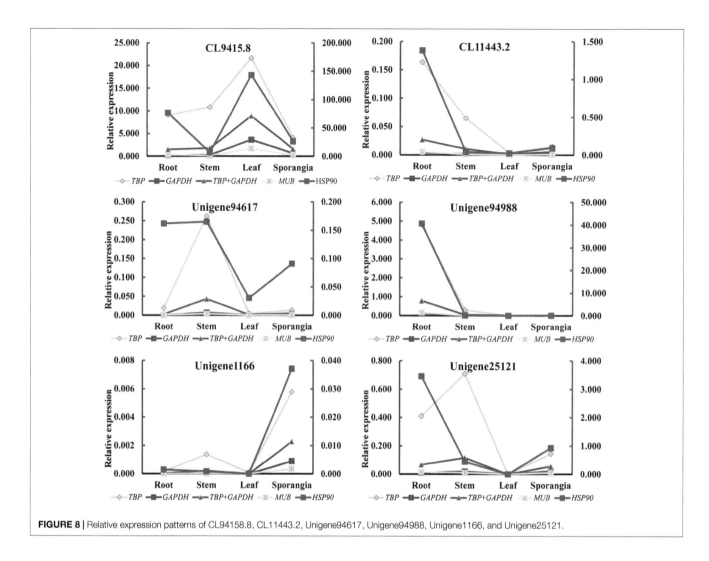

FIGURE 8 | Relative expression patterns of CL94158.8, CL11443.2, Unigene94617, Unigene94988, Unigene1166, and Unigene25121.

L/ODC (Unigene94988) were the same. To further validate, Unigene94617, a homologous gene of Unigene94988, and four cytochrome P450 genes (CL9415.8, CL1143.2, Unigene1166, and Unigene25121) proposed to participate in HupA biosynthesis (Yang et al., 2017) were employed for the normalization. All reference genes, with exception of *HSP90*, acquired a similar expression pattern for all targeted genes. Hence, only *HSP90* was unsuitable for qRT-PCR normalization in all tissues of *H. serrata*, which suggested that RNA-seq-assisted selection was a useful method for selecting suitable reference genes. Previous studies in *Arabidopsis thaliana*, *Coffeea arabica*, *Gossypium hirsutum,* and *Chrysanthemum* showed that the novel reference genes exhibited better performance than traditional reference genes (Czechowski et al., 2005; Cruz et al., 2009; Artico et al., 2010; Qi et al., 2016). Taken all together, although we observed some inconsistency on the expression patterns of the some genes in HupA biosynthesis between RNA-seq and qRT-PCR, this might be due to the plant growth condition differences (season and climate) when we collected (**Supplementary Table S1**). The major reason for this is likely due to the seasonal and climatic factors or growth as this plant takes years to grow (Ma et al., 2006).

Similarly, inconsistency was also observed previous reports. In many cases, the gene expressions quantified with different methods were dramatically different (Wang et al., 2006; Marioni et al., 2008; Qin et al., 2013; Rajkumar et al., 2015; Dapas et al., 2017). Due to the lack of successful *in vitro* propagation approach of Lycopodiaceae family, its important to design such functional genomics study from the control climatic conditions and/or established *in vitro* platform. Our lab is currently exploring the approach of *in vitro* propagation of endangered species of Lycopodiaceae family. This study state possible use of housekeeping genes as a stable candidate for qRT-PCR normalization of plants belonging to Lycopodiaceaea family especially *H. serrata*.

CONCLUSION

In this study, we proposed *H. serrata* as a model plant for functional genomics study in the Lycopodiaceae family. The qRT-PCR reference gene normalization in tissues of *H. serrata* showed that *TBP* and *GAPDH* were the two most suitable reference genes. The combination of the two genes as reference genes was accurate for qRT-PCR normalization, as performed in different tissues of *H. serrata* according to the pairwise variation analysis by geNorm program. The reference genes identified and validated here through RNA-seq data for qRT-PCR normalization will facilitate the establishment of standardized qRT-PCR program for other genetically close plants.

AUTHOR CONTRIBUTIONS

YX conceived the research. YX and SW designed the experiments. WY, SW, and MY, performed the experiments. MY and SW

analyzed the data, wrote the manuscript, and coordinated its revision. YX and AJ revised the manuscript. All authors provided helpful discussions and approved the final version.

FUNDING

This work was financially supported by Chinese Academy of Sciences (CAS) (Grant XDB27020203, 153D31KYSB20170121, and 153D31KYSB20160074) and CAS-JIC center of Excellence in Plant and Microbial Sciences (CEPAMS) funding.

REFERENCES

Andersen, C. L., Jensen, J. L., and Ørntoft, T. F. (2004). Normalization of real-time quantitative reverse transcription-PCR data: a model-based variance estimation approach to identify genes suited for normalization, applied to bladder and colon cancer data sets. *Cancer Res.* 64, 5245–5250. doi: 10.1158/0008-5472. CAN-04-0496

Artico, S., Nardeli, S. M., Brilhante, O., Grossi-De-Sa, M. F., and Alves-Ferreira, M. (2010). Identification and evaluation of new reference genes in *Gossypium hirsutum* for accurate normalization of real-time quantitative RT-PCR data. *BMC Plant Biol.* 10:49. doi: 10.1186/1471-2229-10-49

Benca, J. P. (2014). Cultivation techniques for terrestrial clubmosses (Lycopodiaceae): conservation, research, and horticultural opportunities for an early-diverging plant lineage. *Am. Fern J.* 104, 25–48. doi: 10.1640/0002-8444-104.2.25

Bunsupa, S., Hanada, K., Maruyama, A., Aoyagi, K., Komatsu, K., Ueno, H., et al. (2016). Molecular evolution and functional characterization of a bifunctional decarboxylase involved in *Lycopodium* alkaloid biosynthesis. *Plant Physiol.* 171, 2432–2444. doi: 10.1104/pp.16.00639

Bunsupa, S., Katayama, K., Ikeura, E., Oikawa, A., Toyooka, K., Saito, K., et al. (2012). Lysine decarboxylase catalyzes the first step of quinolizidine alkaloid biosynthesis and coevolved with alkaloid production in leguminosae. *Plant Cell* 24, 1202–1216. doi: 10.1105/tpc.112.09 5885

Bustin, S. A. (2000). Absolute quantification of mRNA using real-time reverse transcription polymerase chain reaction assays. *J. Mol. Endocrinol.* 25, 169–193. doi: 10.1677/jme.0.0250169

Cieslak, J., Mackowski, M., Czyzak-Runowska, G., Wojtowski, J., Puppel, K., Kuczynska, B., et al. (2015). Screening for the most suitable reference genes for gene expression studies in equine milk somatic cells. *PLoS One* 10:e0139688. doi: 10.1371/journal.pone.0139688

Cruz, F., Kalaoun, S., Nobile, P., Colombo, C., Almeida, J., Barros, L. M. G., et al. (2009). Evaluation of coffee reference genes for relative expression studies by quantitative real-time RT-PCR. *Mol. Breed.* 23, 607–616. doi: 10.1007/s11032-009-9259-x

Czechowski, T., Stitt, M., Altmann, T., Udvardi, M. K., and Scheible, W. R. (2005). Genome-wide identification and testing of superior reference genes for transcript normalization in Arabidopsis. *Plant Physiol.* 139, 5–17. doi: 10.1104/pp.105.063743

Dapas, M., Kandpal, M., Bi, Y. T., and Davuluri, R. V. (2017). Comparative evaluation of isoform-level gene expression estimation algorithms for RNA-seq and exon-array platforms. *Brief. Bioinform.* 18, 260–269. doi: 10.1093/bib/bbw016

Derveaux, S., Vandesompele, J., and Hellemans, J. (2010). How to do successful gene expression analysis using real-time PCR. *Methods* 50, 227–230. doi: 10.1016/j.ymeth.2009.11.001

Dzaki, N., Ramli, K. N., Azlan, A., Ishak, I. H., and Azzam, G. (2017). Evaluation of reference genes at different developmental stages for quantitative real-time PCR in *Aedes aegypti. Sci. Rep.* 7:43618. doi: 10.1038/srep43618

Gu, C., Chen, S., Liu, Z., Shan, H., Luo, H., Guan, Z., et al. (2011). Reference gene selection for quantitative real-time PCR in *Chrysanthemum* subjected to

biotic and abiotic stress. *Mol. Biotechnol.* 49, 192–197. doi: 10.1007/s12033-011-9394-6

Jain, M. (2009). Genome-wide identification of novel internal control genes for normalization of gene expression during various stages of development in rice. *Plant Sci.* 176, 702–706. doi: 10.1016/j.plantsci.2009.02.001

Jain, M., Nijhawan, A., Tyagi, A. K., and Khurana, J. P. (2006). Validation of housekeeping genes as internal control for studying gene expression in rice by quantitative real-time PCR. *Biochem. Biophys. Res. Commun.* 345, 646–651. doi: 10.1016/j.bbrc.2006.04.140

Kozera, B., and Rapacz, M. (2013). Reference genes in real-time PCR. *J. Appl. Genet.* 54, 391–406. doi: 10.1007/s13353-013-0173-x

Ma, X., and Gang, D. R. (2004). The *Lycopodium* alkaloids. *Nat. Prod. Rep.* 21, 752–772. doi: 10.1039/b409720n

Ma, X., Tan, C., Zhu, D., and Gang, D. R. (2006). A survey of potential huperzine A natural resources in China: the Huperziaceae. *J. Ethnopharmacol.* 104, 54–67. doi: 10.1016/j.jep.2005.08.042

Ma, X., Tan, C., Zhu, D., Gang, D. R., and Xiao, P. (2007). Huperzine A from *Huperzia* species–an ethnopharmacolgical review. *J. Ethnopharmacol.* 113, 15–34. doi: 10.1016/j.jep.2007.05.030

Marioni, J. C., Mason, C. E., Mane, S. M., Stephens, M., and Gilad, Y. (2008). RNA-seq: an assessment of technical reproducibility and comparison with gene expression arrays. *Genome Res.* 18, 1509–1517. doi: 10.1101/gr.079558.108

Martins, M. Q., Fortunato, A. S., Rodrigues, W. P., Partelli, F. L., Campostrini, E., Lidon, F. C., et al. (2017). Selection and validation of reference genes for accurate RT-qPCR data normalization in *Coffea* spp. under a climate changes context of interacting elevated [CO2] and temperature. *Front. Plant Sci.* 8:307. doi: 10.3389/fpls.2017.00307

Niu, X., Qi, J., Zhang, G., Xu, J., Tao, A., Fang, P., et al. (2015). Selection of reliable reference genes for quantitative real-time PCR gene expression analysis in Jute (*Corchorus capsularis*) under stress treatments. *Front. Plant Sci.* 6:848. doi: 10.3389/fpls.2015.00848

Petriccione, M., Mastrobuoni, F., Zampella, L., and Scortichini, M. (2015). Reference gene selection for normalization of RT-qPCR gene expression data from *Actinidia deliciosa* leaves infected with *Pseudomonas syringae* pv. actinidiae. *Sci. Rep.* 5:16961. doi: 10.1038/srep16961

Pfaffl, M. W., Tichopad, A., Prgomet, C., and Neuvians, T. P. (2004). Determination of stable housekeeping genes, differentially regulated target genes and sample integrity: BestKeeper – Excel-based tool using pair-wise correlations. *Biotechnol. Lett.* 26, 509–515. doi: 10.1023/B:BILE.0000019559.84305.47

Pombo, M. A., Zheng, Y., Fei, Z., Martin, G. B., and Rosli, H. G. (2017). Use of RNA-seq data to identify and validate RT-qPCR reference genes for studying the tomato-*Pseudomonas* pathosystem. *Sci. Rep.* 7:44905. doi: 10.1038/srep44905

Qi, S., Yang, L., Wen, X., Hong, Y., Song, X., Zhang, M., et al. (2016). Reference gene selection for RT-qPCR analysis of flower development in *Chrysanthemum morifolium* and *Chrysanthemum lavandulifolium. Front. Plant Sci.* 7:287. doi: 10.3389/fpls.2016.00287

Qin, J., Scheuring, C. F., Wei, G., Zhi, H., Zhang, M. P., Huang, J. J., et al. (2013). Identification and characterization of a repertoire of genes differentially expressed in developing top ear shoots between a superior hybrid and its parental inbreds in *Zea mays* L. *Mol. Genet. Genomics* 288, 691–705. doi: 10.1007/s00438-013-0781-5

Radonic, A., Thulke, S., Mackay, I. M., Landt, O., Siegert, W., and Nitsche, A. (2004). Guideline to reference gene selection for quantitative real-time PCR. *Biochem. Biophys. Res. Commun.* 313, 856–862. doi: 10.1016/j.bbrc.2003.11.177

Rajkumar, A. P., Qvist, P., Lazarus, R., Lescai, F., Ju, J., Nyegaard, M., et al. (2015). Experimental validation of methods for differential gene expression analysis and sample pooling in RNA-seq. *BMC Genomics* 16:548. doi: 10.1186/s12864-015-1767-y

Rutledge, R. G., and Stewart, D. (2008). Critical evaluation of methods used to determine amplification efficiency refutes the exponential character of real-time PCR. *BMC Mol. Biol.* 9:96. doi: 10.1186/1471-2199-9-96

Saito, K., Hirai, M. Y., and Yonekura-Sakakibara, K. (2008). Decoding genes with coexpression networks and metabolomics–'majority report by precogs'. *Trends Plant Sci.* 13, 36–43. doi: 10.1016/j.tplants.2007.10.006

Shivhare, R., and Lata, C. (2016). Selection of suitable reference genes for assessing gene expression in pearl millet under different abiotic stresses and their combinations. *Sci. Rep.* 6:23036. doi: 10.1038/srep23036

Stanton, K. A., Edger, P. P., Puzey, J. R., Kinser, T., Cheng, P., Vernon, D. M., et al. (2017). A whole-transcriptome approach to evaluating reference genes for quantitative gene expression studies: a case study in mimulus. *G3* 7, 1085–1095. doi: 10.1534/g3.116.038075

Tan, Q. Q., Zhu, L., Li, Y., Liu, W., Ma, W. H., Lei, C. L., et al. (2015). A de novo transcriptome and valid reference genes for quantitative real-time PCR in *Colaphellus bowringi*. *PLoS One* 10:e0118693. doi: 10.1371/journal.pone.0118693

Vandesompele, J., De Preter, K., Pattyn, F., Poppe, B., Van Roy, N., De Paepe, A., et al. (2002). Accurate normalization of real-time quantitative RT-PCR data by geometric averaging of multiple internal control genes. *Genome Biol.* 3:RESEARCH0034. doi: 10.1186/gb-2002-3-7-research0034

Wang, H., Chen, S., Jiang, J., Zhang, F., and Chen, F. (2015). Reference gene selection for cross-species and cross-ploidy level comparisons in *Chrysanthemum* spp. *Sci. Rep.* 5:8094. doi: 10.1038/srep08094

Wang, Y. L., Barbacioru, C., Hyland, F., Xiao, W. M., Hunkapiller, K. L., Blake, J., et al. (2006). Large scale real-time PCR validation on gene expression measurements from two commercial long-oligonucleotide microarrays. *BMC Genomics* 7:59.

Wu, S., Fan, Z., and Xiao, Y. (2018). Comprehensive relative quantitative metabolomics analysis of *Lycopodium* alkaloids in different tissues of *Huperzia serrata*. *Synth. Syst. Biotechnol.* 3, 44–55. doi: 10.1016/j.synbio.2017.12.003

Xie, F., Xiao, P., Chen, D., Xu, L., and Zhang, B. (2012). miRDeepFinder: a miRNA analysis tool for deep sequencing of plant small RNAs. *Plant Mol. Biol.* 80, 75–84. doi: 10.1007/s11103-012-9885-2

Xu, B., Lei, L., Zhu, X., Zhou, Y., and Xiao, Y. (2017). Identification and characterization of L-lysine decarboxylase from *Huperzia serrata* and its role in the metabolic pathway of *Lycopodium* alkaloid. *Phytochemistry* 136, 23–30. doi: 10.1016/j.phytochem.2016.12.022

Xu, G., Cai, W., Gao, W., and Liu, C. (2016). A novel glucuronosyltransferase has an unprecedented ability to catalyse continuous two-step glucuronosylation of glycyrrhetinic acid to yield glycyrrhizin. *New Phytol.* 212, 123–135. doi: 10.1111/nph.14039

Yang, M., You, W., Wu, S., Fan, Z., Xu, B., Zhu, M., et al. (2017). Global transcriptome analysis of *Huperzia serrata* and identification of critical genes involved in the biosynthesis of huperzine A. *BMC Genomics* 18:245. doi: 10.1186/s12864-017-3615-8

Zhang, Y. X., Han, X. J., Chen, S. S., Zheng, L., He, X. L., Liu, M. Y., et al. (2017). Selection of suitable reference genes for quantitative real-time PCR gene expression analysis in *Salix matsudana* under different abiotic stresses. *Sci. Rep.* 7:40290. doi: 10.1038/srep40290

Zhao, Q., and Tang, X. C. (2002). Effects of huperzine A on acetylcholinesterase isoforms in vitro: comparison with tacrine, donepezil, rivastigmine and physostigmine. *Eur. J. Pharmacol.* 455, 101–107. doi: 10.1016/S0014-2999(02)02589-X

8

Molecular Authentication of the Medicinal Species of *Ligusticum* (Ligustici Rhizoma et Radix, "Gao-Ben") by Integrating Non-Coding Internal Transcribed Spacer 2 (ITS2) and its Secondary Structure

Zhen-wen Liu[1], Yu-zhen Gao[2] and Jing Zhou[2]*

[1] *CAS Key Laboratory for Plant Diversity and Biogeography of East Asia, Kunming Institute of Botany, Chinese Academy of Sciences, Kunming, China,* [2] *School of Pharmaceutical Sciences and Yunnan Key Laboratory of Pharmacology for Natural Products, Kunming Medical University, Kunming, China*

Correspondence:
Jing Zhou
zhoujing_apiaceae@163.com

Ligustici Rhizoma et Radix (LReR), an important Chinese medicine known as "Gao-ben," refers to *Ligusticum sinense* Oliv. or *Ligusticum jeholense* Nakai et Kitag. However, a number of other species are commonly sold as "Gao-ben" in the herbal medicine market, which may result in a series of quality control problems and inconsistent therapeutic effects. The "Gao-ben" is commonly sold sliced and dried, making traditional identification methods difficult. Here, the mini barcode ITS2 region was examined on 68 samples representing LReR and 7 potential adulterant or substitute species. The results showed 100% success rates of PCR and sequencing and the existence of a barcoding gap. The neighbor-joining (NJ) tree indicated that all the tested samples could be exactly identified. The ITS2 secondary structure revealed a clear difference between true "Gao-ben" and three adulterant species. We therefore recommend the use of ITS2 as a mini barcode for distinguishing between closely or distantly related plant species that may be used in Chinese medicine.

Keywords: apiaceae, DNA barcoding, Ligustici Rhizoma et Radix, ITS2, secondary structures

INTRODUCTION

Apiaceae, the 16th-largest flowering plant family, comprises more than 3,540 species in 446 genera (Mabberley, 1997). It is a well-known and economically important plant family in medicine, spices, vegetables and ornamental gardening. The roots and rhizomes of *Ligusticum sinense* Oliv. or *Ligusticum jeholense* Nakai et Kitag form a widely used traditional Chinese medicine, known as "Ligustici Rhizoma et Radix" (LReR), or "Gao-ben" in Chinese (Commission, 2015). It is commonly used to treat colds, trapped wind, headaches and rheumatic arthralgia (Commission, 2015). It has been reported to exhibit many beneficial properties such as analgesic, antipyretic, anti-inflammatory and anticonvulsive activities, plus antimicrobial and antioxidant effects (Wang et al., 2011). As a result, this herb has attracted more and more attention in the medical field, and have been widely used in clinical therapies.

However, LReR is easily confused with other herbs, causing potential mistakes in treatment. Certain species that are closely related or morphologically similar to LReR are frequently used as local remedies in various regions due to geographical and historical factors. For instance, *Meeboldia yunnanensis* (H. Wolff) Constance & F. T. Pu, *Ligusticum delavayi* Franchet and *Ligusticum pteridophyllum* Franchet are often used in folk medicine in southwestern China, but their function and efficacy are not quite the same (Li et al., 2001). Additionally, *Conioselinum vaginatum* (Spreng.) Thell., *Ligusticum tenuissimum* (Nakai) Kitagawa, *Sium suave* Walter and *Ligusticum acuminatum* Franch. are also sold as "Gao-ben" in medicinal markets. Using morphology-based or chemical identification methods to identify Rhizoma et Radix herbs is difficult, especially when the plant is sliced and dried, as they often are for selling (Hon et al., 2003; Joshi et al., 2004; Xue et al., 2006; Mishra et al., 2016). Therefore, a simple, inexpensive and effective method for distinguishing between the above species is urgently needed.

DNA barcoding is a new taxonomic method that uses one or a few short, standard genomic DNA region(s) for rapid, reliable and effective species identification (Floyd et al., 2002; Hebert et al., 2003). For identifying traditional herbal medicines, however, the commonly used three-barcode system has not always been effective, because matK and *rbc*L are difficult to amplify, especially from powdered products where DNA degradation is very common. The internal transcribed spacer 2 (ITS2) region of nuclear ribosomal DNA might be a promising standardized region to barcode medicinal plants, due to its relatively short length, consistent performance in distinguishing closely related species, and ease of amplification with a single set of universal primers (Chen et al., 2010). In cells, ITS2 has conserved nucleotide motifs which play a role in forming a three dimensional structure, and hence transformation into a functional complex before conversion to a mature rRNA (Hall, 1999; Lalev and Nazar, 1999). Compared with previous sequence alignments based only on nucleotide similarity, the ITS2 conserved nucleotide motifs permit multiple sequence alignments, from which a more homologous overall alignment can be generated (Kjer, 1995; Coleman and Mai, 1997). Additionally, the secondary structure is maintained by the mutual between base-pairs that are canonical (GC, AU), non-canonical stable (GU) and unstable (AC) (Elgavish et al., 2001; Leontis and Westhof, 2001). Theses paired and unpaired ITS2 structures provide extra molecular morphological features that can greatly improve taxonomic classification (Telford et al., 2005; Keller et al., 2010).

In this study, we use ITS2 sequence and secondary structure information to determine whether genuine "Gao-ben" can be distinguished from the most commonly used adulterants and substitutes. We also discuss the possibility that ITS2 might play a regulatory role in the herbal medicine market in the future.

MATERIALS AND METHODS

Plant Materials
A total of 43 samples belonging to eight species, covering the two original species of LReR (*L. sinense* and *L. jeholense*) and seven potential substitutes (*L. tenuissimum*, *L. pteridophyllum*, *L. acuminatum*, *S. suave*, *M. yunnanensis*, and *C. vaginatum*), were collected from fields. Voucher specimens were deposited in the Kunming Institute of Botany, Chinese Academy of Sciences (KUN), and Chengdu Institute of Biology, Chinese Academy of Sciences (CDBI) (**Supplementary Table S1**). To determine possible infraspecific molecular variation, each species was represented by at least two individuals. Furthermore, 25 commercial "Gao-ben" products were purchased from different medicinal markets in China (**Supplementary Table S1**).

Laboratory Protocols
Before DNA extraction, the surface of the medicinal materials was wiped with 75% ethanol, then ground into powder with a grinder. Genomic DNA was extracted using the modified CTAB procedure of Doyle and Doyle (1987). The primers BEL-2 (5′-GATGCGGAGATTGGCCCCCCGTGC -3′) and BEL-3 (5′-GACGCTTCTCCAGACTACAAT -3′) were used to amplify the complete ITS2 region (Chiou et al., 2007). The PCR parameters were as follows: Initial denaturation for 3 min at 94°C, followed by 36 cycles of denaturation (94°, 45 s), annealing (55°C, 1 min) and extension (72°C, 2 min), and a final extension for 7 min at 72°C. Purified PCR products were sequenced in both directions with the primers used for PCR amplification on an ABI 3730 automated sequencer (Applied Biosystems, Foster City, CA, United States) in Sangon Biotech Corporation (Shanghai, China).

Data Analysis
Newly generated sequences were initially edited and assembled using SeqMan of the DNASTAR 5.01 software package (DNASTAR, Inc., Madison, United States). The ITS2 region was annotated using the Hidden Markov Model (HMM) (Keller et al., 2009) to delete the conserved 5.8 and 28S sections (Koetschan et al., 2012). ITS2 secondary structures of all investigated taxa were predicted by homology modeling in the ITS2 Database (identity matrix and 75% threshold for the helix transfer[1]) (Koetschan et al., 2012). This method usually results in several alternative folding patterns for the same ITS2 sequence. The true folding pattern corresponds to the secondary structure model of Mai and Coleman, and was well supported by compensatory base changes (CBCs) and hemi compensatory base changes (hCBCs) revealed by comparisons among related taxa (Mai and Coleman, 1997). Sequences with homologous structure were automatically and synchronously aligned using 4SALE 1.7 (Seibel et al., 2006, 2008). Genetic distances were calculated according to the kimura-2-parameter (K2P) model using MEGA 7.0 software (Kumar et al., 2016). A neighbor-joining (NJ) tree was constructed and bootstrap tests were performed using 1000 replicates to separate the sampled species via MEGA 7.0

[1] http://its2.bioapps.biozentrum.uni-wuerzburg.de/

(Kumar et al., 2016). CBCs are substitutions in two positions that retain pairing, i.e., $G = C \leftrightarrow C = G$, $A = U \leftrightarrow U = A$. The proposed ITS2 secondary structure was examined for CBCs with the CBCAnalyzer option (Wolf et al., 2005) implemented in 4SALE, whereas hCBCs (pair $\leftrightarrow$ non-pair, i.e., $G = C \leftrightarrow G = U$) were observed manually.

RESULTS

Amplification, Sequencing, and Sequences Characteristics

The success rate of the ITS2 PCR amplification and sequencing was 100% (**Table 1**). All high-quality sequences were submitted to GenBank (**Table 1**). The ITS2 sequence showed minor length variation across all samples, ranging from 220 bp (*M. yunnanensis*) to 226 (*S. suave*). The length of 15 *L. sinense* and *L. jeholense* individuals was 222 bp, and the average GC content was 54.9%. The ITS2 sequence lengths of *L. acuminatum*, *L. delavayi*, *L. pteridophyllum*, *L. tenuissimum*, *C. vaginatum*, *M. yunnanensis*, and *S. suave* were 223, 223, 223, 223, 222, 220, and 226 bp, respectively. The corresponding average GC content of these adulterants varied from 53.2 to 57.9%. The aligned length of 227 bp exhibited 84 variable sites, a rate of 37.0% (**Table 1**). Therefore, the ITS2 sequences for the sampled species were relatively variable.

Intra/Interspecific Distance, Barcoding Gap, and NJ Tree

All individuals of *L. sinense* and *L. jeholense* were identical for ITS2, sharing a single haplotype. According to the K2P model, the average interspecific distance between these and the adulterant species was 0.175, with the maximum interspecific distance being 0.337 from *L. delavayi*, and the minimum being 0.059 from *C. vaginatum* (**Table 2** and **Figure 1A**). The NJ tree showed that 15 individual samples were determined to be *L. jeholense* and *L. sinense* clustered together in a highly supported clade (Bootstrap value = 99) that was separated from the commonly used substitutes and adulterants such as *L. pteridophyllum*, *L. acuminatum*, *L. tenuissimum*, *C. vaginatum*, *S. suave*, *M. yunnanensis*, and *L. delavayi* (**Figure 2A**). There was therefore a high interspecific variation and an obvious barcoding gap was noted (**Figure 1B**).

Of the 25 commercial "Gao-ben" products, six samples were identified as LReR, accounting for 24%, while the remainder were

TABLE 1 | ITS2 sequence characters of samples.

	ITS2
Amplification efficiency (%)	100
Sequencing efficiency (%)	100
Length of all taxa (bp)	220–226
Aligned length (bp)	227
G+C content range in all taxa (%)	53.2–57.9
Number (and %) of variable sites in all taxa	84 (37%)

TABLE 2 | Analysis of intra-specific variation and inter-specific divergence of the ITS2 sequences.

K2P genetic distances	Range of genetic distances (mean)
Intra-specific distance of LReR	0.000
Inter-specific distance between LReR – *Conioselinum vaginatum*	0.059–0.059 (0.059)
Inter-specific distance between LReR – *L. acuminatum*	0.064–0.064 (0.064)
Inter-specific distance between LReR – *L. pteridophyllum*	0.070–0.076 (0.073)
Inter-specific distance between LReR – *L. tenuissimum*	0.092–0.092 (0.092)
Inter-specific distance between LReR – *Sium suave*	0.282–0.291 (0.286)
Inter-specific distance between LReR – *Meeboldia yunnanensis*	0.309–0.319 (0.313)
Inter-specific distance between LReR – *L. delavayi*	0.337–0.337 (0.337)

identified as *M. yunnanensis* (12%), and *C. vaginatum* (64%) (**Figure 2B**).

Analysis of the Secondary Structure

ITS2 secondary structures obtained for all species examined fold into the common core structure known for eukaryotes, made up of four helices, the third being the longest (**Supplementary Figures S1A–H**; Mai and Coleman, 1997; Coleman, 2003, 2007, 2015; Schultz et al., 2005). **Figure 3** visualizes a 51% consensus structure. Sequence motifs include a U-U mismatch in helix II, an A-rich conserved spacer between helices II and III, and a UGGU motif 5′ side to the apex of helix III (**Figure 3**). In comparable portions of the secondary structure, most CBCs, and hCBCs observed between LReR and its adulterants are in helices III, I, and II, with a few in helix IV (**Table 3**). *L. sinense*, *L. jeholense*, *L. tenuissimum*, *L. acuminatum*, *C. vaginatum*, and *L. pteridophyllum* form a group without any CBC in conserved ITS2 regions (i.e., in helices II and III), from which the group of *L. delavayi*, *M. yunnanensis*, and *S. Suave* may be distinguished by the presence of at least one CBC in these regions.

DISCUSSION

Identification Capability of ITS2 for LReR

In Chinese Pharmacopeia, only *L. sinense* and *L. jeholense* are listed as LReR for their very similar chemical compositions and the near identical use and efficacy (Commission, 2015). Morphologically, both species share many similar characters, e.g., ternate-2- or 3-pinnate blade, ultimate segment margins irregularly serrate, and long and reflexed styles. Geographically, *L. jeholense* is in northern China, while *L. sinense* occurs more widely, but does not overlap with *L. jeholense* (Sheh and Watson, 2005). Both our present ITS2 (**Table 2**) and unpublished data including *psbA-trn*H, *mat*K, and *rbc*L show no interspecific variation between these two species. Therefore, we consider

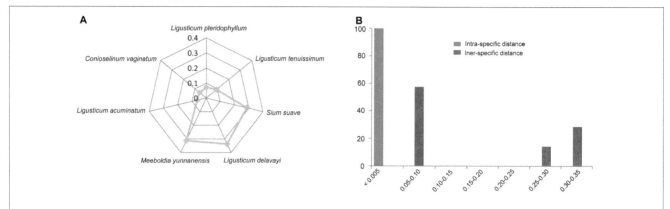

FIGURE 1 | (A) Genetic distances from LReR to its adulterants and substitutes. (B) Relative distribution of interspecific divergence between LReR and its adulterants and substitutes and intraspecific variation in the ITS2 region using K2P genetic distance.

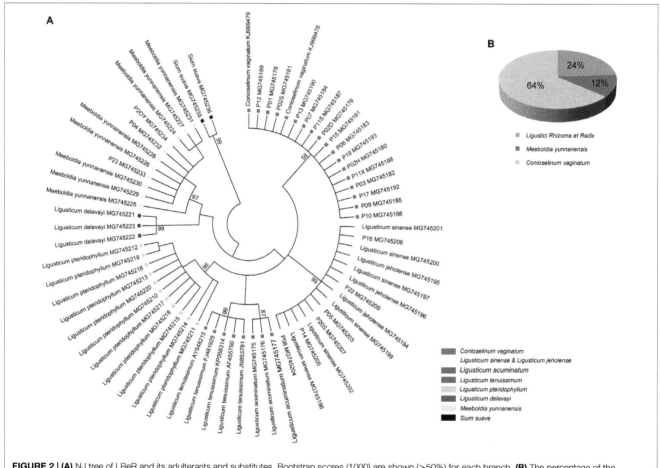

FIGURE 2 | (A) NJ tree of LReR and its adulterants and substitutes. Bootstrap scores (1000) are shown (≥50%) for each branch. (B) The percentage of the commercial "Gao-ben" products identified by barcode ITS2 in this study.

that *L. sinense* and *L. jeholense* are close relatives, or the latter represents a vicariant geographical element.

According to the criterion proposed by Coleman (2003) and coworkers, presence/absence of even a single CBC in the conserved areas of helices II and III of ITS2 is associated with incompatibility/inability to hybridize, thus establishing the boundaries between biological species and populations.

In contrast, hCBCs in the conserved parts as well as changes in the less conserved regions (e.g., in helices I and IV) do not correlate with interbreeding ability. LReR can be distinguished from *L. delavayi*, *M. yunnanensis*, and *S. suave* by at least one CBC in the conserved ITS2 regions (i.e., in helices II and III) (**Table 3** and **Supplementary Figures S1F–H**). *M. yunnanensis* and *L. delavayi* are widely used as "Huang Gao-ben" in Yunnan

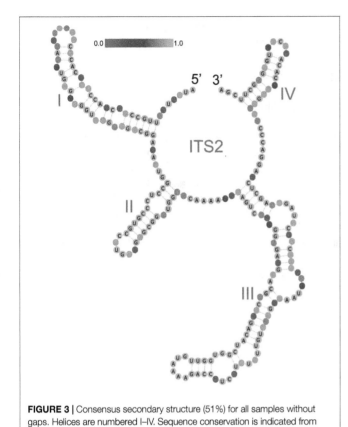

FIGURE 3 | Consensus secondary structure (51%) for all samples without gaps. Helices are numbered I–IV. Sequence conservation is indicated from red/brownish (not conserved) to green (conserved).

analysis indicated that they are phylogenetically distant species (**Figures 1A, 2A** and **Table 2**). Moreover, these three species can be distinguished from the true LReR by the presence of at least one CBC in the conserved ITS2 regions (i.e., in helices II and III) (**Table 3**). Results from epidermal analysis (Zhou and Liu, 2018), together with that from cytological evidence (Zhou et al., 2008) and molecular phylogenetics (Zhou et al., 2009), indicated that these are not close relatives of *L. sinense*. We therefore recommend that *L. delavayi*, *M. yunnanensis*, and *S. Suave* should be marketed under their original herbal medicinal name.

Other genetically close relatives of the LReR plant group include *L. pteridophyllum*, *L. tenuissimum*, *L. acuminatum*, and *C. vaginatum* (**Figures 1A, 2A** and **Table 2**). *L. pteridophyllum* is another herbal medicine widely used in Yunnan in the name of "Hei Gao-ben" and has been regarded as an adulterant of *Peucedanum praeruptorum* Dunn (Rao et al., 1995). In our analysis, all accessions of *L. pteridophyllum* comprised a strongly supported clade, having a sequence divergence value of 0.073 with LReR (**Figures 1A, 2A** and **Table 2**). According to Ye et al. (2004) the chemical composition of *L. pteridophyllum* is similar to LReR, so, considering it as a regional substitute seems to be reasonable. *L. acuminatum* had a sequence divergence value of 0.064 from LReR, for which it is used as a regional substitute in western Sichuan (Sheh and Watson, 2005), so further research is needed to determine whether it can be regarded as an effective "Gao-ben" substitute.

Conioselinum vaginatum, known as "Xinjiang Gao-ben," is found mainly in the Tian and Altai mountains of Xinjiang and western Junggar mountains in central Asia and western Siberia (Sheh and Watson, 2005), and is widely cultivated. Chemical analysis showed that *C. vaginatum* contains 16 compounds, including ligustilide, ferulic acid, and myristic ether, which are the same as in *L. jeholense* (Li, 2013); however, its pharmacological

Province, whereas *S. suave* has also been sold as "Gao-ben" in medicinal markets. It is difficult to distinguish them from LReR when they are dried, sliced, and shredded, but our ITS2

TABLE 3 | Occurrence/frequency of CBCs and hCBCs between LReR (*Ligusticum jeholense/L. sinense*) and its adulterants and substitutes.

Taxa	LReR				Summary
	Helix 1	Helix 2	Helix 3	Helix 4	
L. pteridophyllum		64/91: G-C → G-U	114/173: U-G → C-G		2 hCBCs
L. acuminatum		64/91: G-C → G-U	123/161: U-G → U-A		2 hCBCs
L. tenuissimum	20/42: U-G → C-G	64/91: G-C → G-U	123/161: U-G → U-A		3 hCBCs
L. delavayi	15/49: G-U → A-U	64/91: G-C → G-U	114/173: U-G → C-G		1 CBCs
		73/82: G-C → G-U	119/164: G-U → G-C		5 hCBCs
			123/161: C-G → U-A		
Conioselinum vaginatum		64/91: G-C → G-U	123/161: U-G → U-A		2 hCBCs
Meeboldia yunnanensis	**15/49: G-C → A-U**	64/91: G-C → G-U	110/177: G-C → G-U	203/220: U-G→ C-G	3 CBCs
			114/173: U-A → C-G		3 hCBCs
			123/161: C-G → U-A		
Sium suave	15/49: G-U → A-U		106/184: U-G → C-G		3 CBCs
	21/41: U-G → A-U		110/177: G-C → G-U		5 hCBCs
			115/172: G-U → G-C		
			122/162: A-U → G-C		
			123/161: C-G → U-A		
			124/160: G-U → G-C		

Base pairs displaying CBCs are indicated in bolds.

action remains controversial (Dai, 1988; Li et al., 2013). Given that the annual demand for LReR exceeds 3500 tons, which exceeds the natural production capacity (Ding, 2010), research on the pharmacological efficacy of *C. vaginatum* is urgently needed, to determine whether *C. vaginatum* could be an effective substitute.

Potential Application of ITS2 in the Authentication of Medicinal Materials

The trade in crude drugs has surged globally, generating annual revenues over US $60 billion (Newmaster et al., 2013). There are strong financial incentives for dishonest merchants to use adulterants and substitutes intentionally, leading to treatments not working as advertised, and posing serious risks to the health of consumers (Newmaster et al., 2013). Accurate and rapid species authentication is the best way to combat this. Traditional methods usually require taxonomists, who are few in number, and moreover a fairly complete specimen, meaning they will not work on plant fragments sold as. The ITS2 barcode presented here solves this problem. The ITS2 is region is easy to amplify and sequence, has a short length, and reveals high interspecific variation (Chiou et al., 2007; China Plant Bol Group et al., 2011). While the ITS2 nucleotide sequences evolve quickly, their secondary structures are maintained by certain conserved motifs (Hershkovitz and Zimmer, 1996), which are very useful for sequence alignment (Mai and Coleman, 1997), especially when possible species are spread across many families, as is the case for some Traditional Chinese Medicines (Zhang et al., 2015). Meanwhile, the secondary structures of ITS2 can provide additional molecular morphological characteristics for better species discrimination (Grajales et al., 2007; Gu et al., 2013). Much research has been carried out using ITS2 to regulate the herbal medicine market (Zhang et al., 2015, 2016; Zhao et al., 2015; Zhu et al., 2017), and the current paper shows its effectiveness for LReR or "Gao-ben." Twenty-five commercial "Gao-ben" samples fell into three clades, corresponding to *L. sinense* + *L. jeholense*, *C. vaginatum*, and *M. yunnanensis* (**Figure 2A**). Surprisingly, more than half of the samples were derived from *C. vaginatum*. As mentioned above, whether *C. vaginatum* can be substituted for genuine "Gao-ben" is still controversial. Although *M. yunnanensis* is mainly cultivated and used in Yunnan province in the name of "Huang Gao-ben," its adulteration or substitution can cause confusion in identification and in therapeutic efficacy.

ITS2 has been proved to vary in sequence and secondary structure in a way that highly correlates with species taxonomy. Müller et al. (2007) compared the ITS2 secondary structure of 1373 species to their nearest relatives, and observed that in 93% of cases, if two taxa are different somewhere in their ITS2 by one CBC, they would be classified as different species. This criterion has been less commonly used for herbal medicine authentication. However, in our study, presence of a CBC distinguishes genuine "Gao-ben" from three other species, i.e., *L. delavayi*, *M. yunnanensis*, and *S. suave*, at least the last of which is sometimes sold as "Gao-ben." So, as a rapid, inexpensive, and informative DNA barcode, ITS2 could be widely used to regulate the herbal medicine market.

CONCLUSION

Traditional Chinese medicine is vulnerable to the replacement of the correct and most effective species with others that may be closely or distantly related. ITS2 could be an ideal candidate marker for authentication from both divergences of primary sequences and variations in secondary structures. This method is suitable for the identification of raw medicinal materials, but it is unsuitable for the authentication of heavily processed materials in which DNA degradation frequently occurs. A promising direction suitable for authentication of degraded material would be to combine the next generation sequencing (NGS)-based and species-specific PCR based methods (such as nucleotide signatures). During the process, knowing the secondary structure of ITS2 can help to locate the positions of the short motifs, that is well conserved within the species and develop nucleotide signatures.

AUTHOR CONTRIBUTIONS

Z-wL, Y-zG, and JZ collected the samples and carried out the experiments. Z-wL and JZ analyzed the data, conceived and designed the study, and wrote the manuscript. All authors have read and approved the final manuscript.

FUNDING

This work was supported by the National Natural Science Foundation of China (No. 31460052) and the United Research Foundation of Yunnan Science and Technology Department-Kunming Medical University (No. 2015FB014).

ACKNOWLEDGMENTS

We thank Richard I. Milne from The University of Edinburgh and David E. Boufford from Harvard University Herbaria for language polishing.

SUPPLEMENTARY MATERIAL

FIGURE S1 | Secondary structure of ITS2 in Ligustici Rhizoma et Radix (LReR) and its adulterants and substitutes. **(A)** LReR, **(B)** *L. acuminatum*, **(C)** *L. pteridophyllum*, **(D)** *L. tenuissimum*, **(E)** *Conioselinum vaginatum*, **(F)** *L. delavayi*, **(G)** *Sium suave*, and **(H)** *Meeboldia yunnanensis*. Red and blue arrows show the site of the compensatory base changes (CBCs) and hemi compensatory base changes (hCBCs) between LReR and its adulterants and substitutes, respectively.

TABLE S1 | Detailed information of samples used in this study.

REFERENCES

Chen, S., Yao, H., Han, J., Liu, C., Song, J., Shi, L., et al. (2010). Validation of the ITS2 region as a novel DNA barcode for identifying medicinal plant species. *PLoS One* 5:e8613. doi: 10.1371/journal.pone.0008613

China Plant Bol Group, Li, D. Z., Gao, L. M., Li, H. T., Wang, H., Ge, X. J., et al. (2011). Comparative analysis of a large dataset indicates that internal transcribed spacer (ITS) should be incorporated into the core barcode for seed plants. *Proc. Natl. Acad. Sci. U.S.A.* 108, 19641–19646. doi: 10.1073/pnas.1104551108

Chiou, S. J., Yen, J. H., Fang, C. L., Chen, H. L., and Lin, T. Y. (2007). Authentication of medicinal herbs using PCR-amplified ITS2 with specific primers. *Planta Med.* 73, 1421–1426. doi: 10.1055/s-2007-990227

Coleman, A. W. (2003). ITS2 is a double-edged tool for eukaryote evolutionary comparisons. *Trends Genet.* 19, 370–375. doi: 10.1016/S0168-9525(03)00118-5

Coleman, A. W. (2007). Pan-eukaryote ITS2 homologies revealed by RNA secondary structure. *Nucleic Acids Res.* 35, 3322–3329. doi: 10.1093/nar/gkm233

Coleman, A. W. (2015). Nuclear rRNA transcript processing versus internal transcribed spacer secondary structure. *Trends Genet.* 31, 157–163. doi: 10.1016/j.tig.2015.01.002

Coleman, A. W., and Mai, J. C. (1997). Ribosomal DNA ITS-1 and ITS-2 sequence comparisons as a tool for predicting genetic relatedness. *J. Mol. Evol.* 45, 168–177. doi: 10.1007/PL00006217

Commission, S. P. (2015). *Pharmacopoeia of the People's Republic of China Part I.* Beijing: China Medical Science and Technology Press.

Dai, B. (1988). Comparison of chemical constituents of essential oil from four species of Gaoben (Ligusticum) by GC-MS analysis. *Acta Pharm. Sin.* 23, 361–369.

Ding, L. W. (2010). The depletion price of Ligusticum resources has gone up all the way. *Modern Chin. Med.* 12, 46–48.

Doyle, J. J., and Doyle, J. L. (1987). A rapid DNA isolation procedure for small quantities of fresh leaf issue. *Phytochem. Bull.* 19, 11–15.

Elgavish, T., Cannone, J. J., Lee, J. C., Harvey, S. C., and Gutell, R. R. (2001). AA.AG@Helix. ends: A:A and A:G base-pairs at the ends of 16S and 23S rRNA helices. *J. Mol. Biol.* 310, 735–753. doi: 10.1006/jmbi.2001.4807

Floyd, R., Abebe, E., Papert, A., and Blaxter, M. (2002). Molecular barcodes for soil nematode identification. *Mol. Ecol.* 11, 839–850. doi: 10.1046/j.1365-294X.2002.01485.x

Grajales, A., Aguilar, C., and Sanchez, J. A. (2007).). Phylogenetic reconstruction using secondary structures of internal transcribed spacer 2 (ITS2, rDNA): finding the molecular and morphological gap in Caribbean gorgonian corals. *BMC Evol. Biol.* 7:90. doi: 10.1186/1471-2148-7-90

Gu, W., Song, J., Cao, Y., Sun, Q., Yao, H., Wu, Q., et al. (2013). Application of the ITS2 region for barcoding medicinal plants of selaginellaceae in pteridophyta. *PLoS One* 8:e67818. doi: 10.1371/journal.pone.0067818

Hall, T. A. (1999). BioEdit: a user-friendly biological sequence alignment editor and analysis program for Windows 95/98/NT. *Nucleic Acids Sym. Ser.* 41, 95–98.

Hebert, P. D. N., Cywinska, A., Ball, S. L., and Dewaard, J. R. (2003). Biological identifications through DNA barcodes. *Proc. Biol. Sci.* 270, 313–321. doi: 10.1098/rspb.2002.2218

Hershkovitz, M. A., and Zimmer, E. A. (1996). Conservation patterns in angiosperm rDNA ITS2 sequences. *Nucleic Acids Res.* 24, 2857–2867. doi: 10.1093/nar/24.15.2857

Hon, C. C., Chow, Y. C., Zeng, F. Y., and Leung, F. C. C. (2003). Genetic authentication of ginseng and other traditional Chinese medicine. *Acta Pharm. Sin.* 24, 841–846.

Joshi, K., Chavan, P., Warude, D., and Patwardhan, B. (2004). Molecular markers in herbal drug technology. *Curr. Sci.* 87, 159–165.

Keller, A., Förster, F., Müller, T., Dandekar, T., Schultz, J., and Wolf, M. (2010). Including RNA secondary structures improves accuracy and robustness in reconstruction of phylogenetic trees. *Biol. Direct* 5:4. doi: 10.1186/1745-6150-5-4

Keller, A., Schleicher, T., Schultz, J., Müller, T., Dandekar, T., and Wolf, M. (2009). 5.8S-28S rRNA interaction and HMM-based ITS2 annotation. *Gene* 430, 50–57. doi: 10.1016/j.gene.2008.10.012

Kjer, K. M. (1995). Use of rRNA secondary structure in phylogenetic studies to identify homologous positions: an example of alignment and data presentation from the frogs. *Mol. Phylogenet. Evol.* 4, 314–330. doi: 10.1006/mpev.1995.1028

Koetschan, C., Hackl, T., Müller, T., Wolf, M., Förster, F., and Schultz, J. (2012). ITS2 database IV: interactive taxon sampling for internal transcribed spacer 2 based phylogenies. *Mol. Phylogenet. Evol.* 63, 585–588. doi: 10.1016/j.ympev.2012.01.026

Kumar, S., Stecher, G., and Tamura, K. (2016). MEGA7: molecular evolutionary genetics analysis version 7.0 for bigger datasets. *Mol. Biol. Evol.* 33, 1870–1874. doi: 10.1093/molbev/msw054

Lalev, A. I., and Nazar, R. N. (1999). Structural equivalence in the transcribed spacers of pre-rRNA transcripts in *Schizosaccharomyces pombe*. *Nucleic Acids Res.* 27, 3071–3078. doi: 10.1093/nar/27.15.3071

Leontis, N. B., and Westhof, E. (2001). Geometric nomenclature and classification of RNA base pairs. *RNA* 7, 499–512. doi: 10.1017/S1355838201002515

Li, X. B. (2013). *Study on the Chemical Constituents of Conioselinui Rhizoma et Radix and Quality Evaluation of "Gaoben" Herbs.* [Master/ dissertation].Peking Union Medical College: [Beijing]

Li, X. B., Qi, Y. D., Liu, H. T., Zhang, J., Zhang, Z., Zhang, B. G., et al. (2013). Chemical constituents of *Conioselinum vaginatum*. *Chin. J. Chin. Mater. Med.* 38, 1543–1547.

Li, Y. S., Ye, X. W., Liao, X. R., Zhang, M., and Wang, Z. T. (2001). Textual studies of TCM gaoben (*Ligusticum L.*) habitually prescribing in Yunnan province. *Chin. Tradit. Herbal Drugs* 32, 257–259.

Mabberley, D. J. (1997). *THE PLANT-BOOK: A Portable Dictionary Of The Vascular Plants (2nf Edn).* Cambridge: Cambridge University Press.

Mai, J. C., and Coleman, A. W. (1997). The internal transcribed spacer 2 exhibits a common secondary structure in green algae and flowering plants. *J. Mol. Evol.* 44, 258–271. doi: 10.1007/PL00006143

Mishra, P., Kumar, A., Nagireddy, A., Mani, D. N., Shukla, A. K., Tiwari, R., et al. (2016). DNA barcoding: an efficient tool to overcome authentication challenges in the herbal market. *Plant Biotechnol. J.* 14, 8–21. doi: 10.1111/pbi.12419

Müller, T., Philippi, N., Dandekar, T., Schultz, J., and Wolf, M. (2007). Distinguishing species. *RNA* 13, 1469–1472. doi: 10.1261/rna.617107

Newmaster, S. G., Grguric, M., Shanmughanandhan, D., Ramalingam, S., and Ragupathy, S. (2013). DNA barcoding detects contamination and substitution in North American herbal products. *BMC Med.* 11:222. doi: 10.1186/1741-7015-11-222

Rao, G. X., Liu, Q. X., Dai, Z. J., Yang, Q., and Dai, W. S. (1995). Textual research for the traditional Chinese medicine radix peucedani and discussion of its modern varieties. *J. Yunnan Univ. Tradit. Chin. Med.* 18, 1–6.

Schultz, J., Maisel, S., Gerlach, D., Müller, T., and Wolf, M. (2005). A common core of secondary structure of the internal transcribed spacer 2 (ITS2) throughout the Eukaryota. *RNA* 11, 361–364. doi: 10.1261/rna.7204505

Seibel, P. N., Müller, T., and Dandekar, T. (2008). Synchronous visual analysis and editing of RNA sequence and structure alignments using 4SALE. *BMC Res. Notes* 1:91. doi: 10.1186/1756-0500-1-91

Seibel, P. N., Muller, T., Dandekar, T., Schultz, J., and Wolf, M. (2006). 4SALE - A tool for synchronous RNA sequence and secondary structure alignment and editing. *BMC Bioinform.* 7:498. doi: 10.1186/1471-2105-7-498

Sheh, M. L., and Watson, M. F. (2005). "Apiaceae lindley," in *Flora of China*, eds Z. Y. Wu and P. H. Raven (Beijing: Science Press), 1–205.

Telford, M. J., Wise, M. J., and Gowri-Shankar, V. (2005). Consideration of RNA secondary structure significantly improves likelihood-based estimates of phylogeny: examples from the bilateria. *Mol. Biol. Evol.* 22, 1129–1136. doi: 10.1093/molbev/msi099

Wang, J. H., Xu, L., Yang, L., Liu, Z. L., and Zhou, L. G. (2011). Composition, antibacterial and antioxidant activities of essential oils from *Ligusticum sinense* and *L. jeholense* (Umbelliferae) from China. *Rec. Nat. Prod.* 5, 314–318.

Wolf, M., Friedrich, J., Dandekar, T., and Müller, T. (2005). CBCAnalyzer: inferring phylogenies based on compensatory base changes in RNA secondary structures. *In Silico Biol.* 5, 291–294.

Xue, C. Y., Li, D. Z., Lu, J. M., Yang, J. B., and Liu, J. Q. (2006). Molecular authentication of the traditional Tibetan medicinal plant *Swertia mussotii*. *Planta Med.* 72, 1223–1226. doi: 10.1055/s-2006-951695

Ye, X. W., Zhao, Q., Li, Y. S., Liao, X. R., and Xue, Y. M. (2004). Analysis on chemical constituents of volatile oil from Heigaoben- *Ligusticum pteridophyllum* Franch. *J. Yunnan Univ. Tradit. Chin. Med.* 27, 40–41.

Zhang, W., Yang, S., Zhao, H., and Huang, L. Q. (2016). Using the ITS2 sequence-structure as a DNA mini-barcode: a case study in authenticating the traditional medicine "Fang Feng". *Biochem. Syst. Ecol.* 69, 188–194. doi: 10.1038/s41598-017-09769-y

Zhang, W., Yuan, Y., Yang, S., Huang, J. J., and Huang, L. Q. (2015). ITS2 secondary structure improves discrimination between medicinal "Mu Tong" species when using DNA barcoding. *PLoS One* 10:e0131185. doi: 10.1371/journal.pone.0131185

Zhao, S., Chen, X., Song, J., Pang, X., and Chen, S. (2015). Internal transcribed spacer 2 barcode: a good tool for identifying Acanthopanacis cortex. *Front. Plant Sci.* 6:840. doi: 10.3389/fpls.2015.00840

Zhou, J., Gong, X., Downie, S. R., and Peng, H. (2009). Towards a more robust molecular phylogeny of Chinese *Apiaceae* subfamily *Apioideae*: additional evidence from nrDNA ITS and cpDNA intron (rpl16 and rps16) sequences. *Mol. Phylogenet. Evol.* 53, 56–68. doi: 10.1016/j.ympev.2009.05.029

Zhou, J., and Liu, Z. W. (2018). Comparative morphology of the leaf epidermis in *Ligusticum* (Apiaceae) from china. *Am. J. Plant Sci.* 9, 1105–1123. doi: 10.4236/ajps.2018.96084

Zhou, J., Pu, F. D., Peng, H. J., Pan, Y. Z., and Gong, X. (2008). Karyological studies of ten *Ligusticum* species (Apiaceae) from the hengduan mountains region of china. *Caryologia* 61, 333–341. doi: 10.1080/00087114.2008.10589644

Zhu, R. W., Li, Y. C., Zhong, D. L., and Zhang, J. Q. (2017). Establishment of the most comprehensive ITS2 barcode database to date of the traditional medicinal plant rhodioloa (Crassulaceae). *Sci. Rep.* 7:10051. doi: 10.1038/s41598-017-09769-y

9

Interactions Between Emodin and Efflux Transporters on Rat Enterocyte by a Validated Ussing Chamber Technique

Juan Huang[1], Lan Guo[1], Ruixiang Tan[1], Meijin Wei[1], Jing Zhang[1], Ya Zhao[1], Lu Gong[1], Zhihai Huang[1] and Xiaohui Qiu[1,2]*

[1] The Second Clinical College of Guangzhou University of Chinese Medicine, Guangdong Provincial Hospital of Chinese Medicine, Guangzhou, China, [2] Guangdong Provincial Key Laboratory of Clinical Research on Traditional Chinese Medicine Syndrome, Guangzhou, China

*Correspondence:
Xiaohui Qiu
qiuxiaohui@gzucm.edu.cn

Emodin, a major active anthraquinone, frequently interacts with other drugs. As changes of efflux transporters on intestine are one of the essential reasons why the drugs interact with each other, a validated Ussing chamber technique was established to detect the interactions between emodin and efflux transporters, including P-glycoprotein (P-gp), multidrug-resistant associated protein 2 (MRP2), and multidrug-resistant associated protein 3 (MRP3). Digoxin, pravastatin, and teniposide were selected as the test substrates of P-gp, MRP2, and MRP3. Verapamil, MK571, and benzbromarone were their special inhibitors. The results showed that verapamil, MK571, and benzbromarone could increase digoxin, pravastatin, and teniposide absorption, and decrease their E_r values, respectively. Verapamil (220 μM) could significantly increase emodin absorption at 9.25 μM. In the presence of MK571 (186 μM), the P_{app} values of emodin from M-S were significantly increased and the efflux ratio decreased. With the treatment of emodin (185, 370, and 740 μM), digoxin absorption was significantly decreased while teniposide increased. These results indicated that emodin might be the substrate of P-gp and MRP2. Besides, it might be a P-gp inducer and MRP3 inhibitor on enterocyte, which are reported for the first time. These results will be helpful to explain the drug–drug interaction mechanisms between emodin and other drugs and provide basic data for clinical combination therapy.

Keywords: emodin, P-gp, MRP2, MRP3, Ussing chamber technique

INTRODUCTION

Emodin (1,3,8trihydroxy-6-methylanthraquinone), a major active anthraquinone, is naturally present in some herbs which have been wildly used in Oriental countries, such as *Rheum officinale* Baill., *Polygonum multijiorum* Thunb., *Polygonum cuspidatum* Sieb. Et Zucc., etc. (Dong et al., 2016). In the past decades, emodin has been shown a wide spectrum of biological and pharmacological effects, such as hepatoprotective antiviral, anti-diabetic, anti-bacterial, anti-allergic, anti-osteoporotic, immunosuppressive, and neuroprotective activities (Dong et al., 2016; Monisha et al., 2016). Recent studies have placed emodin back into the limelight, which exhibits a good prospect in anticancer treatment with its anticancer activities against several types of cancer cells, such as lung carcinoma, gastric carcinoma, pancreatic cancer, and breast cancer, with apoptosis, anti-angiogenesis, and anti-proliferation as possible mechanisms of action (Heo et al., 2010; Wei et al., 2013; Li et al., 2014; Cha et al., 2015). Mitoxantrone, a commonly used anticancer drug, is the prodrug of emodin (Riahi et al., 2008).

In recent years, drug–drug interactions between emodin and other drugs attracted more and more researchers' attention. Di et al. (2015) showed that piperine significantly improved the *in vivo* bioavailability of emodin and inhibited glucuronidation metabolism of emodin. Yu et al. (2017) demonstrated that 2,3,5,4'-tetrahydroxystilbene-2-β-D-glucoside could enhance the emodin absorption in a Caco-2 cell culture model. Meanwhile, many studies have shown synergistic effects between emodin and other antineoplastic drugs (Ko et al., 2010; Wang et al., 2010; Tan et al., 2011; Guo et al., 2013). Actually, changes of transporters on intestine affect the absorption characteristics of many drugs, which is one of the essential reasons why the drugs interact with each other. Some researchers have proved that emodin was the substrate of P-glycoprotein (P-gp) and multidrug-resistant associated protein 2 (MRP2; Teng et al., 2007, 2012; Liu et al., 2012). However, there were no reports about the research of emodin direct effects on intestinal transporters.

The Ussing chamber technique has been presently provided a physiologically relevant system for studying transepithelial transport of ion, drugs, and nutrients across various epithelial tissues. In this system, the drugs can be exposed at either mucosal or serosal levels, and therefore the absorption direction (M-S) and secretion direction (S-M) characteristics both can be detected. Furthermore, the usefulness of Ussing chambers for intestinal transport studies has long been recognized, and many researchers regard it as gold standards (Erik et al., 2016). Up to now, studies of P-gp influences in drug intestinal absorption by using this technique have been reported (Ballent et al., 2014; Xiao et al., 2016). However, there were few reports about testing and verifying this technique whether or not suitable for P-gp related studies. Moreover, other efflux transporters studies rarely reported by this technique.

In this study, a validated Ussing chamber technique was established and interaction studies between emodin and three efflux transporters including P-gp, MRP2, and multidrug-resistant associated protein 3 (MRP3) were carried out. To verify this Ussing chamber technique whether or not suitable for transepithelial transport studies related to efflux transporters, P-gp, MRP2, and MRP3 were employed as the typical proteins. Specific substrates and inhibitors were selected to detect P-gp, MRP2, and MRP3 activities and functions under our experimental conditions. Subsequently, interaction studies between emodin and these three efflux transporters were investigated. This is the first time to study the direct influence of emodin on rat intestinal P-gp, MRP2, and MRP3 functions by using this technique. It will be helpful to explain the drug–drug interaction mechanisms between emodin and other drugs and provide basic data for clinical combination therapy.

MATERIALS AND METHODS

Chemicals and Reagents

Standards of digoxin and pravastatin were purchased from Chendu Rui Fensi Biotechnology Co., Ltd. (Chengdu, China). Benzbromarone and teniposide were obtained from Guangzhou Feibo Biotechnology Co., Ltd. (Guangzhou, China). Verapamil, topotecan, etoposide, and MK571 were obtained from Dalian Mellon Biotechnology Co., Ltd. (Dalian, China). Ginsenoside Rg_1 and emodin were purchased from the National Institutes for Food and Drug Control (Beijing, China). Krebs' Ringer bicarbonate (KRB) buffer is composed by 114 mM NaCl, 10 mM Glucose, 1.25 mM $CaCl_2 \cdot 2H_2O$, 1.1 mM $MgCl_2 \cdot 6H_2O$, 5.03 mM KCl, 0.30 mM $NaH_2PO_4 \cdot H_2O$, 1.65 mM Na_2HPO_4, and 25 mM $NaHCO_3$ of pH 6.5 (Huang et al., 2016). Solvents were of HPLC grade and other chemicals used were of analytical grade.

Animals

The specific pathogen-free male Sprague–Dawley rats weighing 220 ± 20 g were obtained from Guangdong Medical Laboratory Animal Center (Guangzhou, China). Before starting the experiments, the rats were kept in an environmentally controlled breeding room (temperature: $22 \pm 1°C$, humidity: 50–70%) and fed standard laboratory food and water for 1 week. The animals were fasted overnight with free access to water before experiments. All animal studies were approved by the Institutional Animal Ethics Committee of Guangdong Provincial Hospital of Chinese Medicine.

Tissue Preparation

The four intestinal segments including duodenum, jejunum, ileum, and colon from anesthetized rats were immediately removed by surgery and washed with KRB solution. Each section of the intestinal segments was then placed in cold (on ice), bubbled ($O_2:CO_2$ 95:5) KRB buffer. The four intestinal segments were then cut into 2 cm pieces, respectively, and serosas were removed by blunt dissection. Peyer's patches were excluded from the experiment by visually identified. The stripped tissues were mounted in chambers with exposed surface area of 0.49 cm^2. Temperature of the chambers was maintained at $37 \pm 0.5°C$. Each of the half-cells in the chambers was filled with 5 mL fresh KRB buffer (pH 6.5). Tissue viability was continuously controlled by potential difference (PD). Tissue with electrical values less than 2 mV was refused (Moazed and Hiebert, 2007; Heinen et al., 2013).

Model Validation for Efflux Transporters' Studies

Digoxin, pravastatin, and teniposide were employed as the test substrates of P-gp, MRP2, and MRP3. Verapamil, MK571, and benzbromarone were inhibitors of these three efflux transporters (**Table 1**; Kool et al., 1999; Zhou et al., 2008; Ellis et al., 2013; Abbasi et al., 2016; Liu et al., 2017). The experiments were started after 30 min equilibration time, by changing

TABLE 1 | The substrates and inhibitors of P-gp, MRP2, and MRP3.

		SRM settings – ion pairs (m/z)				
	substrates			IS		Inhibitors
P-gp	Digoxin	779.147→475.447, 649.548		Ginsenoside Rg1	799.400→637.600	Verapamil
MRP2	Pravastatin	423.232→303.196, 321.138		Topotecan	422.082→320.016, 377.042	MK571
MRP3	Teniposide	674.241→383.235		Etoposide	606.213→229.242	Benzbromarone

The SRM settings of the substrates and specific internal standards (ISs) were performed by LC-MS/MS system.

the KRB buffer on both sides; 5 mL KRB solution with different test compounds was filled in the mucosal or serosal compartment; meanwhile, equal volume fresh buffer was added to the other compartment. In the inhibitory studies, the inhibitors verapamil, MK571, and benzbromarone were added to the mucosal side, respectively; 0.5 mL samples were withdrawn from the receiver compartment every 30 min and replaced with fresh KRB buffer. The bidirectional transport studies with specific inhibitors were assessed to validate this model whether or not suitable for P-gp, MRP2, and MRP3 studies. Samples were stored at –80°C until analysis (Deusser et al., 2013).

Interaction Studies Between Emodin and Efflux Transporters

In this study, the effects of the three efflux transporters on emodin intestinal absorption were investigated. Meanwhile, the influence of emodin on intestinal P-gp, MRP2, and MRP3 functions were also discussed. Solutions with three concentrations (low, middle, and high) of emodin were filled in the mucosal or serosal compartment to measure the bidirectional transport characteristic. In order to observe whether or which efflux transporters involved in emodin intestinal absorption process, verapamil, MK571, and benzbromarone were added to the mucosal side, respectively. In the emodin impact experiments, digoxin, pravastatin, and teniposide were employed as P-gp, MRP2, and MRP3 substrates.

Changes of the bidirectional transport characteristic were measured before and after adding emodin to the mucosal side.

Preparation of Perfusate Samples

Frozen samples were adequately vortexed after thawing at the room temperature; 10 μL suitable IS solution was added to 200 μL samples; 200 μL methanol was added after a thorough vortex mixing for 30 s. The mixtures were then vortexed for 30 s and centrifuged at 15,000 rpm for 30 min. Finally, 5 μL of supernatant was injected into the LC-MS/MS system.

Liquid Chromatographic and Mass Spectrometric Conditions

The quantifications of the compounds were performed by the TSQ Quantum Ultra Triple Quadrupole LC-MS/MS system from Thermo Fisher Scientific. Chromatography was carried out using an Agilent Poroshell 120 SB-C18 (2.7 μm, 2.1 mm × 100 mm) column with a Phenomenex AFO-8497 C_{18} pre-column, operating at 30°C. Adaptive gradient elution methods were applied for the analytes. The flow rate of the mobile phase was kept at 0.2 mL min^{-1}. Flow was directed to the ion spray interface. All measurements were carried out in negative ESI mode. Ion spray voltage was -2500 V. Vaporizer and capillary temperatures were set at 250 and 350°C,

TABLE 2 | The P_{app} of the test substances in perfused rat intestinal segments.

P_{app} (× 10^{-5} cm/s)	Segments	M-S		S-M	
		Control	With inhibitor	Control	With inhibitor
Digoxin (P-gp)	Duodenum	7.25 ± 3.28	4.53 ± 2.32	18.55 ± 14.38	7.97 ± 3.22
	Jejunum	5.78 ± 1.12	11.86 ± 5.85*	26.96 ± 12.49	9.64 ± 8.64*
	Ileum	4.31 ± 1.50	19.12 ± 9.05*	22.78 ± 13.60	15.71 ± 10.82
	Colon	6.31 ± 3.31	18.94 ± 3.43**	13.70 ± 6.63	19.11 ± 4.01
Pravastatin (MRP2)	Duodenum	12.45 ± 6.73	7.79 ± 1.48	28.73 ± 16.52	11.25 ± 5.27
	Jejunum	14.62 ± 3.94	10.70 ± 2.68	49.60 ± 22.56	12.72 ± 3.34**
	Ileum	12.23 ± 5.25	12.45 ± 6.79	67.84 ± 32.52	22.45 ± 14.09**
Teniposide (MRP3)	Jejunum	1.40 ± 0.44	3.72 ± 0.97**	3.35 ± 1.40	1.31 ± 0.64**
	Ileum	1.26 ± 0.77	2.80 ± 1.95	2.45 ± 1.00	1.03 ± 0.29*
	Colon	1.60 ± 1.11	2.83 ± 0.84	2.13 ± 1.19	0.83 ± 0.19*

*Digoxin (25 μM), pravastatin (47 μM), and teniposide (60 μM) were employed as the test substrates of P-gp, MRP2, and MRP3. Verapamil (220 μM), MK571 (186 μM), and benzbromarone (470 μM) were inhibitors of P-gp, MRP2, and MRP3. Each column represents the mean with SD of five measurements (*p < 0.05 and **p < 0.01, compared to the control according to independent samples t-test).*

respectively. Auto sampler temperature was set at 10°C. Sheath gas and aux gas were set at 30 and 15 Arb, respectively. The selective reaction monitoring (SRM) transitions were at m/z 268.934→225.047 for emodin and m/z 779.147→475.447 for ginsenoside Rg_1 [internal standard (IS)]. Other SRM settings

and specific IS are shown in **Table 1**. Peak integrations and calibrations were carried out using LC Quan 2.5.2 software from Thermo Fisher Scientific. All the data were within the acceptable limits to meet the guidelines for bioanalytical methods.

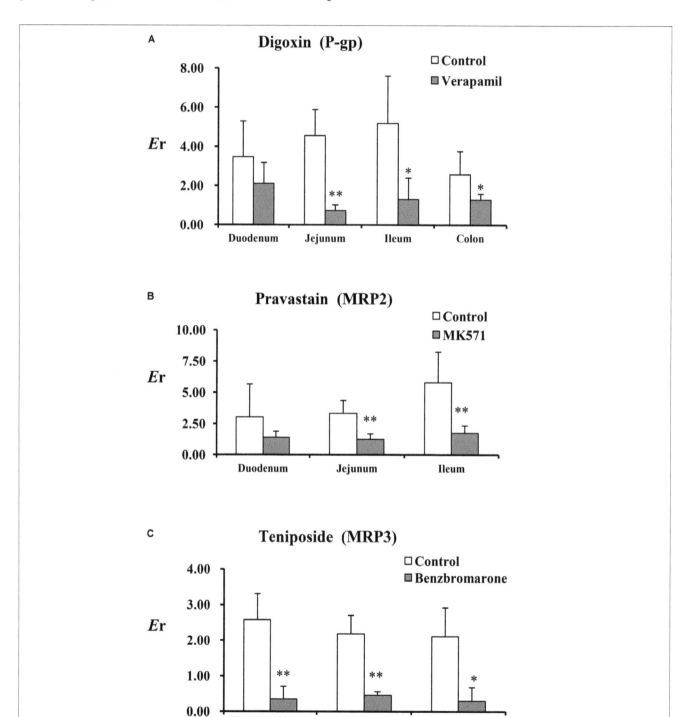

FIGURE 1 | The Er of the test substances in perfused rat intestinal segments. **(A)** Digoxin, **(B)** pravastatin, and **(C)** teniposide were employed as the test substrates of P-gp, MRP2, and MRP3. Verapamil, MK571, and benzbromarone were inhibitors of P-gp, MRP2, and MRP3. Each bar represents the mean with SD of five measurements (*$p < 0.05$ and **$p < 0.01$, compared to the control according to independent samples t-test).

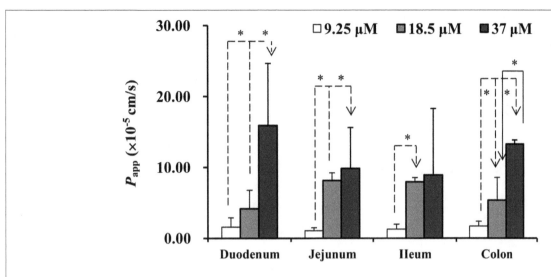

FIGURE 2 | The P_{app} of emodin from mucosal to the serosal side in different intestinal segments. Experiments were conducted at three concentrations (9.25, 18.5, and 36.5 μM). Each bar represents the mean with SD of five measurements (*$p < 0.05$, statistically significant differences among different concentrations, according to a one-way ANOVA test).

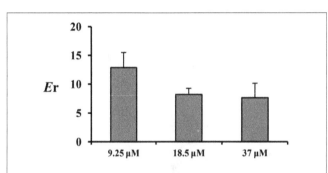

FIGURE 3 | The E_r of emodin in jejunum at three concentrations (9.25, 18.5, and 37 μM). Each bar represents the mean with SD of five measurements.

Data Analysis

The Q (accumulative quantity), P_{app} (apparent permeability), E_r (efflux ratio), P_r (P_{app} ratio), and E_{rr} (E_r ratio) across the excited rat intestinal segments in the Ussing chamber were calculated using the following equations (Li et al., 2012; Huang et al., 2016):

$$Q = 5C_n + 0.5 \sum_{i=1}^{n-1} C_i \qquad (1)$$

$$P_{app} = \frac{dQ/dt}{A \cdot C_0} \qquad (2)$$

$$E_r = \frac{P_{S-M}}{P_{M-S}} \qquad (3)$$

$$P_r = P_{app}/P_{app\,(control)} \qquad (4)$$

$$E_{rr} = E_r/E_{r\,(control)} \qquad (5)$$

where C_n (nM) is the concentration of the drug at the time point (n), Q (nM) is the accumulated absorption amount, A is the exposed surface area of the intestine (0.49 cm^2), dQ/dt (nM·s^{-1}) is the amount of the drug transported, and C_0 (nM) is the initial concentration of the test drug. Experiments were performed in batches, so control groups were set as one for each batch.

Statistical Analyses

The data are presented as the mean ± SD for all experiments. Independent samples t-test was applied to compare the means between treatments. One-way ANOVA with LSD (equal variances assumed) or Danett T3 (equal variances not assumed) multiple comparison (*post hoc*) tests were used to evaluate statistical differences. A p-value of less than 0.05 was considered statistical significance.

RESULTS

The PD Values for Rat Intestinal Segments

After 30 min equilibration time, PD was 7.16 ± 1.59, 7.23 ± 2.18, 6.50 ± 0.75, and 4.12 ± 0.69 mV for duodenum, jejunum, ileum, and colon, respectively. Obviously, the PD values were higher for small intestine segments under this experimental condition. In general, the PD slightly decreased by time when the chambers with small amount drugs (<200 μM).

Model Validation for Efflux Transporters' Studies Were Employed as the Test Substrates of P-gp, MRP2, and MRP3

The P_{app} and Er values of the test substances (digoxin, pravastatin, and teniposide) are summarized in **Table 2** and **Figure 1**. The results showed that the inhibitors, including verapamil, MK571, and benzbromarone, could significantly increase the absorption of the aforesaid substances and inhibit their secretion, and thus their Er values were decreased. In P-gp

validation study, the concentrations of the inhibitor (verapamil) were set at 220 and 440 µM for the small intestine segments and colon, respectively. It was observed that verapamil could

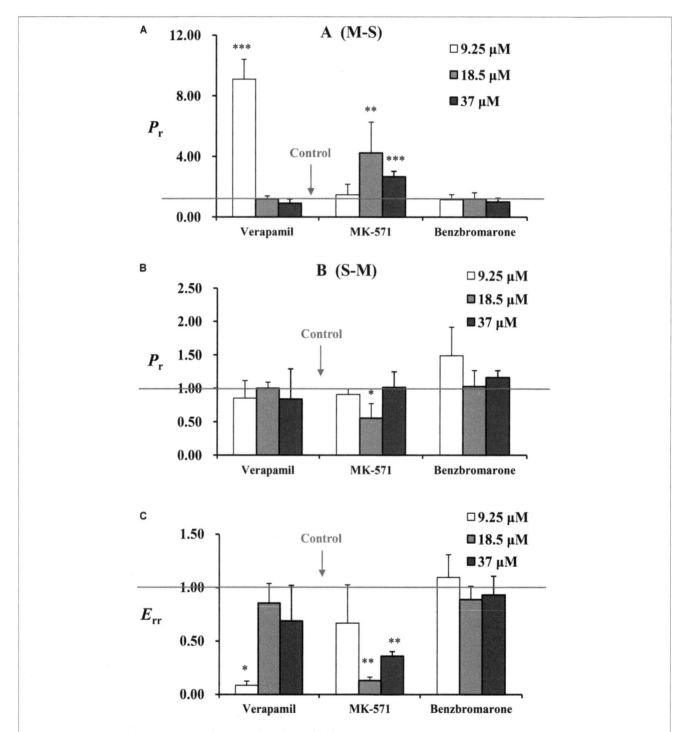

FIGURE 4 | The P_r from **(A)** M-S and **(B)** S-M and **(C)** E_{rr} of emodin at three concentrations (9.25, 18.5, and 37 µM) in jejunum. Experiments were performed in the presence of verapamil (220 µM), MK571 (186 µM), and benzbromarone (470 µM). The three inhibitors were loaded onto the mucosal side, respectively. For the experiments were performed in batches, control groups were set as one for each batch. The result represents the ratio of P_{app} or E_r between without or with inhibitor. Each bar represents the mean with SD of five measurements (*$p < 0.05$, **$p < 0.01$, and ***$p < 0.001$, compared to the control according to independent samples t-test).

TABLE 3 | The P_{app} from M-S and S-M of digoxin (25 μM), pravastatin (47 μM), and teniposide (60 μM) in the presence of emodin.

P_{app} (×10^{-5} cm/s)		Control	Emodin concentration (μM)		
			185	370	740
Digoxin	M-S	9.16 ± 4.10	5.58 ± 2.98	4.90 ± 1.28	2.04 ± 0.76**
	S-M	15.19 ± 4.39	25.66 ± 4.76*	46.09 ± 19.06*	14.16 ± 2.97
Pravastatin	M-S	6.45 ± 2.79	12.28 ± 1.99	10.63 ± 4.03	9.38 ± 2.87
	S-M	8.22 ± 4.04	7.03 ± 1.98	9.08 ± 1.27	10.48 ± 2.73
Teniposide	M-S	6.94 ± 1.75	6.32 ± 0.59	5.25 ± 0.73	9.11 ± 2.73
	S-M	8.18 ± 1.59	5.61 ± 0.57*	3.12 ± 1.32**	4.11 ± 0.62**

Emodin was loaded onto the mucosal side at three concentrations (185, 370, and 740 μM). Each column represents the mean with SD of five measurements (*p < 0.05 and **p < 0.01, compared to the control according to a one-way ANOVA with post hoc test).

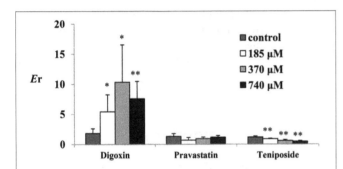

FIGURE 5 | The E_r of digoxin (25 μM), pravastatin (47 μM), and teniposide (60 μM) in the presence of emodin. Emodin was loaded onto the mucosal side at three concentrations (185, 370, and 740 μM). Each bar represents the mean with SD of five measurements (*p < 0.05 and **p < 0.01, compared to the control according to independent samples t-test).

significantly inhibit the effect of P-gp protein on jejunum, ileum, and colon. However, it was showed no statistic difference on duodenum after adding the inhibitor. These may be related to the distribution characteristic of P-gp on rat enterocyte. In MRP2 and MRP3 validation studies, the inhibitors MK571 (186 μM) and benzbromarone (470 μM) were also displayed significant inhibition effect on both jejunum and ileum. These results indicated that the Ussing chamber technique could be used to investigate the role of P-gp, MRP2, and MRP3 in drug intestinal transport studies. Though the distribution characteristics of the effluxes were different, both jejunum and ileum were suitable for the study. Finally, jejunum was chosen for further studies because of the most stable data it revealed during model validation research.

The Absorption Characteristics of Emodin

The absorption characteristics of emodin at three concentrations (9.25, 18.5, and 37 μM) in different intestinal segments were investigated. The intestinal absorption rates of emodin displayed no regioselectivity whereas the P_{app} values from M-S were very low at the lowest concentration (**Figure 2**). These indicated that some efflux transporters may involved in emodin intestinal transport. The E_r values of emodin in jejunum were all more than five at the three concentrations, pointing out that efflux

transporters were involved in emodin intestinal absorption (**Figure 3**).

Interaction Studies Between Emodin and Efflux Transporters

Transport studies were performed in the presence of P-gp, MRP2, and MRP3 inhibitors (verapamil, MK571, and benzbromarone) to determine the effect of these effluxes on the transport of emodin. The data are summarized in **Figure 4**. Verapamil (220 μM) could markedly increase emodin absorption and decrease the efflux ratio at 9.25 μM. In the presence of the MRP2 efflux transporter inhibitor MK571 (186 μM), the P_{app} values of emodin from mucosal to the serosal side were significantly increased and the efflux ratio decreased. However, no significant differences were observed in the presence of benzbromarone. These results indicated that emodin might be the substrate of P-gp and MRP2.

To investigate the role of emodin on the efflux transporters P-gp, MRP2, and MRP3 functions on rat enterocyte, digoxin, pravastatin, and teniposide were carried out for transport studies in the presence of emodin. With the treatment of emodin, the P_{app} values of digoxin from M-S significantly decreased while those from S-M increased. Thus, the E_r values of digoxin were significant higher after adding emodin. The date are summarized in **Table 3** and **Figure 5**. These results indicate that emodin could enhance P-gp function on rat jejunum. In the presence of emodin, the P_{app} from S-M and E_r of the MRP3 substrate teniposide remarkably decreased, indicating that emodin might be an MRP3 inhibitor. No significant differences were observed in the P_{app} and E_r values of pravastatin after emodin added.

DISCUSSION

Emodin, a potential antineoplastic drug, has been proved to have drug–drug interactions with many other drugs whereas the mechanisms have not yet to be discovered. Our results showed that emodin was the substrate of P-gp and MRP2, which is consistent with the literature reported (Teng et al., 2012; Zhang et al., 2012). Furthermore, we found that emodin might be a P-gp inducer and MRP3 inhibitor on enterocyte, which has not been reported in the literature before. However, verapamil only promoted emodin intestinal absorption at a low concentration; this is probably due to the fact that emodin itself is a P-gp inducer. MRP3, an efflux transporter, mainly distributes in liver, intestine, and adrenal glands, while most researches focused on its function and expression on liver. It is involved in the enterohepatic circulation of non-sulfated and sulfated bile salts such as glycocholates and taurocholates (Keppler, 2014, 2017). Our results showed that emodin might not be a substrate of MRP3 whereas it could inhibit MRP3 function on enterocyte, which indicated that the role of MRP3 should not be ignored in intestine. We consider that emodin might regulate MRP3 function by influencing the upstream proteins or kinases. Furthermore, we believe that oral administration of emodin would affect bile transport to some extent.

In this study, we used the Ussing chamber technique to evaluate the interactions between emodin and efflux transporters, which is regarded as gold standards for drug transport studies. The use of a living and intact intestinal tissue is more realistic than cell cultures and provides many advantages. The intestinal tissues are likely to express all the transporters and the enzymes at the same "physiological" level of expression. Moreover, the data obtained through rat intestine can be directly correlated to *in vivo* experiments that will be conducted in the same animal model (Mazzaferro et al., 2012; Sjögren et al., 2016). However, samples withdrawn from the receiver compartment often at very low concentration. With the development of LC-MS/MS technology, the amount of test compounds can easier to be detected. Besides, the procedure for tissue preparation is a technically challenging technique. KRB solution should be filtered with 0.22 μm filter and the removed intestine tissue should be placed in the cold KBR solution with gas in incessancy. Preparation must be done on ice carefully for it takes time and is associated with risks of tissue damage.

Although emodin has multiple pharmacological activities, its toxicity has attracted more and more attention in recent years. However, emodin treatment is a double-edged sword.

It showed protective effect on alcoholic liver injury while hepatotoxicity appeared with high doses and long-term drug delivery (Dong et al., 2009; Wang et al., 2011; Liu et al., 2014). We suspect that the changeable role of emodin may be related to the variation of intestinal environment, including intestinal transporters, structures, microorganisms, and so on. Therefore, it requires further study to find out the changes of environment *in vivo* and emodin disposition characteristics during long-term administration process.

CONCLUSION

In the present study, we have shown that the Ussing chamber technique was suitable for P-gp, MRP2, and MRP3 related studies on rat enterocyte. On the basis of this technique, we discovered that emodin might be the substrate of P-gp and MRP2, but not MRP3. Besides, emodin could decrease digoxin and increase teniposide absorption on rat intestine, indicating that emodin might be a P-gp inducer and MRP3 inhibitor.

AUTHOR CONTRIBUTIONS

JH and XQ designed the project. JH, LaG, RT, and MW performed the experiments. JH, LaG, RT, and XQ analyzed the data. JH, JZ, YZ, LuG, ZH, and XQ wrote the manuscript.

FUNDING

This research was supported by the National Natural Science Foundation of China (No. 81373967) and Science and Technology Planning Project of Guangdong Province (No. 2017B030314166).

REFERENCES

Abbasi, M. M., Valizadeh, H., Hamishehkar, H., and Zakeri-Milani, P. (2016). Inhibition of P-glycoprotein expression and function by anti-diabetic drugs gliclazide, metformin, and pioglitazone in vitro and in situ. *Res. Pharm. Sci.* 11, 177–186.

Ballent, M., Maté, L., Virkel, G., Sallovitz, J., Viviani, P., Lanusse, C., et al. (2014). Intestinal drug transport: ex vivo evaluation of the interactions between ABC transporters and anthelmintic molecules. *J. Vet. Pharmacol. Ther.* 37, 332–337. doi: 10.1111/jvp.12112

Cha, T. L., Chuang, M. J., Tang, S. H., Wu, S. T., Sun, K. H., Chen, T. T., et al. (2015). Emodin modulates epigenetic modifications and suppresses bladder carcinoma cell growth. *Mol. Carcinog.* 54, 167–177. doi: 10.1002/mc.22084

Deusser, H., Roqoll, D., Scheppach, W., Volk, A., Melcher, R., and Richling, E. (2013). Gastrointestinal absorption and metabolism of apple polyphenols ex vivo by the pig intestinal mucosa in the Ussing chamber. *Biotechnol. J.* 8, 363–370. doi: 10.1002/biot.201200303

Di, X., Wang, X., Di, X., and Liu, Y. (2015). Effect of piperine on the bioavailability and pharmacokinetics of emodin in rats. *J. Pharm. Biomed. Anal.* 115, 144–149. doi: 10.1016/j.jpba.2015.06.027

Dong, M. X., Jia, Y., Zhang, Y. B., Li, C. C., Geng, Y. T., Zhou, L., et al. (2009). Emodin protects rat liver from CCl₄- induced fibrogenesis *via* inhibition of hepatic stellate cells activation. *World J. Gastroenterol.* 15, 4753–4762.

Dong, X., Fu, J., Yin, X., Cao, S., Li, X., Lin, L., et al. (2016). Emodin: a review of its pharmacology, toxicity and pharmacokinetics. *Phytother. Res.* 30, 1207–1218. doi: 10.1002/ptr.5631

Ellis, L. C., Hawksworth, G. M., and Weaver, R. J. (2013). ATP-dependent transport of statins by human and rat MRP2/Mrp2. *Toxicol. Appl. Pharmacol.* 269, 187–194. doi: 10.1016/j.taap.2013.03.019

Erik, S., Johanna, E., Charlotta, V., Breitholtz, K., and Hilgendorf, C. (2016). Excised segments of rat small intestine in Ussing chamber studies: a comparison of native and stripped tissue viability and permeability to drugs. *Int. J. Pharm.* 505, 361–368. doi: 10.1016/j.ijpharm.2016.03.063

Guo, J., Li, W., Shi, H., Xie, X., Li, L., Tang, H., et al. (2013). Synergistic effects of curcumin with emodin against the proliferation and invasion of breast cancer cells through upregulation of miR-34a. *Mol. Cell. Biochem.* 382, 103–111. doi: 10.1007/s11010-013-1723-6

Heinen, C., Reuss, S., Saaler-Reinhardt, S., and Langguth, P. (2013). Mechanistic basis for unexpected bioavailability enhancement of polyelectrolyte complexes incorporating BCS class III drugs and carrageenans. *Eur. J. Pharm. Biopharm.* 85, 26–33. doi: 10.1016/j.ejpb.2013.03.010

Heo, S. K., Yun, H. J., Noh, E. K., and Park, S. D. (2010). Emodin and rhein inhibit LIGHT-induced monocytes migration by blocking of ROS production. *Vascul. Pharmacol.* 53, 28–37. doi: 10.1016/j.vph.2010.03.002

Huang, J., Zhang, J., Bai, J. Q., Bai, J., Xu, W., Wu, D., et al. (2016). LC-MS/MS Determination and interaction of the main components from the traditional Chinese drug pair Danshen-Sanqi based on rat intestinal absorption. *Biomed. Chromatogr.* 30, 1928–1934. doi: 10.1002/bmc.3768

Keppler, D. (2014). The roles of MRP2, MRP3, OATP1B1, and OATP1B3 in conjugated hyperbilirubinemia. *Drug Metab. Dispos.* 42, 561–565. doi: 10.1124/dmd.113.055772

Keppler, D. (2017). Progress in the molecular characterization of hepatobiliary transporters. *Dig. Dis.* 35, 197–202. doi: 10.1159/000450911

Ko, J. C., Su, Y. J., Lin, S. T., Jhan, J. Y., Ciou, S. C., Cheng, C. M., et al. (2010). Emodin enhances cisplatin-induced cytotoxicity via down-regulation of ERCC1 and inactivation of ERK1/2. *Lung Cancer* 69, 155–164. doi: 10.1016/j.lungcan.2009.10.013

Kool, M., van der Linden, M., de Haas, M., Scheffer, G. L., de Vree, J. M., Smith, A. J., et al. (1999). MRP3, an organic anion transporter able to transport anti-cancer drugs. *Proc. Natl. Acad. Sci. U.S.A.* 96, 6914–6919.

Li, H., Jin, H. E., Shim, W. S., and Shim, C. K. (2012). An improved prediction of the human in vivo intestinal permeability and BCS class of drugs using the in vitro permeability ratio obtained for rat intestine using an Ussing chamber system. *Drug Dev. Ind. Pharm.* 39, 1515–1522. doi: 10.3109/03639045.2012.714787

Li, W. Y., Ng, Y. F., Zhang, H., Guo, Z. D., Guo, D. J., Kwan, Y. W., et al. (2014). Emodin elicits cytotoxicity in human lung adenocarcinoma A549 cells through inducing apoptosis. *Inflammopharmacology* 22, 127–134. doi: 10.1007/s10787-013-0186-4

Liu, W., Feng, Q., Li, Y., Ye, L., Hu, M., and Liu, Z. (2012). Coupling of UDP-glucuronosyltransferases and multidrug resistance associated proteins is responsible for the intestinal disposition and poor bioavailability of emodin. *Toxicol. Appl. Pharmacol.* 265, 316–324. doi: 10.1016/j.taap.2012.08.032

Liu, Y., Chen, X., Qiu, M., Chen, W., Zeng, Z., and Chen, Y. (2014). Emodin ameliorates ethanol-induced fatty liver injury in mice. *Pharmacology* 94, 71–77. doi: 10.1159/000363413

Liu, Y., Liu, B., Zhang, Y., Peng, Y., Huang, C., Wang, N., et al. (2017). Intestinal absorption mechanisms of 2'-deoxy-2'-β-fluoro-4'-azidocytidine, a cytidine analog for AIDS treatment, and its interaction with P-glycoprotein, multidrug resistance-associated protein 2 and breast cancer resistance protein. *Eur. J. Pharm. Sci.* 105, 150–158. doi: 10.1016/j.ejps.2017.05.009

Mazzaferro, S., Bouchemal, K., Skanji, R., Gueutin, C., Chacun, H., and Ponchel, G. (2012). Intestinal permeation enhancement of docetaxel encapsulated into methyl-β-cyclodextrin/poly (isobutylcyanoacrylate) nanoparticles coated with thiolated chitosan. *J. Control Release* 162, 568–574. doi: 10.1016/j.jconrel.2012.08.005

Moazed, B., and Hiebert, L. M. (2007). An in vitro study with an Ussing chamber showing that unfractionated heparin crosses rat gastric mucosa. *J. Pharmacol. Exp. Ther.* 322, 299–305. doi: 10.1124/jpet.106.116939

Monisha, B. A., Kumar, N., and Tiku, A. B. (2016). Emodin and its role in chronic diseases. *Adv. Exp. Med. Biol.* 928, 47–73. doi: 10.1007/978-3-319-41334-1_3

Riahi, S., Reza Ganjali, M., Dinarvand, R., Karamdoust, S., Bagherzadeh, K., and Norouzi, P. (2008). A theoretical study on interactions between mitoxantrone as an anticancer drug and DNA: application in drug design. *Chem. Biol. Drug Des.* 71, 474–482. doi: 10.1111/j.1747-0285.2008.00653.x

Sjögren, E., Eriksson, J., Vedin, C., Breitholtz, K., and Hilgendorf, C. (2016). Excised segments of rat small intestine in Ussing chamber studies: a comparison of native and stripped tissue viability and permeability to drugs. *Int. J. Pharm.* 505, 361–368. doi: 10.1016/j.ijpharm.2016.03.063

Tan, W., Lu, J., Huang, M., Li, Y., Chen, M., Wu, G., et al. (2011). Anti-cancer natural products isolated from Chinese medicinal herbs. *Chin. Med.* 6:27. doi: 10.1186/1749-8546-6-27

Teng, Z., Yuan, C., Zhang, F., Huan, M., Cao, W., Li, K., et al. (2012). Intestinal absorption and first-pass metabolism of polyphenol compounds in rat and their transport dynamics in Caco-2 cells. *PLoS One* 7:e29647. doi: 10.1371/journal.pone.0029647

Teng, Z. H., Zhou, S. Y., Ran, Y. H., Liu, X. Y., Yang, R. T., Yang, X., et al. (2007). Cellular absorption of anthraquinones emodin and chrysophanol in human intestinal Caco-2 cells. *Biosci. Biotechnol. Biochem.* 71, 1636–1643.

Wang, J. B., Zhao, H. P., Zhao, Y. L., Jin, C., Liu, D. J., Kong, W. J., et al. (2011). Hepatotoxicity or hepatoprotection? Pattern recognition for the paradoxical effect of the Chinese herb *Rheum palmatum* L. in treating rat liver injury. *PLoS One* 6:e24498. doi: 10.1371/journal.pone.0024498

Wang, W., Sun, Y. P., Huang, X. Z., He, M., Chen, Y. Y., Shi, G. Y., et al. (2010). Emodin enhances sensitivity of gallbladder cancer cells to platinum drugs via glutathion depletion and MRP1 downregulation. *Biochem. Pharmacol.* 79, 1134–1140. doi: 10.1016/j.bcp.2009.12.006

Wei, W. T., Lin, S. Z., Liu, D. L., and Wang, Z. H. (2013). The distinct mechanisms of the antitumor activity of emodin in different types of cancer. *Oncol. Rep.* 30, 2555–2562. doi: 10.3892/or.2013.2741

Xiao, Q., Yang, W., Wang, D., Chen, L., Yuan, L., Ding, Y., et al. (2016). Factors limiting the extent of absolute bioavailability of pradefovir in rat. *Xenobiotica* 46, 913–921. doi: 10.3109/00498254.2015.1133866

Yu, Q., Jiang, L. L., Luo, N., Fan, Y. X., Ma, J., Li, P., et al. (2017). Enhanced absorption and inhibited metabolism of emodin by 2, 3, 5, 4'-tetrahydroxystilbene -2-O-β-D-glucopyranoside: possible mechanisms for Polygoni Multiflori Radix-induced liver injury. *Chin. J. Nat. Med.* 15, 451–457. doi: 10.1016/S1875-5364(17)30067-5

Zhang, Y., Wang, P., Wang, J. R., Yu, Y. P., and Meng, X. L. (2012). Study of intestinal absorption of emodin in one-way intestinal perfusion rat model. *Tradit. Chin. Drug Res. Clin. Pharmacol.* 23, 286–290.

Zhou, S. F., Wang, L. L., Di, Y. M., Xue, C. C., Duan, W., Li, C. G., et al. (2008). Substrates and inhibitors of human multidrug resistance associated proteins and the implications in drug development. *Curr. Med. Chem.* 15, 1981–2039.

10

Detection of Cistanches Herba (*Rou Cong Rong*) Medicinal Products Using Species-Specific Nucleotide Signatures

Xiao-yue Wang[1], Rong Xu[1], Jun Chen[1], Jing-yuan Song[1], Steven-G Newmaster[2], Jian-ping Han[1]*, Zheng Zhang[1]* and Shi-lin Chen[3]

[1] Key Laboratory of Bioactive Substances and Resources Utilization of Chinese Herbal Medicine, Ministry of Education, Institute of Medicinal Plant Development, Chinese Academy of Medicinal Science and Peking Union Medicinal College, Beijing, China, [2] NHP Research Alliance, Biodiversity Institute of Ontario (BIO), University of Guelph, Guelph, ON, Canada, [3] Key Laboratory of Beijing for Identification and Safety Evaluation of Chinese Medicine, Institute of Chinese Materia Medica, China Academy of Chinese Medical Sciences, Beijing, China

*Correspondence:
Jian-ping Han
jphan@implad.ac.cn
Zheng Zhang
zhangzheng321@126.com

Cistanches Herba is a medicinal plant that has tonification properties and is commonly used in Asia. Owing to the imbalance between supply and demand, adulterants are frequently added for profit. However, there is no regulatory oversight because quality control tools are not sufficient for identifying heavily processed products. Thus, a novel molecular tool based on nucleotide signatures and species-specific primers was developed. The ITS2 regions from 251 Cistanches Herba and adulterant samples were sequenced. On the basis of SNP sites, four nucleotide signatures within 30~37 bp and six species-specific primers were developed, and they were validated by artificial experimental mixtures consisting of six different species and different ratios. This method was also applied to detect 66 Cistanches Herba products on the market, including extracts and Chinese patent medicines. The results demonstrated the utility of nucleotide signatures in identifying adulterants in mixtures. The market study revealed 36.4% adulteration: 19.7% involved adulteration with *Cynomorium songaricum* or *Cistanche sinensis*, and 16.7% involved substitution with *Cy. songaricum, Ci. sinensis,* or *Boschniakia rossica*. The results also revealed that *Cy. songaricum* was the most common adulterant in the market. Thus, we recommend the use of species-specific nucleotide signatures for regulating adulteration and verifying the quality assurance of medicinal product supply chains, especially for processed products whose DNA is degraded.

Keywords: Cistanches Herba, Chinese patent medicine, nucleotide signature, degraded DNA, medicine quality control

INTRODUCTION

Cistanches Herba (*Rou Cong Rong*) is a well-known Pharmacopoeia-recorded medicine in Asia (Chinese Pharmacopoeia Commission, 2015; Japan Pharmacopeial Convention, 2016); this medicine is derived from the dried succulent stems of *Cistanche deserticola* Y. C. Ma or *Cistanche tubulosa* (Schenk) Wight. Cistanches Herba has been used for more than 3,000 years as a superior tonic, as it is not toxic and can be taken for long periods of time (Li et al., 2016). Furthermore, Cistanches Herba was bestowed with the honor of being named "Desert Ginseng" because of its great medicinal value, especially in strengthening male sexual function (Zhang and Su, 2014; Gu et al., 2016). There are more than 100 Chinese patent medicines recorded in the Chinese Pharmacopoeia Commission (2015) and in other local official promulgated standards (Wang et al., 2012). As the population of elderly individuals increases, there is considerable demand for Cistanches Herba and its medicinal products. However, raw material resources are becoming increasingly scarce. In fact, the two original species of Cistanches Herba have been added to the China Plant Red Data Book as state-protected wild plants (category II) (Fu, 1991). The medicinal materials on the market are mainly cultivated in northwestern China.

Owing to the considerable imbalance between the supply and demand of Cistanches Herba, many adulterants have entered the market; these adulterants are inconsistent with standards and can threaten drug security. The known adulterants include the dried succulent stems of *Cynomorium songaricum* Rupr. (Cynomorii Herba, *Suo Yang* in Chinese), *Cistanche sinensis* Beck, *Orobanche coerulescens* Stephan, and *Boschniakia rossica* (Cham. et Schlecht.) Fedtsch. et Flerov (Sun et al., 2012). These adulterants have morphological characteristics similar to those of Cistanches Herba, making traditional taxonomic identification difficult, particularly after the material is processed into medicinal products. Microscopic identification is not available because Cistanches Herba has no definitive or unique microscopic characteristics. Current analytical chemistry tools are not sufficient for detecting adulteration of Cistanches Herba because similar compounds also exist within the known adulterants *Ci. salsa* (Lei et al., 2001; Chen et al., 2007) and *Ci. sinensis* (Liu et al., 2013). Therefore, the development of a rapid molecular method for the authentication of Cistanches Herba and its products is urgently needed for proper quality control systems in Chinese patent medicine and other medicinal product industries.

Chen et al. first suggested internal transcribed spacer 2 (ITS2) as a universal barcode for medicinal plants (Chen et al., 2010). Sun et al. verified the ITS2 region as a preferable DNA barcode for identifying Cistanches Herba and its adulterants (Sun et al., 2012). However, ITS2 cannot be used to distinguish Chinese patent medicine with degraded DNA. Recently, an increasing number of studies have shown that the "mini barcode" is a useful method for amplifying degraded DNA (Hajibabaei et al., 2006; Meusnier et al., 2008; Dubey et al., 2011; Lo et al., 2015). However, nucleotide signatures are more appropriate than mini barcodes, as the formers refer to one or more nucleotides that are unique to one species and can be effectively utilized by many molecular techniques, such as DNA probes, microfluidics and loop-mediated isothermal amplification (de Boer et al., 2015). Han et al. developed nucleotide signatures for *Panax ginseng*, *Angelica sinensis* and *Lonicera japonica* and successfully identified the associated Chinese patent medicines (Liu et al., 2016; Wang et al., 2016a; Gao et al., 2017).

The goal of our research focused on the development of nucleotide signatures for the identification of adulterants in

functional products containing Cistanches Herba. Specifically, we (1) developed four nucleotide signatures and six specific primer pairs for differentiating authentic Cistanches Herba and known adulterants, (2) validated the four nucleotide signatures in experiments including mixtures of known taxonomic vouchers used to prepare Cistanches Herba products that contain both authentic and adulterated ingredients, and (3) performed a market survey of 66 Cistanches Herba products via their nucleotide signatures.

MATERIALS AND METHODS
Sample Collection and Preparation
In total, 251 samples were collected from Inner Mongolia, Xinjiang, and Ningxia, among other areas; these samples included 214 Cistanches Herba and 37 adulterants and are detailed in **Supplementary Table S1**. Corresponding voucher samples were validated by taxonomists and deposited in the Herbarium of the Institute of Medicinal Plant Development, Chinese Academy of Medical Sciences, Beijing, China. A total of 35 batches of powders, slices and extracts of Cistanches Herba were purchased from online stores and brick-and-mortar drugstores in Beijing and Chengdu (**Table 1**). In total, 31 batches of Chinese patent medicine containing Cistanches Herba were purchased from different drugstores (**Table 2**), and the declared compositions of different Chinese patent medicines are shown in **Supplementary Table S3**. The different morphological characteristics of different dose forms are shown in **Figure 1**.

Mixed samples: Powders of *Ci. deserticola*, *Ci. tubulosa*, *Cy. songaricum*, *Ci. sinensis*, *B. rossica*, and *O. coerulescens* were artificially mixed in different combinations (at a ratio of 1:1) before extraction. The details of these mixed samples are shown in the legend of **Figure 3**. In addition, the powders of four adulterants were mixed with the genuine *Ci. deserticola* at different weight ratios: 10:1, 50:1, 100:1, 200:1, 500:1, 1000:1, 2000:1, 5000:1, 10000:1, 15000:1, 20000:1, 25000:1, 30000:1, 40000:1, 50000:1 and 60000:1 (**Table 3**). And the two genuine products are mixed in the same proportions.

Decoction: Slices of *Ci. deserticola* and *Cy. songaricum* were used to prepare the decoction. The slices (10 g) were boiled in 300 mL of double-distilled water for 30, 60, 90, 120, 150, 180, 210, and 240 min and then used for DNA extraction.

DNA Extraction, Polymerase Chain Reaction (PCR) Amplification and Sequencing
Specimens, decoction, and mixed samples: The samples (40–50 mg) were ground into fine powders via a Retsch MM400 laboratory mixer mill (Retsch Co., Germany) at a frequency of 30 Hz. The genomic DNA was subsequently extracted with a Plant Universal Genomic DNA Kit (Tiangen Biotech Beijing Co., China) according to the manufacturer's instructions. ITS2 was amplified by the universal primers 2F/3R (Chen et al., 2010).

Extract and Chinese patent medicines: Samples (40–50 mg) were collected into a tube and then ground via a Retsch MM400 laboratory mixer mill (Retsch Co.). Ten samples were collected

TABLE 1 | Sample information and identification results of the 35 powders, medicinal slices, and extract.

Sample No.	Latin name of medicinal materials	Sample type	Collection site	Collection approach	Identification result
YC01	Cistanches Herba	Medicinal slices	Beijing	Offline	*Cynomorium songaricum*
YC05	Cistanches Herba	Medicinal slices	Chengdu, Sichuan	Offline	*Cistanche deserticola*
YC06	Cistanches Herba	Medicinal slices	Chengdu, Sichuan	Offline	*Cistanche tubulosa*
YC09	Cistanches Herba	Medicinal slices	Chengdu, Sichuan	Offline	*Cistanche deserticola*
YC11	Cistanches Herba	Medicinal slices	Chengdu, Sichuan	Offline	*Cistanche tubulosa*
YC13	Cistanches Herba	Medicinal slices	Chengdu, Sichuan	Offline	*Salvia miltiorrhiza*
YC17	Cistanches Herba	Medicinal slices	Chengdu, Sichuan	Offline	*Cistanche tubulosa*
YC24	Cistanches Herba	Medicinal slices	Anhui Bozhou Herb Market	Offline	*Cistanche deserticola*
YC25	Cistanches Herba	Medicinal slices	Anhui Bozhou Herb Market	Offline	*Cistanche deserticola*
YC26	Cistanches Herba	Medicinal slices	Anhui Bozhou Herb Market	Offline	*Cistanche tubulosa*
YC27	Cistanches Herba	Medicinal slices	Anhui Bozhou Herb Market	Offline	*Cistanche deserticola*
YC28	Cistanches Herba	Medicinal slices	Anhui Bozhou Herb Market	Offline	*Cistanche deserticola*
YC29	Cistanches Herba	Medicinal slices	Anhui Bozhou Herb Market	Offline	*Cistanche deserticola*
YC30	Cistanches Herba	Medicinal slices	Anhui Bozhou Herb Market	Offline	*Cistanche tubulosa*
YC31	Cistanches Herba	Medicinal slices	Anhui Bozhou Herb Market	Offline	*Cistanche deserticola*
YC32	Cistanches Herba	Medicinal slices	Anhui Bozhou Herb Market	Offline	*Cistanche deserticola*
YC33	Cistanches Herba	Medicinal slices	Anhui Bozhou Herb Market	Offline	*Cistanche tubulosa*
YC34	Cistanches Herba	Medicinal slices	Anhui Bozhou Herb Market	Offline	*Cistanche deserticola*
YC35	Cistanches Herba	Medicinal slices	Anhui Bozhou Herb Market	Offline	*Cistanche deserticola*
YC36	Cistanches Herba	Medicinal slices	Anhui Bozhou Herb Market	Offline	*Cistanche deserticola*
YC37	Cistanches Herba	Medicinal slices	Anhui Bozhou Herb Market	Offline	*Cistanche deserticola*
YC38	Cistanches Herba	Medicinal slices	Anhui Bozhou Herb Market	Offline	*Cistanche deserticola*
YC39	Cistanches Herba	Medicinal slices	Anhui Bozhou Herb Market	Offline	*Cistanche tubulosa*
YC40	Cistanches Herba	Medicinal slices	Anhui Bozhou Herb Market	Offline	*Cistanche tubulosa*
YC41	Cistanches Herba	Medicinal slices	Anhui Bozhou Herb Market	Offline	*Cistanche tubulosa*
YC42	Cistanches Herba	Medicinal slices	Anhui Bozhou Herb Market	Offline	*Cistanche tubulosa*
YC43	Cistanches Herba	Medicinal slices	Anhui Bozhou Herb Market	Offline	*Cistanche tubulosa*
YC03	Cistanches Herba	Powder	Anhui Bozhou Herb Market	Online	*Cynomorium songaricum*
YC04	Cistanches Herba	Powder	Anhui Bozhou Herb Market	Online	*Cistanche deserticola, Cistanche tubulosa, Cynomorium songaricum, Cistanche sinensis*
YC18	Cistanches Herba	Powder	Anhui Bozhou Herb Market	Online	*Cistanche deserticola, Cistanche tubulosa, Cynomorium songaricum, Cistanche sinensis*
YC19	Cistanches Herba	Powder	Anhui Bozhou Herb Market	Online	*Cistanche tubulosa, Cynomorium songaricum, Cistanche sinensis*
YC20	Cistanches Herba	Powder	Anhui Bozhou Herb Market	Online	*Cistanche deserticola, Cistanche tubulosa, Cynomorium songaricum*
YC21	Cistanches Herba	Powder	Anhui Bozhou Herb Market	Online	*Cistanche deserticola, Cistanche tubulosa, Cynomorium songaricum, Cistanche sinensis*
YC22	Cistanches Herba	Powder	Anhui Bozhou Herb Market	Online	*Cistanche sinensis, Cistanche tubulosa, Cynomorium songaricum*
YC23	Cistanches Herba	Extract	Dalian, Liaoning	Online	*Cistanche sinensis*

in parallel per batch. The Chinese patent medicine powder was washed with 700 μL of prewash buffer [100 mM Tris-HCl, pH 8.0; 20 mM ethylenediaminetetraacetic acid (EDTA), pH 8.0; 700 mM NaCl; 2% polyvinylpyrrolidone (PVP)-40; and 0.4% β-mercaptoethanol] several times until the supernatant was clear and colorless, after which the mixture was centrifuged at 7500 × g for 5 min at room temperature. The precipitate was subsequently used to extract the genomic DNA via the Plant Universal Genomic DNA Kit (Tiangen Biotech Beijing Co.) according to the manufacturer's instructions. In the end, DNA from each batch was concentrated into one tube.

Six species-specific primer pairs—SYF1/SYR1, HMRCF/HMRCR, GHRCF/GHRCR, CCRF/CCRR, SCRF/SCRR, and LDF/LDR—were designed via Primer Premier

TABLE 2 | Identification results of Chinese patent medicines based on the nucleotide signatures.

Sample no.	Sample name	Collection site	Collection approach	Identification results of the related species
ZCY16	Shihu Yeguang pills	Beijing	Offline	*Cynomorium songaricum, Cistanche deserticola*
ZCY26	Shihu Yeguang pills	Beijing	Offline	*Cynomorium songaricum*
ZCY29	Wenweishu particles	Shanghai	Online	*Cynomorium songaricum*
ZCY33	Shihu Yeguang pills	Taiyuan, Shanxi	Online	*Cynomorium songaricum, Cistanche tubulosa*
ZCY34	Shihu Yeguang pills	Shaoguan, Guangdong	Online	*Cistanche tubulosa*
ZCY35	Sanbao capsules	Shaoguan, Guangdong	Online	*Cynomorium songaricum, Cistanche deserticola, Cistanche sinensis*
ZCY40	Kangguzhi Zengsheng pills	Shaoguan, Guangdong	Online	*Cynomorium songaricum*
ZCY41	Kanggu Zengsheng pills	Shaoguan, Guangdong	Online	*Cynomorium songaricum, Cistanche tubulosa*
ZCY44	Shihu Yeguang pills	Changsha, Hunan	Online	*Cynomorium songaricum*
ZCY48	Shihu Yeguang pills	Beijing	Online	*Cynomorium songaricum*
ZCY51	Shihu Yeguang pills	Dezhou, Shandong	Offline	*Cistanche tubulosa*
ZCY53	Shihu Yeguang pills	Dezhou, Shandong	Offline	*Cistanche deserticola*
ZCY55	Shihu Yeguang pills	Dezhou, Shandong	Offline	*Boschniakia rossica*
ZCY56	Shihu Yeguang pills	Dezhou, Shandong	Offline	*Cistanche tubulosa*
ZCY57	Shihu Yeguang pills	Guangzhou, Guangdong	Offline	*Boschniakia rossica*
ZCY58	Shihu Yeguang pills	Guangzhou, Guangdong	Online	*Cistanche tubulosa*
ZCY63	Yucong Qiangshen capsules	Guangzhou, Guangdong	Online	*Cistanche deserticola, Cistanche tubulosa*
ZCY64	Shihu Yeguang pills	Shenzhen, Guangdong	Offline	*Cynomorium songaricum, Cistanche deserticola*
ZCY65	Shihu Yeguang pills	Shenzhen, Guangdong	Offline	*Cistanche deserticola*
ZCY66	Wenweishu capsules	Beijing	Offline	*Cistanche deserticola*
ZCY69	Shihu Yeguang pills	Wenzhou, Zhejiang	Online	*Cistanche deserticola, Cistanche tubulosa*
ZCY70	Shihu Yeguang pills	Jiaxing, Zhejiang	Online	*Cistanche deserticola, Cistanche tubulosa*
ZCY71	Shihu Yeguang pills	Jiaxing, Zhejiang	Online	*Cistanche tubulosa*
ZCY72	Shihu Yeguang pills	Guangzhou, Guangdong	Offline	*Cistanche tubulosa*
ZCY74	Shihu Yeguang pills	Kunming, Yunnan	Online	*Cynomorium songaricum, Cistanche tubulosa*
ZCY79	Sanbao capsules	Dongguan, Guangdong	Online	*Cynomorium songaricum*
ZCY85	Shihu Yeguang pills	Bozhou, Anhui	Offline	*Cistanche tubulosa*
ZCY92	Shihu Yeguang pills	Chengdu, Sichuan	Offline	*Cistanche tubulosa*
ZCY94	Sanbao capsules	Chengdu, Sichuan	Offline	*Cynomorium songaricum, Cistanche deserticola, Cistanche sinensis*
ZCY95	Shihu Yeguang pills	Chengdu, Sichuan	Offline	*Cistanche tubulosa*
ZCY96	Shihu Yeguang pills	Chengdu, Sichuan	Offline	*Cistanche tubulosa*

6.0 software (Premier Co., Canada) to amplify Cistanches Herba and its adulterants (the details are shown in **Table 4**). PCR was performed in a 50 μL-volume reaction containing 1 μL of KOD FX (Toyobo Co., Japan), 25 μL of 2 × PCR buffer, 10 μL of dNTPs (2 mM), 1.5 μL of each primer (10 μM), and 4 μL (~50 ng) of DNA template; the remaining volume consisted of double-distilled water. The reactions were performed by a thermal cycler (Veriti™ 96-Well Thermal Cycler, Applied Biosystems Co., USA); the thermal programs are listed in **Table 4**. The PCR products were examined via 3% agarose gel electrophoresis and purified for bidirectional sequencing with an ABI 3730XL sequencer (Applied Biosystems Co.) in accordance with the Sanger sequencing method. Then, the sensitivity of the six primers was tested via the quantitative real-time PCR (qRT-PCR) assay with a CFX96 Real-time System (Bio-rad Lab., USA). The cycle thresholds were automatically calculated by the system via the "PCR Baseline Subtracted Curve Fit" model. qRT-PCR was performed in a 15 μL-volume reaction containing 7.5 μL of SYBR® *Premix Ex Taq*™ (Tli RNaseH Plus) (Takara Bio Co., Japan), 1.0 μL of each primer (10 μM), and 1.0 μL of DNA template with the remaining volume consisting of double-distilled water. The qRT-PCR was performed with three technical replicates based on which standard error was calculated.

Sequence analysis: The sequences were edited and manually assembled via CodonCode Aligner 5.1.4 (CodonCode Co., USA).

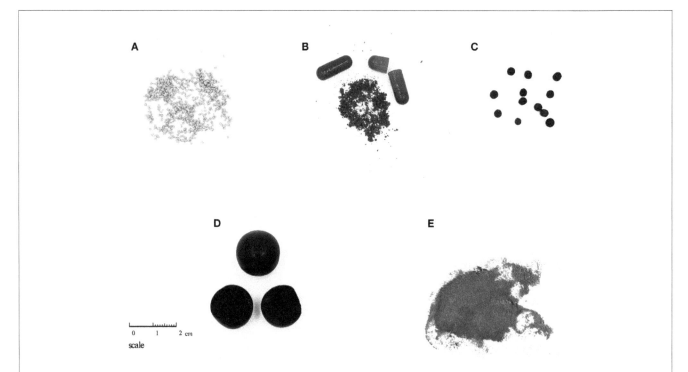

FIGURE 1 | Different morphological characteristics of different dose forms of Cistanches Herba products. **(A)** Particles (ZCY29, Wenweishu particles); **(B)** Capsules (ZCY35, Sanbao capsules); **(C)** Water honeyed pills (ZCY70, Shihu Yeguang pills); **(D)** Large honeyed pills (ZCY48, Shihu Yeguang pills); **(E)** Extracts (YC23).

ITS sequences from GenBank were annotated via the Hidden Markov model (HMM) to obtain the ITS2 sequences (Keller et al., 2009). The sequences were then aligned by MEGA 5.0 software via the "Muscle" alignment method (Edgar, 2004; Tamura et al., 2011).

RESULTS

Development of Nucleotide Signatures and Species-Specific Primer Pairs for Cistanches Herba and Adulterants

The PCR amplification and sequencing success rates of the 251 samples were 100% when the primer pair 2F/3R was used. The aligned length of the *Cy. songaricum* ITS2 sequences was 229 bp (**Supplementary Figure S1**). Analysis of the sequences from the herbarium species and those of closely related species retrieved from GenBank (**Supplementary Table S2**) revealed two single nucleotide polymorphism (SNP) sites for *Cy. songaricum*. On the basis of the SNPs, one *Cy. songaricum*-specific 30-bp nucleotide signature (5′-caattatttg aggtgcattg taagaagcgt-3′) was developed (**Figure 2A**). Basic Local Alignment Search Tool (BLAST) results in NCBI demonstrated that this nucleotide signature was unique to *Cy. songaricum* (**Table 5**). With the similar analysis of the sequences from closely related species, one to two SNPs were discovered from *Ci. sinensis*, *B. rossica* and *O. coerulescens*. On the basis of the SNPs, the nucleotide signatures for the other three adulterants were also developed similarly, including a 34 bp signature (5′-cgatggtctc ccgtgcgcga

ggatgcacgg ccgg-3′) for *Ci. sinensis*, a 37 bp signature (5′-acactggcct cccgtgcgca acgacgtgcg gccggtc-3′) for *B. rossica*, and a 31 bp signature (5′-gtctgtcgtg tcggatggtg ttgcttgttg g-3′) for *O. coerulescens* (**Figures 2B–D**). BLAST analysis in NCBI also revealed that these nucleotide signatures were specific and not present in any other species (**Table 5**).

Cistanches Herba and its adulterants could be amplified simultaneously from mixtures via the 2F/3R universal primer pair. Thus, we designed species-specific primers for nucleotide signature amplification by aligning the ITS2 sequences. Four specific primer pairs—SYF1/SYR1, CCRF/CCRR, SCRF/SCRR, and LDF/LDR—were designed to amplify the nucleotide signatures of *Cy. songaricum*, *B. rossica*, *Ci. sinensis*, and *O. coerulescens*, respectively (**Table 4**). The lengths of the amplicons were 123, 72, 131, and 71 bp, respectively.

In addition, a total of 214 ITS2 sequences from experimental Cistanches Herba materials were analyzed. Two short specific primers—HMRCF/HMRCR and GHRCF/GHRCR for *Ci. deserticola* and *Ci. tubulosa*, respectively—were designed to amplify the short regions of the degraded samples(**Table 4**). The lengths of the amplicons were 132 and 134 bp, respectively.

Validation of the Nucleotide Signature and Species-Specific Primer Method Based on Artificial Mixtures and Decoction

The amplification efficiencies of the new primer pairs were validated from the mixture. PCR products were obtained via each primer pair for each targeted species, as shown

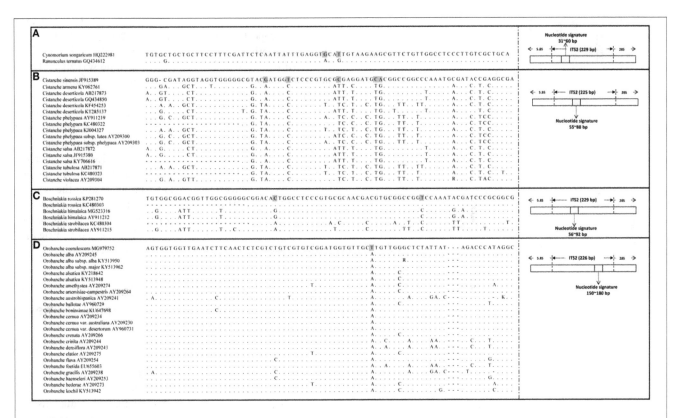

FIGURE 2 | DNA sequence alignment results and SNP sites of the four nucleotide signatures. **(A)** Alignment of *Cynomorium songaricum* nucleotide signature with its region location in ITS2; **(B)** Alignment of *Cistanche sinensis* nucleotide signatures with its region location in ITS2; **(C)** Alignment of *Boschniakia rossica* nucleotide signature with its region location in ITS2; **(D)** Alignment of *Orobanche coerulescens* nucleotide signature with its region location in ITS2. The highlighted regions represent nucleotide signature regions and the marked bases represent the SNP sites of each nucleotide signature, the dots represent identical nucleotides.

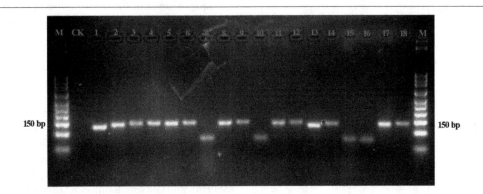

FIGURE 3 | Gel image of the products of PCR amplification of the mixed powders. With the exception of the lanes marked M (marker) and CK (negative control), the other 13 lanes contain the PCR products of the mixtures. Lanes 1–3 are a mixture of *Cy. songaricum*, *Ci. deserticola* and *Ci. tubulosa* amplified with the primers SYF1/SYR1, HMRCF/HMRCR, and GHRCF/GHRCR, respectively; lanes 4–6 are a mixture of *Ci. sinensis*, *Ci. deserticola*, and *Ci. tubulosa* amplified with the primers SCRF/SCRR, HMRCF/HMRCR, and GHRCF/GHRCR, respectively; lanes 7–9 are a mixture of *B. rossica*, *Ci. deserticola*, and *Ci. tubulosa* amplified with the primers CCRF/CCRR, HMRCF/HMRCR, and GHRCF/GHRCR, respectively; lanes 10–12 are a mixture of *O. coerulescens*, *Ci. deserticola*, and *Ci. tubulosa* amplified with the primers LDF/LDR, HMRCF/HMRCR, and GHCRF/GHRCR, respectively; and lanes 13–18 are a mixture of *Cy. songaricum*, *Ci. sinensis*, *B. rossica*, *O. coerulescens*, *Ci. deserticola*, and *Ci. tubulosa* with the primers SYF1/SYR1, SCRF/SCRR, CCRF/CCRR, LDF/LDR, HMRCF/HMRCR, and GHCRF/GHRCR, respectively.

in **Figure 3**. For instance, the fifth mixture sample is a mixture of Cistanches Herba and its four adulterants, and each species could be amplified with the primers SYF1/SYR1, SCRF/SCRR, CCRF/CCRR, LDF/LDR, HMRCF/HMRCR, and GHRCF/GHRCR. Moreover, the amplification regions were

sequenced, and the nucleotide signatures were observed within the target sequences. Furthermore, to measure the sensitivity, mixtures of two of the six samples were created at different weight ratios and the sample with lower proportion was amplified by specific primer pairs via qRT-PCR. As shown in **Table 3**,

TABLE 3 | qRT-PCR Cq values with standard deviation for mixtures at different sample weight ratios.

Detected species	Sample composition of mixture	Cq values with standard deviation of different sample weight ratios							
		10:1	50:1	100:1	200:1	500:1	1000:1	2000:1	5000:1
Cy. songaricum	Ci. deserticola: Cy. songaricum	24.92 ± 0.188	27.1 ± 0.022	27.81 ± 0.147	29.24 ± 0.394	30.47 ± 0.304	31.39 ± 0.561	31.42 ± 0.406	32.46 ± 0.862
Ci. sinensis	Ci. deserticola: Ci. sinensis	23.64 ± 0.078	26.00 ± 0.101	27.07 ± 0.155	28.26 ± 0.109	29.46 ± 0.066	30.47 ± 0.125	31.36 ± 0.101	33.36 ± 0.190
B. rossica	Ci. deserticola: B. rossica	18.27 ± 0.138	21.32 ± 0.821	22.28 ± 0.033	25.78 ± 0.031	26.25 ± 0.031	27.22 ± 0.052	29.33 ± 0.823	30.45 ± 0.262
O. coerulescens	Ci. deserticola: O. coerulescens	19.07 ± 0.022	21.34 ± 0.030	22.53 ± 0.105	23.77 ± 0.111	25.16 ± 0.089	26.36 ± 0.098	27.30 ± 0.164	29.25 ± 0.049
Ci. tubulosa	Ci. deserticola: Ci. tubulosa	24.05 ± 0.145	26.93 ± 0.176	27.97 ± 0.044	29.56 ± 0.161	30.60 ± 0.338	31.18 ± 0.090	32.25 ± 0.122	33.70 ± 0.222
Ci. deserticola	Ci. tubulosa: Ci. deserticola	23.93 ± 0.165	25.06 ± 0.155	26.25 ± 0.093	28.05 ± 0.085	29.07 ± 0.163	30.04 ± 0.194	31.82 ± 0.107	32.90 ± 0.424

Detected species	Sample composition of mixture	10000:1	15000:1	20000:1	25000:1	30000:1	40000:1	50000:1	60000:1
Cy. songaricum	Ci. deserticola: Cy. songaricum	34.48 ± 0.255	35.83 ± 0.328	None	None	None	None	None	None
Ci. sinensis	Ci. deserticola: Ci. sinensis	34.33 ± 0.214	35.45 ± 0.125	36.26 ± 0.756	None	None	None	None	None
B. rossica	Ci. deserticola: B. rossica	31.98 ± 0.804	32.79 ± 0.361	33.80 ± 0.550	35.46 ± 0.886	37.08 ± 0.162	None	None	None
O. coerulescens	Ci. deserticola: O. coerulescens	30.01 ± 0.260	31.36 ± 0.284	32.84 ± 0.338	33.52 ± 0.215	36.38 ± 0.459	36.16 ± 0.509	None	None
Ci. tubulosa	Ci. deserticola: Ci. tubulosa	34.90 ± 0.603	35.95 ± 0.470	36.48 ± 0.501	None	None	None	None	None
Ci. deserticola	Ci. tubulosa: Ci. deserticola	35.17 ± 0.183	35.23 ± 0.544	36.25 ± 0.279	None	None	None	None	None

cq values of *B. rossica* or *O. coerulescens* could be obtained even the proportion of samples was 30000:1 or 40000:1, and the amplification results of *Ci. sinensis, Ci. tubulosa,* and *Ci deserticola* could be detected when the ratio was 20000:1. But no detectable results could be obtained for *Cy. songaricum* when it constituted the proportion of 20000:1.

To verify whether the nucleotide signature method functions with processed materials, decoctions of *Ci. deserticola* and *Cy. songaricum* were prepared. The results showed that the short barcode from *Ci. deserticola* could be amplified, even after the samples were boiled for 210 min. In addition, the nucleotide signature of *Cy. songaricum* could be amplified after the samples were boiled for 150 min, while no PCR products were detected after the samples were boiled for 210 or 240 min (**Figure 4**). The sequencing results demonstrated that the short nucleotide signature was successfully obtained from the decoction.

Market Survey of Adulteration via Nucleotide Signature and Specific Primers

The above method was applied for the detection of Cistanches Herba products on the market. Thirty five batches of Cistanches Herba slices, powders and extracts were amplified and sequenced by using six designed specific primers (the agarose gel electrophoresis results are shown in **Supplementary Figure S2** and the sequences are listed in **Supplementary Data Sheet 1**). Analysis of the sequences via their nucleotide signatures revealed that five batches of slices were authentic. One slice batch and one powder batch were substituted with *Cy. songaricum*, and one extract was substituted with *Ci. sinensis*. The other six batches of powders were mixtures: five were adulterated with *Cy. songaricum* and *Ci. sinensis*, and one was adulterated with *Cy. songaricum* (**Table 1**). In addition, one slice batch was substituted with *Salvia miltiorrhiza*.

The Cistanches Herba in Chinese patent medicines is subjected to various processes that make authentication difficult. The ability of the six primer pairs to amplify the species-specific nucleotide signature regions from the Chinese patent medicines was tested (the agarose gel electrophoresis results are shown in **Supplementary Figure S2**). Most Chinese patent medicines contain components of different types of species. For example, Shihu Yeguang pills (ZCY34) contain 25 ingredients, including Cistanches Herba (*Rou Cong Rong*), Dendrobii Caulis (*Shi Hu*), and Ginseng Radix et Rhizoma (*Ren Shen*). From these ingredients, Cistanches Herba could be amplified specifically via the primer pair GHRCF/GHRCR. Direct sequencing of the PCR products revealed very clean traces. However, a visible band could not be obtained with the primer pair HMRCF/HMRCR.

Another example is Kangguzhi Zengsheng pills (ZCY44). There are eight ingredients in addition to Cistanches Herba in this Chinese patent medicine, but there were no visible bands obtained by either GHRCF/GHRCR or HMRCF/HMRCR, which meant that no Cistanches Herba was present. However, the adulterant region of *Cy. songaricum* was successfully amplified by the specific primer pair SYF1/SYR1. The sequencing results demonstrated the short nucleotide signature of *Cy. songaricum* was successfully obtained.

TABLE 4 | Primers used for PCR amplification and sequencing.

Primer pair	Primer name	Direction	Primer sequences (5'-3')	Amplicon size	Target species	Thermal program
1	SYF1	Forward	CTCAATGTGCTGCTGCTT	123	Cy. songaricum	94°C for 2 min;
	SYR1	Reverse	AGACTTACCGCTCACAATG			98°C for 10 s,
2	HMRCF	Forward	CCTTTAGGGTGATACTTAGGT	132	Ci. deserticola	50°C for 30 s,
	HMRCR	Reverse	CAGCACGAGAGTTGAGAG			68°C for 15 s, 35 cycles;
3	GHRCF	Forward	TTCTGGGACAATGCTTAGG	134	Ci. tubulosa	
	GHRCR	Reverse	CGACACGAGAGTTGAGTT			
4	SCRF	Forward	ATATGGGCGATAGGTAGGT	131	Ci. sinensis	
	SCRR	Reverse	GACAGCACGAGAGTTGAG			
5	CCRF	Forward	CGGTCCAAATACGATCCC	72	B. rossica	
	CCRR	Reverse	GACAGCACGAGAGTTGAG			
6	LDF	Forward	ATCTTCAACTCTCGTCTGTC	71	O. coerulescens	
	LDR	Reverse	CTCGTGCCTATGGGTCTA			

TABLE 5 | BLAST results of the four conserved nucleotide regions.

Source species of nucleotide signature	Blasted result in NCBI	Number of the species	Max score	Total score	Query cover (%)	E-value	Ident (%)
Cynomorium songaricum	Cynomorium songaricum	29	60.0	60.0	100	1e−06	100
	Bacillus subtilis strain	3	44.1	44.1	73	0.085	100
	Ranunculus ternatus	1	44.1	44.1	100	0.085	93
	Spirometra erinaceieuropaei	1	42.1	42.1	83	0.34	96
	Laccaria bicolor	1	40.1	40.1	66	1.3	100
Cistanche sinensis	Cistanche sinensis	4	63.9	63.9	100	5e−08	100
Boschniakia rossica	Boschniakia rossica	7	69.4	69.4	100	2e−09	100
	Boschniakia himalaica	2	60.2	60.2	94	1e−06	97
Orobanche coerulescens	Orobanche coerulescens	7	58.4	58.4	100	1e−06	100

By seeking the nucleotide signatures developed in this study, we found that 15 of 31 Chinese patent medicines labeled as containing Cistanches Herba instead contained adulterants, including eight counterfeit ingredients and seven adulterants (**Table 2**). For example, six batches were replaced with Cy. songaricum, including three batches of Shihu Yeguang pills, one batch of Kangguzhi Zengsheng pills, one batch of Sanbao capsules, and one batch of Wenweishu particles.

Moreover, different batches from the same manufacturer produced somewhat different results. For example, among three batches from one manufacturer (ZCY16, ZCY69, and ZCY71), one batch comprised a mixture of Ci. deserticola and Cy. songaricum, one batch comprised a mixture of Ci. deserticola and Ci. tubulosa, and one batch contained only Ci. tubulosa. Two batches from another manufacturer (ZCY44 and ZCY70) also differed: one batch contained Cy. songaricum, whereas the other batch contained Ci. deserticola and Ci. tubulosa.

Cistanches Herba was detected in 23 of the 31 Chinese patent medicines tested (**Table 2**), and only 16 samples were authentic, e.g., without adulterants or counterfeit ingredients. Ci. tubulosa was detected in 16 batches of Chinese patent medicines, and Ci. deserticola was detected in 10 batches. O. coerulescens was not detected in any of the products (**Table 2**).

DISCUSSION

Necessity of Developing a New Method for Monitoring Commercially Available Medicinal Products Containing Cistanches Herba

Cistanches Herba is a tonic that is widely used in restorative Chinese patent medicines and other medicinal products. However, the quality control of Chinese patent medicines presents great challenge due to the diversity and complexity of the ingredients. Due to the lack of regulatory oversight, there is considerable opportunity for product adulteration or counterfeiting. In addition, all products should be processed in accordance with the Pharmacopoeia or other standards; adulterating or counterfeiting is not permitted during processing. Thus, varieties of quality control methods have been established, such as multi-heart-cutting two-dimensional liquid chromatography (Yao et al., 2015), near-infrared reflectance spectroscopy (Zhang and Su, 2014; Zhang et al., 2015) and liquid chromatography-mass spectrometry (Wang et al., 2016b). However, the analytical chemistry methods currently in the Chinese Pharmacopoeia Commission (2015) cannot be used to authenticate all of the ingredients in Chinese patent medicines or to detect the presence of adulterant ingredients. Moreover,

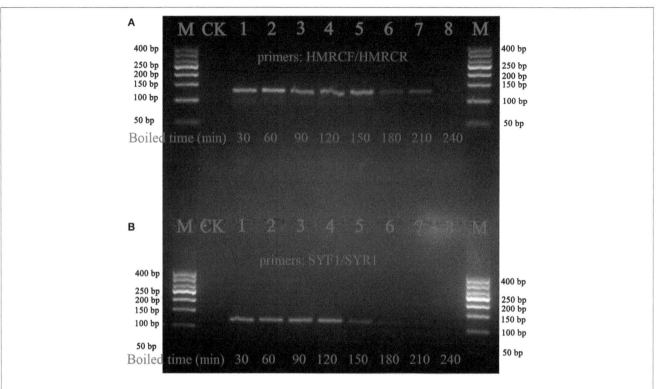

FIGURE 4 | Gel images of the PCR amplifications of the boiled samples of *Ci. deserticola* and *Cy. Songaricum*. **(A)** *Ci. deserticola*; **(B)** *Cy. Songaricum*. With the exception of the lanes marked M (marker) and CK (negative control), the remaining 8 lanes contain the PCR products from the samples boiled for 30, 60, 90, 120, 150, 180, 210, and 240 min, respectively.

studies have shown that targeted metabolites in plants are altered during product processing, resulting in considerable variability in test results or complete failure of test methods (Ananingsih et al., 2013). Thus, molecular tools such as species-specific nucleotide signatures are poised to reinforce quality control systems against the risk of fraudulent product substitution and adulteration and inclusion of unlabeled ingredients.

Although ITS/ITS2 is considered a high-efficiency tool for the identification of herbal medicines, these sequences cannot be amplified from highly processed samples (Newmaster et al., 2013; de Boer et al., 2015). Wang et al. reported that ITS2 could not be amplified from Angelicae Sinensis Radix extract or decoctions boiled for more than 120 min (Wang et al., 2016a). According to traditional technologies and the Chinese Pharmacopoeia Commission (2015), Cistanches Herba is always highly processed to increase its medicinal efficacy; these processes, include oven drying, salting and steaming with wine (Zou et al., 2017), which lead to DNA degradation. In addition, various excipients are added during processing, such as honey, starch, and dextrin. If these excipients are not removed completely, the purity of DNA will be affected. For example, the following manufacturing process is used to generate Cistanches Herba-containing Sanbao capsules: "Boil the medicinal slices for 1.5 h twice, combine the decoctions and filter the mixture. Concentrate the filtrate to a relative density of 1.20~1.25 (at 80°C). Add other ground powders and combine them to obtain a homogeneous mixture. Next, dry the mixture at 60°C, and then grind it into a fine

powder." However, after the production process described above, there could be difficulties during the DNA extraction of Chinese patent medicines, and long fragments might not be amplified from the degraded DNA, which would prevent the identification of adulterants. Thus, to ensure the quality and purity of DNA, we added additional steps before the genomic DNA extraction, including washing with prewash buffer and eluting ten parallel tubes into one tube for each batch.

Although all the Chinese patent medicines used in the present study contained 6–25 ingredients, the primer pairs developed could specifically amplify the sequences of the adulterants in these Chinese patent medicines. Direct sequencing of the PCR products showed clean trace files. Thus, this nucleotide signature method is capable of identifying both authentic species ingredients and adulterants and should broaden the application of DNA-based molecular diagnostic tools for market supervision.

Nucleotide Signatures for the Effective Identification of Cistanches Herba Products

Molecular tools that utilize PCR technology are very promising for medicinal product authentication within quality control systems. The successful application of the primers for identifying DNA-degraded adulterants from Cistanches Herba suggests that a PCR-based detection method could be used widely. In the Chinese herbal medicine market, the price of authentic

Cistanches Herba species ingredients is more than five times higher than the prices of its adulterants. Our results showed that *Cy. songaricum* is the most common adulterant of Cistanches Herba on the market, followed by *Ci. sinensis*. *Cy. songaricum* was added because these medicines share similar morphological characteristics. In addition, the chemical composition of *Ci. sinensis* is similar to that of Cistanches Herba. As quality control markers for Cistanches Herba extracts, echinacoside and acteoside can be inexpensively extracted from *Ci. sinensis*. Thus, some pharmaceutical factories use *Ci. sinensis* as a substitute in the production of Cistanches Herba extracts. Taken together, the results of this study indicate that there is considerable fraud in the market for medicinal products.

Adulteration in Chinese patent medicine is similar to that found in other countries. Similar levels of adulteration have been recorded in North America (Newmaster et al., 2013), Europe (Raclariu et al., 2017), and Asia (Cheng et al., 2014; Shanmughanandhan et al., 2016; Gao et al., 2017). In this study, the adulterated rate of Chinese patent medicines was approximately 48.4%, with only 16 of the 31 samples being authentic Cistanches Herba. In addition, we speculated that the different results produced in products from the same manufacturer could be attributed to differences in the qualities of the different batches of Chinese medicine materials. Therefore, to control the quality of Chinese patent medicines, the raw materials should be authenticated before being processed into products.

Adulteration of Cistanches Herba has traditionally been associated with issues of supply and demand of raw materials. *Ci. deserticola* and *Ci. tubulosa* are the two original plants currently used to formulate Cistanches Herba. However, *Ci. deserticola* is the only original species in traditional authentic Cistanches Herba listed in the Chinese Pharmacopoeia Commission (2000), in which *Ci. tubulosa* is identified as an adulterant. Owing to the shortage of *Ci. deserticola* resources, *Ci. tubulosa* has been listed as a supplement in the Chinese Pharmacopoeia since 2005 (Jiang and Tu, 2009). Until recently, the prices of these herbs have markedly differed; *Ci. tubulosa* has been much less expensive than *Ci. deserticola* because there is a much larger supply of the former. Here, our results showed that *Ci. tubulosa* is more widely used in commercially available Cistanches Herba products.

In conclusion, the nucleotide signatures and PCR-based methods developed in this study may serve as useful tools for the medicinal product industry to authenticate ingredients and detect adulterants in Cistanches Herba products. In accordance of the sensitivity result, even if the proportion of adulterant was one in ten thousand, it can be detected via qRT-PCR. It means that once a nucleotide signature is detected in Cistanches Herba-containing functional products, it could be identified as an adulterant or counterfeit ingredient. A novel solution for detecting counterfeit ingredients or adulterated Cistanches Herba was provided that was not previously available via chemical detection methods in the Chinese Pharmacopoeia. In addition, this method could be used to validate increasing types of medicine and to broaden the applications of DNA-based molecular diagnostic tools for market supervision.

AUTHOR CONTRIBUTIONS

JH conceived the study and participated in its design. XW, RX, and JC contributed samples and performed the experiments. XW analyzed the data. XW, JH, ZZ, S-GN, JS, and SC drafted the manuscript. All authors have read and approved the final manuscript.

FUNDING

This work was supported by the National Natural Science Foundation of China [grant number 81673552], the CAMS Innovation Fund for Medical Sciences [grant number 2016-I2 M-3-016], and the United Fund Key Project of the National Natural Science Foundation of China [grant number U1403224].

ACKNOWLEDGMENTS

We would like to thank our colleagues who helped with the sample collection, identification, laboratory work and manuscript preparation, including Chaokui Sun, Dianyun Hou, and Piao Zhang.

SUPPLEMENTARY MATERIAL

Supplementary Figure S1 | The alignment result of ITS2 sequence from six species.

Supplementary Figure S2 | Agarose gel electrophoresis of all samples.

Supplementary Table S1 | Sampling information of Cistanches Herba and its adulterants.

Supplementary Table S2 | Sequence information of related species downloaded from GenBank.

Supplementary Table S3 | The declared compositions of different Chinese patent medicine samples.

Supplementary Data Sheet S1 | All the sequences obtained in this study.

REFERENCES

Ananingsih, V. K., Sharma, A., and Zhou, W. (2013). Green tea catechins during food processing and storage: a review on stability and detection. *Food Res. Int.* 50, 469–479. doi: 10.1016/j.foodres.2011.03.004

Chen, H., Jing, F. C., Li, C. L., Tu, P. F., Zheng, Q. S., and Wang, Z. H. (2007). Echinacoside prevents the striatal extracellular levels of monoamine neurotransmitters from diminution in 6-hydroxydopamine lesion rats. *J. Ethnopharmacol.* 114, 285–289. doi: 10.1016/j.jep.2007.07.035

Chen, S., Yao, H., Han, J., Liu, C., Song, J., Shi, L., et al. (2010). Validation of the ITS2 region as a novel DNA barcode for identifying medicinal plant species. *PLoS ONE* 5:e8613. doi: 10.1371/journal.pone.0008613

Cheng, X., Su, X., Chen, X., Zhao, H., Bo, C., Xu, J., et al. (2014). Biological ingredient analysis of traditional Chinese medicine preparation based on highthroughput sequencing: the story for Liuwei Dihuang Wan. *Sci. Rep.* 4:5147. doi: 10.1038/srep05147

Chinese Pharmacopoeia Commission. (2000). *Pharmacopoeia of the People's Republic of China. Part I.* Beijing: China Medical Science Press.

Chinese Pharmacopoeia Commission. (2015). *Pharmacopoeia of the People's Republic of China. Part I.* Beijing: China Medical Science Press.

de Boer, H. J., Ichim, M. C., and Newmaster, S. G. (2015). DNA barcoding and pharmacovigilance of herbal medicines. *Drug Saf.* 38, 611–620. doi: 10.1007/s40264-015-0306-8

Dubey, B., Meganathan, P. R., and Haque, I. (2011). DNA mini-barcoding: an approach for forensic identification of some endangered Indian snake species. *Forensic. Sci. Int. Genet.* 5, 181–184. doi: 10.1016/j.fsigen.2010.03.001

Edgar, R. C. (2004). MUSCLE: multiple sequence alignment with high accuracy and high throughput. *Nucleic Acids Res.* 32, 1792–1797. doi: 10.1093/nar/gkh340

Fu, L. (1991). *China Plant Red Data Book. Part I.* Beijing: Science Press, 502.

Gao, Z., Liu, Y., Wang, X., Song, J., Chen, S., Ragupathy, S., et al. (2017). Derivative technology of DNA barcoding (nucleotide signature and SNP double peak methods) detects adulterants and substitution in Chinese patent medicines. *Sci. Rep.* 7:5858. doi: 10.1038/s41598-017-05892-y

Gu, C. M., Yang, X. Y., and Huang, L. F. (2016). Cistanches Herba: a neuropharmacology review. *Front. Pharmacol.* 7:289. doi: 10.3389/fphar.2016.00289

Hajibabaei, M., Smith, M. A., Janzen, D. H., Rodriguez, J. J., Whitfield, J. B., and Hebert, P. D. N. (2006). A minimalist barcode can identify a specimen whose DNA is degraded. *Mol. Ecol. Notes* 6, 959–964. doi: 10.1111/j.1471-8286.2006.01470.x

Japan Pharmacopeial Convention. (2016). *The Japanese Pharmacopoeia, 17th Edn.* Tokyo: The Ministry of Health, Labour and Welfare of Japan, 1831–1832.

Jiang, Y., and Tu, P. F. (2009). Analysis of chemical constituents in *Cistanche* species. *J. Chromatogr.* A 1216, 1970–1979. doi: 10.1016/j.chroma.2008.07.031

Keller, A., Schleicher, T., Schultz, J., Müller, T., Dandekar, T., and Wolf, M. (2009). 5.8S-28S rRNA interaction and HMM-based ITS2 annotation. *Gene* 430, 50–57. doi: 10.1016/j.gene.2008.10.012

Lei, L., Yang, F., Zhang, T., Tu, P., Wu, L., and Ito, Y. (2001). Preparative isolation and purification of acteoside and 2'-acetyl acteoside from *Cistanches salsa* (C.A. Mey.) G. Beck by high-speed counter-current chromatography. *J. Chromatogr.* A 912, 181–185. doi: 10.1016/S0021-9673(01)00583-0

Li, Z., Lin, H., Gu, L., Gao, J., and Tzeng, C. M. (2016). Herba Cistanche (Rou Cong-Rong): one of the best pharmaceutical gifts of traditional Chinese medicine. *Front. Pharmacol.* 7:41. doi: 10.3389/fphar.2016.00041

Liu, X. M., Li, J., Jiang, Y., Zhao, M. B., and Tu, P. F. (2013). Chemical constituents from *Cistanche sinensis* (Orobanchaceae). *Biochem. Syst. Ecol.* 47, 21–24. doi: 10.1016/j.bse.2012.09.003

Liu, Y., Wang, X., Wang, L., Chen, S., Pang, X., and Han, J. (2016). A nucleotide signature for the identification of American ginseng and its products. *Front. Plant Sci.* 7:319. doi: 10.3389/fpls.2016.00319

Lo, Y. T., Li, M., and Shaw, P. C. (2015). Identification of constituent herbs in ginseng decoctions by DNA markers. *Chin. Med.* 10:1. doi: 10.1186/s13020-015-0029-x

Meusnier, I., Singer, G. A., Landry, J. F., Hickey, D. A., Hebert, P. D., and Hajibabaei, M. (2008). A universal DNA mini-barcode for biodiversity analysis. *BMC Genomics* 9:214. doi: 10.1186/1471-2164-9-214

Newmaster, S. G., Grguric, M., Shanmughanandhan, D., Ramalingam, S., and Ragupathy, S. (2013). DNA barcoding detects contamination and substitution in North American herbal products. *BMC. Med.* 11:222. doi: 10.1186/1741-7015-11-222

Raclariu, A. C., Mocan, A., Popa, M. O., Vlase, L., Ichim, M. C., Crisan, G., et al. (2017). *Veronica officinalis* product authentication using DNA metabarcoding and HPLC-MS reveals widespread adulteration with *Veronica chamaedrys*. *Front. Pharmacol.* 8:378. doi: 10.3389/fphar.2017.00378

Shanmughanandhan, D., Ragupathy, S., Newmaster, S. G., Mohanasundaram, S., and Sathishkumar, R. (2016). Estimating herbal product authentication and adulteration in India using a vouchered, DNA-based biological reference material library. *Drug Saf.* 39, 1211–1227. doi: 10.1007/s40264-016-0459-0

Sun, Z. Y., Song, J. Y., Yao, H., and Han, J. P. (2012). Molecular identification of Cistanches Herba and its adulterants based on nrITS2 sequence. *J. Med. Plants Res.* 6, 1041–1045. doi: 10.5897/JMPR11.1115

Tamura, K., Peterson, D., Peterson, N., Stecher, G., Nei, M., and Kumar, S. (2011). MEGA5: molecular evolutionary genetics analysis using maximum likelihood, evolutionary distance, and maximum parsimony methods. *Mol. Biol. Evol.* 28, 2731–2739. doi: 10.1093/molbev/msr121

Wang, Q., Song, W., Qiao, X., Ji, S., Kuang, Y., Zhang, Z. X., et al. (2016b). Simultaneous quantification of 50 bioactive compounds of the traditional Chinese medicine formula Gegen-Qinlian decoction using ultra-high performance liquid chromatography coupled with tandem mass spectrometry. *J. Chromatogr.* A 1454, 15–25. doi: 10.1016/j.chroma.2016.05.056

Wang, T., Zhang, X. Y., and Xie, W. Y. (2012). *Cistanche deserticola* YC Ma, "Desert ginseng": a review. *Am. J. Chin. Med.* 40, 1123–1141. doi: 10.1142/S0192415X12500838

Wang, X., Liu, Y., Wang, L., Han, J., and Chen, S. (2016a). A nucleotide signature for the identification of Angelicae Sinensis Radix (Danggui) and its products. *Sci. Rep.* 6:34940. doi: 10.1038/srep34940

Yao, C. L., Yang, W. Z., Wu, W. Y., Da, J., Hou, J. J., Zhang, J. X., et al. (2015). Simultaneous quantitation of five Panax notoginseng saponins by multi heart-cutting two-dimensional liquid chromatography: method development and application to the quality control of eight Notoginseng containing Chinese patent medicines. *J. Chromatogr.* A 1402, 71–81. doi: 10.1016/j.chroma.2015.05.015

Zhang, C., and Su, J. (2014). Application of near infrared spectroscopy to the analysis and fast quality assessment of traditional Chinese medicinal products. *Acta. Pharm. Sin.* B 4, 182–192. doi: 10.1016/j.apsb.2014.04.001

Zhang, W., Qu, Z., Wang, Y., Yao, C., Bai, X., Bian, S., et al. (2015). Near-infrared reflectance spectroscopy (NIRS) for rapid determination of ginsenoside Rg1 and Re in Chinese patent medicine Naosaitong pill. *Spectrochim. Acta. A Mol. Biomol. Spectrosc.* 139, 184–188. doi: 10.1016/j.saa.2014.11.111

Zou, P., Song, Y., Lei, W., Li, J., Tu, P., and Jiang, Y. (2017). Application of 1H NMR-based metabolomics for discrimination of different parts and development of a new processing workflow for *Cistanche deserticola*. *Acta. Pharm. Sin.* B 7, 647–656. doi: 10.1016/j.apsb.2017.07.003

11

Genome-Wide Identification and Characterization of *Salvia miltiorrhiza* Laccases Reveal Potential Targets for Salvianolic Acid B Biosynthesis

Qing Li[1†], Jingxian Feng[1†], Liang Chen[1], Zhichao Xu[2], Yingjie Zhu[3], Yun Wang[1], Ying Xiao[1], Junfeng Chen[1], Yangyun Zhou[1], Hexin Tan[4], Lei Zhang[4,5*] and Wansheng Chen[1*]

[1] Department of Pharmacy, Changzheng Hospital, Second Military Medical University, Shanghai, China, [2] Institute of Medicinal Plant Development, Chinese Academy of Medical Sciences, Peking Union Medical College, Beijing, China, [3] Institute of Chinese Materia Medica, China Academy of Chinese Medical Sciences, Beijing, China, [4] Department of Pharmaceutical Botany, School of Pharmacy, Second Military Medical University, Shanghai, China, [5] State Key Laboratory of Subtropical Silviculture, Zhejiang A & F University, Hangzhou, China

Correspondence:
Lei Zhang
zhanglei@smmu.edu.cn
Wansheng Chen
chenwansheng@smmu.edu.cn

[†] These authors have contributed equally to this work

Laccases are widely distributed in plant kingdom catalyzing the polymerization of lignin monolignols. Rosmarinic acid (RA) has a lignin monolignol-like structure and is converted into salvianolic acid B (SAB), which is a representatively effective hydrophilic compound of a well-known medicinal plant *Salvia miltiorrhiza* and also the final compound of phenolic acids metabolism pathway in the plant. But the roles of laccases in the biosynthesis of SAB are poorly understood. This work systematically characterizes *S. miltiorrhiza* laccase (SmLAC) gene family and identifies the SAB-specific candidates. Totally, 29 laccase candidates (SmLAC1-SmLAC29) are found to contain three signature Cu-oxidase domains. They present relatively low sequence identity and diverse intron–exon patterns. The phylogenetic clustering of laccases from *S. miltiorrhiza* and other ten plants indicates that the 29 SmLACs can be divided into seven groups, revealing potential distinct functions. Existence of diverse *cis* regulatory elements in the *SmLAC*s promoters suggests putative interactions with transcription factors. Seven *SmLAC*s are found to be potential targets of miR397. Putative glycosylation sites and phosphorylation sites are identified in SmLAC amino acid sequences. Moreover, the expression profile of *SmLAC*s in different organs and tissues deciphers that 5 *SmLAC*s (*SmLAC7/8/20/27/28*) are expressed preferentially in roots, adding the evidence that they may be involved in the phenylpropanoid metabolic pathway. Besides, silencing of *SmLAC7*, *SmLAC20* and *SmLAC28*, and overexpression of *SmLAC7* and *SmLAC20* in the hairy roots of *S. miltiorrhiza* result in diversification of SAB, signifying that *SmLAC7* and *SmLAC20* take roles in SAB biosynthesis. The results of this study lay a foundation for further elucidation of laccase functions in *S. miltiorrhiza*, and add to the knowledge for SAB biosynthesis in *S. miltiorrhiza*.

Keywords: *Salvia miltiorrhiza*, laccase, genome-wide, bioinformatics, salvianolic acid B

Abbreviations: ABA, abscisic acid; GA, gibberellins; LAC, laccase; MeJA, methyl jasmonate; RA, rosmarinic acid; SA, salicylic acid; SAB, salvianolic acid B.

INTRODUCTION

Laccase (*p*-diphenol: dioxygen oxidoreductase, EC.1.10.3.2), originally found in *Rhus vernicifera*, widely exists in fungi, bacteria, insects and plants (Yoshida, 1883; Wang et al., 2015). As a multicopper glycoprotein oxidase, laccase (LAC) mainly works in catalyzing one-electron oxidation of a wide range of substrates, coupled with the reduction of oxygen to water (Mot and Silaghi-Dumitrescu, 2012). LACs typically contain three conserved Cu-oxidase sites, named Type 1 (T1), Type 2 (T2), and binuclear Type 3 (T3) Cu sites respectively. When a substrate is bound and oxidized at T1, an electron is released and transferred to T2/T3 trinuclear copper cluster (TNC), consequently the free hydrogens are combined with molecule oxygens (O_2) and reduced to water molecules (H_2O) (Jones and Solomon, 2015). Due to the ability of oxidizing a variety of substrates, such as phenols, aromatic amines and metal ions, LACs have the potential to be used in industrial processes (Forootanfar and Faramarzi, 2015).

In recent years, great achievements have been made on the studies of LACs in lignin biosynthesis in plants (Liang et al., 2006a; Berthet et al., 2011; Cesarino et al., 2013; Zhao et al., 2013). In *Arabidopsis*, through T-DNA insertional mutagenesis, Berthet et al. (2011) found that the xylem was collapsed and the soluble constituents were detected in both laccase 4 (*AtLAC4*) and laccase 17 (*AtLAC17*) knockout mutants. By knocking down *AtLAC4* and *AtLAC17* along with *AtLAC11* (laccase 11), Zhao et al. (2013) observed serious physiological changes in the living plants, such as growth inhibition, narrowed stems and lack of lignified vascular bundles, indicating that *AtLAC11* may also be involved in the lignin polymerization. In addition to their functions in lignin biosynthesis (Cai et al., 2006; Liang et al., 2006a,b; Berthet et al., 2011; Zhao et al., 2013), LACs may perform other roles as some LACs are expressed in non-woody tissues and participate in oxidation of flavonoids (Pourcel et al., 2007; Turlapati et al., 2011).

Salvia miltiorrhiza (Dan-Shen) is one of the most commonly used medicinal plants in traditional Chinese medicine for treatment of cardiovascular and cerebrovascular diseases. Salvianolic acid B (SAB) is a representatively effective hydrophilic compound in *S. miltiorrhiza*. According to Chinese pharmacopeia (Chinese Pharmacopoeia Commission, 2015), it is also the quality control component of *S. miltiorrhiza*. Understanding the biosynthetic pathway of SAB will help improve the quality of *S. miltiorrhiza* by breeding improvement or quality control during the growth of *S. miltiorrhiza*. It will also benefit the metabolic engineering in *S. miltiorrhiza* such as increasing the abundance of SAB in the plant for extraction. Based on our studies of the biosynthetic pathway of salvianolic acids (**Figure 1**), a similar pathway to that of lignin and flavonoids, we suspected that LACs in the plant might be candidates in catalyzing rosmarinic acid (RA) to SAB (Di et al., 2013). In fact, five candidate LACs (SMil_00009266, SMil_00023004, SMil_00000484, SMil_00003461, and SMil_00018228) were claimed to participate in the salvianolic acids pathway (Xu Z. et al., 2016) in *S. miltiorrhiza*. However,

SMil_00000484, SMil_00003461 and SMil_00018228 are non-members of LAC family. SMil_00000484 is a monocopper oxidase-like protein while SMil_00003461 and SMil_00018228 are both L-ascorbate oxidase homologs.

Under the umbrella of *S. miltiorrhiza* genome data, 80 LACs were annotated (Xu H. et al., 2016; Xu Z. et al., 2016). However, confirmation is required in urgent since not only could the annotation of LACs be easily mixed with other multi-copper oxidases and peroxidases, but the functions of LACs also vary in plants. Since there is no comprehensive analysis of LAC multigene family in *S. miltiorrhiza*, the aim of this work is to characterize *S. miltiorrhiza* laccases (SmLACs), with the long-term goal to identify *bona fide* LACs involved in SAB biosynthesis. For this purpose, we characterized the annotated LACs in *S. miltiorrhiza* through a genome-wide comprehensive analysis of the gene family including analysis of the gene structures, protein domains as well as putative promoter *cis* regulatory elements. A phylogenetic tree was constructed using the neighbor-joining method. In addition, the expression patterns of *SmLAC* genes were evaluated and confirmed by quantitative real-time PCR. Silencing and overexpression of the candidate *SmLACs* in the hairy roots of *S. miltiorrhiza* were carried out to detect the variation of SAB. To sum up, 29 LAC candidates were identified in *S. miltiorrhiza* genome. All of them have conserved copper-binding domains but are different in gene structures, indicating similar genetic origin but divergent biological functions. The potential regulation mechanism of *SmLAC* genes by transcription factors, miRNAs and phosphorylation were discussed. Five *SmLACs* (*SmLAC7/8/20/27/28*) are assumed to be involved in the SAB biosynthetic pathway. Besides, silencing of *SmLAC7*, *SmLAC20* and *SmLAC28*, and overexpression of *SmLAC7* and *SmLAC20* in the hairy roots of *S. miltiorrhiza* resulted in diversification of SAB accumulation.

MATERIALS AND METHODS

Genome-Wide Characterization of Laccase Genes in *S. miltiorrhiza*

Based on the annotation of *S. miltiorrhiza* genome, all the peptide sequences contained Cu-oxidase domains were extracted with related coding sequences. The peptide sequences were then verified while blasted in NCBI[1] and checked on the Conserved Domain Database in the same website. Sequences with three typical Cu-oxidase domains were classified as LAC candidates after exclusion of L-ascorbate oxidase homologs and monocopper oxidase-like proteins.

The various physical and chemical characteristics of all the candidate SmLAC proteins were analyzed using the ProtParam tool[2]. Putative signal peptide cleavage sites were predicted by

---

[1] https://blast.ncbi.nlm.nih.gov/Blast.cgi?PROGRAM=blastp&PAGE_TYPE=BlastSearch&LINK_LOC=blasthome

[2] http://web.expasy.org/protparam

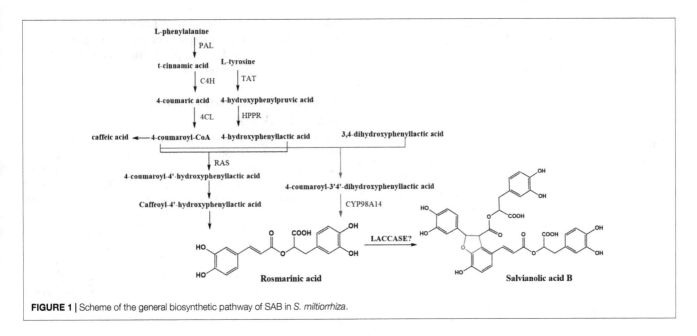

FIGURE 1 | Scheme of the general biosynthetic pathway of SAB in *S. miltiorrhiza*.

SignalP 4.1 server[3] (Petersen et al., 2011). WoLF PSORT server[4] and TargetP 1.1 server[5] were used to predict the subcellular localization of the mature SmLAC proteins, respectively. Potential glycosylation sites and phosphorylation sites were separately analyzed through online NetNGlyc 1.0 Server[6], YinOYang 1.2 server[7], and NetPhos 2.0 Sever[8]. Visualization of the intron-exon structure of *SmLAC* genes was conducted by Gene Structure Display Server (GSDS 2.0)[9] based on each coding sequence and corresponding genomic sequence. Sequence similarity of SmLAC proteins was obtained with alignment in ClustalX 2[10], and the conserved sites were checked manually for their corresponding amino acid residues, which were shaded by GeneDoc software (Nicholas et al., 1997). Secondary structure predictions of SmLACs were performed with Secondary Structure Prediction Method (SOPMA[11]) (Combet et al., 2000). All the performance was carried out with default settings.

Pairwise Distances, Phylogenetic and MEME Motif Analyses

The amino acid sequence alignments of SmLACs were performed using ClustalW implemented in the MEGA 5.05 software with p-distance settings. Phylogenetic and molecular evolutionary genetics analyses were performed using the Neighbor-Joining (NJ) method (Saitou and Nei, 1987) with pairwise deletion option in MEGA 5.05 and 1000 bootstrap replicates. The bootstrap

values above 50% were added to the tree branches generated from the original dataset. Conserved motifs in the complete amino acid sequences of SmLACs were identified using MEME (Multiple EM for Motif Elicitation[12]) (Bailey et al., 2006) with the maximum number of motifs setting at 10.

Prediction of miR397 Target Laccase Genes and *in silico* Analysis of *SmLAC* Promoter Sequences

The transcript sequences of the candidate *SmLACs* were uploaded to web-based psRNATarget server[13] for identification of potential targets corresponding to the ptr-miR397a and ssl-miR397. Sequences with a cut-off score ≤ 5 were chosen as putative targets.

PlantCARE (Plant *cis*-Acting Regulatory Elements[14]) was appointed to investigate the promoter sequences of *S. miltiorrhiza* LACs for potential *cis*-acting regulatory elements. The identified elements were sort out based on their reported functions.

Methyl Jasmonate Treatment

Methyl jasmonate (MeJA) was dissolved in ethanol and added into the culture medium of hairy root at the final concentration of 0.1mM for 0, 4, 8, 16, and 24 h, respectively. Three independent biological replicates for each group were performed.

Transcript Abundance of Laccases in Different Organs and Tissues of *S. miltiorrhiza*

To get insight into the transcript abundance of *SmLAC* genes, the Illumina and PacBio RNA-Seq data provided by Xu et al. (2015) was utilized. The RNA-Seq expression profile data were generated

---

[3]http://www.cbs.dtu.dk/services/SignalP/

[4]http://www.genscript.com/psort/wolf_psort.html

[5]http://www.cbs.dtu.dk/services/TargetP/

[6]http://www.cbs.dtu.dk/services/NetNGlyc/

[7]http://www.cbs.dtu.dk/services/YinOYang/

[8]http://www.cbs.dtu.dk/services/NetPhos/

[9]http://gsds.cbi.pku.edu.cn/index.php

[10]http://www.ebi.ac.uk/Tools/clustalw2/

[11]http://npsa-pbil.ibcp.fr/cgi-bin/npsa_automat.pl?page=/NPSA/npsa_sopma.html

[12]http://meme-suite.org/tools/meme

[13]http://plantgrn.noble.org/psRNATarget/?function=3

[14]http://bioinformatics.psb.ugent.be/webtools/plantcare/html/

using different organs of mature *S. miltiorrhiza* at blooming stage, including roots, stems, leaves and flowers. The periderm, phloem and xylem of roots were also included. At least three biological replicates for each kind of organ and tissue were used. Finally, the heat map of *SmLAC* gene expression patterns was constructed using the log2 transformed and normalized expression level data in Multi Experiment Viewer (MeV).

Plant Materials

The plant of *S. miltiorrhiza* was grown at the medicinal botanical garden of Second Military Medical University in Shanghai, China. It was identified by Professor Hanming Zhang. The fresh leaves, stems and roots of the plant were treated with liquid nitrogen immediately after collection, and then stored at $-80°C$ for subsequently use. At least three biological duplicate samples of each organ were collected.

The hairy roots were derived after the infection of 60-day-old *S. miltiorrhiza* leaves with *Agrobacterium tumefaciens* C58C1, and stocked in 1/2 MS solid medium at 25°C in the dark. They were harvested from the culture medium at the 60th day after been transferred into liquid medium, and as much as 0.2 g of harvested hairy roots were used for total RNA isolation. The rest hairy roots were dried at 40°C in an oven until constant dry weight was reached.

Preparation of RNA and cDNA

Total RNA of *S. miltiorrhiza* was isolated from stored roots, stems and leaves respectively using the *TransZol* Up Plus RNA Kit (TransBionovo Co., Ltd., Beijing, China). The integrity and quality of the RNA were confirmed by 1% agarose gels stained with ethidium bromide, and the RNA concentration was determined by a Nanodrop 2000 spectrophotometer (Thermo, Waltham, MA, United States). One μg of RNA for each sample was used for reverse transcription following the *TransScript* First-Strand cDNA Synthesis SuperMix operating procedures (TransBionovo Co., Ltd., Beijing, China).

Quantitative Real-Time PCR

Quantitative real-time PCR was performed on a TaKaRa TP800 PCR system (TaKaRa, Japan) using *TransStart* Top Green qPCR SuperMix Kit (TransBionovo Co., Ltd., Beijing, China) according to the manufacturer's instructions with three technical replicates. Primer Express 3.0[15] was used to design the gene-specific primers (see **Supplementary Table 1**) for each *SmLAC*. Specificity of each primer pair was verified by 2% agarose gels and dissociation curve analysis. The transcript abundance of each *SmLAC* gene was normalized to *SmACTIN* as control and compared with roots as reference using $2^{-\Delta\Delta Ct}$ method.

Construction of Recombinant Vectors

The candidate *SmLAC* cDNAs were cloned from S. *miltiorrhiza* through *pEASY*-Blunt Zero Cloning Vector (TransBionovo Co., Ltd., Beijing, China) respectively according to the manufacturer's instructions. Then the fragments of cloned *SmLACs* without the termination codons were PCR amplified using Primer 1 F/R and

---

[15]http://primer3.ut.ee/

Primer 2 F/R (see **Supplementary Table 2**) respectively. They were cleaved with the correspondent restriction enzymes, and cloned into pCambia-1300 or pPHB-flag vectors to yield the RNAi or overexpression vectors.

Extraction and Analysis of Phenolic Acids

The dried hairy roots were ground into powder, and 1 mL methanol: water (70:30, v/v) per 10 milligrams of powder was added into each sample. The mixture was sonicated for 30 min, 3 times with an output amplitude 50%. The solution was centrifuged at 13000 rpm for 10 min in an Eppendorf centrifuge 5418R rotor, and the supernatant was diluted with the same solvent to 5 mL per milliliter. Then the extract solution was filtered through a 0.2 μm organic membrane. Liquid chromatography-MS/MS (LC-MS/MS) was carried out to analyze the metabolites content using a triple-quadrupole mass spectrometer (Agilent G6410A). The separation was performed on a 2.1 × 50 mm 2.5 μm C18 column (Waters). The mobile phase consisted of acetonitrile: water (60:40 v/v).

RESULTS

Genome-Wide Identification of Laccases in *S. miltiorrhiza*

To identify LAC genes in *S. miltiorrhiza* at the genome level, the genome database and the genome annotation information of *S. miltiorrhiza* were downloaded from http://www.ndctcm.org/shujukujieshao/2015-04-23/27.html (Xu H. et al., 2016). According to the annotation information, 80, 80 and 79 genes models were identified containing Cu-oxidase, Cu-oxidase_2 and Cu-oxidase_3 domain respectively, which are the typical domains of LACs (see **Supplementary Table 3**).

After combining the Cu-oxidase domain contained genes, 101 sequences were obtained. They were then blasted in NCBI and checked on via the Conserved Domain Database in NCBI. The results showed that 32 genes were non-laccases, and 40 ones were partial laccases because of low quality sequencing or assembling, and only 29 were full-length LACs (see **Supplementary Table 4**). SMil_00000484, SMil_00003461, and SMil_00018228 are all Cu-oxidase domain contained genes, but they are not LACs as mentioned in previous studies (Xu Z. et al., 2016). SMil_00000484 is a monocopper oxidase-like protein while SMil_00003461 and SMil_00018228 are both L-ascorbate oxidase homologs.

The 29 full-length LACs of *S. miltiorrhiza* [named SmLAC1 to SmLAC29 randomly (see **Supplementary Text 1**)] were applied for bioinformatics analysis. Generally, SmLACs consist of 500–600 amino acids (aa) and most between 560 and 580 aa. The molecular masses of the 29 SmLAC proteins range from circa 57.15 kDa (SmLAC15) to 67.70 kDa (SmLAC16) and the predicted theoretical isoelectric points (pI) range from 5.83 (SmLAC12) to 9.47 (SmLAC17). The signal peptide prediction showed that 23 of the SmLACs had a 20–30 aa length signal peptide at the N-terminus, indicating that most SmLACs are probably secreted proteins. This agrees with McCaig's finding that most plant LACs have a cleavable N-terminal signal peptide targeting themselves to the secretory pathway (McCaig et al., 2005). The subcellular prediction showed that most of SmLAC proteins are localized in the secretory pathway and a few of them in mitochondria (SmLAC17 and SmLAC23) or nucleus (SmLAC5), indicating that most SmLACs are extracellular proteins. In addition, variable N- or O-glycosylation sites and phosphorylation sites were predicted to present in all SmLAC proteins, indicating potential post-translational modifications (**Table 1**).

Gene Structure Analysis of S. miltiorrhiza Laccase Family

The gene structure of SmLACs was investigated by using Gene Structure Display sever (**Figure 2**). The number of exons in the 29 SmLACs varied from 4 to 9, indicating a diverse intron-exon pattern within SmLAC genes. In general, there were 17 genes containing 5 introns, 6 genes containing 6 introns, 3 genes containing 4 introns and 2 genes containing 3 introns. Gene

SmLAC16 contained 8 introns. It is noteworthy that all the genes consisted of an intron phase 0 at the initiating terminal (except SmLAC16 and SmLAC17) and an intron phase 1 at the C-terminal, which indicates that they are relatively conserved.

The secondary structures of SmLACs were predicted on SOPMA. The results showed that random coil element was the main unit in SmLACs, followed by extended strand and α-helix (see **Supplementary Table 5**). The proportion of the α-helix structure in the 29 SmLACs ranges from 12.74% (SmLAC26) to 21.43% (SmLAC5), and the β-turn structure ratio from 8.66% (SmLAC18) to 12.63% (SmLAC25). The extended strand and random coil are from 26.52% (SmLAC15) to 32.23% (SmLAC18), and 39.27% (SmLAC10) to 46.90% (SmLAC26) respectively.

Protein Sequence Similarity Analysis

Protein sequence similarity of the 29 SmLACs was first carried out through sequence comparisons. According to the result of sequence alignment (**Figure 3**), the highly conserved residues with 4 coordinated copper atoms were found, except SmLAC5 which lacks the T1 copper binding site (H-C-H) near the

TABLE 1 | Physical, chemical characterization and the prediction of signal peptide and protein location of 29 SmLACs.

Designate name	Sequence ID	Amino acid length (aa)	MW (kD)	pI	Signal peptide length (aa)	Cleavage site	Protein location	Potential glycosylation sites		Potential phosphorylation sites		
								N-glyc	O-glyc	Serine	Threonine	Tyrosine
SmLAC1	SMil_00001393	573	64.64	6.79	24	VHA-LV	Secretory	4	8	18	16	6
SmLAC2	SMil_00001395	575	64.80	6.79	24	VDA-LV	Secretory	5	12	20	12	9
SmLAC3	SMil_00006361	564	62.37	9.45	23	AMA-KL	Secretory	10	10	13	17	9
SmLAC4	SMil_00008399	573	63.12	9.21	28	ANA-IT	Secretory	12	8	13	23	5
SmLAC5	SMil_00008533	588	64.86	8.91	–	–	Nuclear	9	15	17	18	6
SmLAC6	SMil_00009265	523	59.04	8.38	22	VHG-KI	Secretory	7	8	16	12	8
SmLAC7	SMil_00009266	562	63.21	6.21	22	VHG-KI	Secretory	9	8	19	16	8
SmLAC8	SMil_00009822	557	60.73	9.29	21	VDG-AV	Secretory	7	12	19	20	3
SmLAC9	SMil_00011367	579	66.22	8.46	–	–	Extracellular	5	5	23	17	8
SmLAC10	SMil_00012308	573	63.31	8.54	24	VHG-IK	Secretory	8	8	19	17	6
SmLAC11	SMil_00013111	571	63.98	6.55	21	VHA-VV	Secretory	5	11	20	15	10
SmLAC12	SMil_00017786	562	63.39	5.83	26	VNA-SI	Secretory	4	8	14	22	10
SmLAC13	SMil_00019237	548	62.46	8.62	–	–	Extracellular	5	6	20	15	7
SmLAC14	SMil_00020653	562	62.95	8.84	23	VKA-SD	Secretory	6	6	19	13	8
SmLAC15	SMil_00020657	528	57.15	9.21	25	VDS-RI	Secretory	5	19	19	20	3
SmLAC16	SMil_00021274	595	67.70	8.22	–	–	Extracellular	3	9	24	16	7
SmLAC17	SMil_00021810	593	65.11	9.47	–	–	Mitochondrial	9	9	24	16	8
SmLAC18	SMil_00022417	543	60.48	9.27	23	ANA-ET	Secretory	8	16	14	21	8
SmLAC19	SMil_00023003	565	63.50	7.29	26	SYA-MT	Secretory	11	8	13	21	13
SmLAC20	SMil_00023004	568	63.37	6.46	26	IHA-KT	Secretory	11	13	23	21	8
SmLAC21	SMil_00023210	551	61.77	6.42	30	VHA-VV	Secretory	5	12	14	17	7
SmLAC22	SMil_00023712	577	63.50	9.17	30	ASC-IT	Secretory	15	11	16	23	9
SmLAC23	SMil_00023714	556	63.33	8.05	-	-	Mitochondrial	4	5	22	16	11
SmLAC24	SMil_00023969	542	59.61	9.05	25	AEA-IT	Secretory	11	7	12	21	6
SmLAC25	SMil_00024180	570	62.14	5.99	24	ASA-RI	Secretory	12	12	17	20	7
SmLAC26	SMil_00025257	565	63.23	6.62	26	SHA-AT	Secretory	11	12	19	18	7
SmLAC27	SMil_00026282	559	61.10	8.87	22	VES-RV	Secretory	11	14	16	28	4
SmLAC28	SMil_00028093	575	65.09	8.02	28	VHA-LV	Secretory	2	10	20	20	7
SmLAC29	SMil_00028534	566	62.21	8.54	24	ASA-AI	Secretory	11	13	20	28	5

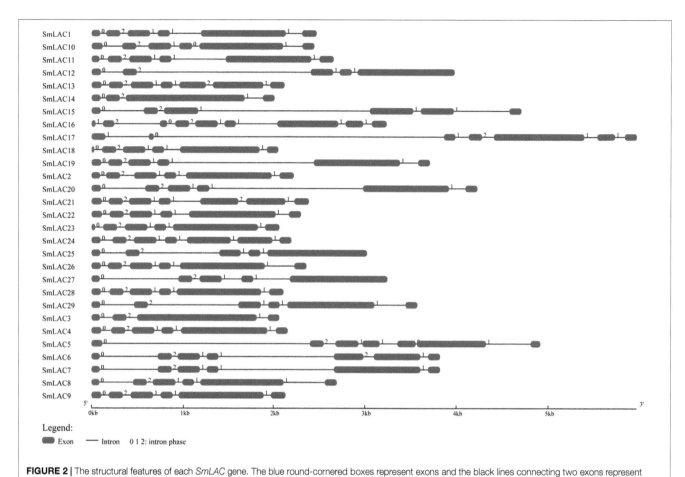

FIGURE 2 | The structural features of each *SmLAC* gene. The blue round-cornered boxes represent exons and the black lines connecting two exons represent introns. The numbers above the line are the intron phase.

C-terminus. It was believed that the axial ligand near the T1 copper binding site (H-C-H-X3-H-X3-G-[LMI(F)]) proximal to the C-terminus partially influenced LAC redox potential (Turlapati et al., 2011). Functions of SmLAC5 might be different and need further examination.

Pairwise sequence similarities among the predicted 29 peptide sequences of SmLACs ranged from a low of 39.7% (SmLAC10 vs. SmLAC16) to a high of 98.2% (SmLAC9 vs. SmLAC13) (see **Supplementary Table 6**). For most ones, the identity percentage varied from 40 to 70%. SmLAC9 and SmLAC13 are examples of closely related proteins sharing amino acid identity greater than 98% that may represent within-species alleles.

Phylogenetic Analysis and Conserved Motifs Identification

To obtain the evolutionary relationships among the 29 SmLACs and other LACs from 10 selected plants (*Zea mays*, *Nicotiana tabacum*, *Populus trichocarpa*, *Pinus taeda*, *Gossypium arboreum*, *Glycine max*, *Acer pseudoplatanus*, *Liriodendron tulipifera*, *A. thaliana* and *Oryza sativa*), a neighbor-joining tree was constructed by MEGA 5.05 with 1000 bootstrap reconstruction and pairwise deletion gaps/missing data treatment and clustered into seven phylogenetic groups (**Figure 4**). Both group I and

II contained 3 SmLACs respectively. Group III consisted of 4 SmLACs. There were 1, 2 and 1 SmLACs in group IV, V, and VI, respectively. Group VII included nearly half of the total SmLACs (15 SmLACs).

It is commonly accepted that proteins usually bear similar functions in their respective species if they share a high degree of sequence similarity. Although the functions of SmLACs are unknown, our construction of the SmLACs phylogenetic tree with different plants can help to derive the functions of SmLACs and lay a solid foundation for future functional studies. As shown in **Figure 4**, SmLAC10 shares 100% similarity with AtLAC6 and SmLAC14 shares 99% similarity with AtLAC15, strongly suggesting that SmLAC10 and SmLAC14 may have similar functions with AtLAC6 and AtLAC15 respectively. AtLAC15 is known involving in lignin synthesis, seed germination, root elongation (Liang et al., 2006a), oxidizing epicatechin into the oligomers as well as the synthesis of flavonoids in the seed coat of *A. thaliana* (Pourcel et al., 2005), SmLAC14 therefore may have the same functions in *S. miltiorrhiza*'s development. It was reported that when *AtLAC8* was knocked out, the flowering of plant was delayed and the number of the leaves was decreased (Cai et al., 2006). SmLAC25 and SmLAC29 are close to AtLAC8 in the phylogenetic tree, they might play similar roles in controlling the flowering and leaves growth of *S. miltiorrhiza* as AtLAC8

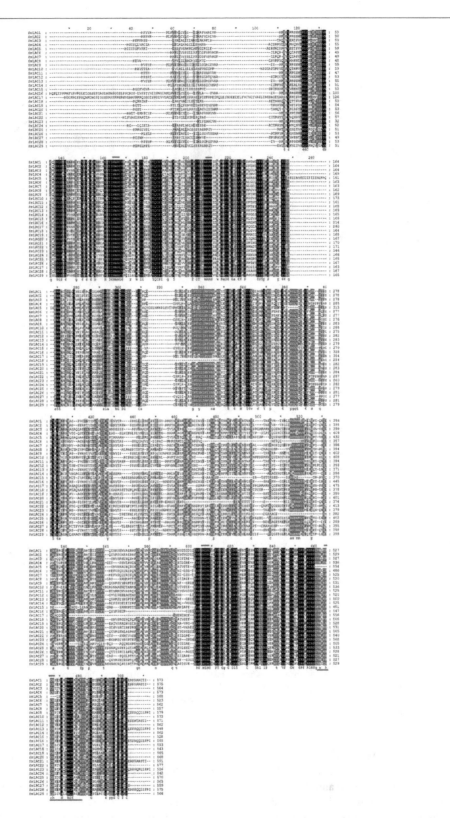

FIGURE 3 | Alignment of amino acid sequences of SmLACs. Dark boxes refer to amino acid identity or similarity between the 29 sequences. Bars placed at the top of the sequences correspond to the four highly conserved ligands for copper whereas the bar placed on the bottom corresponds to the blue copper oxidase signature. Amino acid residue number is indicated on the right side of the figure for each protein.

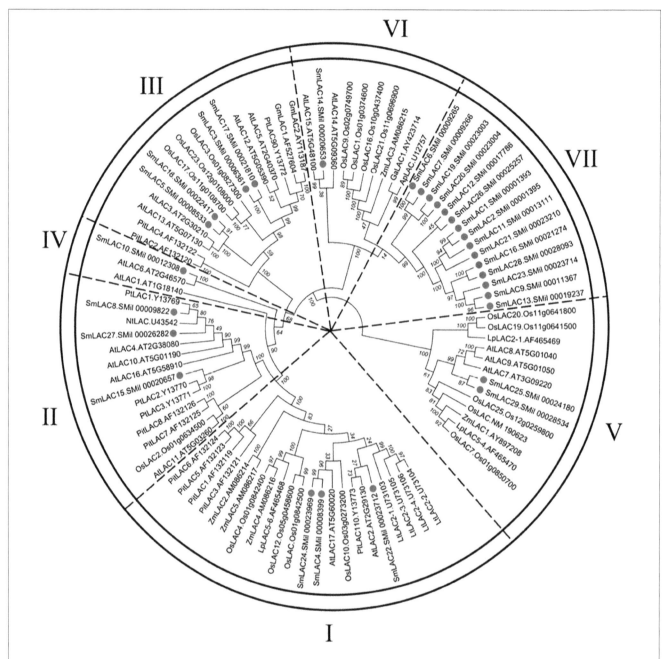

FIGURE 4 | Neighbor-Joining (NJ) phylogenetic tree of laccases from *S. miltiorrhiza* and other 10 plants. The amino acid sequences are aligned using ClustalW, and the phylogenetic tree is constructed using neighbor-joining criteria in MEGA 5.05. The values on the branches are bootstrap proportions, which indicate the percentage values for obtaining this particular branching in 1000 repetitions of the analysis. Only bootstrap values larger than 50% support are indicated. The letters (I–VII) represent the main groups. The red dots represent laccases from *S. miltiorrhiza*.

does in *Arabidopsis*. SmLAC4 and SmLAC24 are the closest homologs to AtLAC17 (up to 90% similarity), which was strongly expressed in *Arabidopsis*'s stems and participated in lignin synthesis (mainly participate in guaiacol radical accumulation) (Berthet et al., 2011), indicating that SmLAC4 and SmLAC24 may participate in *S. miltiorrhiza*'s lignin synthesis too. SmLAC22 is close to AtLAC2, whose function is related to root elongation in *Arabidopsis* (Cai et al., 2006). Group VII contains 15 SmLACs but without any members from other species, indicating that

they might have species specificity and drive the unknown functions in *S. miltiorrhiza*.

To further analyze the sequence features of these 29 SmLAC proteins, a conserved motif search was conducted by MEME (**Figure 5**). The result suggested that most SmLAC proteins in the same group have similar motifs. Members in group IV, V, and VI contained 10 different types of conserved motifs. Eleven SmLACs in group VII held 10 kinds of motifs, while the rest four contained 9 motifs. Eight types of conserved

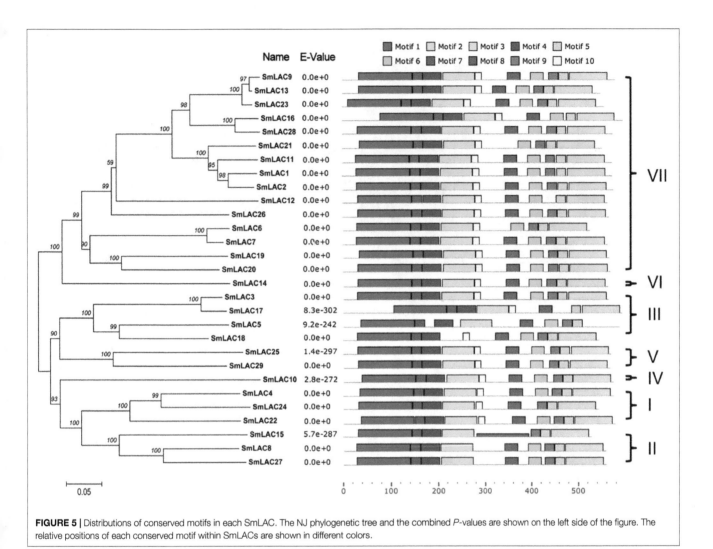

FIGURE 5 | Distributions of conserved motifs in each SmLAC. The NJ phylogenetic tree and the combined *P*-values are shown on the left side of the figure. The relative positions of each conserved motif within SmLACs are shown in different colors.

motifs were found in some members of group II and group III (SmLAC15/5/17).

Prediction of Diverse *cis* Regulatory Elements in SmLAC Promoters

Various numbers of putative *cis*-acting elements, including the core CAAT box and TATA box, were detected in the promoters of each *S. miltiorrhiza* LAC genes by PlantCARE (see **Supplementary Table 7**). All 29 SmLAC promoter sequences have many light responsive elements, such as G-box (Argüello Astorga and Herrera Estrella, 1998), revealing an essential role of SmLACs in plant morphogenesis. Besides, there are three types of representative DNA regulatory elements: stress responsive elements responding to diverse abiotic (anaerobic induction, defense and stress, cold and dehydration, heat stress, low temperature, drought, and wound) and biotic (fungal elicitor) stresses; hormone responsive elements involved in response to various plant hormones, such as ABA, MeJA, GA, SA, auxin, and ethylene; tissue specific expressed elements related to meristem-, endosperm-, seed- or shoot-specific activation and regulation.

Moreover, two classes of MYB binding site elements (MBS I and MBS II), which are the flavonoid biosynthetic genes regulation sites were discovered in the promoters of five SmLAC genes (*SmLAC3/9/10/13/28*).

Seven *SmLACs* Were Found to Be Potential Targets of miR397

It is reported that ptr-miR397a is a negative regulator of LAC genes in *Populus trichocarpa* (Lu et al., 2013). Since miR397 sequence of *S. miltiorrhiza* was not available, ptr-miR397a from *P. trichocarpa* was used to search the transcript sequences of the 29 candidate *SmLACs*, and 7 *SmLACs* (*SmLAC8/24/4/27/5/25/29*) were predicted to be the potential ptr-miR397a targets (see **Supplementary Table 8**). Ssl-miR397 of *Salvia sclarea*, which is the congener plant of *S. miltiorrhiza* from the same genus, was also used to search the 29 *SmLACs* transcript sequences, the same seven *SmLACs* turned out to be the potential ssl-miR397 targets. Thus, *SmLAC8/24/4/27/5/25/29* may be negatively regulated by miR397 in *S. miltiorrhiza*.

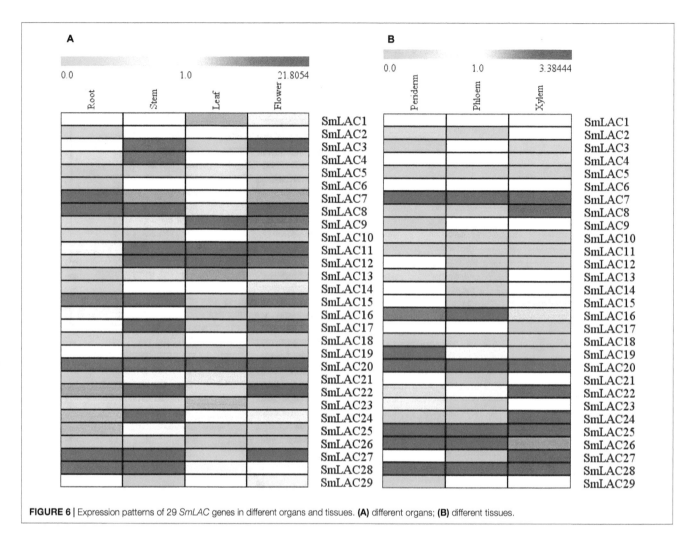

FIGURE 6 | Expression patterns of 29 *SmLAC* genes in different organs and tissues. **(A)** different organs; **(B)** different tissues.

Differential Expression Profiles of *SmLACs* in Different Organs and Tissues

The relative constitutive abundance of the 29 *SmLACs* was quantified in roots, stems, leaves and flowers through Illumina and PacBio sequencing technology (Xu et al., 2015). Besides, the abundance of *SmLACs* in different tissue parts of roots including periderm, phloem and xylem was also tested. The expression level of each *SmLAC* was estimated according to RPKM (reads per kilobase per million) values and presented in the heatmap in **Figure 6**. The results showed that the expression levels of the 29 *SmLACs* varied with organs. For instance, *SmLAC7/8/20/27/28* were highly expressed in roots while *SmLAC3/8/11/12/15/17/20/22/24/27/28* were highly expressed in stems. *SmLAC9/11/12/20* were highly expressed in leaves, and *SmLAC3/8/20/22/27* were highly expressed in flowers. The expression level of *SmLAC20* was high in all the four organs. *SmLAC8* and *SmLAC27* were highly expressed in roots, stems and flowers. However, the expression level of 5 *SmLACs* (*SmLAC5/10/18/19/26*) was very low in the four organs.

As to the three different tissues of roots, 5 *SmLACs* (*SmLAC7/20/25/26/28*) displayed the highest transcript

abundance in all xylem, epidermis and periderm. *SmLAC16* was found to be highly expressed in phloem followed by periderm and xylem. *SmLAC19* was highly expressed in periderm and more than in phloem and xylem. *SmLAC8/22/24/27* were highly expressed in xylem. These results indicated the functional conservation and diversity of *SmLACs*.

Confirmation of Five Highly Expressed *SmLACs* in Roots

Transcript abundance of a gene often correlates to its function. Considering the fact that hydrophilic compounds such as SAB of *S. miltiorrhiza* are more in roots than in other organs, the highly expressed five *SmLACs* (*SmLAC7/8/20/27/28*) in roots may participate in salvianolic acids biosynthesis. To verify their expression levels, real-time PCR was performed (**Figure 7**) and the results showed that the expression levels of *SmLAC8*, *SmLAC27* and *SmLAC28* were higher in stems than in roots and leaves. The expression level of *SmLAC7* was high in roots, followed by stems and leaves. It was consistent with its expression in the heatmap. *SmLAC20* exhibited a high expression pattern in leaves and its expression in stems was much lower than that in roots and in leaves.

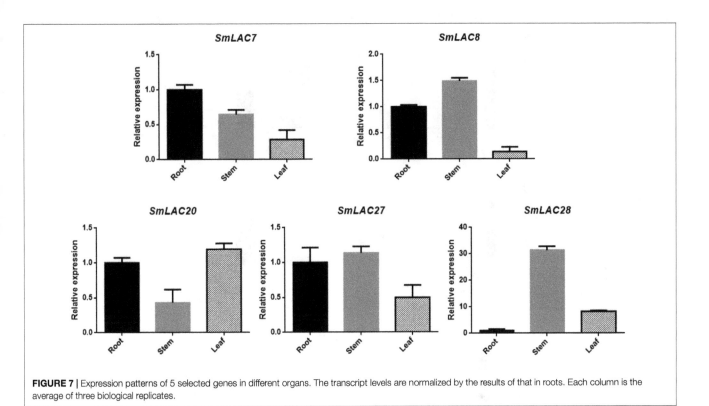

FIGURE 7 | Expression patterns of 5 selected genes in different organs. The transcript levels are normalized by the results of that in roots. Each column is the average of three biological replicates.

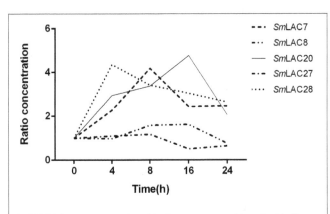

FIGURE 8 | Relative expression of the 5 target genes subjected to MeJA treatment. The expression levels are normalized to corresponding values of MeJA treatments at 0 h. Each data point is the average of three biological replicates.

Effects of Methyl Jasmonate on Expression of the Five Targeted *SmLACs*

Methyl jasmonate (MeJA) has been used in plant cell engineering for inducing gene expression (Xiao et al., 2009). Previous studies have shown that genes in the metabolic pathway of *S. miltiorrhiza* can be significantly induced by MeJA and thus increase the content of SAB (Xiao et al., 2009). In order to obtain preliminary information about the effect of MeJA on *SmLACs*, different expression levels of the five *SmLACs* in MeJA treated hairy roots at different times, including 0, 4, 8, 16, and 24 h were analyzed through real-time PCR using

gene-specific primers (see **Supplementary Table 1**). The results (**Figure 8**) showed that *SmLAC7*, *SmLAC20* and *SmLAC28* were significantly induced by MeJA, and the expressions of the genes were increased more than 3-fold. *SmLAC28* reached its peak at the 4th hour, while the maximum expressions of *SmLAC7* and *SmLAC20* appeared at the 8th and the 16th hour. However, there was no significant arising trend in *SmLAC8* and *SmLAC27*.

Silencing of *SmLAC7*, *SmLAC20*, and *SmLAC28* in Hairy Roots of *S. miltiorrhiza*

To explore the roles of MeJA responded genes (*SmLAC7*, *SmLAC20* and *SmLAC28*) in phenolic acid synthetic pathway in *S. miltiorrhiza*, RNAi transgenic hairy roots were generated by RNAi strategy under the control of the CaMV35S promoter. Real-time PCR was performed to confirm the transcript levels of these genes (**Figure 9A**). In contrast with the wild type (WT) line, the transcript levels of *SmLAC7*, *SmLAC20*, and *SmLAC28* were all decreased in the RNAi lines (**Figure 9A**). It also resulted in reductions of RA and SAB content in the *SmLAC7* or *SmLAC20* silenced lines (**Figure 9C**). The content of RA and SAB in the negative control (NC) line was dramatically different with the WT line. Since the NC line was induced by *A. tumefaciens* with the empty vector of RNAi, the accumulation of compounds might be affected. Therefore, the NC line was used as control. Compared to NC, the average reduction of SAB was 87% in line *SmLAC20*, 29.6% and 7.45% in line *SmLAC7* and SmLAC28, respectively (**Figure 9C**).

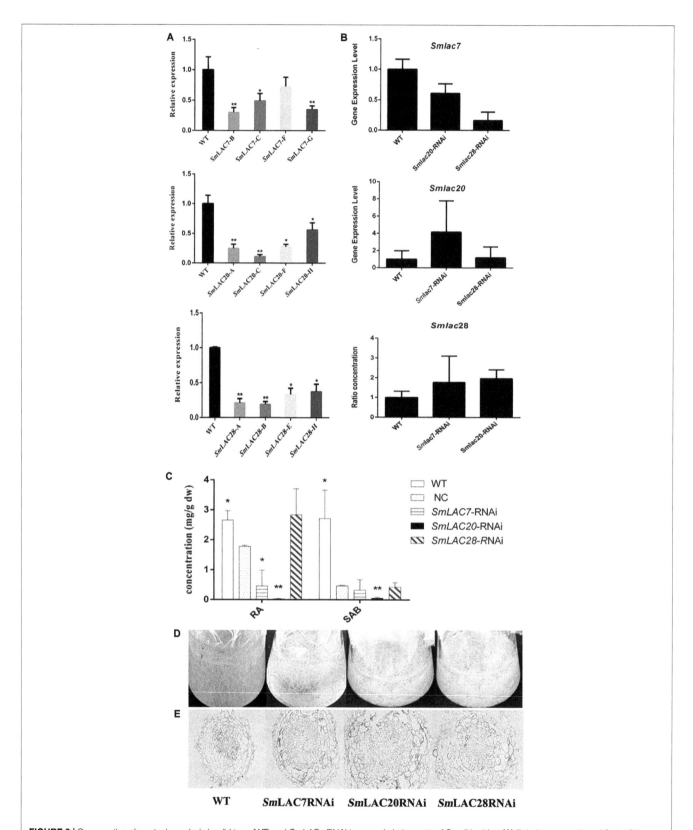

FIGURE 9 | Comparative phenotypic analysis in wild type (WT) and *SmLACs*-RNAi transgenic hairy roots of *S. miltiorrhiza*. **(A)** Relative expression of *SmLAC7*, *SmLAC20*, and *SmLAC28* in WT and their correspondent lines of RNAi hairy roots. **(B)** The average transcript level of *SmLAC7*, *SmLAC20*, and *SmLAC28* in fellow RNAi hairy roots. The fellow groups are named on the horizontal axis. **(C)** The content of RA and SAB in the experimental hairy root cultures. The statistical differences are compared with NC. **(D)** Effects of laccases RNAi on the biomass of hairy root cultures. **(E)** Cross sections of hairy roots. The level of significance obtained by using the Student *t*-test is marked by the following: *$P < 0.05$, **$P < 0.01$, means ± SD, $n = 3$.

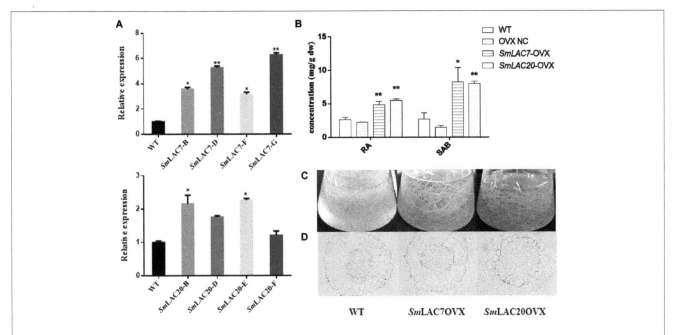

FIGURE 10 | Comparative phenotypic analysis in wild type (WT) and *SmLACs* overexpressed transgenic hairy roots of *S. miltiorrhiza*. **(A)** Relative expression of *SmLAC7* and *SmLAC20* in WT and their correspondent lines of overexpression hairy roots. **(B)** The content of RA and SAB in the experimental hairy root cultures. **(C)** Effects of laccases overexpressed on the biomass of hairy root cultures. The statistical differences are compared with NC. **(D)** Cross sections of hairy roots. The level of significance obtained by using the Student *t*-test is marked by the following: *$P < 0.05$, **$P < 0.01$, means $\pm$ SD, $n = 3$.

Besides, the transcriptional expression levels of the other two genes showed different performance in every single RNAi line. In *SmLAC7* silence line, the expression levels of *SmLAC20* and *SmLAC28* were higher than that in WT (4.18 folds and 1.78 folds respectively for the most), while in silence lines *SmLAC20* and *SmLAC28*, the expression of *SmLAC7* was lower than that in WT (about 0.6 folds and 0.16 folds of that in WT, respectively). However, the behavior of *SmLAC20* in *SmLAC28* silence line did not show obvious discrepancy when contrasted with that in WT, even though *SmLAC28* in *SmLAC20* silence line could reach to 1.97 folds compared with that in WT (**Figure 9B**).

To further investigate the putative impact of the transgenes at lignin biosynthesis, the vascular development of the hairy roots was inspected. The cross sections of hairy roots of both wild type and RNAi samples were dyed by Safranine O-Fast green FCF. The diameters of the transgenic cultures were much greater than that of the WT ones, so was the width of xylem (**Figure 9E**). More significantly, the xylem cells in RNAi samples appeared larger and looser than that in WT samples. There existed holes in the middle of the RNAi samples except the *SmLAC28* silence line. What's more, the biomass of the hairy roots with *SmLACs* silenced in shake-flask cultures exhibited an obviously decreasing growth trend after 30 days cultivation compared with the wild type (**Figure 9D**).

Overexpression of *SmLAC7* and *SmLAC20* in Hairy Roots of *S. miltiorrhiza*

SmLAC7, *SmLAC20*, and *SmLAC28* were all overexpressed in *S. miltiorrhiza* hairy roots. However, hairy roots with *SmLAC28* overexpressed didn't grow well and were excluded during this analysis. To explore the *in vivo* roles of *SmLAC7* and *SmLAC20* in SAB biosynthesis pathway, their transcript levels were determined by real-time PCR and showed strikingly increase in the transgenic lines (**Figure 10A**), accordingly, the contents of RA and SAB (**Figure 10B**). The accumulation of SAB in *SmLAC20* overexpressed line was 5.45 folds higher than that of NC. It was 5.61 folds higher in *SmLAC7* overexpressed line than the NC one.

Unlike the LACs silencing lines, the *SmLAC7* and the *SmLAC20* overexpressed lines (**Figures 10C,D**) showed increased biomass, as well as larger diameter of vascular compared to WT lines. Interestingly, the lignification degree in LACs overexpressed hairy root lines was increased compared with the wild type. The area of xylem in the *SmLAC20* overexpressed lines turned to be larger than that in the wild type (**Figure 10D**).

DISCUSSION

As a multigene family, LACs widely exist in fungi, bacteria, plants and animals. Because of their special catalytic properties, function variations have been found in fungi and bacteria. However, functions of plant LACs are still poorly understood. Recent studies in structural and functional genomics in higher plant model species such as *Arabidopsis* revealed 17 LACs which are involved in stress response and lignin biosynthesis (Turlapati et al., 2011). The availability of the whole genome sequences of *S. miltiorrhiza* facilitates a comprehensive characterization of LAC genes in the commonly used herb. Here, we identified and characterized 29 LAC candidates in

S. miltiorrhiza. They all exhibit the typical characteristics of three conserved Cu-oxidase domains, four signature sequences and 12 housed copper ligands.

Through utilization of a number of bioinformatics methods, we systematically analyzed all the 29 SmLACs. Although they all share similar coding domain structures, their sequence similarities are relatively low and intron–exon structures are quite different. Further differences in terms of number of amino acids and values of *pI*, implicate potentially functional divergence. In agreement with previous reports on *Arabidopsis* LACs (Turlapati et al., 2011), we find out that *S. miltiorrhiza* LAC genes are mostly located in the secretory pathway and contain glycosylation sites ensuring protein stability, folding, and formation of the cell wall.

Based on the phylogenetic relationships of *S. miltiorrhiza* and other ten plants, 29 SmLACs are mainly distributed into seven groups. The group VII contains 15 LACs all from *S. miltiorrhiza*, suggesting that these 15 SmLACs might hold species specificity. The homology of SmLAC8 and SmLAC27 is very close to AtLAC4. Also both SmLAC4 and SmLAC24 are just next to AtLAC17 in the phylogenetic tree. Since the two AtLACs function in lignin synthesis (Berthet et al., 2011; Zhao et al., 2013), we anticipate that all the four SmLAC4/8/24/27 participate in the synthesis of lignin in *S. miltiorrhiza*. This could be supported by the potential involvement of MYB58 in regulating *SmLAC4/8/24/27* since *SmLAC4/8/24/27* promoters contain the MYB binding site (MBS). MYB members MYB58 and MYB63 are known transcription activators in lignin biosynthesis, and MYB58 is particularly capable of activating *AtLAC4* (Zhou et al., 2009).

SmLACs may be negatively regulated by miR397. In *P. trichocarpa*, overexpressed ptr-miR397a negatively regulates LAC genes and decreases lignin content (Lu et al., 2013). We contrast the 29 *SmLACs* with ptr-miR397a and ssl-miR397 one by one and find out that 7 *SmLACs* (*SmLAC4/5/8/24/25/27/29*) can be combined with miR397 tightly, reflecting miR397's roles in regulating the expressions of *SmLACs*.

Expressions of the 29 LACs are tissues and organs dependent as supported by the analysis of transcriptome sequencing. We also observed SAB is mainly accumulated in the roots and the accumulation is positively correlated with the overexpressions of *Smlac7/8/20/27/28*, thus we speculate that these LACs may be involved in the synthesis of lignin and salvianolic acid in roots. This is supported by a combination of an early report that the content of SAB as well as RA are affected by MeJA (Xiao et al., 2009) and our current result that MeJA responsiveness motifs appear in the promoters of more than half *SmLACs* (*SmLAC1/3/4/5/6/7/8/9/12/13/14/15/19/20/21/23/24/25/27*), including the four highly expressed genes (*SmLAC7/8/20/27*) in roots. And indeed, MeJA significantly affected the expressions of *SmLAC7*, *SmLAC20*, and *SmLAC28* based on the results of real-time PCR on MeJA treated hair roots of *S. miltiorrhiza*. What's more, when the LAC in poplar is inhibited, its lignin

component is not changed, but the phenolic metabolites are altered (Ranocha et al., 2002). This indicates that the highly expressed genes in roots likely participate in the biosynthesis of secondary metabolites in the phenylpropanoid pathway. Therefore, the three MeJA affected and highly expressed genes in roots were chosen for further study to illustrate their roles in the biosynthesis of SAB.

As expected, the contents of SAB in both *SmLAC7* and *SmLAC20* silenced lines were lower than in the wild type and negative control. Conversely, in the *SmLACs* overexpressed transgenic hairy root lines, SAB content increased with the expression of LACs. These observations strongly support that both *SmLAC7* and *SmLAC20* participate in the synthesis progress of SAB despite the exact SAB biosynthesis mechanism remains to be revealed.

In short, we comprehensively characterized LACs of *S. miltiorrhiza* and analyzed their molecular regulation functions. The results provide a solid ground for further exploring LACs in *S. miltiorrhiza* and other species as well. Our work adds to the knowledge for unveiling the formation of SAB and demonstrates a promising future in *S. miltiorrhiza* metabolic regulation in quality control.

AUTHOR CONTRIBUTIONS

QL and JF conceived the study. QL participated in data mining, data analysis, and proofreading the manuscript. JF performed the RNAi and overexpression experiment and wrote the manuscript. LC carried out the qRT-PCR experiment. ZX and YZhu provided the genome and transcription information of *S. miltiorrhiza*. YW, YZhou, and HT prepared the figures. YX initiated the project. JC helped to analysis the data. LZ participated in the design of the study. WC helped to conceive the study and participated in its design and coordination. All authors read and approved the final manuscript.

FUNDING

This work was financially supported by the National Natural Science Foundation of China (31770329, 81325024, 81603220, 81303160, and 81673529) and the State Key Laboratory of Subtropical Silviculture, Zhejiang A & F University (2018FR003 and ZY20180206).

ACKNOWLEDGMENTS

We are greatly acknowledge Prof. Shilin Chen (China Academy of Chinese Medical Sciences), Prof. Jingyuan Song and Hongmei Luo (Peking Union Medical College) for kindly providing the genome data and transcription profiling of *S. miltiorrhiza*.

Genome-Wide Identification and Characterization of Salvia miltiorrhiza Laccases Reveal Potential Targets...   129

REFERENCES

Argüello Astorga, G., and Herrera Estrella, L. (1998). Evolution of light-regulated plant promoters. *Annu. Rev. Plant Physiol. Plant Mol. Biol.* 49, 525–555. doi: 10.1146/annurev.arplant.49.1.525

Bailey, T. L., Williams, N., Misleh, C., and Li, W. W. (2006). Meme: discovering and analyzing DNA and protein sequence motifs. *Nucleic Acids Res.* 34, W369–W373.

Berthet, S., Demont-Caulet, N., Pollet, B., Bidzinski, P., Cézard, L., Bris, P. L., et al. (2011). Disruption of LACCASE4 and 17 results in tissue-specific alterations to lignification of *Arabidopsis thaliana* stems. *Plant Cell* 23, 1124–1137. doi: 10.1105/tpc.110.082792

Cai, X., Davis, E. J., Ballif, J., Liang, M., Bushman, E., Haroldsen, V., et al. (2006). Mutant identification and characterization of the laccase gene family in *Arabidopsis*. *J. Exp. Bot.* 57, 2563–2569. doi: 10.1093/jxb/erl022

Cesarino, I., Araújo, P., Sampaio Mayer, J. L., Vicentini, R., Berthet, S., Demedts, B., et al. (2013). Expression of *SofLAC*, a new laccase in sugarcane, restores lignin content but not S:G ratio of *Arabidopsis* lac17 mutant. *J. Exp. Bot.* 64, 1769–1781. doi: 10.1093/jxb/ert045

Chinese Pharmacopoeia Commission. (2015). *The Pharmacopoeia of People's Republic of China 2015*, 1st Edn, Vol. 1. Beijing: China Medical Science Press, 76–77.

Combet, C., Blanchet, C., Geourjon, C., and Deléage, G. (2000). NPS@: network protein sequence analysis. *Trends Biochem. Sci.* 25, 147–150. doi: 10.1016/s0968-0004%2899%2901540-6

Di, P., Zhang, L., Chen, J., Tan, H., Xiao, Y., Dong, X., et al. (2013). ^{13}C tracer reveals phenolic acids biosynthesis in hairy root cultures of *Salvia miltiorrhiza*. *ACS Chem. Biol.* 8, 1537–1548. doi: 10.1021/cb3006962

Forootanfar, H., and Faramarzi, M. A. (2015). Insights into laccase producing organisms, fermentation states, purification strategies, and biotechnological applications. *Biotechnol. Prog.* 31, 1443–1463. doi: 10.1002/btpr.2173

Jones, S. M., and Solomon, E. I. (2015). Electron transfer and reaction mechanism of laccases. *Cell. Mol. Life Sci.* 72, 869–883. doi: 10.1007/s00018-014-1826-6

Liang, M., Davis, E., Gardner, D., Cai, X., and Wu, Y. (2006a). Involvement of *AtLAC15* in lignin synthesis in seeds and in root elongation of *Arabidopsis*. *Planta* 224, 1185–1196. doi: 10.1007/s00425-006-0300-6

Liang, M., Haroldsen, V., Cai, X., and Wu, Y. (2006b). Expression of a putative laccase gene, *ZmLAC1*, in maize primary roots under stress. *Plant Cell Environ.* 29, 746–753. doi: 10.1111/j.1365-3040.2005.01435.x

Lu, S., Li, Q., Wei, H., Chang, M. J., Tunlaya-Anukit, S., Kim, H., et al. (2013). Ptr-mir397a is a negative regulator of laccase genes affecting lignin content in *Populus trichocarpa*. *Proc. Natl. Acad. Sci. U.S.A.* 110, 10848–10853. doi: 10.1073/pnas.1308936110

McCaig, B. C., Meagher, R. B., and Dean, J. F. D. (2005). Gene structure and molecular analysis of the laccase-like multicopper oxidase (LMCO) gene family in *Arabidopsis thaliana*. *Planta* 221, 619–636. doi: 10.1007/s00425-004-1472-6

Mot, A. C., and Silaghi-Dumitrescu, R. (2012). Laccases: complex architectures for one-electron oxidations. *Biochemistry* 77, 1395–1407. doi: 10.1134/S0006297912120085

Nicholas, K. B., Nicholas, H. B. Jr., and Deerfield, D. W. (1997). GeneDoc: analysis and visualization of genetic variation. *EMBNEW News* 4:14.

Petersen, T. N., Brunak, S., von Heijne, G., and Nielsen, H. (2011). Signalp 4.0: discriminating signal peptides from transmembrane regions. *Nat. Methods* 8, 785–786. doi: 10.1038/nmeth.1701

Pourcel, L., Routaboul, J. M., Cheynier, V., Lepiniec, L., and Debeaujon, I. (2007). Flavonoid oxidation in plants: from biochemical properties to physiological functions. *Trends Plant Sci.* 12, 29–36. doi: 10.1016/j.tplants.2006.11.006

Pourcel, L., Routaboul, J. M., Kerhoas, L., Caboche, M., Lepiniec, L., and Debeaujon, I. (2005). TRANSPARENT TESTA10 encodes a laccase-like enzyme involved in oxidative polymerization of flavonoids in *Arabidopsis* seed coat. *Plant Cell* 17, 2966–2980. doi: 10.1105/tpc.105.035154

Ranocha, P., Chabannes, M., Chamayou, S., Danoun, S. D., Jauneau, A., Boudet, A. M., et al. (2002). Laccase down-regulation causes alterations in phenolic metabolism and cell wall structure in poplar. *Plant Physiol.* 129, 145–155. doi: 10.1104/pp.010988

Saitou, N., and Nei, M. (1987). The neighbor-joining method: a new method for reconstructing phylogenetic trees. *Mol. Biol. Evol.* 4, 406–425.

Turlapati, P. V., Kim, K. W., Davin, L. B., and Lewis, N. G. (2011). The laccase multigene family in *Arabidopsis thaliana*: towards addressing the mystery of their gene function(s). *Planta* 233, 439–470. doi: 10.1007/s00425-010-1298-3

Wang, J., Feng, J., Jia, W., Chang, S., Li, S., and Li, Y. (2015). Lignin engineering through laccase modification: a promising field for energy plant improvement. *Biotechnol. Biofuels* 8:145. doi: 10.1186/s13068-015-0331-y

Xiao, Y., Gao, S., Di, P., Chen, J., Chen, W., and Zhang, L. (2009). Methyl jasmonate dramatically enhances the accumulation of phenolic acids in *Salvia miltiorrhiza* hairy root cultures. *Physiol. Plant* 137, 1–9. doi: 10.1111/j.1399-3054.2009.01257.x

Xu, H., Song, J., Luo, H., Zhang, Y., Li, Q., Zhu, Y., et al. (2016). Analysis of the genome sequence of the medicinal plant Salvia miltiorrhiza. *Mol. plant* 9, 949–952.

Xu, Z., Luo, H., Ji, A., Zhang, X., Song, J., and Chen, S. (2016). Global identification of the full-length transcripts and alternative splicing related to phenolic acid biosynthetic genes in *Salvia miltiorrhiza*. *Front. Plant Sci.* 7:100. doi: 10.3389/fpls.2016.00100

Xu, Z., Peters, R. J., Weirather, J., Luo, H., Liao, B., Zhang, X., et al. (2015). Full-length transcriptome sequences and splice variants obtained by a combination of sequencing platforms applied to different root tissues of *Salvia miltiorrhiza* and tanshinone biosynthesis. *Plant J.* 82, 951–961. doi: 10.1111/tpj.12865

Yoshida, H. (1883). Chemistry of lacquer (urushi). Part I. Communication from the chemical society of tokio. *J. Chem. Soc.* 43, 472–486. doi: 10.1039/ct8834300472

Zhao, Q., Nakashima, J., Chen, F., Yin, Y., Fu, C., Yun, J., et al. (2013). Laccase is necessary and nonredundant with *peroxidase* for lignin polymerization during vascular development in *Arabidopsis*. *Plant Cell* 25, 3976–3987. doi: 10.1105/tpc.113.117770

Zhou, J., Lee, C., Zhong, R., and Ye, Z. (2009). MYB58 and MYB63 are transcriptional activators of the lignin biosynthetic pathway during secondary cell wall formation in *Arabidopsis*. *Plant Cell* 21, 248–266. doi: 10.1105/tpc.108.063321

12

Medicinal Plant Analysis: A Historical and Regional Discussion of Emergent Complex Techniques

Martin Fitzgerald[1], Michael Heinrich[2] and Anthony Booker[1,2]*

[1] *Herbal and East Asian Medicine, School of Life Sciences, College of Liberal Arts and Sciences, University of Westminster, London, United Kingdom,* [2] *Pharmacognosy and Phytotherapy, UCL School of Pharmacy, London, United Kingdom*

*Correspondence:
Anthony Booker
a.booker@westminster.ac.uk

The analysis of medicinal plants has had a long history, and especially with regard to assessing a plant's quality. The first techniques were organoleptic using the physical senses of taste, smell, and appearance. Then gradually these led on to more advanced instrumental techniques. Though different countries have their own traditional medicines China currently leads the way in terms of the number of publications focused on medicinal plant analysis and number of inclusions in their Pharmacopoeia. The monographs contained within these publications give directions on the type of analysis that should be performed, and for manufacturers, this typically means that they need access to more and more advanced instrumentation. We have seen developments in many areas of analytical analysis and particularly the development of chromatographic and spectroscopic methods and the hyphenation of these techniques. The ability to process data using multivariate analysis software has opened the door to metabolomics giving us greater capacity to understand the many variations of chemical compounds occurring within medicinal plants, allowing us to have greater certainty of not only the quality of the plants and medicines but also of their suitability for clinical research. Refinements in technology have resulted in the ability to analyze and categorize plants effectively and be able to detect contaminants and adulterants occurring at very low levels. However, advances in technology cannot provide us with all the answers we need in order to deliver high-quality herbal medicines and the more traditional techniques of assessing quality remain as important today.

Keywords: herbal medicine, medicinal plant, analysis, quality, pharmacopoeia, complexity, advances

INTRODUCTION

Medicinal plants have been a resource for healing in local communities around the world for thousands of years. Still it remains of contemporary importance as a primary healthcare mode for approximately 85% of the world's population (Pešić, 2015), and as a resource for drug discovery, with 80% of all synthetic drugs deriving from them (Bauer and Brönstrup, 2014). Concurrently, the last few hundred years has seen a prolific rise in the introduction, development, and advancement of herbal substances analysis. Humans have been identifying and selecting medicinal plants and foods based on organoleptic assessment of suitability and quality for thousands of years, but it is only in the span of the last seven decades since the invention of basic analytical techniques, e.g., paper chromatography, that has seen rapid development from sight, touch, and smell to using sophisticated instrumentation. Though this mechanization of the senses has appeared relatively recently, historically conceptual expansion has been building throughout the scientific revolution, outwards toward the universe and inwards to a scale below recognition capable with a human eye, leading to development of some of the earliest analytical tools assisting the senses, the telescope and microscope. From the initial discovery of new microscopic worlds, through structural, chemical, and atomic levels, the sensitivity and range of human perception has been extended and enhanced.

Rapid progress is especially evident considering that the concept of a laboratory was only formally formed in Europe during the early 1600s. First as an extension of philosophers', doctors', and scientists' workrooms, it becomes a space to study nature and gather empirical evidence (Wilson, 1997), where studies could be conducted at the analyst's convenience rather than at specific times when daylight or weather permitted. This was a small but important step towards more formalized analytical investigations.

In modern analysis, single techniques such as paper chromatography and much earlier colorimetry appeared. It was followed by a greater range and wider application of these techniques until early hyphenations such as LC-UV emerged, culminating more recently in multiple combinations of multi-hyphenated instrumentation, availing of the analytical advantages inherent in each individual technique. The emergence of hyphenated analytical techniques in many aspects is analogous to the organoleptic synthesis that occurs when selecting a medicinal plant; viewing, smelling and tasting it to use combinations of different senses, increasing the points of reference/statistical degrees of freedom to improve the probability of correctly identifying and assessing its quality. The emergence and application of these hyphenated techniques only became possible and useful as computer systems and data management tools developed, enabling rapid and selective synthesis of information from the large amount of instrumental and analytical data signals generated.

Probably the single greatest influence in recent times in the advancement of the analysis of herbal materials (and arguably analysis generally) is, though, how large amounts of data can be collected, assimilated, and used more meaningfully in human readable forms. Similar to the historical advancements in combinatorial hyphenated instrumentation, now combinatorial data processing techniques like fingerprinting, metabolomic profiling, and pattern recognition algorithms have emerged, further increasing analytical capabilities, while reducing operator time and expertise required. This trend has further accelerated the pace and rate of advancement of analytical techniques and has led to an increase in the pace and capability of the associated research. In this paper, we analyze publication trends and pharmacopoeial developments in order to better understand the role and progression of analytical techniques. Since their initial discovery and development, with

a particular focus on China, an Asian country with both deep cultural and long-term historical roots in plant medicine, to more modern day developments and applications.

PUBLICATION TRENDS

Increasing interest in medicinal plant research and analysis is reflected in the number of recent publications, with more than a three-fold increase from 4,686 publications during the year 2008 to 14,884 in 2018. Output published during the 8 years of the present decade alone outnumbered all those combined before 2000, since the included database records began in 1800 (**Figure 1**).

The largest proportion of publications cited in current databases over the last 10 years for medicinal plant analysis reports are in the disciplines of pharmacology and pharmacy (**Figure 2**). With plant sciences, biochemical molecular biology and agriculture research following closely behind, together comprising almost 70% of the total publications.

REGIONAL TRENDS—LAST 10 YEARS

The majority (about 58%) of medicinal plant analysis publications in the last 10 years have collectively emerged from mainland China, India, USA, and South Korea (**Figure 3**). This may be an expression of the strong medicinal plant traditions in Asia in addition to the USA's dominant presence as an international user of herbal products (Hu et al., 2013). The major East Asian regions, in particular, China, Japan, South Korea, together with Taiwan, contribute more than half of the total citations (55%). This may be indicative of the rapid economic progress and technological capability of these countries. China is the major contributor, with a 15% increase in its dominance of research outputs in the last 10 years. This influence has also been seen in the effect of China's growing involvement in aiding the development of pharmacopoeias around the world and as a leader in the analysis of Chinese medicinal plants (**Figure 3**).

REGULATION AND A CHANGING ANALYTICAL LANDSCAPE

From a regulatory perspective, the pharmacopoeial requirements are the central reference point for the analysis of medicinal plants. Though internationally many pharmacopoeias exist, the most comprehensive of these relating to herbal medicinal materials is the Chinese Pharmacopoeia (ChP). The current ChP introduced in 2015 is the 10th iteration presented in three volumes and includes 5,608 drugs, a 10-fold increase from its first edition in 1953. More than half of the current monographs (Hamid-Reza et al., 2013, 598) relate to CHM specifically including raw plants, slices, herbal mixtures, and oils. A noticeable inclusion in the current version compared with the previous version is the addition of 400 herbal mixtures (Qian et al., 2010).

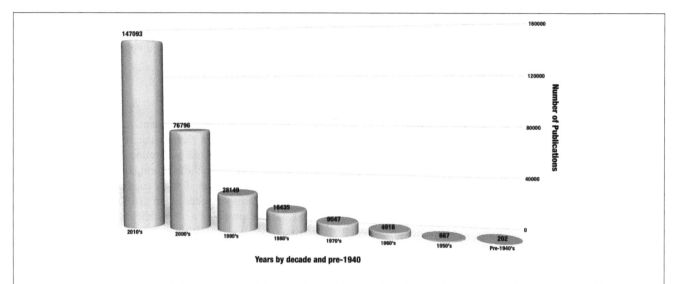

FIGURE 1 | The herbal substance analysis publications trend since search records began in 1800. A keyword search was conducted using the combination "medicinal plant" OR "herbal medicine" AND "analysis" chosen for the maximum retuned records after exploring a list of similar topic and combination of keywords such as "photochemical analysis," "traditional medicine," and "herbal." The Web of Science or collection, KCI- Korean Journal database, MEDLINE®, Russian Science Citation index, and SciELO Citation index databases were included in the search.

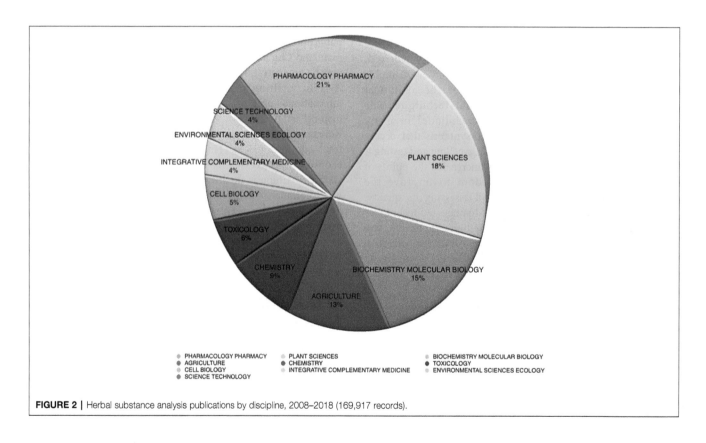

FIGURE 2 | Herbal substance analysis publications by discipline, 2008–2018 (169,917 records).

PHARMACOPOEIA MONOGRAPHS— THEIR INFLUENCES AND CHALLENGES

Though more recently the ChP is playing an increasing role in influencing medicinal plant analysis, the development of the ChP has been heavily influenced by Western pharmacopoeias.

Historically the identification, preparation, and analysis of medicinal plants were based on classic texts such as the Shengnong Bencao Jing (Shengnong Materia Medica, 25–220 CE), where the category and quality of 365 plants and 113 prescriptions were assessed by taste. Organoleptic sensing of bitterness, sweetness, saltiness, and even neutral tastes were

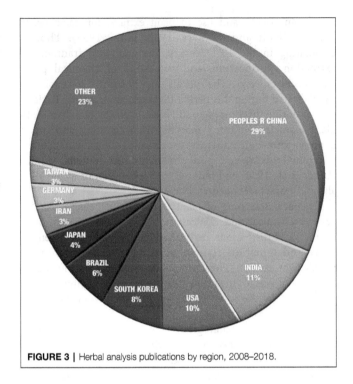

FIGURE 3 | Herbal analysis publications by region, 2008–2018.

thought to indicate the function and application of the medicine. Arguably, the most influential Chinese pharmacy monograph is the Bencao Gangmu (Compendium of Materia Medica, 1368–1644 CE) containing 1,892 plant descriptions and 11,096 prescriptions sorted in 16 divisions and 60 orders, emphasizing appearance, taste, and odor as a key to authentication and quality.

However, the main precursor to the modern format of the current Chinese Pharmacopoeia was printed in the 1930s with 670 drugs. Even at this early stage, the then dominant Western powers such as Britain, Germany, America, and Japan found challenges in understanding and forming consensus for recognizing, categorizing, and assuring the quality of Chinese medical materials. At this time a difficulty emerged in securing materials for the more Western styled "scientifically run" hospitals. Initially it was though that as Japan had adopted a translation of the German pharmacopoeia in 1886, the Chinese could follow suit using the British Pharmacopoeia, which in 1927 had been translated into Chinese as a joint effort by the London and British Chambers of Commerce. However, some differences in opinion between the four occupiers had to be first resolved.

Many of the technological demands necessary to produce and maintain the pharmacopoeial standards required by the Americans was beyond the ability and technological capability of the Chinese at that time. America had recently just printed a Chinese translation of its United States Pharmacopeia (10th edition) published in 1926. The strict American standards for aconite, digitalis, adrenalin, and insulin were purported to be managed by new or foreign trained pharmacists (Read, 1930). Preparations such as liniments found in the British and U.S. Pharmacopoeias were included in the Chinese version. Syrups such as those of codeine and glucose and tinctures of cannabis

were from the British influence. Foreign residents in China found it difficult to ingest local food and stated an "extensive need for bowel remedies." Therefore, drugs of the time, albuminis, aspidium, and emetin, were included. Vaccines for diphtheria, tetanus, and smallpox were maintained through the instruction of the USP.

German chemists had already gained a reputation for the isolation of chemical compounds, many of which were used medicinally and were already included in the Japanese Pharmacopoeia such as oxalic acid, pyrogallic acid, and bromine. Therefore, the existing German-Japanese analytical methods were generally utilized for these areas, which comprised about 25% of the new Chinese Pharmacopoeia. Whereas more British and American derived analytical methods and preparations were included for vegetable- and animal-based materials.

Agreement over the correct translation and naming of chemical compounds also proved problematic, e.g. when attempting to resolve disagreement between German-Latin and Anglo-American descriptions such as "natrium chloratum" and "sodii chloridum." The shared Latin common language elements aided European and American common understanding; however, translation into Chinese was troublesome. A potentially easier route would have been to adopt the Japanese Pharmacopoeia names and descriptions, often possessing the same Asian (Hanzi) character as that in China, however, this was resisted due to the strong nationalistic sentiment at the time in mainland China (Read, 1930).

Though the Japanese favored direct foreign phonetic transliterated terms for drugs, about 60 original Chinese *materia medica* entries had persisted in the Japanese Pharmacopoeia including entries for camphor, ginger, aloes, cardamom, and star anise.

Difficulty in plant identification and common naming was not confined to Asia. During the early 1900s period of European and American political expansion, attempts were being made in Europe to catalogue multilingual terms for similar plants such as the publication of "the illustrated polyglot dictionary of plants names" in Latin, Arabic, Armenian, English, French, German, Italian, and Turkish languages (Bedevian, 1936), cataloguing 3,657 plants in eight languages.

CHRONOLOGY OF PHARMACOPOEIAL DEVELOPMENTS IN CHINA

1900–1949

Medicinal plant publications during the early 1900s, before the formation of the People's Republic of China in 1949, were greatly influenced by the previous "age of exploration." Many scientific societies were set up by explorers, their peers, and investors as forums to communicate knowledge and acknowledge ownership of findings and discoveries (Fyfe and Moxham, 2016). The rise in fashion of the "gentleman scholar" engaging in academic pursuits supported the occupation of writing. During this time, many publications focused on the identification and classification of ethnic/indigenous medical plants, such as Aztec medicinal plants still in use in modern Mexico (Braubach, 1925; Heinrich et al., 2014), Algonquians from nowadays, Canada, (Speck, 1917), Micronesians (St John, 1948), Babylonians and Assyrians, (Jastrow, 1914), Native American Indian tribes (Castetter et al., 1935), Persia, (Garrison, 1933) and India, (Chopra, 1933). Publications in English describing the history and use of Chinese medicine in the context of Western orthodox also appeared (Chan, 1939).

Post-1949

Periods of advancements in TCM research after 1949 to the present day have been described as occurring in three defined phases lasting about 20 years each. The first was 1950–1970, springing from the rapid development of TCM in universities, research, and hospitals in China during this time. The second phase took place during 1980–2000s, where we see the construction of legal, economic, and scientific networks. The third phase, from 2000 to date, is defined by a focus on elucidating the scientific basis and scientific clinical practice of TCM using cross-disciplinary and global collaborations (Xu et al., 2013).

1950–1969
Political Context

This period immediately followed the formation of the People's Republic of China and saw a rise in nationalism and political introspection. International relationships cooled and a closer connection with the Soviet Union was officially forged with the Sino-Soviet Treaty of Friendship, Alliance, and Mutual Assistance in 1950.

Regulatory and Pharmacopoeial Developments

This period saw the launch of the first edition of the People's Republic of China Pharmacopoeia (ChP) in Chinese launched in 1953. It contains 531 monographs and mainly retains the information of the previous precursor published in the 1930s, compiled from foreign influences. It guided both identification and quantification of synthetic drugs and medicines together in one issue. Some crude herbal materials were listed, but not in analytical detail. Internationally post-World War II, good-will fostered a sense of cooperation and collaboration. This was also reflected by the World Health Organization's release of the international pharmacopoeia (Ph. Int) issued by the World Health Organization in 1951, produced in two volumes. It contained 344 monographs and 84 tests, with an aim to provide a harmonized international reference for pharmacopoeial methods. The first European Pharmacopoeia Ph. Eur. was produced in 1967, with a more European focus, but combining many common elements of the long-existing British Pharmacopoeia and the United States Pharmacopeia.

Medicinal Plant Research and Analytical Development

Research publication output during the 1950s was varied but the most cited publication trends concerned identification of plant species using electron microscopy (Watson, 1958), the use of plant tissue staining methods (Bergeron and Singer, 1958;

Fernstrom, 1958), and use of plant extracts for colorimetric analysis (Holt and Withers, 1958; Lillie, 1958). Though originating in the 19th century, the analytical tradition of extraction, purification, and separation of chemical plant components, e.g., the alkaloids, became increasingly sophisticated during this period (Svoboda et al., 1959). Toxicity studies during this time were still basic, exposing mainly mice to plant extracts and using mortality rate counting and organ biopsy and cell station techniques, e.g., quercetin, podophyllotoxin, and podophyllin extract toxicity studies (Leiter et al., 1950) and induced liver lesions with Pyrrolizidine alkaloid extracts (Schoental, 1959).

Chemical screening of plants for their medicinal effects in various chemical and clinical trials is featured (Farnsworth, 1966) as did their use in derivatized forms for the treatment of nerve inflammation (Jancso et al., 1967) and in human metabolism studies (Pletscher, 1968). Studies into the use of medicinal plants for their potential use in cancer treatments were encouraged by the first isolation of paclitaxel from the pacific yew, *Taxus brevifolia* Nutt.

Older basic chromatographic techniques that had been already in use remained commonly used analytical techniques, e.g., paper chromatography applied to the analysis of common broom [*Cytisus scoparius* (L.) Link.] (Jaminet, 1959) and in medicinal plant quality control (Paris and Viejo, 1955). Separation of alkaloids e.g. in *Duboisia myoporoides* R. Br. (Hills and Rodwell, 1951) remained a common interest and the analysis of other important metabolites including scilliroside in red squill, *Drimia maritima*. (L.) Stearn (Dybing et al., 1954). An investigation of *Cannabis sativa* L. for its antibacterial activity was also conducted during this timeframe (Krejci, 1958).

Much of the medicinal plant research of this period concerned the extraction and isolation of single compounds from plants. Basic colorimetric tests, UV-visible and infrared spectroscopy, and paper chromatography had previously supported this type of analysis. Spectroscopic techniques such as UV-Vis spectrometry with chart recorders had been in use since the 1920s (Hardy, 1938). These were being increasingly used for quantitative applications, such as in the analysis of glucoside in walnuts and monitoring the chemical composition of plants in relation to seasonal variations (Daglish, 1950).

However, the 1950–1970s was a golden period for the development of analytical technology. A time when the techniques of mass spectrometry (MS), nuclear magnetic resonance (NMR) spectroscopy, and gas chromatography (GC) techniques had come of age. Mass spectrometry, which had been invented in the late 1800s and used in a more analytical form during the 1910s, had now come into a relatively more advanced era. It was during the period 1950-1970 that the ion trap technique was developed, for which Dehmelt and Paul later received a Noble prize. The Purcell and Bloch groups at Harvard and Stanford University, respectively, developed NMR techniques and in 1952 also received a Nobel Prize (in Physics). In 1952, Archer John Porter Martin and Richard Synge also shared a Nobel Prize (in chemistry) for inventing partition chromatography, the basis of modern GC. Gas–liquid separations solved the problem of separating sugar-based molecules, which tended to bond with traditional stationery phases such as silica and volatile compounds, such as volatile oils, which are lost through evaporation during collection, preparation, and analysis. GC was applied for the first time to resolve 17 difficult to separate plant glycosides from a broad range of chemical classes, including phenolic, coumarin, isocoumarin, isoflavone, anthraquinone, cyanogenic, isothiocyanate, and monoterpene (Furuya, 1965), 15 kinds of valerian sesquiterpenoids in valerianaceous plant oils (Furuya and Kojima, 1967), and the extraction and analysis of rose oil (Minkov and Trandafilov, 1969).

Publications included well-applied examples where visible, ultra-violet (UV), and infrared (IR) spectral data were combined to elucidate structural characteristics of plants while undergoing chemical degradation, e.g., the stereochemical discrimination of lignin components paulownin and isopaulownin from *Paulownia tomentosa* Steud. (Takahashi and Nakagawa, 1966), the alkaloids of the Orchidaceae (Lüning et al., 1967), and terpenoids of *Zanthoxylum rhetsa* DC (Mathur et al., 1967).

MS was also used side-by-side with NMR, resulting in the structural elucidation of key metabolites, e.g., the characterization of the opium papaverrubine alkaloids and their *N*-methyl derivatives in the genus *Papaver* (Brochmann-Hanssen et al., 1968), the analysis of three new coumestan derivatives from the root of licorice, *Glycyrrhiza* spp., (Shibata and Saitoh, 1968), and the isolation and purification of polyprenols from the leaves of *Aesculus hippocastanum* L. (horse chestnut) (Wellburn et al., 1967).

Up to this time, China had played a very marginal role in international research and development activities, a situation that was to change significantly in the following period.

1970–1989
Political Context
1971 saw China's introspection from the Mao era revert to more external international engagement with the "People's Republic of China" (PRC) elected as a permanent member of the United Nations' General Assembly. This followed the American government's extension of political relations with PRC after the Richard Nixon presidential visit that catalyzed an "Opening up to the West" phase in Chinese history. This opening began in 1978, orchestrated by the interim leader Deng Xiaoping, who initiated support for wide sweeping economic reforms. On a local level this manifested as individuals within China being allowed to make personal economic decisions, with the tightly governed communes being dissolved. Rural markets were replaced by open markets, resulting in a dramatic increase in international trade, supporting Xiaoping's wish to fund economic growth from foreign investment. In the context of medicine, China's ambition to look outward was highlighted over a decade earlier by a University College London anatomy Professor, Derrick James, when a British delegation visited China in 1954 and in his subsequent Lancet article outlined China's intention to introduce a more scientific, modernized TCM (James, 1955).

As international trade from China expanded, so did the trade in medicinal plants from Asia and with it, increased access for

Chinese scientists to modern analytical instrumentation. Internally by the mid-1980s, 25 Chinese medicine colleges were formed in a reportedly scientific and modern style with an almost 30-fold increase of TCM hospital beds to 2.5 million since the formation of the state in 1949 (Cai, 1988).

Regulatory and Pharmacopoeial Developments
The establishment in 1985 of the China State Administration of Traditional Chinese Medicine began the formal organization of TCM research and development nationally and internationally, sowing the seeds for the formal cooperative global links that would provide the backbone for the future of international Chinese medicinal plant research. China's motivation to secure international links was also manifest in the publication of the PRC's first dual Chinese and English language Pharmacopoeia, ChP, 4th edition in 1997, which began its new 5-year publication cycle trend.

Medicinal Plant Research and Analytical Developments
The newly fostered R&D investment and cooperation during this period globally is represented by the leap in sophistication and complexity of the research published, with a shift from basic to more advanced biochemical investigations and more emphasis focused on disease and diagnosis strategies such as in cancer and infectious disease. The most widely cited articles of this time include advanced biomedical research on Forskolin, from the roots of *Plectranthus barbatus* Andrews as a diterpene activator in nucleotide metabolism. Even though basic biochemical equipment and colorimetric methods and spectrometric enzymatic assays were used, a more complex understanding of plant metabolites is apparent (Seamon et al., 1981).

This is also evident in the investigation of lectins as cell recognition molecules and their involvement in a wide range of molecular processes and potential pathologies, e.g., in metabolic regulation, viral, and bacterial infection processes (Sharon and Lis, 1989). In addition to plants playing a role as phytochelants in complexing heavy metals (Grill et al., 1985 and Grill et al., 1987), licorice was studied in greater depth using a conceptually new approach of assessing the mineral-corticoid activity of licorice and its role in sodium retention (Stewart et al., 1987) and the radical scavenging properties of its flavonoids (Hatano et al., 1988).

Awareness of plants having a role in cancer with both causative and curative effects emerged, with a highly cited review of potential causes of esophageal cancer in China. Particular concerns were linked to effects of fungal growth and associated nitrosamines due to poor storage conditions (Mingxin et al., 1980). This was a precursor to later studies on aflatoxins, which are now acknowledged as causing serious health problem linked to poor storage and processing. From a therapeutic perspective, the interest in antileukemia and anti-tumor agents, e.g., in *Taxus brevifolia* Nutt. stem bark, first investigated some decades before, continued and ultimately resulted in the introduction of a completely new therapeutic approach (Wani et al., 1971).

One of the landmark discoveries in medicinal plant history was reported to the west during this period. The antimalaria effect of artemisinin, derived from *Artemisia annua* L., for which the Chinese scientist Youyou Tu later received a Nobel Prize in Medicine (Klayman, 1985), described a conceptual shift in the approach to treating malaria, illustrating both a change in approach from using quinoline-based drugs, which parasites were showing increasing resistance to, and paving the way for the development of new classes of drugs e.g. with potential in antiviral and anticancer treatment (Su and Miller, 2015).

1990–2008
Political Context
This period in China was characterized largely by economic, political, and academic success delivering on the earlier aspirations of Deng Xiaoping through focused planning and the tight administrative grip of three successive presidents (Chairpersons) and state administration. An unusually high-performing economy producing more than a 10% sustained gross domestic profit (GDP) created a stable base for China to successfully join the world trade organization in 2001, marking its arrival on the world stage as a competent economic power and its transition to a market economy (Morrison, 2013). This, however, came with challenges to families and the environment.

On a local level as communes of the last decades had dissolved, a system of "household responsibility" was adapted as a kind of contract that guaranteed agricultural family holdings to provide a certain level of food (and herb) output (Ash, 1988). This ensured that levels of agricultural production were optimized for the land available. Because families were now allowed to sell grown products in an open market that mirrored the economic national trend, food and medicinal herbs began to take on more distinct financial attributes. This combined with mass migration of rural workers to rapidly developing industrialized cities away from countryside homes without sufficient locally produced food in urban surrounds created a situation of widespread supply and demand, leading to new value chains for food and medicinal plant products, along with potential motivation for the substitution or adulteration of these products.

Regulatory and Pharmacopoeial Developments
As industrialization occurred so too did environmental pollution, with increased volume and concentration of raw materials and waste presenting greater potential for pollution of medicinal plant material. The PRC at this stage had gone through a period of prolonged political stability. Economic policy became more flexible and governance developed an increasingly regulatory role compared with that of previous, more rigid enforcement. Regulation and safety testing of medical products saw further guidance through the production of four further volumes of the ChP in both Chinese and English culminating in the 8th edition in 2005, listing 3,217 monographs, almost double that of the 1990 edition. This period saw China's confidence increase and extend to regulatory and guidance aspects, with the ChP undergoing the greatest leap in analytical sophistication and rate of change to date. The 1990 edition was a

significant step in the acceptance and introduction of modern instrumental analytical techniques for standard herbal substance testing. Since the 1985 edition, specific identification tests were introduced using mainly thin layer chromatography (TLC). Now chromatogram images of the crude and test samples were included and required for testing. Basic identification was expanded to require quantitation where high-performance liquid chromatography (HPLC) and GC were now included for the first time and TLC extended for content analysis. More instrumental techniques replaced older ones such as the introduction of spectrophotometric determination of the alkaloid content of berberine, which had been gravimetrically analyzed in previous editions. Quantification moved from measuring simpler marker components to more specific active compounds like anthroquinone from He Shou Wu, *Polygonum multiflorum* Thunb [now *Reynoutria multiflora* (Thunb.) Moldenke]. The 2000 edition introduced assays for residues of organic chlorine pesticides for Gan Cao, *Glycyrrhiza uralensis* Fisch. ex DC. and Huang Qi, *Astragalus membranaceus* Fisch. ex Bunge (Kwee, 2002). Another leap occurred in the 2005 edition with an expansion of the acceptance of HPLC-MS, LC-MS-MS, and DNA molecular markers and chemical fingerprinting, setting the stage for 21st century pharmacopoeial trends and the ChP as a central global influence for the analysis of medicinal plants.

Medicinal Plant Research and Analytical Developments
The fruition of investment in external academic relations from the "opening up" phase and internal support for the now formed TCM structures of the previous decades state initiatives were borne out by the publication output in this period, with a six-fold increase in output compared with that of the previous equivalent 20-year period. Much of the output from this time demonstrated a refinement of thought around the effect of plant compounds on humans as a holistic system rather than the more singular metabolic pathway thinking of previous years. It also shows a tremendous emphasis on obtaining large datasets especially of the known metabolites and a wide exploration of acclaimed effects. Whole plant extracts and combinations of metabolites rather than single ones became a core theme, as became a medicinal plant's effect on longer term health and preventative medicine. This ignited a resurgence of interest in the analysis of medicinal plants as a source of lead compounds for drug discovery.

The role of medical plants in coronary disease analysis becomes topical during this phase, e.g., long-term studies on elderly demonstrating the reduced risk of death from sustained flavonoids intake *via* inhibition of the oxidation of low-density lipoprotein (Hertog et al., 1993). More sophisticated quantitative analysis and differentiation appeared during this time such as HPLC of mulberry leaves containing four varieties of flavonoids (including rutin and quercetin), and their antioxidant properties (Zhishen et al., 1999). Flavonoid coronary disease risk prevention and cancer roles were advanced by the characterization and analysis studied in a wide range of fruits, seeds, oils, wines, and tea (Middleton et al., 2000). A greater awareness of the potency and efficacy of drugs and medicinal plants became evident as in the studies and analysis of the effect of fluorine on drug binding and potency (Purser et al., 2008). Cancer research also demonstrated further advances through combining previous findings on receptor binding with advancements in DNA extraction, amplification techniques, and cloning techniques. Resveratrol became a key area of interest for its chemoprotective effects (Jang et al., 1997).

Many of the most cited publications of these two decades were detailed reviews, which brought together the findings of previous research on individual plant research.

21st Century

China's growing influence was marked in 2011 with the Chinese State Administration of TCM (SATCM) forming an official relationship with the European Directive on the Quality of Medicines (EDQM) to share expertise and knowledge in addition to raising the standards of testing in China and Europe through cooperation. These include translation of historical TCM documents, information relating to preparation of products, process, and sourcing. Europe, seen as an aggregate, has an approximately 16% representation in the last decades' research output, higher than the USA. The European Pharmacopoeia (Ph Eur) manages CHM's by allowing importation of CHM's to countries who have signed up to the European Pharmacopoeia convention. Currently there are 43 CHMs included in the Ph Eur, 8th edition, 34 from the Ph Eur TCM Working Party, 21 of which have been included as full monographs (Wang and Franz, 2015). New Ph Eur CHM monographs are being developed based, in part, on the ChP. This was facilitated by a working party on TCM (Ph Eur WP) and was officially introduced in 2005. It included 38 member states with a delegation from the EU (a representative from DG Health & Food Safety and the European Medicines Agency). Additional observers are composed of 27 countries/regions/organizations [which include 7 European countries, the Taiwan Food and Drug Administration (TFDA), and World Health Organization (WHO)] (EDQM, 2017). The WHO, through participation in the PhEur, additionally has led efforts to develop a harmonized international pharmacopoeia (WHO, 2018).

The monographs for medicinal plants in Ph Eur have developed from standard western drug monographs with an emphasis on chemical and physical testing, while those in the ChP have formed from revisions of older traditional texts.

As pharmacopoeial monographs expand and develop, so too does the range and complexity of analytical methods and analytical hardware needed to meet the regulatory demands and expectations of quality.

These emerging research trends and pharmacopoeial directives have paved the way for the development of a broad range of analytical techniques, mainly centering around the use of liquid chromatography (LC), GC, MS, and established UV/visible spectrophotometric techniques.

We present a selection of these analytical techniques and give examples of their applications in the analysis of medicinal plants and medicinal plant products.

Analytical Hardware, Attested and Emerging Methods
High-Performance Liquid Chromatography

HPLC is one of the most developed and widely used analytical techniques. It is built on a historical knowledge base amassed from TLC and optical chemistry experience. HPLC chromatography elements rely on similar principles of TLC/HPTLC, where separation of components is dependent on selective affinities to stationary supports and liquid phases.

Detection employs a photomultiplier system able to detect individual wavelengths of light, a range (spectrum) and/or multiple simultaneous wavelengths in its different iterations, combined in an enclosed automated instrument system with sample injectors; this has significantly increased the precision and reproducibility of the chromatography when compared with older chromatographic methods. The widespread use of HPLC has made it more affordable for laboratories. High operator skill level is not required; it is robust and sensitive to low level detection and is particularly used for the quantification of components (active substances and adulterants).

HPLC applied to herbal products is well developed, and it has been successfully applied to the analysis of complex mixtures of similar compounds, both for the separation of individual compounds and for the differentiation of medicinal plant species. The high resolution of the technique has supported the development of the concept of a characteristic "fingerprint" developed for medicinal plants and herbal products to aid identification and authentication, e.g., Li et al. (2010) demonstrated differentiation of the same type of medicinal plant product from 40 different manufacturers, while simultaneously separating nine marker chemical compounds (berberine, aloe-emodin, rhein, emodin, chryso- phanol, baicalin, baicalein, wogonoside, and wogonin).

High-Performance Thin Layer Chromatography

HPTLC has become a common addition to the method section of new monographs, replacing the widely used TLC tests; it has shown to be a reliable and reproducible method of analysis that provides essential information regarding the compositional quality of an herbal substance.

Some advantages of this technique include low cost and a relatively simple test method. It does not require advanced sample preparation methods or high levels of expertise. Sample amounts are relatively small, and it is a more sensitive technique compared with HPLC, well suited to detecting contaminants. However, some disadvantages are that the reproducibility is dependent on a variety of external factors, and although more sensitive than HPLC, it is not able to sufficiently detect compounds at very low concentrations (PPB) where LC-MS (or HPTLC-MS) may be more suitable. HPTLC relies on the same principle as TLC and uses similar TLC plates and mobile phases, although relatively small amounts of solvents are required compared with standard TLC. The process of adding the sample to plates (spotting) has been made more reproducible and precise by spraying the sample onto the plate to form a band of compound rather than a spot. Retention factors for individual compounds are more reproducible due to controlled humidity during development. Derivatizing the analysis plates is completed mainly by machine and the visualization is captured by modern camera systems connected to powerful software. The software allows further manipulation of images to optimize visualization in a way that would be very difficult chemically. Another advantage is that the HPTLC system can be easily linked to a scanning densitometer; this not only allows for more precise quantitative work to be carried out but also the data can be exported for multivariate analysis. It is likely that more of the monographs with TLC requirements will be upgraded to HPTLC in the future.

Gas Chromatography

GC in respect to medicinal plant analysis is mainly used for the analysis of compounds with higher volatility, e.g., compounds found within essential oils, and more volatile adulterants, e.g., pesticides. While single GC column chromatography and its hyphenated derivatives have been use for many years, 1991 saw the introduction of 2D-GC or GC x GC, where the eluents of a standard separation are trapped and recirculated for another round of separation. This allows not only greater resolution and better separation but also the ability to purge undesired or interfering compounds so that more specific areas of the separation can be targeted (Liu and Philips, 1991). This led the way for multidimensional gas chromatography (MDGC) and the advances of the modules and valve systems that trap, control, and divert sample streams. These improvements extend to the thermal control and valve systems allowing greater thermal flow and split streaming (Bahaghighat et al., 2019). One key problem with GC is the introduction of sample into a gas stream. Historically squeezing, boiling, and later distillation of herbal materials were used for the collection and production of volatile compounds such as oils. However, the inherent instability of volatile components and losses as well as the poor recovery of these substances presented difficulties. This situation has somewhat been overcome by advances in extraction techniques such a solvent-free microwave extraction, e.g., for citrus peel oils [Citrus sinensis (L.) Osbeck]. No solvents or water are necessary for high recoveries with this method, and it allows for highly efficient, compatible sample introduction without the need for interfering solvents (Aboudaou et al., 2018). This sample extraction method commonly known as headspace analysis for GC has undergone many iterations (Gerhardt et al., 2018). It has now developed to the stage where it is increasingly used for bacterial and microorganism detection such as in Commiphora species (Rubegeta et al., 2018).

Microextraction techniques are essential for the introduction of small sample volumes into the GC gas stream. Needle-based extraction techniques have the advantage of automation, ease of interface to other instruments, and compatibility with miniaturization. Advances in solid phase dynamic extraction (SPDE), In-tube extraction (ITEX), and needle trap extraction (NTE) have refined the use of these techniques for natural and herbal compounds (Kędziora-Koch and Wasiak, 2018), e.g., SPDE and ITEX for pesticide residues in dried herbs (Rutkowska et al., 2018), herbal mint aromas compounds in

commercial wine (Picard et al., 2018), and volatiles in Chinese herbal formula Baizhu Shaoyao San (Xu et al., 2018).

Supercritical Fluid Chromatography

Another liquid-based chromatographic technique based on pressurized low viscosity (supercritical) fluids, often carbon dioxide, is supercritical fluid chromatography (SFC). Since its introduction by Klesper in 1962, it has made large advances mainly due to improvements in its initially troublesome instrumentation (Desfontaine et al., 2015). Its main advantage over other techniques is in its usefulness for separating complex components characteristic of natural compounds. Selection of the correct conditions of SFC mobiles phases and modifiers can be finely tuned across a wide range of polarities from non-polar to polar allowing a broad selection of separations (Gao et al., 2010). Early analysis of natural products with SFC was when it was first hyphenated with gas chromatography (King, 1990). Recently, it has been more fully developed to analyze a range of natural compounds in herbal substances, notably, focusing on terpenes, phenolics, flavonoids, alkaloids, and saponins. This has been achieved with hyphenation to MS, diode array detectors, SFC-ELSD, in addition to the development of novel stationary phases such as cyanopropyl, pentaflouro phenyl (PFP), and imidazolyl. An example of this is with the separation of coumarins in Angelica dahurica (Hoffm.) Benth. & Hook.f. ex Franch. & Sav. roots and anthraquinones in rhubarb root (Pfeifer et al., 2016).

Near-Infrared Spectroscopy

Although commonly used within industry since the 1990's, near-infrared (NIR) spectroscopy was not the method of choice for medicinal plant analysis mainly due to overlapping peaks making interpretation of data problematic, and consequently, it never became the instrumentation of choice within the quality control laboratory in the same way that HPLC and TLC developed. However, with the addition of new computational software, NIR is re-emerging as an affordable and useful analytical technique used in the analysis of medicinal plants and has been particularly favored by Chinese companies in routine quality control analysis due to its ability to both rapidly differentiate between species and provide quantitative information on metabolite content (Li et al., 2013; Zhang and Su, 2014).

As with HPTLC and NMR data, NIR also provides an opportunity for multivariate analysis and it appears capable of resolving very small variations in metabolite content. It is argued that more traditional TLC or HPLC techniques can be more subjective in the data interpretation stage and require a high degree of operator skill and that NIR is more suitable for high volume analysis in the routine quality control laboratory (Wang and Yu, 2015). However, this has partly been addressed by the introduction of the fully automated systems available for HPTLC analysis and the inclusion of scanning densitometry equipment that reduce the need for operator interpretation. The main advantages of NIR appear to be the preservation of sample integrity, little sample preparation needed, and no need for solvents, and it has shown to perform well comparable to HPLC for species differentiation and quantification of metabolites (Chan et al., 2007). Probably the main drawback in NIR compared with other methods, and especially, TLC, HPTC, LC-MS is in its sensitivity and some reports suggest that this technique may only be suitable for detecting compounds that exist at a concentration above 0.1% (Lau et al., 2009). Another consideration is that variation in NIR data is dependent both on the chemical and physical properties of the sample, with the physical properties, e.g., particle size, having greater effects on the variation than the chemical. Therefore, before multivariate analysis can take place some pre-treatment of the spectral data is necessary, e.g., to reduce baseline noise, light scattering, and consequently enhance any chemical variation in the sample set (Chen et al., 2008). Some advantages of NIR certainly are apparent, although it may not be appropriate for all situations and all types of samples. The technology has made a huge leap forward since its first introduction and now it needs to establish itself more widely as a useful tool in the quality analysis of medicinal plants.

Hyphenated Techniques

Combinations of techniques with modern developments in metabolomic analysis and computational pattern recognition programs open up a wider scope of applications to medicinal plant analysis. Tandem combinations of analytical instrumentation such as MS with HPLC has proved a productive route to expanding analytical medicinal plant applications. Not only in identification and fingerprinting but further chemical characterization of individual compounds e.g., Liu et al. (2011), characterized a spectrum of alkaloid components in the Chinese herb Ku Shen (*Sophora flavescens* Aiton). Further combinations and permutations of MS and NMR in combination with HPTLC have been demonstrated, such as the detection of acetylcholinesterase inhibitors in galbanum in a search for natural product drug candidates (Hamid-Reza et al., 2013), and mass spectroscopy (MS) HPTLC-MS shown for *Ilex vomitoria* Aiton with the use of a sampling probe following HPTLC combined with MS with Electrospray Ion Trap (Ford and Van Berkel., 2004) and *Hydrastis canadensis* L., with HPLTLC-MS atmospheric pressure chemical ionization (Van Berkel et al., 2007).

Analytical combinations including ESI-IT-TOF/MS-HPLC-DAD-ESI-MS have been demonstrated for the analysis of coumarin patterns in Angelica polymorpha Maxim. roots (Liu et al, 2011) and multihyphenated techniques such as SPE-LC-MS/MS-ABI quadrupole trap have been used for the analysis of six major flavones in *Scutellaria baicalensis* Georgi (Fong et al., 2014) and 38 saponins in the roots *of Helleborus niger* L. by LC-ESI-IT-MS (Duckstein et al., 2014).

Merging the separation ability of HPTLC or HPLC with the analysis power of NMR and MS has significant benefits for analyzing complex samples in complex matrices such a blood, soil, and plants. However, each technique also possesses its inherent disadvantages. MS being complex, expensive, and time-consuming, requiring high analytical skill levels, it may not be suitable for a general quality assurance laboratory. Though powerful, extensive method development and post analysis data processing is required when applied to natural

compounds with broad complex compositions in contrast to simpler synthesized pharmaceutical ingredients. Similarly, NMR is also expensive and sensitive to variations in sample preparation and composition. It is not fully applicable to all natural compound samples and signals generated from NMR analysis often overlap making data analysis for individual compounds problematic. However, the relative speed, rich information output, and insight into the overall composition of medicinal plants from both MS and NMR far outweigh the disadvantages. These techniques allow the detection of compounds into the parts per billion analytical range (MS) and allow a detailed fingerprint of metabolites across differing polarities (NMR) and so for research and for larger companies they are highly applicable analytical hardware.

METABOLOMICS

Pharmacopoeial methods focus on authentication and quality of herbal materials; however, metabolomics allow us to go a step beyond authentication and look in more detail at a broad range of secondary metabolites. By coupling analytical data to multivariate software, this allows us to develop statistical models to firstly differentiate between species but also to get a better idea of a typical metabolite composition for a particular species. The advantage of this is that it can help to inform any laboratory test or clinical intervention. There has been great emphasis on making sure that any experiment or intervention uses plant material that is authenticated, with a herbarium specimen deposited. However, the requirements do not stipulate that a good representative of the species should be used. This is where metabolomics can provide essential information—by collecting a wide range of samples from different geographical locations, altitudes, growing conditions, it allows us to map their metabolite differences and highlight how diverse or how similar metabolite composition is. When an experiment is performed, we have the choice to use a specimen that may be typical, i.e., contains an average composition or we can look at compositions that are atypical, containing greater amounts of specific metabolites or even different metabolites. Moreover, if a particular experiment produces positive results and we want to reproduce the data, a metabolomic model allows us to choose species that have a similar composition.

This approach has important economic implications as a detailed understanding of metabolomic analysis allows us to inform industry as to how to grow plants that will be of the best composition and so help to support local livelihoods of farmers and primary processors in developing economies, e.g., Chachacoma (*Senecio nutans Sch. Bip.*) cultivation in the high altitude regions of Chile where metabolomics has helped to establish the best altitude for growing plants with the highest content of the anti-inflammatory acetophenone (Lopez et al., 2015).

This strategy also has applications in product development, where metabolomics can help to determine the quality of products based on their metabolite content, e.g., *Curcuma longa* L. (Turmeric products) (Booker et al., 2014), and also help to provide evidence that can lead to value addition of a product and greater confidence in its quality and safety.

NANOPARTICLES

Nanoparticles 1–100 nm sized ions or organic/inorganic molecules have proven to be important in the development of new analytical testing (Tao et al., 2018), occupying the analytical regions of space between the ionic dimensions and small molecules.

Recent developments in nanoparticle research has led to an increased focus on chemo-bio sensing, as DNA has become the most used biological molecule to functionalize nanoparticles. Nanoparticles have provided many advantages to more consistent and specific testing including providing a more reproducible stable matrix for research and development, more controllable and reliable basis for designing and conjugating to functional molecules, and a wide rebate of flexibility for purification, selection, and modification of analytes. Nanoparticles have been used in creating a biological bar code for trace analysis of mycotoxins in Chinese herbs e.g. conjugated nanoparticles with DNA fragments to bind and target Chinese medicinal plants, e.g., Jue Ming Zi [Cassia seeds—*Senna obtusifolia* (L.) H.S.Irwin & Barneby], Yuan Zhi (*Polygala tenuifolia* Willd.), and Bai Zi Ren [*Platycladus orientalis* (L.) Franco] (Yu et al., 2018).

THE FUTURE

The next steps in analytical advancement in combination with technological improvements will most likely occur in the realm of artificial intelligence. Neural networks have already shown promise in consumer electronics and online search engine optimization. Self-learning algorithms have been in development for decades, with great potential for the application of self-synthesizing, auto-creating, and auto-adapting algorithms, which can optimally recognize and synthesize analytical data into meaningful and useful patterns. This goes beyond what a single human mind could hope to achieve in lifetimes, now possible in seconds with current and more so with future technology. This extends not only the human potential of thinking and observation but also prediction and design. This could potentially play a role in self-design of analytical instrumentation and its modules, self-optimizing of methods in real-time, saving time that would perhaps take an analyst weeks or months of human work-hours to complete.

The greatest challenge with AI is its opacity and computational complexity. With self-learning systems already

self-generating codes and pathways that would take decades for a single human to decode and understand, if ever possible. This presents a great challenge for use in reproducible, validated quality-driven, audit-trailed regulated orientated environments. This is where natural compounds such as herbal substances can play a significant role i.e. data from the same plants species with variable composition can help verify the input and outputs of complex analysis and recognition software. In AI-driven systems, natural substances are ideal candidates for testing the analytical attributes such as accuracy, precision, and robustness of whole AI-instrumentation systems.

CONCLUSIONS

As pharmacopoeial requirements continue to develop and instrumental technology advances, it is clear that we will be able to delve further and further into the chemical composition of medicinal plants and develop more advanced techniques for the detection and quantification of adulterants and contaminants. However, it should be considered that although these technological advances give us this opportunity, more traditional organoleptic analysis also provides us with essential sensory information regarding medicinal plant quality.

We have shown the emergence and historical importance of complex analytical techniques used in medicinal plant analysis. However, any analytical approach, can only provide a partial perspective on complex multicomponent preparations. So future improvements in this area may not entirely rely on developing ever more complex analytical techniques, but in implementing best practice throughout all stages of the production and supply of herbal medicines.

AUTHOR CONTRIBUTIONS

AB wrote the sections on applications of metabolomics, NIR, parts of the introduction, and conclusions. MF wrote most of the instrumentation, trends in publications and history, part of the introduction and conclusions. MH contributed towards the methodological design of the study and assisted with the data analysis.

FUNDING

MF scholarship is funded by Brion Research Group (Sun Ten Pharmaceutical Co) and Herbprime, UK.

REFERENCES

Aboudaou, M., Ferhat, M. A., Hazzit, M., Ariño, A., and Djenane, D. (2018). Solvent free-microwave green extraction of essential oil from orange peel (Citrus sinensis L.): effects on shelf life of flavored liquid whole eggs during storage under commercial retail conditions. [Preprint]. Available at: https://www.preprints.org/manuscript/201801.0055/v12018010055 (Accessed August 15, 2018). doi: 10.20944/preprints201801.0055.v1

Ash, R. F. (1988). The evolution of agricultural policy. *China Quart.* 116, 529–555. doi: 10.1017/S0305741000037887

Bahaghighat, H. D., Freye, C. E., and Synovec, R. E. (2018). Recent advances in modulator technology for comprehensive two dimensional gas chromatography. *TrAC Trends In Anal. Chem.* 113, 379–391. doi: 10.1016/j.trac.2018.04.016

Bauer, A., and Brönstrup, M. (2014). Industrial natural product chemistry for drug discovery and development. *Natural Prod. Rep.* 31 (1), 35–60. doi: 10.1039/C3NP70058E

Bedevian, A. K. (1936). *Illustrated polyglottic dictionary of plant names in Latin, Arabic, Armenian, English, French, German, Italian and Turkish languages, including economic, medicinal, poisonous and ornamental plants and common weeds* (Egypt: Medbouly Library Press). (Reprint: 1994)

Bergeron, J. A., and Singer, M. (1958). Metachromasy: an experimental and theoretical reevaluation. *J. Cell Biol.* 4 (4), 433–457. doi: 10.1083/jcb.4.4.433

Booker, A., Frommenwiler, D., Johnston, D., Umealajekwu, C., Reich, E., and Heinrich, M. (2014). Chemical variability along the value chains of turmeric (Curcuma longa): a comparison of nuclear magnetic resonance spectroscopy and high performance thin layer chromatography. *J. Ethnopharmacol.* 152 (2), 292–301. doi: 10.1016/j.jep.2013.12.042

Braubach, C. (1925). Medicinal plants of the aztecs which are still in common use in Mexico. *J. Am. Pharmaceut. Assoc.* 14 (6), 498–505. doi: 10.1002/jps.3080140610

Brochmann-Hanssen, E., Hirai, K., Nielsen, B., Pfeifer, S., Mann, I., and Kühn., L. (1968). Opium alkaloids VI. Isolation of N-methyl-14-O-desmethylepiporphyroxine. *J. pharmaceut. Sci.* 57 (1), 30–35. doi: 10.1002/jps.2600570106

Cai, J. F. (1988). Integration of traditional Chinese medicine with Western medicine - Right or wrong. *Soc. Sci. Med.* 27 (5), 521–529. doi: 10.1016/0277-9536(88)90376-0

Castetter, E. F., Underhill, R. M., Opler, M. E., Bell, W. H., and Grove, A. R. (1935). *Ethnobiological studies in the American Southwest* (Vol. 1) (Mexico: University of New Mexico Press). doi: 10.1525/aa.1937.39.3.02a00180

Chan, C.-O., Chu, C.-C., Mok, D. K.-W., and Chau, F.-T. (2007). Analysis of berberine and total alkaloid content in Cortex Phellodendri by near infrared spectroscopy (NIRS) compared with high-performance liquid chromatography coupled with ultra-visible spectrometric detection. *Anal. Chimica Acta* 592 (2), 121–131. doi: 10.1016/j.aca.2007.04.016

Chan, L. (1939). A brief history of Chinese herbs and Medicine. *Bull. Torrey Bot. Club* 66 (8), 563–568. doi: 10.2307/2480844

Chen, Y., Xie, M. Y., Yan, Y., Zhu, S. B., Nie, S. P., Li, C., et al. (2008). Discrimination of Ganoderma lucidum according to geographical origin with near infrared diffuse reflectance spectroscopy and pattern recognition techniques. *Anal. Chimica Acta* 618 (2), 121–130. doi: 10.1016/j.aca.2008.04.055

Chopra, R. N. (1933). "Indigenous Drugs of India," in *Their Medical and Economic Aspects. Indigenous Drugs of India. Their Medical and Economic Aspects* (Calcutta: The Art Press (1933)). doi: 10.1001/jama.1933.02740210065038

Daglish, C. (1950). The isolation and identification of a hydrojuglone glycoside occurring in the walnut. *Biochem. J.* 47 (4), 452. doi: 10.1042/bj0470452

Desfontaine, C., Guillarme, D., Francotte, E., and Nováková, L. (2015). Supercritical fluid chromatography in pharmaceutical analysis. *J. pharmaceut. Biomed. Anal.* 113, 56–71. doi: 10.1016/j.jpba.2015.03.007

Duckstein, S. M., Lorenz, P., Conrad, J., and Stintzing, F. C. (2014). Tandem mass spectrometric characterization of acetylated polyhydroxy hellebosaponins, the principal steroid saponins in Helleborus niger L. roots. *Rapid Commun. In Mass Spectrometry* 28 (16), 1801–1812. doi: 10.1002/rcm.6959

Dybing, F., Dybing, O., and Jensen, K. B. (1954). Detection of scilliroside in organic material. *Acta Pharmacol. Toxicol.* 10 (2), 93–100. doi: 10.1111/j.1600-0773.1954.tb01326.x

EDQM. (2017). European Regulations for Medicines Place and Role of the European Pharmacopoeia in Europe - Ph. Eur. Concept. EDQM Symposium on Microbiology 10-11 October 2017. [online] Strasbourg: 8. Available at: https://www.edqm.eu/sites/default/files/european_regulations_for_medicines-cathie_vielle-october2017.pdf (Accessed August 15, 2018).

Farnsworth, N. R. (1966). Biological and phytochemical screening of plants. *J. Pharmaceut. Sci.* 55 (3), 225–276. doi: 10.1002/jps.2600550302

Fernstrom, R. C. (1958). A durable Nissl stain for frozen and paraffin sections. *Stain Technol.* 33 (4), 175–176. doi: 10.3109/10520295809111844

Fong, S., Kau, Y., Wong, Y. C., and Zuo, Z. (2014). Development of a SPE-LC/MS/MS method for simultaneous quantification of baicalein, wogonin, oroxylin A and their glucuronides baicalin, wogonoside and oroxyloside in rats and its application to brain uptake and plasma pharmacokinetic studies. *J. Pharmaceut. Biomed. Analysis* 97, 9–23. doi: 10.1016/j.jpba.2014.03.033

Ford, M. J., and Van Berkel, G. J. (2004). An improved thin-layer chromatography/mass spectrometry coupling using a surface sampling probe electrospray ion

trap system. *Rapid Commun. In Mass Spectrom.* 18 (12), 1303–1309. doi: 10.1002/rcm.1486

Furuya, T., and Kojima, H. (1967). Gas-liquid chromatography of valerian sesquiterpenoids. *J. Chromatography A.* 29, 341–348. doi: 10.1016/s0021-9673(00)92676-1

Furuya, T. (1965). Gas-liquid chromatography of plant glycosides. *J. Chromatography A.* 18, 152–156. doi: 10.1016/s0021-9673(01)80333-2

Fyfe, A., and Moxham, N. (2016). Making public ahead of print: meetings and publications at the Royal Society, 1752–1892. *Notes Records: R. Soc. J. History Sci.* 70 (4), 361–379.

Gao, L., Zhang, J., Zhang, W., Shan, Y., Liang, Z., Zhang, L., et al. (2010). Integration of normal phase liquid chromatography with supercritical fluid chromatography for analysis of fruiting bodies of Ganoderma lucidum. *J. Separation Sci.* 33 (23–24), 3817–3821. doi: 10.1002/jssc.201000453

Garrison, F. H. (1933). Persian Medicine and Medicine in Persia: A geomedical survey. *Bull. History Med.* 1, 129.

Gerhardt, N., Birkenmeier, M., Schwolow, S., Rohn, S., and Weller, P. (2018). Volatile-compound fingerprinting by headspace-gas-chromatography ion-mobility spectrometry (HS-GC-IMS) as a benchtop alternative to 1H NMR profiling for assessment of the authenticity of honey. *Anal. Chem.* 90 (3), 1777–1785. doi: 10.1021/acs.analchem.7b03748

Grill, E., Winnacker, E. L., and Zenk, M. H. (1985). Phytochelatins: the principal heavy-metal complexing peptides of higher plants. *Science* 230 (4726), 674–676. doi: 10.1126/science.230.4726.674

Grill, E., Winnacker, E. L., and Zenk, M. H. (1987). Phytochelatins, a class of heavy-metal-binding peptides from plants, are functionally analogous to metallothioneins. *Proc. Natl. Acad. Sci.* 84 (2), 439–443. doi: 10.1073/pnas.84.2.439

Hamid-Reza, A., Scherer, U., Kaehlig, H., Hettich, T., Schlotterbeck, G., Reich, E., et al. (2013). Combination of bioautography with HPTLC–MS/NMR: a fast identification of acetylcholinesterase inhibitors from galbanum. *Phytochem. Anal.* 24 (4), 395–400. doi: 10.1002/pca.2422

Hardy, A. C. (1938). History of the design of the recording spectrophotometer. *JOSA* 28 (10), 360–364. doi: 10.1364/josa.28.000360

Hatano, T., Kagawa, H., Yasuhara, T., and Okuda, T. (1988). Two new flavonoids and other constituents in licorice root: their relative astringency and radical scavenging effects. *Chem. Pharmaceut. Bull.* 36 (6), 2090–2097. doi: 10.1248/cpb.36.2090

Heinrich, M., Frei Haller, B., and Leonti, M. (2014). A perspective on natural products research and ethnopharmacology in Mexico: the eagle and the serpent on the prickly pear cactus. *J. Natural Prod.* 77 (3), 678–689. doi: 10.1021/np4009927

Hertog, M. G., Feskens, E. J., Kromhout, D., Hollman, P. C. H., and Katan, M. B. (1993). Dietary antioxidant flavonoids and risk of coronary heart disease: the Zutphen Elderly Study. *Lancet* 342 (8878), 1007–1011. doi: 10.1016/0140-6736(93)92876-u

Hills, K. L., and Rodwell, C. N. (1951). Variation in the alkaloids of clones of northern Duboisia myoporoides R. *Br. Aust. J. Biol. Sci.* 4 (4), 486–499. doi: 10.1071/bi9510486

Holt, S. J., and Withers, R. F. J. (1958). V. An appraisal of indigogenic reactions for esterase localization. *Proc. R. Soc. Lond. Ser. B-Biol. Sci.* 148 (933), 520–532. doi: 10.1098/rspb.1958.0043

Hu, Y., Scherngell, T., Man, S. N., and Wang, Y. (2013). Is the United States still dominant in the global pharmaceutical innovation network? *PloS One* 8 (11), e77247. doi: 10.1371/journal.pone.0077247

James, D. W. (1955). Chinese medicine. *Lancet* 265 (6873), 1068–1069. doi: 10.1016/s0140-6736(55)91135-1

Jaminet, F. (1959). Comparative study of planimetric and densitometric methods on quantitative paper chromatography. Application to the determination of the alkaloids and the amines of Genista (Sarothamnus scoparius L.). *Pharm. Acta Helvetiae* 34, 571–584.

Jancso, N., Jancsó-Gábor, A., and Szolcsanyi, J. (1967). Direct evidence for neurogenic inflammation and its prevention by denervation and by pretreatment with capsaicin. *Br. J. Pharmacol. Chemother.* 31 (1), 138–151. doi: 10.1111/j.1476-5381.1967.tb01984.x

Jang, M., Cai, L., Udeani, G. O., Slowing, K. V., Thomas, C. F., Beecher, C. W., et al. (1997). Cancer chemopreventive activity of resveratrol, a natural product derived from grapes. *Science* 275 (5297), 218–220. doi: 10.1126/science.275.5297.218

Jastrow, M. (1914). The medicine of the Babylonians and Assyrians. *Proc. R. Soc. Med. Sect. Hist. Med.* 109–176. doi: 10.1177/003591571400701610

Kędziora-Koch, K., and Wasiak, W. (2018). Needle-based extraction techniques with protected sorbent as powerful sample preparation tools to gas chromatographic analysis: trends in application. *J. Chromatography A.* 1565, 1–18. doi: 10.1016/j.chroma.2018.06.046

King, J. W. (1990). Applications of capillary supercritical fluid chromatography-supercritical fluid extraction to natural products. *J. Chromatogr. Sci.* 28 (1), 9–14. doi: 10.1093/chromsci/28.1.9

Klayman, D. L. (1985). Qinghaosu (artemisinin): an antimalarial drug from China. *Science* 228 (4703), 1049–1055. doi: 10.1126/science.3887571

Krejci, Z. (1958). Hemp (Cannabis sativa) antibiotic drugs. II. Method & results of bacteriological experiments & preliminary clinical experience. *Die Pharmazie.* 13 (3), 155–166.

Kwee, S. H. (2002). The development of the Chinese Pharmacopoeia. *PEFOTS News Pan Eur. Fed. TCM Sci.* 2 (1), 15.

Lau, C. C., Chan, C. O., Chau, F. T., and Mok, D. K. W. (2009). Rapid analysis of Radix puerariae by near-infrared spectroscopy. *J. Chromatography A.* 1216 (11), 2130–2135. doi: 10.1016/j.chroma.2008.12.089

Leiter, J., Downing, V., Hartnell, J. L., and Shear, M. J. (1950). Damage induced in sarcoma 37 with podophyllin, podophyllotoxin alpha-peltatin, beta-peltatin, and quercetin. *J. Natl. Cancer Inst.* 10, 1273–1293. doi: 10.1093/jnci/10.6.1273

Li, Y., Wu, T., Zhu, J., Wan, L., Yu, Q., Li, X., et al. (2010). Combinative method using HPLC fingerprint and quantitative analyses for quality consistency evaluation of an herbal medicinal preparation produced by different manufacturers. *J. Pharmaceut. Biomed. Anal.* 52 (4), 597–602. doi: 10.1016/j.jpba.2010.01.018

Li, W., Cheng, Z., Wang, Y., and Qu, H. (2013). Quality control of Lonicerae Japonicae Flos using near infrared spectroscopy and chemometrics. *J. Pharmaceut. Biomed. Analysis* 72, 33–39. doi: 10.1016/j.jpba.2012.09.012

Lillie, R. D. (1958). The Nile blue reaction of peptic gland zymogen granules: the effect of methylation and alkali demethylation. *J. Histochem. Cytochem.* 6 (2), 130–132. doi: 10.1177/6.2.130

Liu, G., Dong, J., Wang, H., Hashi, Y., and Chen, S. (2011). Characterization of alkaloids in Sophora flavescens Ait. by high-performance liquid chromatography–electrospray ionization tandem mass spectrometry. *J. Pharmaceut. Biomed. Analysis* 54 (5), 1065–1072. doi: 10.1016/j.jpba.2010.12.024

Liu, Z., and Phillips, J. B. (1991). Comprehensive two-dimensional gas chromatography using an on-column thermal modulator interface. *J. Chromatogr. Sci.* 29 (6), 227–231. doi: 10.1093/chromsci/29.6.227

Lopez, N., Booker, A., Simirgiotis, M., León, G., Alfaro-Lira, S., Salas, C. O., et al. (2015). Metabolomic variation in Senecio graveolens (Asteraceae) in altitudinal populations. *Planta Med.* 81 (16), 72. doi: 10.1055/s-0035-1565449

Lüning, B., Lundin, C., Garegg, P. J., Haug, A., and Hagen, G. (1967). Studies on orchidaceae alkaloids. VI. Synthesis and relative configuration of 5,7-dimethyloctahydroindolizines. *Acta Chem. Scand.* 21, 2136–2142. doi: 10.3891/acta.chem.scand.21-2136

Mathur, R. K., Ramaswamy, S. K., Rao, A. S., and Bhattacharyya, S. C. (1967). Terpenoids—CVIII: Isolation of an oxidodiol from Zanthoxylum rhetsa. *Tetrahedron* 23 (5), 2495–2498. doi: 10.1016/0040-4020(67)80086-3

Middleton, E., Kandaswami, C., and Theoharides, T. C. (2000). The effects of plant flavonoids on mammalian cells: implications for inflammation, heart disease, and cancer. *Pharmacol. Rev.* 52 (4), 673–751.

Minkov, E., and Trandafilov, T. (1969). Stabilization of liquid systems by means of surface-active substances. Solubilization and extraction of rose oil. *Die Pharmazie* 24 (6), 327.

Mingxin, L., Ping, L., and Baorong, L. (1980). Recent progress in research on esophageal cancer in China. *Adv. Cancer Res.* 173–249. doi: 10.1016/s0065-230x(08)60671-5

Morrison, W. M. (2013). *China,s Economic Rise: History, Trends, Challenges, and Implications for the United States* (Washington: Congressional Research Service:), 22–24.

Paris, R., and Viejo, J. P. (1955). Identification des drogues simples et contrôle des médicaments végétaux par chromatographie sur papier. *Presse Medicale* 63 (39), 833–834.

Pešić, M. (2015). Development of natural product drugs in a sustainable manner. Brief for United Nations Global Sustainable Development Report 2015.

Available at: https://sustainabledevelopment.un.org/content/documents/6544118_Pesic_Development%20of%20natural%20product%20drugs%20in%20a%20%20sustainable%20manner.pdf. (Accessed August 15, 2018).

Pfeifer, I., Murauer, A., and Ganzera, M. (2016). Determination of coumarins in the roots of Angelica dahurica by supercritical fluid chromatography. *J. Pharmaceut. Biomed. Analysis* 129, 246–251. doi: 10.1016/j.jpba.2016.07.014

Picard, M., Franc, C., de Revel, G., and Marchand, S. (2018). Dual solid-phase and stir bar sorptive extraction combined with gas chromatography-mass spectrometry analysis provides a suitable tool for assaying limonene-derived mint aroma compounds in red wine. *Anal. Chimica Acta* 1001, 168–178. doi: 10.1016/j.aca.2017.11.074

Pletscher, A. (1968). Metabolism, transfer and storage of 5-hydroxytryptamine in blood platelets. *Br. J. Pharmacol. Chemother.* 32 (1), 1–16. doi: 10.1111/j.1476-5381.1968.tb00423.x

Purser, S., Moore, P. R., Swallow, S., and Gouverneur, V. (2008). Fluorine in medicinal chemistry. *Chem. Soc. Rev.* 37 (2), 320–330. doi: 10.1039/b610213c

Qian, Z. Z., Dan, Y., Liu, Z., and Peng, Y. (2010). Pharmacopoeia of the People's Republic of China (2010 edition): a milestone in development of China's healthcare. *Chin. Herb. Medicines* 2 (2), 157–160.

Read, B. E. (1930). The Chinese Pharmacopoeia. *Can. Med. Assoc. J.* 23 (4), 568.

Rubegeta, E., Ahmad, A., Kamatou, G. P. P., Sandasi, M., Sommerlatte, H., and Viljoen, A. M. (2018). Headspace analysis, antimicrobial and anti-quorum sensing activities of seven selected African Commiphora species. *South Afr. J. Bot.* 122, 522–528. doi: 10.1016/j.sajb.2018.03.001

Rutkowska, E., Łozowicka, B., and Kaczyński, P. (2018). Modification of multiresidue QuEChERS protocol to minimize matrix effect and improve recoveries for determination of pesticide residues in dried herbs followed by GC-MS/MS. *Food Anal. Methods* 11 (3), 709–724. doi: 10.1007/s12161-017-1047-3

Schoental, R. (1959). Liver lesions in young rats suckled by mothers treated with the pyrrolizidine (Senecio) alkaloids, lasiocarpine and retrorsine. *J. Pathol. Bacteriol.* 77, 485–495. doi: 10.1002/path.1700770220

Seamon, K. B., Padgett, W., and Daly, J. W. (1981). Forskolin: unique diterpene activator of adenylate cyclase in membranes and in intact cells. *Proc. Natl. Acad. Sci.* 78 (6), 3363–3367. doi: 10.1073/pnas.78.6.3363

Sharon, N., and Lis, H. (1989). Lectins as cell recognition molecules. *Science* 246 (4927), 227–234. doi: 10.1126/science.2552581

Shibata, S., and Saitoh, T. (1968). The chemical studies on the oriental plant drugs. XIX. Some new constituents of licorice root. The structure of Licoricidin. *Chem. Pharmaceut. Bull.* 16 (10), 1932–1936. doi: 10.1248/cpb.16.1932

Speck, F. G. (1917). Medicine practices of the northeastern Algonquians, in: Proceedings of Nineteenth International Congress of Americanists. 1917, 303–321.

St John, H. (1948). Report on the flora of Pingelap Atoll, Caroline Islands, Micronesia, and observations on the vocabulary of the native inhabitants. *Pacific Plant Sci.* 2, 96–113.

Stewart, P., Valentino, R., Wallace, A. M., Burt, D., Shackleton, C. L., and Edwards, C. W. (1987). Mineralocorticoid activity of liquorice: 11-beta-hydroxysteroid dehydrogenase deficiency comes of age. *Lancet* 330 (8563), 821–824. doi: 10.1016/S0140-6736(87)91014-2

Su, X. Z., and Miller, L. H. (2015). The discovery of artemisinin and the Nobel Prize in Physiology or Medicine. *Sci. China Life Sci.* 58 (11), 1175–1179. doi: 10.1007/s11427-015-4948-7

Svoboda, G. H., Neuss, N., and Gorman, M. (1959). Alkaloids of Vinca rosea Linn. (Catharanthus roseus G. Don.) V. Preparation and characterization of alkaloids. *J. Am. Pharmaceut. Assoc.* 48 (11), 659–666. doi: 10.1002/jps.3030481115

Takahashi, K., and Nakagawa, T. (1966). Studies on constituents of medicinal plants. VIII. The stereochemistry of paulownin and isopaulownin. *Chem. Pharmaceut. Bull.* 14 (6), 641–647. doi: 10.1248/cpb.14.641

Tao, Y., Gu, X., Li, W., and Cai, B. (2018). Fabrication and evaluation of magnetic phosphodiesterase-5 linked nanoparticles as adsorbent for magnetic dispersive solid-phase extraction of inhibitors from Chinese herbal medicine prior to ultra-high performance liquid chromatography-quadrupole time-of-flight mass spectrometry analysis. *J. Chromatography A.* 1532, 58–67. doi: 10.1016/j.chroma.2017.11.062

Van Berkel, G. J., Tomkins, B. A., and Kertesz, V. (2007). Thin-layer chromatography/desorption electrospray ionization mass spectrometry: investigation of goldenseal alkaloids. *Anal. Chem.* 79 (7), 2778–2789. doi: 10.1021/ac0622330

Wang, M., and Franz, G. (2015). The role of the European Pharmacopoeia (Ph Eur) in quality control of traditional Chinese herbal medicine in European member states. *WJTCM* 1, 5–15. doi: 10.15806/j.issn.2311-8571.2014.0021

Wang, P., and Yu, Z. (2015). Species authentication and geographical origin discrimination of herbal medicines by near infrared spectroscopy: a review. *J. Pharmaceut. Analysis* 5 (5), 277–284. doi: 10.1016/j.jpha.2015.04.001

Wani, M. C., Taylor, H. L., Wall, M. E., Coggon, P., and McPhail, A. T. (1971). Plant antitumor agents. VI. Isolation and structure of taxol, a novel antileukemic and antitumor agent from Taxus brevifolia. *J. Am. Chem. Soc.* 93 (9), 2325–2327. doi: 10.1021/ja00738a045

Watson, M. L. (1958). Staining of tissue sections for electron microscopy with heavy metals. *J. Cell Biol.* 4 (4), 475–478. doi: 10.1083/jcb.4.4.475

Wellburn, A. R., Stevenson, J., Hemming, F. W., and Morton, R. A. (1967). The characterization and properties of castaprenol-11,-12 and-13 from the leaves of Aesculus hippocastanum (horse chestnut). *Biochem. J.* 102 (1), 313. doi: 10.1042/bj1020313

WHO. (2018). Index of world pharmacopoeias and pharmacopoeial authorities. Working document QAS/11.453/Rev.10. [online] Geneva: Available at:http://www.who.int/medicines/publications/pharmacopoeia/index-of-pharmacopoeias_17012018.pdf. (Accessed 28 July 2018).

Wilson, C. (1997). *The invisible world: early modern philosophy and the invention of the microscope* (Princeton: Princeton University Press).

Xu, Q., Bauer, R., Hendry, B. M., Fan, T. P., Zhao, Z., Duez, P., et al. (2013). The quest for modernisation of traditional Chinese medicine. *BMC Complement. Altern. Med.* 13 (1), 132. doi: 10.1186/1472-6882-13-132

Xu, Y., Cai, H., Cao, G., Duan, Y., Pei, K., Zhou, J., et al. (2018). Discrimination of volatiles in herbal formula Baizhu Shaoyao San before and after processing using needle trap device with multivariate data analysis. *R. Soc. Open Sci.* 5 (6), 171987. doi: 10.1098/rsos.171987

Yu, Y. Y., Chen, Y. Y., Gao, X., Liu, Y. Y., Zhang, H. Y., and Wang, T. Y. (2018). Nanoparticle based bio-bar code technology for trace analysis of aflatoxin B1 in Chinese herbs. *J. Food Drug Analysis* 26 (2), 815–822. doi: 10.1016/j.jfda.2017.11.003

Zhang, C., and Su, J. (2014). Application of near infrared spectroscopy to the analysis and fast quality assessment of traditional Chinese medicinal products. *Acta Pharm. Sin. B.* 4 (3), 182–192. doi: 10.1016/j.apsb.2014.04.001

Zhishen, J., Mengcheng, T., and Jianming, W. (1999). The determination of flavonoid contents in mulberry and their scavenging effects on superoxide radicals. *Food Chem.* 64 (4), 555–559. doi: 10.1016/s0308-8146(98)00102-2

13

Goji Who? Morphological and DNA Based Authentication of a "Superfood"

Sascha Wetters*, Thomas Horn and Peter Nick

Molecular Cell Biology, Karlsruhe Institute of Technology, Karlsruhe, Germany

*Correspondence:
Sascha Wetters
sascha.wetters@kit.edu

"Goji" (*Lycium barbarum* and *Lycium chinense*) is a generic name for medical plants with a long historical background in the traditional Chinese medicine. With the emerging trend of "Superfoods" several years ago, Goji berries soon became an established product in European countries and not only are the most popular product of traditional Chinese medicine outside of China but to this day one of the symbols of the entire "Superfood" trend. However, since Goji is an umbrella term for different plant species that are closely related, mislabeling and adulterations (unconsciously or purposely) are possible. We carefully verified the identity of Goji reference plant material based on morphological traits, mainly floral structures of several inflorescences of each individual, in order to create a robust background for the downstream applications that were used on those reference plants and additionally on commercial Goji products. We report morphological and molecular based strategies for the differentiation of *Lycium barbarum* and *Lycium chinense*. The two different Goji species vary significantly in seed size, with an almost double average seed area in *Lycium chinense* compared to *Lycium barbarum*. Differences could be traced on the molecular level as well; using the psbA-trnH barcoding marker, we detected a single nucleotide substitution that was used to develop an easy one-step differentiation tool based on ARMS (amplification refractory mutation system). Two diagnostic primers used in distinct multiplex PCRs yield a second diagnostic band in a subsequent gel electrophoresis for *Lycium barbarum* or *Lycium chinense*, respectively. Our ARMS approach is a strong but simple tool to trace either of the two different Goji species. Both the morphological and the molecular analysis showed that all of the tested commercial Goji products contained fruits of the species *Lycium barbarum* var. *barbarum*, leading to the assumption that consumer protection is satisfactory.

Keywords: Goji, superfood, food diagnostics, *Lycium barbarum*, *Lycium chinense*, molecular authentication, ARMS

INTRODUCTION

A rising concern for health and an aging society seem to be important driving forces for the boom of "Superfoods" in Europe with a rapid sequence of new products entering a dynamic and further growing market. Germany ranks second (behind the United States) with respect to the import of products that are labeled as "Superfood" (Mintel, 2018). Every season new products are trending and advertised as "Superfoods." Current trends are, for instance, basil seeds, or even varieties of cabbage, *Brassica oleracea* L., that have been in use in Germany for more than 500 years (Baumann et al., 2001) but currently experience a revival as "Superfood," e.g., kale (*Brassica oleracea* var. *acephala*) Šamec et al., 2018. Some of these "Superfoods," such as Chia seeds or Goji berries have in the meantime turned into established products that can be obtained in almost every supermarket or even in discounters as well. This hype of "Superfoods" is expected to continue, which can be seen in the sales numbers, that for Chia doubled from 2015 to 2016 to a volume around 23 million Euro in Germany alone (Statista, 2018a) and are still growing. Among the "Superfoods," Wolfberries, or "Goji" rank among the leading products. "Goji" is the generic name for different plant species from the genus *Lycium*, belonging to the Solanaceae family. "Goji" represents the most popular product of traditional Chinese medicine outside of China (Chinadaily, 2018), the Western vernacular name "Goji" derives from the Chinese term *gou qi* (Potterat, 2010). In traditional Chinese medicine different plants, mainly *Lycium barbarum* L. and *Lycium chinense* Mill. are described under the umbrella term *gou qi* and have both been used for more than 2,000 years (Burke et al., 2005). Though exotic, Goji berries were already used in Europe before the introduction of the Novel Food Regulation (1997) to an extent that it did not fall under the Novel Food Legislation. However, this actually holds true only for the species *Lycium barbarum*. Several years ago, "Goji" berries were marketed as one of the first so called "Superfoods" and praised in advertisements and newspapers for miraculous properties (Latimes, 2018). Although it is already some time back that "Goji" berries became popular, they are still appreciated and bought for the perceived health effects, and continue to lead the charts for the most popular "Superfoods" (Statista, 2018b). Also in the news coverage of "Superfoods," "Goji" is inevitably used as example and almost can be considered as symbol for the entire trend (SWR, 2018). While numerous reports refer to high levels of antioxidants, vitamins, minerals, or proteins that are claimed to account for the positive effects of such "Superfoods," it has to be kept in mind that numerous traditional food plants harbor comparable levels of these healthy ingredients, rendering the term "Superfood" rather ambiguous. The combination of media hype with vernacular nomenclature (that had been separated from its traditional context) conceals the fact that it is often unclear, what plant is actually found in the package sold as "Goji." Therefore, it is important to focus on the actual plants hidden behind the term "Superfood Goji." The Flora of China distinguishes among others between *Lycium barbarum* (宁夏枸杞, *ning xia gou qi*), *Lycium chinense* (枸杞, *gou qi*), and *Lycium ruthenicum* Murray (黑果枸杞, *hei guo gou qi*, also called "Black Goji") (Efloras, 2018). These plants are thorny shrubs (common name boxthorn) with heights up to three meters, small inconspicuous purple flowers and orange to red fruits (black for *Lycium ruthenicum*) that reach up to two centimeters in length. Especially *Lycium barbarum* and *Lycium chinense* are very similar with respect to morphology and phylogenetic relationship. Moreover, they grow in the same habitat, are harvested at the same time (usually from August to October) and have both been used in traditional medicine

all over East Asia since thousands of years (Potterat, 2010). Because of their important role in traditional Chinese medicine, the fruits of "Goji" have been intensively investigated with respect to their bioactive compounds (reviewed in Potterat, 2010; Amagase and Farnsworth, 2011; Masci et al., 2018), as well as for their anatomical and histochemical features (Konarska, 2018). While both species are marketed to a conspicuous extent, the Pharmacopoeia of the People's Republic of China lists only *Lycium barbarum* as the official drug (Zhonghua Renmin Gongheguo wei sheng bu yao dian wei yuan hui, 2000), and also the Novel Food Catalogue of the EU allows the usage of only *Lycium barbarum* as food or food ingredient (Europa, 2018). Because of these legal constraints, providers of Goji Berries claim that their commercial products that are offered outside of Asia exclusively contain fruits of *Lycium barbarum* (Potterat, 2010). However, not all commercial Goji products are properly labeled with the scientific name. Usually the generic name "Goji" is accompanied by additional Western vernacular names, such as Boxthorn, Wolfberry, Chinese Wolfberry, or Matrimony Wine which does not really contribute to consumer safety (Blaschek et al., 1993). Considering how closely related these species are, this nomenclatural nonchalance and partially also ignorance will easily create mislabeling. A simple and robust one-step differentiation method based on molecular markers derived from carefully determined reference plants is needed. Such a marker has to be robust enough to be amenable to processed samples, since "Goji" is often sold as powder, and even for dry fruits it is very hard to trace back to the originating plant(s).

DNA barcoding is an important identification tool that was first used for animal identification done by amplification of the mitochondrial COI1 gene (Hebert et al., 2003). This approach has meanwhile been developed for plants as well. A number of different marker regions are commonly used, but still there is no universal region that fulfills all the desired criteria, that are: the simple amplification of the respective region with one primer pair, an adequate size to perform bidirectional sequencing without additional primer, and the condition for maximal discrimination power between species (Hollingsworth et al., 2009). The plastid psbA-trnH spacer region that is flanked by the highly conserved psbA and trnH genes is one of the most frequently used DNA barcodes and widely accepted as reliable, because of its high variance that can be used for discrimination down to the species level (Kress et al., 2005). The region has been especially valuable for phylogenetic and taxonomic studies of the genus *Solanum* from the Solanaceae family, where an estimated 96.5% (projected from a small sample range) of the species can be differentiated with this marker (Pang et al., 2012). While DNA barcoding requires sequencing, discrimination of two species with a known sequence can make use of sequence polymorphisms that can be translated into a specific pattern. Amplification of the rbcL barcode followed by restriction with appropriate enzymes has been used successfully to discriminate two Australian Myrtaceae that are commercialized under the same vernacular name "Lemon Myrtle" (Horn et al., 2012). Alternatively, such barcodes can be used to design a duplex PCR, where a diagnostic third primer located in the center of the amplicon will produce a diagnostic band in addition to the full-length barcode (Horn et al., 2014). To improve the discriminative power of this approach, the diagnostic primer is designed using the amplified refractory mutation system (ARMS) strategy, where even single base-pair substitutions in sequences can be detected by design of a 3'-end destabilized primer, which is added to the full-length primer pair. As a result, this duplex PCR yields a second, smaller amplicon that can be detected as a second band in the subsequent gel electrophoresis. Originally developed for the detection of mutations (Old, 1992), this method can be used to discriminate two closely related species using a single PCR leading to a specific fingerprint that can be visualized by gel electrophoresis. In the past, this ARMS approach had been successfully used to discriminate closely related Lamiaceae species to safeguard against adulteration in commercial products (Horn et al., 2014), or to discover adulteration of Bamboo Tea by Chinese Carnations in consequence of a false translation of a Chinese vernacular name into English (Horn and Häser, 2016). As contribution to consumer safety and quality control, we are reporting a method to validate the identity of "Goji" in commercial products. Our approach is based on carefully authenticated reference plants for different *Lycium* species that are validated by taxonomical characterization which forms the base for downstream morphological and molecular analysis of those *Lycium barbarum* and *Lycium chinense* accessions, development of a diagnostic assay, and application of this assay to clarify the identity of commercial products sold as "Superfood Goji."

MATERIALS AND METHODS

Plant Specimens

A set of 15 accessions of *Lycium* was analyzed in this study (**Table 1**). The set included two specimens of *Lycium barbarum*, one of Asian origin and one commercially available in Germany, and seven specimens of *Lycium chinense* that were all cultivated and are maintained in the Botanic Garden of the Karlsruhe Institute of Technology. Fruits from *Lycium ruthenicum* were obtained from China. To get insight into the phylogenetic relations of *Lycium barbarum* and *Lycium chinense*, four additional *Lycium* species were cultivated, including specimens of the Mediterranean (*Lycium europaeum* L.) and South American (*Lycium chilense* Bertero and *Lycium ameghinoi* Speg.) regions. In addition, the DNA of one South African specimen (*Lycium oxycarpum* Dunal) was included into the study. This set of 15 *Lycium* specimens was complemented by a set of 17 "Goji" commercial products that were obtained as dried fruits from different sources (**Table 2**), making in total 32 accessions.

Identification of Reference Specimens

The identity of specimens was verified by taxonomical identification using appropriate taxonomic keys (Flora of China (Efloras, 2018), Schmeil/Fitschen: The Flora of Germany and the neighboring countries, 95th edition (Schmeil and Fitschen, 2011). In detail, we documented floral traits (i.e., pubescense of corolla, undulation of calyx, length of corolla

tube) from 30 inflorescences of each of the *L. barbarum* and *L. chinense* accessions to eliminate errors in determination that might occur when looking only at a single flower. The observed characteristics were documented digitally (Stereolupe 420, Leica, Bensheim, Germany).

Seed Analysis

Fruits of the cultivated plants were harvested and the seeds phenotyped quantitatively. 30 seeds of each *Lycium barbarum*, *Lycium chinense* and *Lycium ruthenicum* accession, as well as from all of the commercial "Goji" products were excised from at least five different fruits and digital images recorded (Stereolupe 420, Leica, Bensheim, Germany). The digital images of the seeds were analyzed using the program SmartGrain (Tanabata et al., 2012). With this software many parameters like area size or length-to-width ratio of seeds can be measured, after the digital image of the seeds is loaded into the program, and the scale bar is calibrated by the "set scale" tool. SmartGrain automatically detects the objects of the image, or the seeds can be picked manually as well. To evaluate and illustrate the obtained data as boxplots R Studio version 3.2.0 was used.

DNA Barcoding

DNA from fresh leaves of reference plants (using 60 mg of starting material) and dried fruits of commercial products (using 120 mg of starting material) was isolated using the Invisorb® Spin Plant Mini Kit (Stratec Biomedical AG). The quality and quantity of isolated DNA was evaluated by spectrophotometry (NanoDrop, Peqlab), and DNA concentration was diluted to 50 ng/μl to be used as template in PCR.

A 30 μl reaction volume containing 20.4 μl nuclease free water (Lonza, Biozym), onefold Thermopol Buffer (New England Biolabs), 1 mg/ml bovine serum albumin, 200 μM dNTPs (New England Biolabs), 0.2 μM of forward and reverse primer (see Primer list, **Table 3**), 100–150 ng DNA template and three units of Taq polymerase (New England Biolabs) was used to amplify the marker sequences.

Thermal cycler conditions for the amplification of the psbA-trnH intergenic spacer region included initial denaturation at 95°C for 2 min; following 33 cycles at 94°C for 1 min, 56°C for 30 s, 68°C for 45 s; ending with an extension of 68°C for 5 min.

The PCR was subsequently evaluated by agarose gel electrophoresis using NEEO ultra-quality agarose (Carl Roth, Karlsruhe, Germany). DNA was visualized using SYBRsafe (Invitrogen, Thermo Fisher Scientific, Germany) and blue light excitation. The fragment size was determined using a 100 bp size standard (New England Biolabs). Amplified DNA was purified for subsequent sequencing using the MSB® Spin PCRapace kit (Stratec). Sequencing was outsourced to Macrogen Europe (Netherlands) or GATC (Germany).

The quality of the obtained sequences was examined with the program FinchTV Version 1.4.0[1]. To get a more robust result, the marker region was sequenced from two directions. The resulting two sequences were merged for each accession.

---

[1]https://digitalworldbiology.com/FinchTV

TABLE 1 | *Lycium* reference specimens, overview of identity and origin.

Accession ID	ID KIT	Taxon	Provider/Origin	GenBank ID for psbA-trnH *igs*
Lb01	1470	*L. barbarum*	Phytocomm/Taiwan	KY570934
Lb02	5548	*L. barbarum*	Phytocomm/Germany	KY570933
Lc01	5549	*L. chinense**	Fa. Ruehlemanns/Germany	KY570941
Lc02	5550	*L. chinense**	BGU Hohenheim/Germany	KY570940
Lc03	5551	*L. chinense*	IPK Gatersleben/North Korea	KY570939
Lc04	5552	*L. chinense*	IPK Gatersleben/China	KY570942
Lc05	5553	*L. chinense*	FBGU Goettingen/Germany	KY570936
Lc06	6815	*L. chinense*	NIBIO/Japan	KY570938
Lc07	6967	*L. chinense*	China	KY570937
Lr01	9176	*L. ruthenicum*	Dr. Peijie Gong/China	MH713864
Le01	7064	*L. europaeum*	BGU Lautaret/Morocco	KY570943
Le02	8213	*L. europaeum*	JBU Grenoble/Morocco	MH713865
Lo01	7067	*L. chilense*	BGU Lautaret/Argentina	KY570935
Lo02	8211	*L. ameghinoi*	JBU Grenoble/Argentina	KY570932
Lo04	8352	*L. oxycarpum*	Dr. Max Seyfried/South Africa	KY570945

**Received as Lycium barbarum, determined as Lycium chinense.*

TABLE 2 | Commercial Goji products obtained from different sources.

Accession ID	KIT ID	Name	Provider	GenBank ID for psbA-trnH *igs*
Gp01	8603	Goji Product 1	HANOJU Deutschland GmbH	KY683015
Gp02	8604	Goji Product 2	Krauterhaus Sanct Bernhard KG	KY683014
Gp03	8619	Goji Product 5	Grubauer's Gewurze & Teeversand	KY683022
Gp04	8620	Goji Product 6	Feng Juan (China)	KY683021
Gp05	8621	Goji Product 7	Feng Juan (China)	KY683020
Gp06	8622	Goji Product 8	Feng Juan (China)	KY683019
Gp07	8623	Goji Product 9	Feng Juan (China)	KY683023
Gp08	8691	Goji Product 10	Edeka	KY683026
Gp09	8692	Goji Product 11	Alnatura	KY683025
Gp10	8693	Goji Product 12	Edeka	KY683024
Gp11	8694	Goji Product 13	Phytocomm	KY683017
Gp12	8695	Goji Product 14	Phytocomm	KY683016
Gp13	8696	Goji Product 15	VitFrisch	KY683018
Gp16	9310	Goji Product 16	Dr. Peijie Gong	MH713866
Gp17	9293	Goji Product 17	Dr. Peijie Gong	MH713867
Gp18	9307	Goji Product 18	Jumbo store (Netherlands)	MH713868
Gp19	9308	Goji Product 19	Raw organic food	MH713869

Phylogenetic Analysis

For the sequence alignment and the phylogenetic analysis the program MEGA7 (Version 7.0.14) with the integrated tree explorer was used (Kumar et al., 2016). The Sequences were aligned using the Muscle algorithm of MEGA7 (Edgar, 2004). Alignments were trimmed to the first nucleotide downstream of the forward primer and the nucleotide preceding the reverse primer. With the same software, the evolutionary relationships were inferred by using the neighbor-joining algorithm with a bootstrap value that was based on 1,000 replicates (Felsenstein, 1985; Saitou and Nei, 1987). The species *Nolana werdermannii* was chosen as an outgroup, since the genus *Nolana* is a

sister taxon to the Lycieae (Levin and Miller, 2005). The psbA-trnH spacer region sequence for *N. werdermannii* (GenBank: FJ189604) was obtained from the NCBI database.

ARMS Diagnostics

A single nucleotide difference in psbA-trnH intergenic spacer sequences of *L. barbarum* and *L. chinense* was used to design a diagnostic primer to clearly discriminate these two closely related species in an one-step duplex-PCR protocol.

The primer was designed with the Primer3Plus webtool (Untergasser et al., 2012). A thymine in position 265 of the psbA-trnH multiple sequence alignment in *Lycium barbarum* is

TABLE 3 | Primer list.

Name	5′ → 3′ sequence	Purpose	Design
psbA[U]	GTTATGCATGAACG TAATGCTC	Amplification of the psbA-trnH spacer region	Sang et al., 1997
trnH[U]	CGCGCATGGTGGAT TCACAATCC		Tate and Simpson, 2003
LB_265T_fw[d]	GCATTTATTCATGAT TGAGTATTCTATTCTT	Additional diagnostic band in *Lycium barbarum*	Current study
LC_265T_fw[d]	CATTTATTCATGATT GAGTATTCTATTCTG	Additional diagnostic band in *Lycium chinense*	Current study

U, universal primers; d, diagnostic primer for ARMS. For the diagnostic primers the decisive nucleotide is underlined.

substituted by a guanine in the other *Lycium* species. Thymine was placed at the 3′-end of the diagnostic primer and an additional nucleotide was exchanged in the 3′-region, to prevent the binding of the primer to the other *Lycium* species. With this design, this diagnostic primer (LB_265T_fw) should only be able to bind to the *Lycium barbarum* accessions. Since the region surrounding this nucleotide substitution is very AT-rich, the primer length had to be increased to 31 nucleotides in order to reach an appropriate annealing temperature.

Based on the same strategy, a second diagnostic primer (LC_265T_fw) was designed that should only bind to the psbA-trnH spacer region template of *Lycium chinense*.

These diagnostic primers were then used in combination with the universal psbA and trnH primers (see primer list, **Table 3**) in distinct duplex-PCRs. Usage of either LB_265T_fw or LC_265T_fw ought to yield an additional second diagnostic band of 290 bp in only one of the species while in the other species only the full-length amplicon with a length of 546 base pairs would be visible after the gel electrophoresis. We tested this prediction and validated the predicted readout experimentally (**Figure 6**).

RESULTS

Morphology of Floral Organs Clearly Delineate the Two Main "Goji" Species

To assess the validity of morphological traits that are used to delineate the main species behind "Goji," we assessed three morphological features that are used to discriminate *Lycium barbarum* and *Lycium chinense* (Reference Flora of China) across 30 inflorescences collected from the reference plants (**Figures 1, 2**). An elongated corolla tube and glabrescence of corolla blades as distinctive traits of *Lycium barbarum* (**Figure 1A**) were consistently found over all investigated 30 inflorescenses collected from each of the two reference plants. In contrast, for all reference plants of *Lycium chinense* all corolla blades were densely pubescent at the margin (**Figure 2A**), and the corolla tube was distinctively shorter than the corolla lobes (**Figure 1A**). Thus, both of these traits could be validated to differentiate *Lycium barbarum* and *Lycium chinense* specimens. Opposed to this, the third feature reported to discriminate the

two species, the number of calyx lobes (**Figure 1B**), was not consistent over all flowers of *Lycium chinense*. Depending on the accession, between 6.7% (in accessions 5551 and 6815) and 23.3% (in accession 5550) of the *Lycium chinense* flowers had a two-lobed calyx, which is usually characteristic for *Lycium barbarum*. In fact, without any exception, all flowers of our *Lycium barbarum* accessions had a calyx that was two-lobed. The Flora of China additionally lists different varieties of *Lycium barbarum* and *Lycium chinense*, respectively. However, all of the available reference plants were determined as either *Lycium barbarum* var. *barbarum* or *Lycium chinense* var. *chinense*.

Seed Size Can Be Used to Discriminate the Two "Goji" Species

Since "Goji" is traded as fruit, we were searching for morphological traits that can be inspected in fruits and allow to discriminate the two types of "Goji" berries. We noted that the seeds of *Lycium barbarum* var. *barbarum* and *Lycium chinense* var. *chinense* differ significantly in size (**Figure 2B**), and we quantified this trait by measuring cross-section areas (**Figure 3**). The two available accessions of *Lycium barbarum* var. *barbarum* showed cross sections that were less than half of those seen in the seven investigated *Lycium chinense* var. *chinense* (<2.5 mm^2 as compared to almost 5 mm^2). Although the intraspecific variation in *Lycium chinense* var. *chinense* was more pronounced, even the accessions with smaller seeds were clearly bigger than seeds from *Lycium barbarum* var. *barbarum* plants. The single available accession of *Lycium ruthenicum* had small seeds that are comparable to the values of the two *Lycium barbarum* var. *barbarum* sizes, but it is easy to delineate those fruits, due to their black pericarp. With an average boxplot median of 2.62 mm^2 all the investigated commercial Goji products had seed sizes that were comparable to *Lycium barbarum* var. *barbarum*, with low variance between the different commercial samples; the lowest median was Goji product 2 (2.22 mm^2), and the highest median was Goji product 19 (2.88 mm^2), suggesting that these "Goji" products indeed contained *Lycium barbarum*.

psbA-trnH Spacer Phylogeny Clearly Distinguishes *Lycium* Species

To probe the phylogenetic relationship of the three different "Goji" species (*Lycium barbarum* var. *barbarum*, *Lycium chinense* var. *chinense* and *Lycium ruthenicum*) and the tested commercial products (abbreviated as Gp in **Figure 4**) in comparison to *Lycium* accessions from Europe and the New World, we used a 510-bp region of the psbA-trnH marker including the variable intergenic spacer (**Figure 4**). Although this universal psbA-trnH spacer region is one of the most variable DNA barcodes, we found only small differences between those three obviously closely related species. The only difference between *Lycium barbarum* var. *barbarum* and *Lycium chinense* var. *chinense* was one nucleotide substitution at site 265 with a thymine for *Lycium barbarum* var. *barbarum* and a guanine for *Lycium chinense* var. *chinense* and *Lycium ruthenicum* (**Figure 5A**). As already

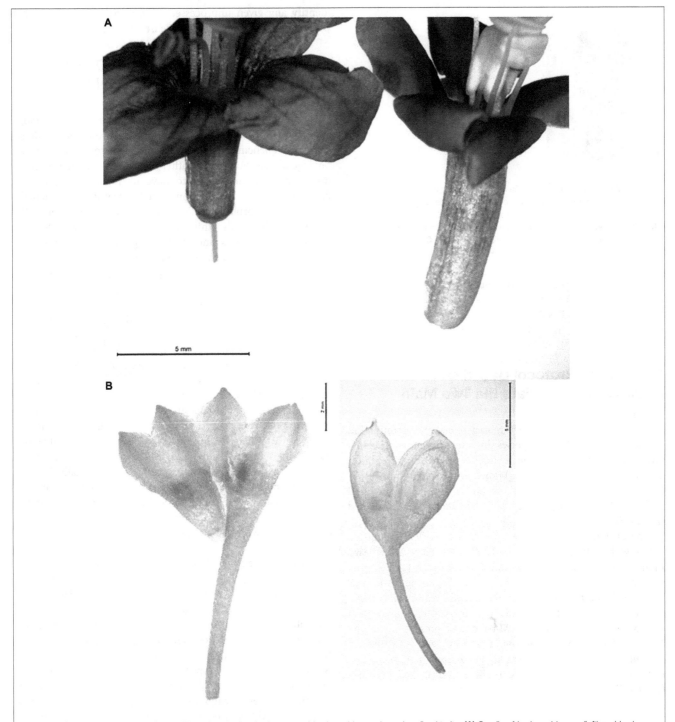

FIGURE 1 | Two morphological traits to differentiate *Lycium barbarum* and *Lycium chinense* based on floral traits. **(A)** Corolla of *Lycium chinense* (left) and *Lycium barbarum* (right). The flora of china mentioned difference in corolla tube length is clearly visible; for *Lycium barbarum* the corolla tube is obviously longer than the corolla lobes. **(B)** Opened and flattened calyx of *Lycium chinense* (left) and *Lycium barbarum* (right). *Lycium chinense* is usually three to five lobed, whereas *Lycium barbarum* has only two lobes. Compared to the corolla tube length this trait is not 100% consistent.

seen for seed size (**Figure 3**), the commercial "Goji" products all clustered with *Lycium barbarum* by sharing the informative thymine at position 265. The three Asian species are closely related to each other and clearly clustered separately from the two tested species from South America, as well as from the two species from Europe and South Africa (**Figure 4**). *Lycium ruthenicum* had an additional substitution from thymine to guanine at site 358 and an additional nine nucleotide insert at site 450, that was neither present in *Lycium barbarum*, nor in *Lycium chinense*. All accessions of *L. barbarum* var.

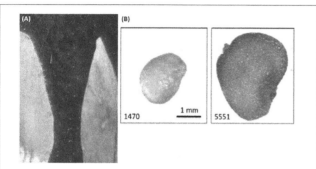

FIGURE 2 | (A) Comparison of corolla lobe pubescence in *Lycium chinense* (left) and *Lycium barbarum* (right). The corolla lobes of the latter are glabrescent, while *Lycium chinense* corolla lobes are finely haired.
(B) Difference in seed size can be seen with the bare eye in some cases, with significant smaller seeds of *Lycium barbarum*. See **Figure 3**.

barbarum and *L. chinense* var. *chinense* were identical within the respective species. The variations were exclusively interspecific. This single nucleotide substitution was used to design a strategy based on ARMS to discriminate *Lycium barbarum* from *Lycium chinense*.

A One-Step Protocol Based on ARMS Allows to Differentiate the Two Main "Goji" Species

To develop an assay that allows an easy one-step discrimination of the two main "Goji" species in unprocessed commercial samples, we used the single nucleotide polymorphism at position 265 of the *psbA-trnH* spacer (**Figure 5A**) to apply an ARMS based-strategy. Two diagnostic primers – LB_265T_fw and LC_265T_fw – with complementary readouts were designed (**Figure 5B**).

The diagnostic LB_265T_fw primer yielded clear diagnostic bands with a fragment length of 290 base pairs at the two *Lycium barbarum* var. *barbarum* accessions and all of the Goji products (**Figure 6A**), while this diagnostic band was absent in *Lycium chinense* var. *chinense* and *Lycium ruthenicum*. Conversely, adding the LC_265T_fw diagnostic primer in a duplex-PCR, the diagnostic 290-band was present in all the *Lycium chinense* var. *chinense* accessions and the *Lycium ruthenicum* sample, but absent in the *Lycium barbarum* var. *barbarum* reference plants and the commercial Goji products (**Figure 6B**).

DISCUSSION

In the current work, we have developed an one-step assay to discriminate two closely related, but distinct species of *Lycium* that are used in traditional Chinese medicine and are currently booming in Europe and US as so called "Superfood" under the common vernacular name of "Goji berries." Based on validated plant material, we have developed morphological and molecular traits that allow to differentiate between both species, and we have developed a robust one-step PCR-based assay that can reliably

identify any given unprocessed commercial product as either *Lycium barbarum* or *Lycium chinense*.

Identity Matters: Any Assay Is Only as Good as the Reference Material Is Reliable

It is a time where the possibilities of plant molecular biology appear to be overwhelming, including huge throughput of whole-genome sequencing, mapping of gene regulatory networks and phylogenomics; however, a rather ancient nevertheless essential discipline of botany starts to have its renaissance (Ledford, 2018). Although it is often considered as trivial task, to actually look at and morphologically determine the plant that is the subject of the study, this task is far from trivial. Surveys of misdeterminations and mislabeling in herbaria, botanical gardens, and germplasm collections show that between 10 and 20% of accessions are not what they are supposed to be (Goodwin et al., 2015).

Even for DNA barcoding, the correct determination of the used reference plant material is a necessary precondition for the validity of the outcome. This requirement is even more important for medicinal plants or plants that are *en vogue* because of their promised health effects. The power of the determination key is crucial to have a robust background for all subsequent experiments. Unfortunately in many keys terms with a low degree of certainty like "about" or "usually" are used, that can be interpreted differently by different taxonomists. This is also true for the otherwise high-quality Flora of China, that was mainly used in this study. For the discrimination of *Lycium barbarum* and *Lycium chinense* terms such as "usually 2-lobed" can be found in this key. To avoid uncertainties in determining a plant species, different morphological traits should be applied, if possible. The Flora of China lists three different traits to distinguish between the two *gou qi* species, *Lycium barbarum* and *Lycium chinense*.

Regarding the close relation of those two species, the common usage of both species in traditional Chinese medicine and the expectation of consumers to get the correct plants in the purchased products, the importance of correct determination is undoubtedly urgent. For the discrimination of closely related plant species, the evaluation of floral morphology traits should be central, since they are most likely linked with the reproductive isolation between these species. With the combination of the different floral traits, corolla pubescence, length of corolla tube and the number of calyx lobes, an impeccable discrimination of the two widely used Goji species could be done for the available reference plants. However, the corolla traits were more robust and therefore more reliable compared to those of the calyx, since there was variability in the features of the calyx in a considerable number of investigated inflorescences of *Lycium chinense*. The importance of evaluating an appropriate number of flowers becomes obvious, because phenomena like phenotypic plasticity or changes due to environmental factors can influence the appearance of single plant organs. For instance, differences in the velocity of polar auxin transport as they might occur depending on light quantity and quality are expected

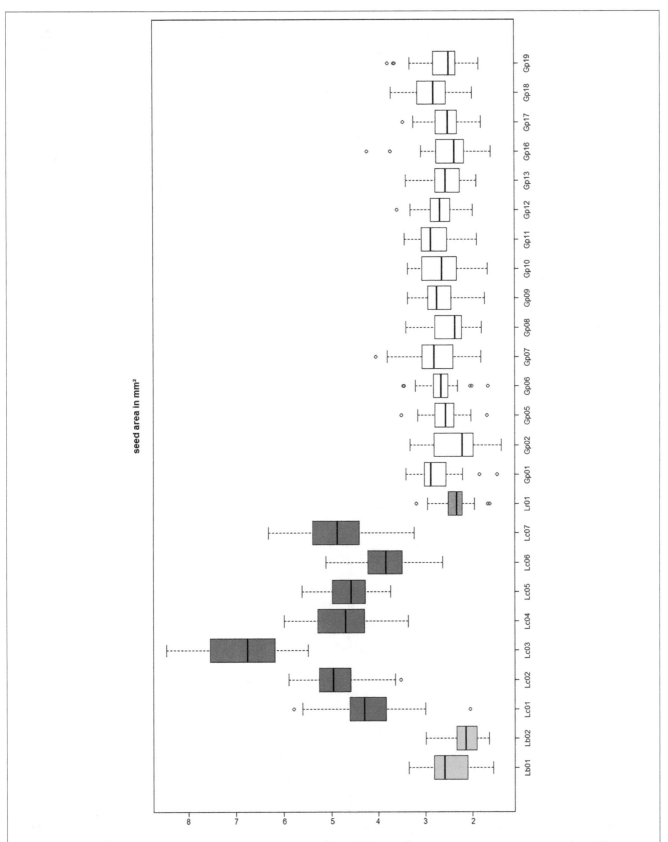

FIGURE 3 | Lb, *Lycium barbarum* var. *barbarum*; Lc, *Lycium chinense* var. *chinense;* Lr, *Lycium ruthenicum;* Gp, commercial Goji product. Seed size evaluation of the reference plants *Lycium barbarum* var. *barbarum* (green), *Lycium chinense* var. *chinense* (red) and *Lycium ruthenicum* (dark gray). Those values are compared to
(Continued)

FIGURE 3 | Continued
the commercial Goji products (white). The median of the *Lycium barbarum* var. *barbarum* reference plants is between 2 and 3 mm^2, whereas the *Lycium chinense* var. *chinense* seeds are significantly bigger in area size with a median between 4 and 6 mm^2. *Lycium ruthenicum* seeds are smaller again, with a median slightly bigger than 2 mm^2. The commercial Goji products have boxplots medians ranging from 2 and 3 mm^2, similar to *Lycium barbarum* and *Lycium ruthenicum*.

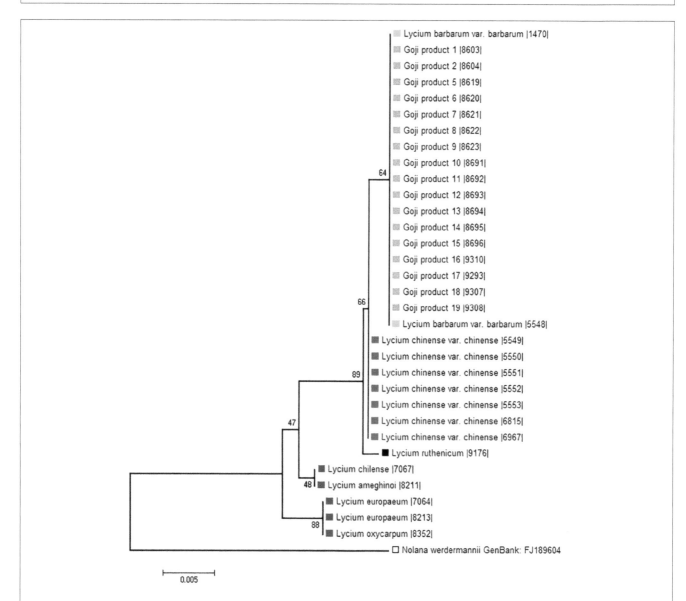

FIGURE 4 | Phylogenetic tree based on psbA-trnH spacer region sequences of morphological identified *Lycium* reference plants and commercial Goji products. The evolutionary history was inferred using the Neighbor-Joining method (Saitou and Nei, 1987). The percentage of replicate trees in which the associated taxa clustered together in the bootstrap test (1,000 replicates) are shown next to the branches (Felsenstein, 1985). There were a total of 532 positions in the final dataset. *Nolana werdermannii* was chosen as outgroup. The reference plants of *Lycium barbarum* var. *barbarum* (green), *Lycium chinense* var. *chinense* (red) and *Lycium ruthenicum* (black) are labeled with colored squares. The evaluated commercial Goji products are labeled with light gray squares. To put the three different "Goji" species into a context of the *Lycium* genus, species from South America (*Lycium chilense* and *Lycium ameghinoi*, yellow) and Europe (*Lycium europaeum* and *Lycium oxycarpum*, blue) were included into the phylogenetic analysis. The *Lycium barbarum* var. *barbarum* reference plants cluster with the Goji products, while *Lycium chinense* var. *chinense* (that is closest related to *Lycium barbarum*) and *Lycium ruthenicum* have their own clusters.

to modulate the number of apices in the primordial whorl committed to form the calyx (Reinhardt et al., 2003). However, the possibility that the morphospecies *Lycium chinense* might comprise several genetically isolated cryptospecies, should also be kept in mind.

The seed analysis revealed significant differences in the area size of *Lycium barbarum* var. *barbarum* and *Lycium chinense* var. *chinense* specimens. Thus, besides the prior described differences in the reproductive organs the two species can be distinguished by the size of their dispersal units. All the

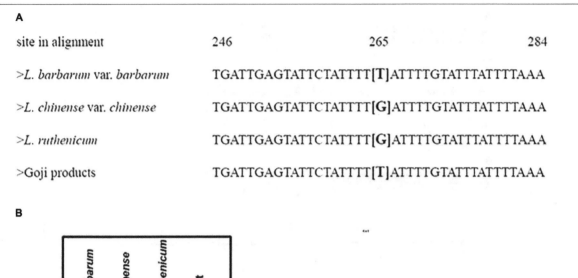

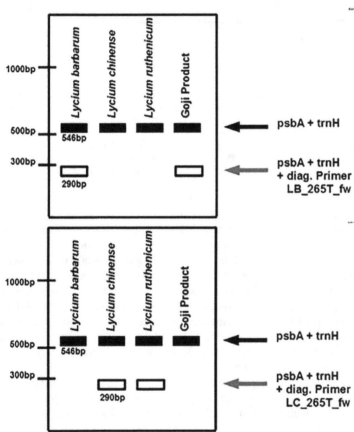

FIGURE 5 | (A) Partial depiction of the multiple sequence alignment of different reference plants. The decisive nucleotide that is used for designing the diagnostic primers is located at site 265 in the alignment of the psbA-trnH spacer regions of the respective samples. *Lycium barbarum* var. *barbarum* and the commercial Goji products have a thymine at this site, whereas *Lycium chinense* var. *chinense* and *Lycium ruthenicum* have a guanine. **(B)** Predicted banding pattern of the psbA-trnH spacer region fragment and the diagnostic fragments after the ARMS-based multiplex PCR. Left: using the diagnostic primer for tracing *Lycium barbarum* var. *barbarum*. Right: using the diagnostic primer for tracing *Lycium chinense* var. *chinense* and *Lycium ruthenicum*.

seeds of the tested commercial Goji products had similar boxplots medians compared to the two *Lycium barbarum* var. *barbarum* reference plants, wherefore we conclude that all the investigated commercial Goji products are actually fruits of the *ningxia gou qi* (*Lycium barbarum*). The boxplot median of the commercial products is comparable to *Lycium ruthenicum* as well; however, since the fruits of *Lycium*

barbarum and *Lycium chinense* differ in size and especially in color from *Lycium ruthenicum*, surrogation by this species is unlikely.

"Goji Berries" Are *Lycium barbarum*

The evaluated commercial Goji products of this study were obtained from a many different companies and different

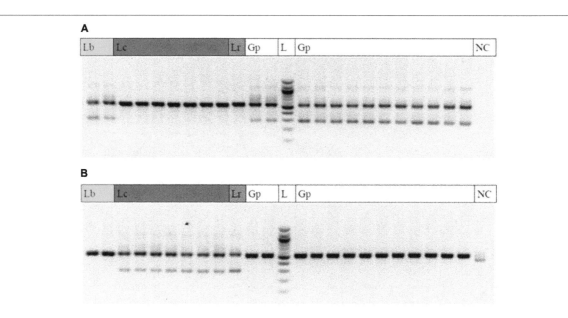

FIGURE 6 | Gel electrophoresis result of the multiplex ARMS PCRs. Lb, *Lycium barbarum* var. *barbarum;* Lc, *Lycium chinense* var. *chinense;* Lr, *Lycium ruthenicum;* Gp, commercial Goji product; L, 100 bp ladder; NC, negative control. **(A)** PCR with the universal psbA and trnH primers and the additional LB_265T_fw diagnostic primer to trace *Lycium barbarum* var. *barbarum.* A clear double band occurs with the *Lycium barbarum* var. *barbarum* reference plants (lines 1 and 2) and all of the tested Goji products (Lines 11, 12, and 14–24). The second (diagnostic) band is absent in *Lycium chinense* var. *chinense* reference plants (lines 3–9) and *Lycium ruthenicum* (line 10). Line 13 is a 100 bp ladder. The last lane is the negative control. **(B)** PCR with the universal psbA and trnH primers and the additional LC_265T_fw diagnostic primer to trace *Lycium chinense* var. *chinense.* When using this additional primer a second band is visible for all the *Lycium chinense* var. *chinense* reference plants (lines 3–9) and *Lycium ruthenicum* (line 10). This band is absent in *Lycium barbarum* var. *barbarum* and the commercial Goji products.

geographic origin. Nevertheless, all of the investigated products seem to originate from *Lycium barbarum* var. *barbarum* plants. Asian companies claim to sell only the *ningxia gou qi* (*Lycium barbarum*) as "Goji" in commercial products outside of China. Our results suggest that the consumer protection seems to be quite satisfactory in this respect, and that the "correct" products are sold on the German market. However, the pronounced difference in price for otherwise comparable "Goji" products indicates that consumer protection has to consider additional aspects of quality assessment. In this context, it should be noted that in China, "Goji" is marketed in different quality grades termed "super," "king," "special," and "Grade A," (EzineArticles, 2018) whereby the grade is linked with berry size. In other words, berries of *Lycium chinense* would be sold at higher prize. Thus, the fact that only the small *Lycium barbarum* berries were found in the commercial products sampled in Germany might therefore have a different explanation from a efficient system of consumer protection: the smaller berries from *Lycium barbarum* are less attractive for consumers in China (except for the few knowledgeable professionals that know about their medicinal value) and therefore are preferentially exported to Europe and the United States, where they still can be sold at high price. While the commercial Goji products as well as the *Lycium barbarum* var. *barbarum* reference plants show a fairly homogenous seed size, there is significant intraspecific variation in seed size among the accessions of *Lycium chinense* var. *chinense.* Since the measured seeds were chosen randomly and the sample size was sufficient, the likelihood that this variation is caused by sampling bias is rather

low, which means that the differences in size must have genetic or developmental reasons. There are some reports that the chromosome number of *Lycium chinense* varies from $2n = 24$ to 36 or even 48 (Tropicos, 2018), which would mean that there exist cryptospecies within *Lycium chinense.* This might also be a possible factor for the observed variability seen in calyx lobing between the different accessions of this species. The enlargement of seed size in *Lycium chinense* might therefore be linked with allopolyploidy. However, for the closely related Asian Goji species the literature regarding karyotypes is surprisingly scarce.

During the past years, the phylogenetic relations within the genus *Lycium* and its biogeographic background has been intensively studied. One of the surprising outcomes was the paraphyletic nature of *Lycium* (Fukuda, 2001; Levin and Miller, 2005). Different barcoding marker regions were used and combined for the genus to which Goji belongs, ranging from the more common rbcL, matK, trnF–trnH, psbA-trnH to conserved ortholog sequences (COS) regions (Levin and Miller, 2009). For our morphologically validated species we choose the sequences of the highly variable chloroplast psbA-trnH spacer region to find small differences in sequences that can be utilized for a simple one-step test to discriminate *Lycium barbarum* and *Lycium chinense.* However, we wanted to link our data into the context of the *Lycium* genus as well. We found three well separated clades corresponding to the three biogeographic regions. The East Asian "Goji" species were closely related, and formed a separate clade distinct from the other Old-World and the clade from New-World species of *Lycium*. Of course, for a biogeographic and in-depth phylogenetics approach many independent regions should be evaluated for a large set of species to receive a robust tree. However, as mentioned above this has been done extensively and our main goal was to find informative single-nucleotide polymorphisms that can be used to differentiate between the two "Goji" species *Lycium barbarum* and *Lycium chinense* by a one-step ARMS assay. The reliance on DNA based-methods is crucial, since the flowers of a commercial Goji product can obviously not be traced back, and some commercial Goji products are processed as powders as well.

Authentication by ARMS Provides an Innate Positive Control for DNA Quality and PCR Quality

Based on the single nucleotide substitution between *Lycium barbarum* and *Lycium chinense* two diagnostic ARMS primers could be designed to trace either of the species. In both of the *Lycium barbarum* var. *barbarum* reference plants using the LB_265T_fw primer, and in all of the seven *Lycium chinense* var. *chinense* reference primer using the LC_265T_fw primer, the desired second diagnostic band could be amplified in distinct multiplex PCR approaches. The results of this molecular approach strengthen the data of the seed analysis, because for all commercial Goji products there was an additional diagnostic band, when using the LB_265T_fw primer. Thus, all of the investigated commercial Goji products were authenticated morphologically and by molecular markers to be *Lycium barbarum* var. *barbarum*. The advantage of this ARMS approach is the implemented positive control of the universal psbA-trnH spacer region band in the gel. This control displays that the extracted DNA is actually of good quality and, more importantly, that the region of interest is present and the discrimination occurs exclusively because of the nucleotide substitution between the two species. Apart from the practical application of the discrimination for two closely related species of commercial importance, we'd like to highlight the importance of morphology and taxonomy and the endangered art of looking at plants in order to really understand them.

While considerable effort has been invested into the evaluation of bioactive compounds of Goji (Chang and So, 2008), to our knowledge this is the first case, where a robust one-step discrimination for these closely (from an evolutionary, cultural-historic and medicinal point of view) related "Goji" species has been developed. Previous studies have used RAPD fingerprinting and the downstream Sequence characterized amplified region (SCAR) strategy (Zhang et al., 2001; Sze et al., 2008). A disadvantage of RAPD in authentication is its limited reproducibility and reliability as fingerprint patterns are strongly dependent on sample quality and DNA integrity. Despite these drawbacks RAPD is a rapid and cost effective method that continues to be used today (Krishnan et al., 2017), especially for authentication approaches combined with downstream SCAR markers (Mei et al., 2017). RAPD-based SCAR markers yield reproducible binary results, and this method

has been used successfully for "Goji" (Sze et al., 2008), ginseng (*Panax ginseng* C.A. Mey.) (Wang et al., 2001), saffron (*Crocus sativus* L.) (Torelli et al., 2014), and others. The validation by SCAR at first sight seems easier to interpret, because only a single band has to be assessed. However, missing bands after gel electrophoresis could also be caused by problems with DNA purity or integrity, or likewise with suboptimal conditions of the PCR. Both problems are avoided by the ARMS approach, because the full-length amplicon serves as an inbuilt positive control to calibrate presence or absence of the additional diagnostic band. ARMS has been successfully used for authentication of several TCM taxa, including *Curcuma* (Sasaki et al., 2002), *Alisma* (Li et al., 2007) and *Rheum* (Yang et al., 2004). The authors emphasize the efficiency and reproducibility of this method. We realize that the ARMS application has its disadvantages as well, i.e., if it is applied to "Goji" products that are processed as powders, one would need to extend the one-step protocol and use both diagnostic primers to examine whether only *Lycium barbarum*, only *Lycium chinense* or both species are present in the respective sample. For strongly degraded DNA that might derive from extraction of processed powder products the amplification of the relatively long psbA-trnH spacer region might be difficult, meaning the internal control that is the advantage of this ARMS approach might suffer in quality. However, most of the commercial "Goji" products are sold as unprocessed dried fruits, for which the presented method easily can be applied. The ARMS approach shown in this study is not limited to superfoods like "Goji," but equally applicable to other fields of nutrition, and has the potential to be an important tool for consumer safety and quality control when it comes to discriminating "real" ingredients from surrogate species. The public availability of sequences for a large number of different plant taxa in NCBI GenBank makes it easy to design ARMS primers for prospective projects, and in many cases removes the need for initial sequencing to design new ARMS primers. However, we want to emphasize that only sequences from correctly identified herbarium vouchered material should be used for the highly sensitive ARMS method.

AUTHOR CONTRIBUTIONS

PN and TH contributed to the idea, topic, background information, and experiment planning. SW carried out the shown experiments under the lab supervision of TH. PN and SW wrote the manuscript.

ACKNOWLEDGMENTS

We acknowledge support by Deutsche Forschungsgemeinschaft and Open Access Publishing Fund of Karlsruhe Institute of Technology. We also acknowledge the staff of the Botanical Garden of the KIT for their excellent support.

REFERENCES

Amagase, H., and Farnsworth, N. R. (2011). A review of botanical characteristics, phytochemistry, relevance in efficacy and safety of *Lycium barbarum* fruit (Goji). *Food Res. Int.* 44, 1702–1717. doi: 10.1016/j.foodres.2011.03.027

Baumann, B., Baumann, H., and Baumann-Schleihauf, S. (2001). *Die Kräuterbuch Handschrift des Leonhart Fuchs*, 1st Edn. Stuttgart: Ulmer Verlag.

Blaschek, W., Hänsel, R., Keller, K., Reichling, J., Rimpler, H., and Schneider, G. (1993). *Hagers Handbuch der pharmazeutischen Praxis: Drogen E–O*, Vol. 5. Berlin: Springer Verlag.

Burke, D. S., Smidt, C. R., and Vuong, L. T. (2005). Momordica cochichinensis, *Rosa roxburghii*, wolfberry, and sea buckthorn – highly nutritional fruits supported by tradition and science. *Curr. Top. Nutraceutical. Res.* 3, 259–266.

Chang, R. C., and So, K. F. (2008). Use of anti-aging herbal medicine, *Lycium barbarum*, against aging-associated diseases. What do we know so far? *Cell. Mol. Neurobiol.* 28, 643–652. doi: 10.1007/s10571-007-9181-x

Chinadaily (2018). Available at: http://www.chinadaily.com.cn/business/2015-10/20/content_22228738.htm

Edgar, R. C. (2004). MUSCLE: multiple sequence alignment with high accuracy and high throughput. *Nucleic Acids Res.* 32, 1792–1797. doi: 10.1093/nar/gkh340

Efloras (2018). Available at: http://www.efloras.org/florataxon.aspx?flora_id=2&taxon_id=119146

Europa (2018). Available at: http://ec.europa.eu/food/safety/novel_food/catalogue/search/public/index.cfm

EzineArticles (2018). Available at: http://EzineArticles.com/593234

Felsenstein, J. (1985). Confidence limits on phylogenies: an approach using the bootstrap. *Evolution* 39, 783–791. doi: 10.1111/j.1558-5646.1985.tb00420.x

Fukuda, T. (2001). Phylogeny and biogeography of the Genus *Lycium* (Solanaceae): inferences from chloroplast DNA sequences'. *Mol. Phylogenet. Evol.* 19, 246–258. doi: 10.1006/mpev.2001.0921

Goodwin, Z. A., Harris, D. J., Filer, D., Wood, J. R., and Scotland, R. W. (2015). Widespread mistaken identity in tropical plant collections. *Curr. Biol.* 25, R1057–R1069. doi: 10.1016/j.cub.2015.10.002

Hebert, P. D., Cywinska, A., Ball, S. L., and deWaard, J. R. (2003). Biological identifications through DNA barcodes. *Proc. Biol. Sci.* 270, 313–321. doi: 10.1098/rspb.2002.2218

Hollingsworth, P. M., Forrest, L. L., Spouge, J. L., Hajibabaei, M., Ratnasingham, S., and van der Bank, M. (2009). A DNA barcode for land plants. *Proc. Natl. Acad. Sci. U.S.A.* 106, 12794–12797. doi: 10.1073/pnas.0905845106

Horn, T., Barth, A., Rühle, M., Häser, A., Jürges, G., and Nick, P. (2012). Molecular diagnostics of lemon myrtle (*Backhousia citriodora* versus *Leptospermum citratum*). *Eur. Food Res. Technol.* 234, 853–861. doi: 10.1007/s00217-012-1688-9

Horn, T., and Häser, A. (2016). Bamboo tea: reduction of taxonomic complexity and application of DNA diagnostics based on rbcL and matK sequence data. *PeerJ* 4:e2781. doi: 10.7717/peerj.2781

Horn, T., Völker, J., Rühle, M., Häser, A., Jürges, G., and Nick, P. (2014). Genetic authentication by RFLP versus ARMS? The case of moldavian dragonhead (*Dracocephalum moldavica* L.). *Eur. Food Res. Technol.* 238, 93–104. doi: 10.1007/s00217-013-2089-4

Konarska, A. (2018). Microstructural and histochemical characteristics of *Lycium barbarum* L. fruits used in folk herbal medicine and as functional food. *Protoplasma* 255, 1839–1854. doi: 10.1007/s00709-018-1277-2

Kress, J. W., Wurdack, K. J., Zimmer, E. A., Weigt, L. A., and Janzen, D. H. (2005). Use of DNA barcodes to identify flowering plants. *Proc. Natl. Acad. Sci. U.S.A.* 102, 8369–8374. doi: 10.1073/pnas.0503123102

Krishnan, A., Reshma, J., Cyriac, A., and Sible, G. V. (2017). Estimation of genetic diversity in nutmeg (Myristica fragrans Houtt.) selections using RAPD markers. *Int. J. Plant Sci.* 12, 102–107. doi: 10.15740/HAS/IJPS/12.2/102-107

Kumar, S., Stecher, G., and Tamura, K. (2016). MEGA7: molecular evolutionary genetics analysis version 7.0 for bigger datasets. *Mol. Biol. Evol.* 33, 1870–1874. doi: 10.1093/molbev/msw054

Latimes (2018). Available at: http://articles.latimes.com/2009/aug/05/food/fo-goji5

Ledford, H. (2018). Botanical renaissance. *Nature* 553, 396–398. doi: 10.1038/d41586-018-01075-5

Levin, R. A., and Miller, J. S. (2005). Relationships within tribe *Lycieae* (Solanaceae): paraphyly of *Lycium* and multiple origins of gender dimorphism'. *Am. J. Bot.* 92, 2044–2053. doi: 10.3732/ajb.92.12.2044

Levin, R. A., and Miller, J. S. (2009). The utility of nuclear conserved ortholog set II (COSII) genomic regions for species-level phylogenetic inference in *Lycium* (Solanaceae). *Mol. Phylogenet. Evol.* 53, 881–890. doi: 10.1016/j.ympev.2009.08.016

Li, X., Ding, X., Chu, B., Ding, G., Gu, S., Qian, L., et al. (2007). Molecular authentication of Alisma orientale by PCR-RFLP and ARMS. *Planta Med.* 73, 67–70. doi: 10.1055/s-2006-951746

Masci, A., Carradori, S., Casadei, M. A., Paolicelli, P., Petralito, S., Ragno, R., et al. (2018). *Lycium barbarum* polysaccharides: extraction, purification, structural characterisation and evidence about hypoglycaemic and hypolipidaemic effects. A review. *Food Chem.* 254, 377–389. doi: 10.1016/j.foodchem.2018.01.176

Mei, Z., Khan, M. D. A., Zhang, X., and Fu, J. (2017). Rapid and accurate genetic authentication of *Penthorum* chinense by improved RAPD-derived species-specific SCAR markers. *Biodiversitas* 18, 1243–1249. doi: 10.13057/biodiv/d180349

Mintel (2018). Available at: http://de.mintel.com/pressestelle/deutschland-der-weltweit-zweit-innovativste-markt-fuer-superfoods

Old, J. M. (1992). Detection of mutations by the amplification refractory mutation system (ARMS). *Methods Mol. Biol.* 9, 77–84.

Pang, X., Liu, C., Shi, L., Liu, R., Liang, D., Li, H., et al. (2012). Utility of the trnH-psbA intergenic spacer region and its combinations as plant DNA barcodes: a meta-analysis. *PLoS One* 7:e48833. doi: 10.1371/journal.pone.0048833

Potterat, O. (2010). 'Goji (*Lycium barbarum* and L. chinense): phytochemistry, pharmacology and safety in the perspective of traditional uses and recent popularity'. *Planta Med.* 76, 7–19. doi: 10.1055/s-0029-1186218

Reinhardt, D., Pesce, E. R., Stieger, P., Mandel, T., Baltensperger, K., Bennett, M., et al. (2003). Regulation of phyllotaxis by polar auxin transport. *Nature* 426, 255–260. doi: 10.1038/nature02081

Saitou, N., and Nei, M. (1987). The neighbor-joining method: a new method for reconstructing phylogenetic trees. *Mol. Biol. Evol.* 4, 406–425.

Šamec, D., Urliæ, B., and Salopek-Sondi, B. (2018). Kale (Brassica oleracea var. acephala) as a superfood: review of the scientific evidence behind the statement. *Crit. Rev. Food Sci. Nutr.* doi: 10.1080/10408398.2018.1454400 [Epub ahead of print].

Sang, T., Crawford, D., and Stuessy, T. (1997). Chloroplast DNA phylogeny, reticulate evolution, and biogeography of *Paeonia* (Paeoniaceae). *Am. J. Bot.* 84, 1120–1136. doi: 10.2307/2446155

Sasaki, Y., Fushimi, H., Cao, H., Cai, S. Q., and Komatsu, K. (2002). Sequence analysis of Chinese and Japanese curcuma drugs on the 18S rRNA gene and trnK gene and the application of amplification-refractory mutation system analysis for their authentication. *Biol. Pharm. Bull.* 25, 1593–1599. doi: 10.1248/bpb.25.1593

Schmeil, O., and Fitschen, J. (2011). *Flora Von Deutschland und Angrenzender Länder*, 95th Edn. Wiebelsheim: Quelle & Meyer Verlag.

Statista (2018a). Available at: https://de.statista.com/infografik/10823/umsatz-mit-superfoods-im-deutschen-lebensmitteleinzelhandel/

Statista (2018b). Available at: https://de.statista.com/statistik/daten/studie/722141/umfrage/umfrage-zum-regelmaessigen-kauf-von-superfood-in-deutschland/

SWR (2018). Available at: https://www.swr.de/wissen/gefaelschtes-superfood/-/id=253126/did=21391134/nid=253126/px1w90/index.html

Sze, S. C., Song, J. X., Wong, R. N., Feng, Y. B., Ng, T. B., Tong, Y., et al. (2008). Application of SCAR (Sequence characterized amplified region) analysis to autheticate *Lycium barbarum* (wolfberry) and its alduterants. *Biotechnol. Appl. Biochem.* 51(Pt 1), 15–21. doi: 10.1042/BA20070096

Tanabata, T., Shibaya, T., Hori, K., Ebana, K., and Yano, M. (2012). SmartGrain: high-throughput phenotyping software for measuring seed shape through image analysis. *Plant Physiol.* 160, 1871–1880. doi: 10.1104/pp.112.205120

Tate, J. A., and Simpson, B. B. (2003). Paraphyly of tarasa (Malvaceae) and diverse origins of the polyploid species. *Syst. Bot.* 28, 723–737.

Torelli, A., Marieschi, M., and Bruni, R. (2014). Authentication of saffron (*Crocus sativus* L.) in different processed, retail products by means of SCAR markers. *Food Control* 36, 126–131. doi: 10.1016/j.foodcont.2013.08.001

Tropicos (2018). Available at: http://www.tropicos.org/Name/29600036?projectid=9

Untergasser, A., Cutcutache, I., Koressaar, T., Ye, J., Faircloth, B. C., Remm, M., et al. (2012). Primer3 – new capabilities and interfaces. *Nucleic Acids Res.* 40:e115. doi: 10.1093/nar/gks596

Wang, J., Ha, W. Y., Ngan, F. N., But, P. P., and Shaw, P. C. (2001). Application of sequence characterized amplified region (SCAR) analysis to authenticate panax species and their adulterants. *Planta Med.* 67, 781–783. doi: 10.1055/s-2001-18340

Yang, D. Y., Fushimi, H., Cai, S. Q., and Komatsu, K. (2004). Polymerase chain reaction restriction fragment length polymorphism (PCR-RFLP) and amplification refractory mutation system (ARMS) analyses of medicinally used Rheum species and their application for identification of Rhei Rhizoma. *Biol. Pharm. Bull.* 27, 661–669. doi: 10.1248/bpb.27.661

Zhang, K. Y., Leung, H. W., Yeung, H. W., and Wong, R. N. (2001). Differentiation of *Lycium barbarum* from its related *Lycium* species using random amplified polymorphic DNA'. *Planta Med.* 67, 379–381. doi: 10.1055/s-2001-14310

Zhonghua Renmin Gongheguo wei sheng bu yao dian wei yuan hui (2000). *Pharmacopoeia of The People's Republic of China.* Beijing: Chemical Industry Press.

14

A Practical Quality Control Method for Saponins without UV Absorption by UPLC-QDA

Manjia Zhao[1], Yuntao Dai[1]*, Qi Li[1], Pengyue Li[1], Xue-Mei Qin[2] and Shilin Chen[1]*

[1] Institute of Chinese Materia Medica, China Academy of Chinese Medical Sciences, Beijing, China, [2] Modern Research Center for Traditional Chinese Medicine, Shanxi University, Taiyuan, China

*Correspondence:
Yuntao Dai
ytdai@icmm.ac.cn;
dai_yuntao@live.cn
Shilin Chen
slchen@icmm.ac.cn

Saponins are a class of important active ingredients. Analysis of saponin-containing herbal medicines is a major challenge for the quality control of medicinal herbs in companies. Taking the medicine Astragali radix (AR) as an example, it has been shown that the existing evaporative light scattering detection (ELSD) methods of astragaloside IV (AG IV) has the disadvantages of time-consuming sample preparation and low sensitivity. The universality of ELSD results in an inapplicable fingerprint with huge signals from primary compounds and smaller signals from saponins. The purpose of this study was to provide a practical and comprehensive method for the quality control of the astragalosides in AR. A simple sample preparation method with sonication extraction and ammonia hydrolyzation was established, which shortens the preparation time from around 2 days to less than 2 h. A UPLC-QDA method with the SIM mode was established for the quantification of AG IV in AR. Methanol extract was subjected to UPLC-QDA for fingerprinting analysis, and the common peaks were assigned simultaneously with the QDA. The results showed that with the newly established method, the preparation time for a set of samples was less than 90 min. The fingerprints can simultaneously detect both saponins and flavonoids in AR. This simple, rapid, and comprehensive UPLC-QDA method is suitable for quality assessment of RA and its products in companies, and also provides references for the quality control of other saponin ingredients without UV absorption.

Keywords: saponins, *Astragalus membranaceus*, astragaloside IV, fingerprint, UPLC-QDA

INTRODUCTION

Saponins are of great value in the development of new drugs or functional foods because of their wide distribution and various activities (Monschein et al., 2013). Some commonly used Chinese medicines, including ginseng (*Panax ginseng* C.A. Mey), Notoginseng (*Panax notoginseng*), Astragali radix (*Astragalus membranaceus*), licorice (*Glycyrrhiza*), dioscoreae rhizoma (*Dioscorea opposita* Thunb.), Ophiopogonis radix (*Ophiopogon japonicus*), all contain saponins (Ministry of Public Health of the People's Republic of China, 2015). Therefore, the establishment of a simple and comprehensive quality control method is important for ensuring the quality of products containing saponins.

Because of the complexity of botanical ingredients, quantitative determination of index compounds (or active compounds) and the holistic analysis of fingerprints are widely used for the quality control of herbal medicines (Liu et al., 2007). However, saponins do not produce UV absorption or have terminal absorption. The ultraviolet detection method is used to detect the ultraviolet absorption peak of the compounds, with 203 nm often used as the detection wavelength for saponins (Qi et al., 2006). However, this method has weak sensitivity and low accuracy, and therefore, its usage rate gradually reduced. The existing evaporative light scattering detection (ELSD) method is currently used more as a general-purpose detector for saponins. Although the compounds with no UV absorption have relatively high sensitivity compared with the former, there are still some disadvantages such as insufficient sensitivity (Qi et al., 2008). The high-performance liquid chromatography with mass spectrometry (HPLC-MS) method for the determination of astragalosides has better selectivity and higher sensitivity, but it is relatively expensive and cannot be widely applied. QDA is a modular single quadruple mass detector. It is a small and inexpensive mass spectrometer detector compared with QTOF and a detector with high sensitivity for saponins compared with ELSD (Veryser et al., 2015; Yao et al., 2016). In this study, QDA was used to establish fingerprints and for the quantitative determination of astragalosides.

Astragalosides have important pharmacological functions in Astragali radix (AR) (Ministry of Public Health of the People's Republic of China, 2015), which is one of the best known and widely used herbal medicines. It has been used over 2000 years for its immunomodulating (Huang et al., 2007; Zhang et al., 2009), for antioxidative (Sheih et al., 2011), and for antiinflammatory (Shon and Nam, 2003; Hoo et al., 2010). At present, quality control methods for AR include the determination of astragaloside IV with HPLC-ELSD in the Chinese Pharmacopoeia (Ministry of Public Health of the People's Republic of China, 2015). In this method, sample preparation involves reflux extraction and liquid–liquid separation with *n*-butanol, which may take more than 2 days per sample. In addition, attempts were made to establish fingerprints for saponins by HPLC-ELSD for the overall quality control of AR (Ministry of Public Health of the People's Republic of China, 2015). However, the fingerprint of saponins was overwhelmed by very large peaks from primary components, and the peaks for the saponins were too small because of the universality of the HPLC-ELSD method and the high proportion of primary components. For these reasons, quality control of saponins is time-consuming and lacks specificity or integrity. Hence, a simple, economical, and valid quality control method for AR is urgently required.

Taking AR as an example, the purpose of this study was to establish a simple and integrated quality control method for saponins in order to meet the requirements of product quality supervision during production. The astragaloside content was determined by the SIM mode of ultra-performance liquid chromatography (UPLC-QDA), and the full scanning mode was used to establish the fingerprint of the astragalosides and the main flavonoids in AR. It is a simple, fast, and holistic quality control method for saponins from AR.

MATERIALS AND METHODS

Plants and Chemicals

Commercial samples of AR were collected from different places in China and authenticated as the dry roots of *Astragalus membranaceus* (Fisch.) Bge. var. *mongholicus* (Bge.) Hsiao using DNA barcoding method. The mean content of AG IV in all samples met the requirements of the Chinese Pharmacopoeia (Ministry of Public Health of the People's Republic of China, 2015). A voucher specimen was deposited in the herbarium of the Institute of Chinese Materia Medica, China Academy of Chinese Medical Sciences.

Saponin reference compounds, including astragaloside IV (AG IV, S1), astragaloside III (AG III, S2), astragaloside II (AG II, S3), astragaloside I (AG I, S5), and isoastragaloside I (iAG I, S6), and the internal standard ginsenoside Rg1 (N1), were obtained from the National Institute for the Control of Pharmaceutical and Biological Products. Their purities, as determined by HPLC, were above 98%. The structures of these compounds are shown in **Figure 1**. HPLC-grade acetonitrile (Fisher Scientific, United States), Optima LC-MS grade formic acid (Fisher Scientific, Czechia), and pure water (Wahaha, China) were used in the mobile phase. Other reagents and chemicals were of analytical grade. All solvents and samples were filtered through 0.22 μm membrane filters (Jinteng, Tianjin, China) before injecting into the HPLC.

Astragaloside IV (AG) Analysis
Reference Solution Preparation

Five saponin reference compounds and the internal standard ginsenoside Rg1 were accurately weighed and formulated into

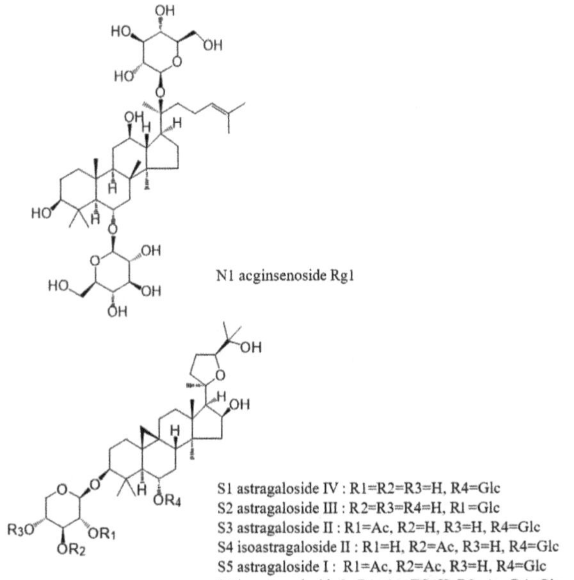

N1 acginsenoside Rg1

S1 astragaloside IV : R1=R2=R3=H, R4=Glc
S2 astragaloside III : R2=R3=R4=H, R1 =Glc
S3 astragaloside II : R1=Ac, R2=H, R3=H, R4=Glc
S4 isoastragaloside II : R1=H, R2=Ac, R3=H, R4=Glc
S5 astragaloside I : R1=Ac, R2=Ac, R3=H, R4=Glc
S6 isoastragaloside I : R1=Ac, R2=H, R3=Ac, R4=Glc
S7 acetylastragaloside I : R1=R2=R3=Ac, R4=Glc

FIGURE 1 | Chemical structure of marker constituents and the internal standard.

standard solutions of 1 mg/mL with methanol and stored at 4°C for further use.

Sample Preparation

The dried roots of AR were milled to a homogeneous powder, and then sieved through a No. 65 mesh. Each powder sample, accurately weighed (2 g), was placed in a 50 mL centrifuge tube and ultrasonicated (40 kHz, 500 W) with 30 mL methanol for 30 min. After being centrifuged (about $3000 \times g$) for 5 min, the methanol solution was filtered. The residue was washed twice with 15 mL methanol, ultrasonicated (40 kHz, 500 W) for 5 min, centrifuged (about $3000 \times g$) for 5 min, and filtered. The filtrate was combined and evaporated with a rotary evaporator, and then the residue was redissolved in 10 mL of 10% (V/V) ammonia solution, shaken from time to time for 10 min, filtered through a membrane filter (0.22 μm), and then injected into the HPLC.

UPLC-QDA Conditions

Chromatographic analysis was performed on a Waters ACQUITY H-Class UPLC® system, equipped with a quaternary solvent manager, sample manager, flow-through needle, high temperature column heater with active preheating, and QDA detector. Chromatographic separation was carried out at 35°C on a BEH Shield RP18 column (2.1 mm × 100 mm, 1.7 μm) (Waters). The mobile phase consisted of 0.1% formic acetonitrile (A) and 0.1% formic acid water (B), using an gradient elution of 5–30% A at 0–3 min, 30–40% A at 3–5 min, 40–100% A at 5–15 min, and 100–5% A at 15–18 min. The sample volume injected was 2.5 μL, and the flow rate was 0.4 mL/min.

The conditions of the electrospray ionization (ESI) source were as follows: ESI in positive mode; capillary voltage, 800 V; fragmentor, 15 V; sampling frequency, 5 Hz; Probe temperature 500°C. Ginsenoside Rg1 was detected in SIM 823.48 Da $[M+Na]^+$ mode at 0–5.5 min; AG IV and AG III were detected in SIM 808.00 Da $[M+Na]^+$ mode at 5.5–8 min; AG II and iAG II were detected in SIM 849.50 Da $[M+Na]^+$ mode at 0–8 min; AG I was detected in SIM 869.50 Da $[M+H]^+$ mode at 0–8 min; iAG I was detected in SIM 891.50 Da $[M+Na]^+$ mode at 0–8 min.

HPLC-ELSD Conditions

Quantitative analysis was performed using a 1200 Series HPLC (Agilent)–ELSD (Alltech 2000 ES). A YMC-Triart C18 column (250 mm × 4.6 mm. D.S-5 μm) was used for the chromatographic separations. The mobile phase consisted of 0.1% formic acetonitrile (A) and 0.1% formic acid water (B), using a gradient elution of 5–10% A at 0–5 min, 10–32% A at 5–10 min, 32–45% A at 10–30 min, 45–95% A at 30–35 min, and 95–20% A at 35–40 min. The injection volume was 20 μL, and the flow rate was 1 mL/min. ELSD was performed with air as the carrier gas at a flow rate of 2.5 L/min, and the nebulizer temperature was set to 100°C.

Method Validation

Calibration Curves, Limits of Detection (LOD) and Quantification (LOQ)

Methanol stock solution of AG IV was prepared and diluted to appropriate concentration ranges (0.008, 0.009, 0.01, 0.06,

0.08, and 0.09 mg/mL) for the construction of calibration curves. The calibration curve was constructed using relative peak area (analyte/internal standard; Y axis), and the concentration of the standard (μg/mL; X axis). The diluted solution of the reference compound was further diluted with methanol to a series of concentrations for the gain of LOD and LOQ. The LOD and LOQ under the present chromatographic conditions were determined at a signal-to-noise (S/N) ratio of 3 and 10, respectively.

Precision, Repeatability, Stability, and Accuracy

Intra-day variations for six successive injections within 1 day were chosen to determine the precision of the developed method. Inter-day variations for three consecutive days were chosen to determine the precision of the developed method. To confirm the repeatability, six different working solutions from the same sample were prepared and analyzed. The sample stability test was determined with one sample during 1 day at 0, 0.5, 1, 2, 4, 8, 16, and 24 h. Over this period, the solution was stored at room temperature.

A recovery test was used to evaluate the accuracy of this method. For this, 1 mL of the above-developed AG IV standard solution of 1 mg/mL was combined with 1 g of the sample, and the mix was extracted as described above in the "Sample Preparation" section. Recovery was determined by comparing the difference between the mass of AG IV of the mix (sample + standard) (M1) and the mass of AG IV in the 1-g sample alone (M2), divided by the mass of AG IV standard added (M3), as shown in Equation (1). Recovery (%) = [(M1–M2)/M3] × 100% (1).

Fingerprint Analysis
Sample Preparation

Each powder sample, accurately weighed (2 g), was placed in a 50 mL centrifuge tube and ultra-sonicated (40 kHz, 500 W) with 30 mL methanol for 30 min. After being centrifuged (about $3000 \times g$) for 20 min, the methanol solution was filtered through a membrane filter (0.22 μm), and then injected into the HPLC.

UPLC-QDA Conditions

Chromatographic separation was carried out at 30°C on a Waters CORTECS T3 column (2.1 mm × 100 mm, 1.6 μm). The mobile phase consisted of 0.1% formic acetonitrile (A) and 0.1% formic acid water (B) using an elution gradient of 2–19% A at 0–2 min, 19–42% A at 2–11.5 min, 42–55% A at 11.5–15 min, 55–65% A at 15–16.5 min, 65–75% A at 16.5–18 min, 75–100% A at 18–22.5 min, and 100–2% A at 22.5–24 min. The sample volume injected was 3 μL, and the flow rate was 0.4 mL/min.

The conditions of the ESI source were as follows: ESI in positive mode; capillary voltage, 800 V; fragmentor, 20 V; sampling frequency, 10 Hz. The QDA analysis worked using full scan mode, and the mass range was set at m/z 450–1200.

Method Validation

Intraday variations for six times within 1 day were chosen to determine the precision of the developed method. To confirm the repeatability, six different working solutions prepared from the same sample were analyzed. The sample stability test was determined with one sample during 1 day. In this period, the solution was stored at room temperature. By using the software "Similarity Evaluation System for Chromatographic Fingerprint of TCM," the "correlation coefficients" and the "relative retention time (RRT)" and "relative peak area (RPA)" of the "common peaks" were calculated. Then the correlation coefficients and the RSD% of the RRT and RPA of common peaks were used as evaluation criterion, which could semi-quantitatively express the chemical properties in the chromatographic profiles of samples.

RESULTS AND DISCUSSION

Optimization of UPLC Systems

Accord to literature, acetonitrile-water with 0.1% formic acid was used as mobile phase (Qi et al., 2009). Two columns were screened as fixed phase for the determination of AG IV in the AR extracts. **Figure 2** shows the total ion chromatograms (TICs) of ESI (+) for the AR extracts separated on different columns. AG IV and AG III did not separate on a CORTECS T3 column, whereas good separation was achieved with a BEH Shield RP18 column (**Figure 2**).

An elution gradient was used for the determination of AG IV, instead of the isocratic elution methods used in Chinese Pharmacopoeia, and most literature (Ministry of Public Health of

the People's Republic of China, 2015). To avoid the interference of other compounds, the elution gradient was set to start with 5–30% of organic solvent for 3 min before the elution of target compounds. A UV spectrum showed that most of the flavonoids compounds were eluted out before the peak of AG IV. The elution gradient was optimized to ensure that the elution of most highly polar compounds took place before the elution of AG IV, avoiding the impact of other compounds on the determination of AG IV.

Optimization of Sample Preparation

Sample preparation of AR in the determination methods of AG IV in the Chinese Pharmacopoeia includes 4-h solid-liquid extraction, liquid–liquid separation with butanol, taking more than 1 day, and column enrichment (Ministry of Public Health of the People's Republic of China, 2015). One sample preparation will take more than 2 days, which is not suitable for monitoring a large number of products in a commercial situation. In this study, sonication extraction methods were used, instead of reflux extraction. The results showed that there was no statistical difference between the sonication and the reflux extraction methods (**Supplementary Table S1**).

After extraction, liquid–liquid separation with butanol and column enrichment were used to separate and enrich astragalosides from the extracts in the methods of Chinese

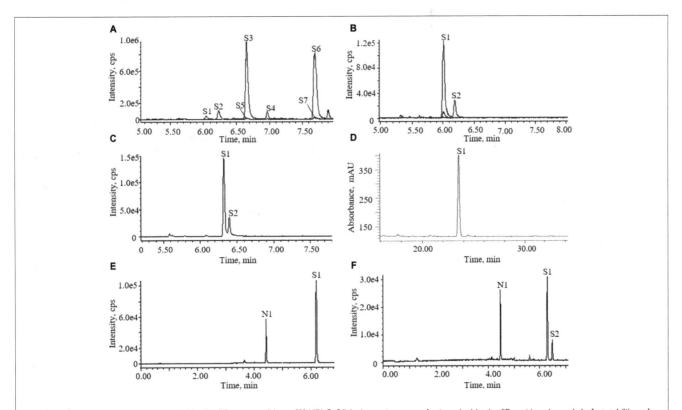

FIGURE 2 | Chromatograms of astragalosides in different conditions: **(A)** UPLC-QDA chromatograms of astragalosides in different ion channels before addition of ammonia; **(B)** UPLC-QDA chromatograms of astragalosides in different ion channels after addition of ammonia; **(C)** UPLC-QDA chromatograms of Astragali radix (AR) extracts separated on CORTECS T3 column; **(D)** HPLC-ELSD chromatograms of AR extracts on YMC C18 column; **(E)** UPLC-QDA chromatograms of standard compounds; **(F)** UPLC-QDA chromatograms of AR samples. (S1) astragaloside IV; (S2) astragaloside III; (S3) astragaloside II; (S4) isoastragaloside II; (S5) astragaloside I; (S6) isoastragaloside I; (S7) acetylastragaloside I; (N1) ginsenoside Rg1.

TABLE 1 | Comparisons the validation parameters of UPLC-QDA with HPLC-ELSD for analysis of astragaloside IV.

	UPLC-QDA	HPLC-ELSD
Retention time (min)	6.15	23.75
Linear	$Y = 29.215X + 0.2772$, $r = 0.999$	$Ln(Y) = 1.535ln(X) + 0.7998$, $r = 0.998$
Linearity range (mg/ml)	0.008–0.09	0.27–0.54
LOD (ng)	8	200
LOQ (ng)	25	500
Intra-day RSD (%) ($n = 6$)	1.96	0.74
Inter-day RSD (%) ($n = 3$)	1.77	0.21
Repeatability RSD (%) ($n = 6$)	2.77	1.56
Stability RSD (%) ($n = 8$)	2.10	1.40
Recovery mean (%)	100.95 (RSD 3.37%)	100.88 (RSD 3.19%)

TABLE 2 | Quantitative analytical results of astragaloside IV in AR samples.

No.	Mean contents ± SD (%) ($n = 3$)
Sample_1	0.19 ± 0.0061
Sample_2	0.21 ± 0.0045
Sample_3	0.22 ± 0.0087
Sample_4	0.15 ± 0.0004
Sample_5	0.04 ± 0.0007
Sample_6	0.08 ± 0.0036
Sample_7	0.14 ± 0.0016
Sample_8	0.16 ± 0.0008
Sample_9	0.14 ± 0.0016
Sample_10	0.10 ± 0.0016
Sample_11	0.19 ± 0.0044
Sample_12	0.25 ± 0.0048
Sample_13	0.09 ± 0.0026
Sample_14	0.23 ± 0.0011
Sample_15	0.19 ± 0.0020

Pharmacopoeia (Ministry of Public Health of the People's Republic of China, 2015). This step was omitted in the sample preparation here and was done in the following UPLC analysis

step, with a graduated wash starting with a high percentage of water elution, as described in the "Materials and Methods" section of this paper. This on-line elution with UPLC, instead of both solvent extraction and off-line column enrichment, saved a significant amount of time and also improved the sample preparation accuracy.

After extraction, ammonia solution was added into the extracts, and the amounts of ammonia compared. The results showed that the peak area of AG IV increased with the amount of ammonia solution, reaching its highest values with 10 mL or more of 10% (V/V) ammonia solution; therefore, 10 mL of 10% (V/V) ammonia solution was used in this study.

One important step for the sample preparation in Chinese Pharmacopoeia was reverse extraction with ammonia. It has proved that the purpose of this step was to transform other saponins into AG IV (Chu et al., 2014). The chromatograms of the astragalosides in different ion channels were recorded before and after the addition of aqueous ammonia treatment (**Figure 2**). They showed that the saponins detectable in the methanol extract of AR were AG IV (S1) and other astragalosides, including AG II (S3), iAG II (S4), AG I (S5), and iAG I (S6). After being processed with ammonia, AG II (S3), iAG II (S4), AG I (S5), and iAG I (S6) all disappeared and transformed into AG IV (S1) (Chu et al., 2014). The results indicated that other astragalosides, except AG III, could be converted into AG IV, and that the amount of AG IV detected was mainly the sum of AG I (S5), iAG I, AG II (S3), and AG IV (S1).

Method Validation and Comparison With HPLC-ELSD

The calibration curve ($Y = 29.215X + 0.2772$) was successfully constructed using relative peak area for the Y axis and the concentration of standard as µg/mL for the X axis. The linearity of analytical response was acceptable with correlation coefficients higher than 0.99 offering a linear dynamic range of about two orders of magnitude. The LOD, LOQ, precision, stability, repeatability, and accuracy of the established methods for the determination of AG IV are summarized in **Table 1** and **Supplementary Table S2**. All results of precision, stability,

TABLE 3 | On-line detected data for assigned compounds in Astragali Radix.

No.	Name	Observed RRT (min)	Relative peak area (RPA)	Observed m/z
F1	Calycosin-7-O-β-D-glucoside	0.85	0.38	469.23
F2	Calycosin-7-O-β-D-glucoside-6″-O-malonate	1.00	1.00	555.11
F3	Formononetin-7-O-β-D-glucoside	1.12	0.18	453.24
F4	9,10-Dimethoxypterocarpan-3-O-β-D-glucoside	1.20	0.73	485.22
F5	Formononetin-7-O-β-D-glucoside-6″-O-malonate	1.28	0.35	539.08
F6	3-Hydroxyl-9,10-dimethoxypterocarpan-7-O-β-D-glucoside-6″-O-malonate	1.34	0.35	571.16
S1	Astragaloside IV	1.71	0.24	807.58
S2	Astragaloside III	1.74	1.47	807.56
S3	Astragaloside II	1.90	1.08	849.54
S4	Isoastragaloside II	2.02	0.25	849.46
S5	Astragaloside I	2.20	1.97	891.53
S6	Isoastragaloside I	2.28	0.09	891.74
S7	Cycloastragenol	2.26	0.02	513.39

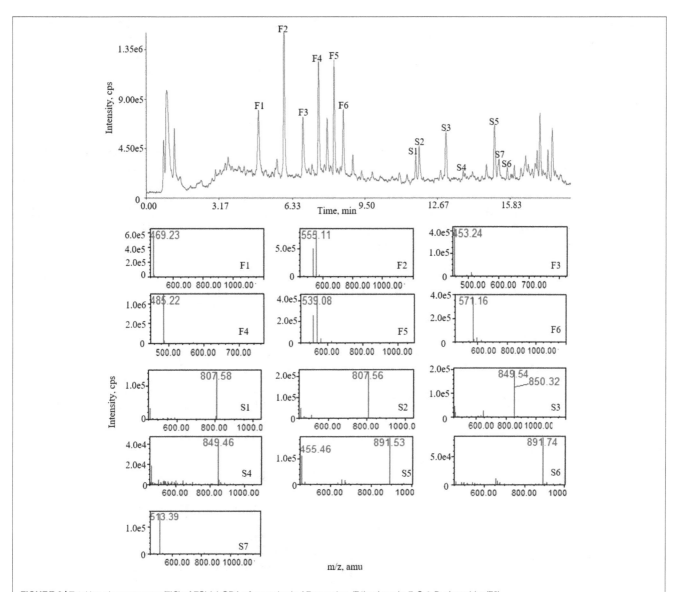

FIGURE 3 | Total ion chromatogram (TIC) of ESI (+) QDA of saponins in AR samples: (F1) calycosin-7-O-β-D-glucoside; (F2) calycosin-7-O-β-D-glucoside-6″-O-malonate; (F3) formononetin-7-O-β-D-glucoside; (F4) 9,10-dimethoxypterocarpan-3-O-β-D-glucoside; (F5) formononetin-7-O-β-D-glucoside-6″-O-malonate; (F6) 3-hydroxy-9,10-dimethoxypterocarpan-7-O-β-D-glucoside-6″-O-malonate; (S1) astragaloside IV; (S2) astragaloside III; (S3) astragaloside II; (S4) isoastragaloside II; (S5) astragaloside I; (S6) isoastragaloside I; (S7) cycloastragenol.

repeatability, and accuracy indicated that this method was valid.

The potential of UPLC-QDA was compared with the performance of HPLC-ELSD. **Table 1** lists the performance index of UPLC-QDA compared with HPLC-ELSD for the analysis of AG IV. LOD and LOQ were seen to be low at 8 and 25 ng, compared with 200 and 500 ng for ELSD, which meant that the sensitivity was greatly improved by the use of UPLC-QDA instead of HPLC-ELSD. The higher sensitivity of UPLC-QDA than that of ELSD was also observed in sample detection. **Figure 2** shows the chromatograms for the sample (d) with HPLC-ELSD and the chromatogram for standard compound (e) and sample (f) with UPLC-QDA. An obvious peak for AG III was observed with the established method, but it was not obvious in the

chromatogram by HPLC-ELSD, which is attributed to the higher sensitivity of QDA than that of ELSD. The linearity range was also broadened with UPLC-QDA than ELSD and UPLC-QDA also showed a notably shortened analysis time. These advantages of UPLC-QDA indicate it successfully quantitative applications in quality analysis of RA. The precision, stability, and repeatability of the established UPLC-QDA method were not as good as the HPLC-ELSD method, but it is acceptable for the determination of AG IV in AR.

The established UPLC-QDA method was investigated for the analysis of AR. Fifteen samples from different batches were analyzed and the analytical contents were summarized in **Table 2**. All the analyses were carried out and repeated three times, and the data were recorded and expressed as the mean AG IV content.

Table 2 shows the means for 15 batches detected with UPLC-QDA, and the results show a successful application of UPLC-QDA method to for the determination of AG IV in different AR sample.

Optimization of UPLC-QDA Conditions for Fingerprint

The elution gradient was optimized to achieve good separation for each peak in a short time. Several different gradients were tried and finally the gradient used in this study was selected, with good separation of each peak.

Validation for Fingerprint Method

The correlation coefficients and the RSD% of the RRT and RPA of common peaks were calculated (**Supplementary Tables S3–S5**). The correlation coefficients of precision were higher than 0.989 and the RSD% of RPA was lower than 5.00. The correlation coefficients of the repeatability test were higher than 0.992 and the RSD% of RPA was lower than 8.00. The correlation coefficients of the stability test were higher than 0.984 and the RSD% of RPA was lower than 6.10, indicating that the sample remained stable for 1 day. All tests for precision, repeatability, and stability indicated that this method was valid and applicable.

Establishment of Fingerprint of Saponins in AR

In this study, 15 samples were analyzed by the newly developed method. The mean chromatogram and correlation coefficients of the samples were calculated by using the similarity software, and it was found that correlation coefficients of AR samples were higher than 0.920, which indicated that all the samples tested have high consistency in quality.

There were 13 "common peaks" existing in the chromatograms for the AR samples, which were assigned with ion mass analyzed with QDA and confirmed with reference compounds. **Figure 3** shows the typical mass spectra for saponins. In the positive ion mode, six of the saponins generated typical $[M+Na]^+$ ions, with mass accuracy at $807.5 + 42$ n ($n = 0$ refers to AG IV, $n = 1$ refers to AG II/iAG II, $n = 2$ refers to AG I/iAG I). The six peaks of the flavonoids generated typical $[M+Na]^+$ ions. The MS data for the six saponins and flavonoids in the positive ion mode are shown in **Table 3**. The RRT and RPA of the common peaks in the 15 samples were calculated and the data of the RPA was shown in **Supplementary Table S6**.

The results shows that the fingerprint method established in this study can simultaneously detect a variety of saponins and flavonoids. In addition, the identities of each compound can be directly established by its mass number.

CONCLUSION

A simple and fast quantification method for AG IV and an overall fingerprint of the main components (astragalosides and flavonoids) in AR have been established with UPLC-QDA. The established method was feasible for comprehensive quality evaluation of RA. The UPLC-QDA exhibits advantages over ELSD in sensitivity, peak assignment and simultaneous detections of components with and without UV absorption in fingerprint. The established methods provide references for the quality control of saponin ingredients without UV absorption. This study therefore provides suitable methods for the practical quality assessment of saponins in commercial situations.

AUTHOR CONTRIBUTIONS

YD, QL, X-MQ, and SC designed the study. MZ did the experiments. YD and MZ wrote the manuscript. All authors gave approval to the final version.

FUNDING

The authors are grateful for the financial support provided by National Science Foundation (81473340 and 81803734), Project of Institute of Chinese Materia Medica, China Academy of Chinese Medical Sciences (ZXKT17048), and Project of China Academy of Chinese Medical Sciences (ZXKT17009 and GH201701).

ACKNOWLEDGMENTS

We would like to thank Waters Technologies (Shanghai) Ltd. providing UPLC-QDA for analysis and Editage (www.editage.cn) for English language editing.

REFERENCES

Chu, C., Liu, E. H., Qi, L. W., and Li, P. (2014). Transformation of astragalosides from radix astragali under acidic, neutral, and alkaline extraction conditions monitored by LC-ESI-TOF/MS. *Chin. J. Nat. Med.* 12, 314–320. doi: 10.1016/s1875-5364(14)60062-5

Hoo, R. L., Wong, J. Y., Qiao, C., Xu, A., Xu, H., and Lam, K. S. (2010). The effective fraction isolated from Radix Astragali alleviates glucose intolerance, insulin resistance and hypertriglyceridemia in db/db diabetic mice through

its anti-inflammatory activity. *Nutr. Metab.* 7:67. doi: 10.1186/1743-7075-7-67

Huang, G. C., Wu, L. S., Chen, L. G., Yang, L. L., and Wang, C. C. (2007). Immuno-enhancement effects of Huang Qi Liu Yi Tang in a murine model of cyclophosphamide-induced leucopenia. *J. Ethnopharmacol.* 109, 229–235. doi: 10.1016/j.jep.2006.07.023

Liu, A. H., Lin, Y. H., Yang, M., Guo, H., Guan, S. H., Sun, J. H., et al. (2007). Development of the fingerprints for the quality of the roots of Salvia miltiorrhiza and its related preparations by HPLC-DAD and LC-MS(n).

J. Chromatogr. B. Analyt. Technol. Biomed. Life Sci. 846, 32–41. doi: 10.1016/j.jchromb.2006.08.002

Ministry of Public Health of the People's Republic of China (2015). *Pharmacopoeia of the People's Republic of China*, Vol. 1, Beijing: Ministry of Public Health of the People's Republic of China, 302–303.

Monschein, M., Ardjomand-Woelkart, K., Rieder, J., Wolf, I., Heydel, B., Kunert, O., et al. (2013). Accelerated sample preparation and formation of astragaloside IV in Astragali Radix. *Pharm. Biol.* doi: 10.3109/13880209.2013.839712 [Epub ahead of print].

Qi, L. W., Cao, J., Li, P., and Wang, Y. X. (2009). Rapid and sensitive quantitation of major constituents in Danggui Buxue tang by ultra-fast HPLC-TOF/MS. *J. Pharm. Biomed. Anal.* 49, 502–507. doi: 10.1016/j.jpba.2008.10.026

Qi, L. W., Wen, X. D., Cao, J., Li, C. Y., Li, P., Yi, L., et al. (2008). Rapid and sensitive screening and characterization of phenolic acids, phthalides, saponins and isoflavonoids in Danggui Buxue Tang by rapid resolution liquid chromatography/diode-array detection coupled with time-of-flight mass spectrometry. *Rapid. Commun. Mass. Spectrom.* 22, 2493–2509. doi: 10.1002/rcm.3638

Qi, L. W., Yu, Q. T., Li, P., Li, S. L., Wang, Y. X., Sheng, L. H., et al. (2006). Quality evaluation of Radix Astragali through a simultaneous determination of six major active isoflavonoids and four main saponins by high-performance liquid chromatography coupled with diode array and evaporative light scattering detectors. *J. Chromatogr. A.* 1134, 162–169. doi: 10.1016/j.chroma.2006.08.085

Sheih, I. C., Fang, T. J., Wu, T. K., Chang, C. H., and Chen, R. Y. (2011). Purification and properties of a novel phenolic antioxidant from Radix astragali fermented by *Aspergillus oryzae* M29. *J. Agric. Food Chem.* 59, 6520–6525. doi: 10.1021/jf2011547

Shon, Y. H., and Nam, K. S. (2003). Protective effect of Astragali radix extract on interleukin 1beta-induced in fl ammation in human amnion. *Phytother. Res.* 17, 1016–1020. doi: 10.1002/ptr.1276

Veryser, L., Taevernier, L., Roche, N., Blondeel, P., and De Spiegeleer, B. (2015). Implementation of a single quad MS detector in high-throughput transdermal research of plant extracts. *J. Pharm. Biomed. Anal.* 115, 594–602. doi: 10.1016/j.jpba.2015.08.016

Yao, C. L., Yang, W., Si, W., Pan, H., Qiu, S., Wu, J., et al. (2016). A strategy for establishment of practical identification methods for Chinese patent medicine from systematic multi-component characterization to selective ion monitoring of chemical markers: shuxiong tablet as a case study. *RSC Adv.* 6, 65055–65066. doi: 10.1039/c6ra10883k

Zhang, R. P., Zhang, X. P., Ruan, Y. F., Ye, S. Y., Zhao, H. C., Cheng, Q. H., et al. (2009). Protective effect of Radix Astragali injection on immune organs of rats with obstructive jaundice and its mechanism. *World J. Gastroenterol.* 15, 2862–2869.

15

Systems Pharmacology Based Strategy for Q-Markers Discovery of HuangQin Decoction to Attenuate Intestinal Damage

Xiao-min Dai[1,2], Dong-ni Cui[1,2], Jing Wang[3], Wei Zhang[4], Zun-jian Zhang[1,2]* and Feng-guo Xu[1,2]*

[1] Key Laboratory of Drug Quality Control and Pharmacovigilance, Ministry of Education, China Pharmaceutical University, Nanjing, China, [2] State Key Laboratory of Natural Medicines, China Pharmaceutical University, Nanjing, China, [3] College of Pharmacy, Shaanxi University of Chinese Medicine, Xianyang, China, [4] State Key Laboratory for Quality Research in Chinese Medicines, Macau University of Science and Technology, Taipa, Macau

*Correspondence:
Feng-guo Xu
fengguoxu@gmail.com
Zun-jian Zhang
zunjianzhangcpu@hotmail.com

The quality control research of traditional Chinese medicine (TCM) is lagged far behind the space of progress in modernization and globalization. Thus the concept of quality marker (Q-marker) was proposed recently to guide the quality investigations of TCM. However, how to discover and validate the Q-marker is still a challenge. In this paper, a system pharmacology based strategy was proposed to discover Q-marker of HuangQin decoction (HQD) to attenuate Intestinal Damage. Using this strategy, nine measurable compounds including paeoniflorin, baicalin, scutellarein, liquiritigenin, norwogonin, baicalein, glycyrrhizic acid, wogonin, and oroxylin A were screened out as potential markers. Standard references of these nine compounds were pooled together as components combination according to their corresponding concentration in HQD. The bioactive equivalence between components combination and HQD was validated using wound healing test and inflammatory factor determination experiment. The comprehensive results indicated that components combination is almost bioactive equivalent to HQD and could serve as the Q-markers. In conclusion, our study put forward a promising strategy for Q-markers discovery.

Keywords: Q-marker, systems pharmacology, traditional Chinese medicine, HuangQin decoction, intestinal damage

INTRODUCTION

Traditional Chinese medicine (TCM) plays a vital role in prevention and treatment of diseases and receives more and more attention (Jiang et al., 2010). Due to its highly complex chemical composition, TCM is confronting a major challenge in quality control research (Yang et al., 2017). In Chinese Pharmacopeia monographs, the quality standards of TCM were usually established based on the absolute quantitation of one or several specific chemical compounds. This approach can only ensure the consistency of the assigned chemical markers. It is often questionable whether these chemical markers are responsible for and directly related to the holistic efficacy of TCM. Many efforts have been made to drive the advance of quality control research of TCM (Tilton et al., 2010; Long et al., 2015; Wang F. et al., 2017). But the proposed strategy or methods are quite complex and not easy to follow. Thus, a standardized and commonly accepted strategy for

TCM quality control research is needed. Recently, the concept of quality marker (Q-marker) was proposed to standardize TCM quality research and to enhance the quality consistency (Liu et al., 2016). However, how to discover and validate the Q-marker is still a huge challenge.

Systems pharmacology is an emerging approach that integrates chemoinformatics, network pharmacology and -omics data. It is a useful tool to achieve a comprehensive insight into the therapeutical mechanism of multi-compound herbs. The public availability of system pharmacology platforms and other bioinformation databases put systems pharmacology-based TCM research strategy into practice (Ru et al., 2014). It has been successfully used to reveal the material basis and the mechanism of Yin-Huang-Qing-Fei capsule (Yu et al., 2017) and rhubarb (Xiang et al., 2015) on the treatment of chronic bronchitis and renal interstitial fibrosis, respectively. Systems pharmacology provides a bridge to link the TCM chemical constituents with the corresponding targets, which would facilitate the Q-markers discovery. Therefore, we proposed a systems pharmacology based strategy (**Figure 1**) for Q-marker discovery. The feasibility of this strategy was tested by taking HuangQin decoction (HQD) as an example.

HuangQin decoction (HQD) is a basic formula listed in *Treatise on Exogenous Febrile Disease* written by Zhongjing Zhang. It has been widely used in China for more than 1800 years on the treatment of gastrointestinal (GI) ailments, including diarrhea, abdominal spasms, vomiting, and nausea (Wang X. et al., 2017). Recent studies have revealed that PHY906, a modified formulation derived from HQD, could ameliorate chemotherapy-induced GI toxicity and enhance the therapeutic efficacy of irinotecan, capecitabine and other antitumor drugs (Lam et al., 2010; Saif et al., 2010; Wang et al., 2011). HQD is constituted with four medicinal herbs, i.e., *Scutellaria baicalensis* Georgi, *Glycyrrhiza uralensis* Fisch, *Paeonia lactiflora* Pall, and *Ziziphus jujuba* Mill. Up to now, it is still unclear that which

ingredients of HQD are active to ameliorate intestinal damage, which significantly limits the establishment of quality standards.

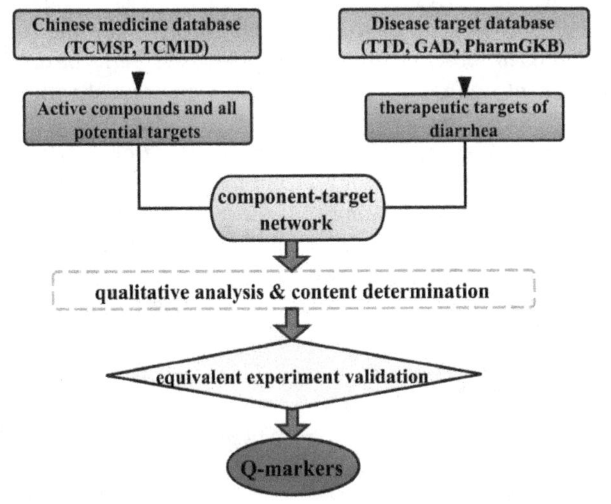

In this paper, we tried to discover the Q-marker of HQD to treat diarrhea using a system pharmacology based strategy. After collecting the active components of HQD and the corresponding therapeutic targets of diarrhea, the component-target (C-T) network was constructed firstly. LC-IT-TOF/MS fingerprint was used to clarify which active compounds actually existed in water decoction of HQD. Then the detectability of selected potential markers were tested and the absolute concentration of measurable components were quantified using HPLC/UV. Bioactive equivalent experiment was performed to evaluate the efficacy of HQD and the combination of selected potential markers from the aspect of alleviating intestinal damage.

MATERIALS AND METHODS

Chemicals and Reagents

Paeoniflorin, baicalin, scutellarein, liquiritigenin, baicalein, glycyrrhizic acid, wogonin, and oroxylin A were purchased from Chengdu Herbpurify Co., Ltd. (Sichuan, China). Glycyrrhizic acid ammonium salt and norwogonin were purchased from ChemFaces (China). All other reagents and solvents were of high performance liquid chromatography (HPLC) grade. Deionized water was purified using a Milli-Q system (Millipore, Bedford, MA, United States). *Scutellaria baicalensis* Georgi (Hebei Province), *Glycyrrhiza uralensis* Fisch (Inner Mongolia of China), *Paeonia lactiflora* Pall (Anhui Province), and *Ziziphus jujuba* Mill (Henan Province) were authenticated by Dr. Ehu Liu (State Key Laboratory of Natural Medicines, China Pharmaceutical University, China).

Collection of Active Ingredients and Diarrhea Targets

The ingredients of the four constitutional herbs, i.e., *Scutellaria baicalensis* Georgi, *Glycyrrhiza uralensis* Fisch, *Paeonia lactiflora* Pall, and *Ziziphus jujuba* Mill in HQD were collected from Traditional Chinese Medicines for Systems Pharmacology Database and Analysis Platform (TCMSP[1]), Traditional Chinese Medicine integrative database (TCMID), TCM Database @ Taiwan, HIT and wide-scale literature mining. Generally, ADME screening was used in previous prediction, which includes series of pharmacokinetic parameters such as oral bioavailability (OB), drug-likeness (DL), and blood–brain barrier (BBB) value (Shen et al., 2016). Considering that our study focused on intestinal damage, the active components might exert therapeutic effect without being absorbed into serum or brain. Thus, we only set DL ≥ 0.05 as criteria to filter out active ingredients as many as possible.

Targets of all effective components in HQD were collected from DrugBank, TCMSP, and STITCH. The targets that are in close relationship with diarrhea were obtained from PharmGKB[2],

FIGURE 1 | Whole framework of Q-markers discovery of TCM based on systems pharmacology and a case of HQD.

---

[1]http://lsp.nwu.edu.cn/tcmsp.php

[2]https://www.pharmgkb.org/

TTD database[3] (Yang et al., 2016) GAD (Genetic Association Database) and OMIM (Online Mendelian Inheritance in Man, up data to 2017). Then UniProt database[4] was employed to standardize the target related genes and to focus on the targets from the human. The genes that are associated with diarrhea and can be targeted by HQD were kept. And then, the Compound-Target (C-T) network were generated and their topological properties were analyzed by Cytoscape 3.4.0.

Active Components Identification in HQD by LC/MS

LC-IT-TOF/MS was used to clarify which active compounds are actually existing in water decoction of HQD. One milliliter of standard decoction HQD (Wang X. et al., 2017) was dissolved in a suitable amount of 80% (v/v) methanol with the assistant dissolve effect of DMSO by ultra-sonication and subsequently centrifuged (16000 rpm, 4°C) for 10 min. The supernatants were filtered and analyzed on a ZORBAX SB-C18 rapid resolution HT (2.1 mm × 100 mm, 1.8 μm) (Agilent Technologies). The mobile phase consisted of 0.1% formic acid (A) and methanol (B). The gradient elution began with 10% B, increased to 45% B in 12 min, further increased to 100% B in 16 min and last for 6 min, and brought back to 10% B in 1 min followed by 10 min of re-equilibration. The mass spectrometry (MS) analysis was performed in a ultrafast LC-ion trap time-of-flight mass spectrometer via electrospray ionization (ESI) interface (SHIMADZU, Japan). The parameters were as follows: ESI (±), nebulizing gas rat, 1.5 L/min; drying gas pressure, 100 kPa; detector voltage, 1.85 kV; interface voltage, −3.5 kV; CDL and heat block temperature, 200°C; ion accumulation time, 30 ms. The mass range was set at m/z 100–1000. The components in HQD were identified by comparing with the reference standards available in our lab or the fragment models in literatures. The results were combined with those identified in PHY906 (Ye et al., 2007).

Potential Markers Quantification in HQD by HPLC/UV

After checking the identified components of HQD in the C-T network, only the common ones were screened out as potential markers. The detectability of these selected potential markers was tested and the absolute concentration of measurable components were quantified using HPLC/UV. After dilution and filtering, HQD was analyzed on an Agilent 1100 series HPLC system (Agilent, United States) using Agilent Zorbax SB-C18 column (250 mm × 4.6 mm, 5 μm). The mobile phase consisted of 0.1% phosphoric acid in water (A) and acetonitrile (B). The gradient elution program was 19–21% B at 0–8 min, 21–35% B at 8–10 min, 35–35% B at 10–18 min, 35–40% B at 18–20 min, 40–40% B at 20–38 min, 40–100% B at 38–43 min. The flow rate was kept at 1.0 ml/min at 30°C. Different detection wavelengths were set for different

compounds. 236 nm for paeoniflorin; 278 nm for baicalin, baicalein, wogonin, liquiritigenin; 250 nm for glycyrrhizic acid ammonium salt; 270 nm for oroxylin A; 340 nm for scutellarein; 280 nm for norwogonin. Standard references of these compounds were pooled together as components combination according to their corresponding concentration in HQD.

Bioactive Equivalence Assessment Between Components Combination and HQD

Cell Culture

Lipopolysaccharide (LPS)-stimulated NCM460 damage (Bhattacharyya et al., 2008) and LPS-stimulated THP-1-derived macrophage inflammation (Perezperez et al., 1995) were used as two cell models to assess the bioactive equivalence between components combination and HQD. NCM460 and THP-1 were obtained from Model Animal Research Center of Nanjing University and Stem Cell Bank of Chinese Academy of Sciences, respectively. Cells were grown at 37°C under a humidified atmosphere with 5% (v/v) CO_2. NCM460 and THP-1 were cultured in Dulbecco's modified Eagle's medium (DMEM) (Boster Biological Technology Co., Ltd.) and Roswell Park Memorial Institute (RIPM) 1640 medium (Gibco-Thermo Fisher Scientific, United States) respectively, containing 10% fetal bovine serum and 1% penicillin-streptomycin (Biological Industries, Israel).

Cell Migration Assay

Collective migration of epithelial cells refers to fundamental physiological processes as an inherent part of embryonic morphogenesis, cancer and wound healing, which can be measured by scratch assay (Das et al., 2015). In colon epithelial monolayer (NCM460), opening of a free surface by scratch-wounding triggers collective movement of the surrounding cells to fill the gap. To assess the effect of medicines on NCM460, we pretreated cells with HQD, components combination and baicalin (corresponding concentrations in 400, 200, 100, 50 μg/ml HQD) for 24 h. After pre-incubation and the 100% cell confluent observed, scratch-wounding was performed. The supernatant was removed and the cells were washed with PBS three times to remove the damaged cells. Then cells were subjected to 1 μg/ml LPS (Lipopolysaccharides from *Escherichia coli* O111:B4, Sigma) for 24 h except the vehicle control group. The images of two migrating epithelial monolayers of NCM460 was captured with an inverted phase contrast microscope (Nikon Eclipse Ti-U), which was used to calculate the % relative cell migration according to the following equation (Buranasukhon et al., 2017).

$$\%\text{Relative migration} = \frac{\text{Area between cells}_{0\,h} - \text{Area between cells}_{24\,h}}{\text{Area between cells}_{0\,h}} \times 100$$

TNF-α and PGE$_2$ Release

To assess the anti-inflammatory effect of HQD, components combination and baicalin, the NCM460 and THP-1-derived macrophages were pretreated for 12 h with medicines. Then, NCM460 were cultured in serum-free DMEM supplemented with LPS(1 μg/ml) for 6 or 12 h, while THP-1-derived macrophages were cultured in serum-free RIPM 1640 supplemented with 1 μg/ml LPS (8 h for TNF-α, 21 h for PGE$_2$) (Padilla et al., 2017). The accumulated TNF-α and PGE$_2$ in the culture medium were measured using commercial ELISA kits [Multisciences(Lianke) Biotech for TNF-α and MEIMIAN for PGE$_2$] according to the manufacturer's instruction.

Statistical Analysis

All data were expressed as mean ± standard deviation (SD). Data were subjected to statistical analysis using Graphpad Prism 5.0 (Graphpad Software, San Diego, CA, United States). One-way analysis of variance (ANOVA) with Dunnett's *post hoc* test was carried out for statistical comparison. In all cases, the value of $P < 0.05$ was considered to be statistical significance.

RESULTS

Collection of HQD Ingredients and Diarrhea Targets

Considering that intestinal tissues and intestinal content play important roles in the occurrence of diarrhea, we selected DL as the only standard to filter active ingredients. The name and Mol ID of 186 ingredients from *Scutellaria baicalensis* Georgi, 111 from *Paeonia lactiflora* Pall, 236 from *Glycyrrhiza uralensis* Fisch, and 226 from *Ziziphus jujube* Mill was shown in **Supplementary Table S1**. The corresponding target that these ingredients act on was screened out based on TCMSP and STITCH database (**Supplementary Table S2**). At the same time, 64 diarrhea-related proteins were found from PharmGKB, TTD, GAD, and OMIM (**Supplementary Table S3**). Only 33 common targets from these two independent search were kept, which were interacted with 208 ingredients of HQD (**Supplementary Table S4**).

Compound-Target Network Construction and Analysis

As small molecules typically exert their bioactive effects through interactions with protein targets. Thus in order to identify the interaction between the filtered 208 compounds and 33 diarrhea targets, a network was established. As we can see from **Figure 2**, 430 compound-target interactions were generated. The node degree represents the connectedness of a node with other nodes and it is the basic quantitative properties of network. The degree of compounds and targets were listed in **Supplementary Table S5**. Among these 33 targets, Prostaglandin G/H synthase 2 (PTGS2, $D = 199$) has the highest degree, followed by Nitric (nitric) oxide synthase (NOS2, $D = 97$), Vascular endothelial growth factor receptor 2 (KDR, $D = 25$), Tumor necrosis factor (TNF, $D = 20$) and so on, which indicated that they played a significant role in the network as the hub target. Wogonin, oroxylin A, and berberine could interacted with PTGS2 and NOS2 simultaneously. Rutin, wogonin, baicalein, and

paeoniflorin could interacted with TNF. The above results clearly elucidated the "multi-component and multi-target" mechanism of HQD and synergistic therapeutical effect on diarrhea.

Active Components Identification and Quantification of HQD

Although above results suggested that 208 ingredients have effects on diarrhea-related targets, it does not mean that all these 208 components are detectable in HQD. The phytochemical components in water decoction of the four constitutional herbs were then identified by LC-IT-TOF/MS fingerprint in ESI positive and negative ion modes (**Supplementary Figure S1**). Totally, 38 compounds in HQD were identified by comparison with available reference standards in our lab or the fragment information in literatures, including 8 from *Glycyrrhiza uralensis* Fisch, 2 from *Paeonia lactiflora* Pall and 28 from *Scutellaria baicalensis* Georgi (**Supplementary Table S6**). Combining these 38 compounds with those identified in PHY906 (Ye et al., 2007), we got 79 compounds. Eleven of them that could be well matched with the C-T network of diarrhea were kept as potential markers.

Quantitative determination results (**Supplementary Figure S2**) demonstrated that except chrysin and rutin, the content of the rest 9 potential markers in HQD was more than Limit of Quantitation (LOQ). The LOQ of chrysin and rutin by HPLC/UV was 66.15 and 45.14 ng, respectively. Therefore, paeoniflorin, baicalin, scutellarein, liquiritigenin, norwogonin, baicalein, glycyrrhizic acid, wogonin, and oroxylin A were screened out as potential markers. Standard references of these 9 compounds were pooled together as components combination according to their corresponding concentration in HQD.

Bioactive Equivalence Assessment Between Components Combination and HQD

Wound healing test and inflammatory factor determination experiment results indicated that HQD showed remarkable protective effects and components combination exerted the same or better effects.

Representative phase-contrast images of control group wound areas at 0 and 24 h following scratching were shown in **Figure 3A**. Quantitative results demonstrated that LPS stimulation resulted in significantly lower cell mobility of NCM460 than the control group ($P < 0.01$). Components combination increased the cell mobility of LPS-stimulated NCM460 with dose-dependent and the effect was better than that of HQD at the same dose (**Figure 3B**). Baicalin (12 μg/mL), one of the most abundant compounds in HQD, showed some activities but could not achieve bioactive equivalence with HQD at the same dose level (400 μg/mL). In addition, LPS stimulation resulted in a substantial increase of TNF-α secretion in NCM460, while pre-incubation of components combination or HQD alleviated the LPS-induced increase of TNF-α. The results of LPS stimulation 6 h suggested that 400 μg/mL components combination had a similar efficacy to 200 μg/mL HQD. With LPS stimulation 12 h, only 200 μg/mL components combination exerted

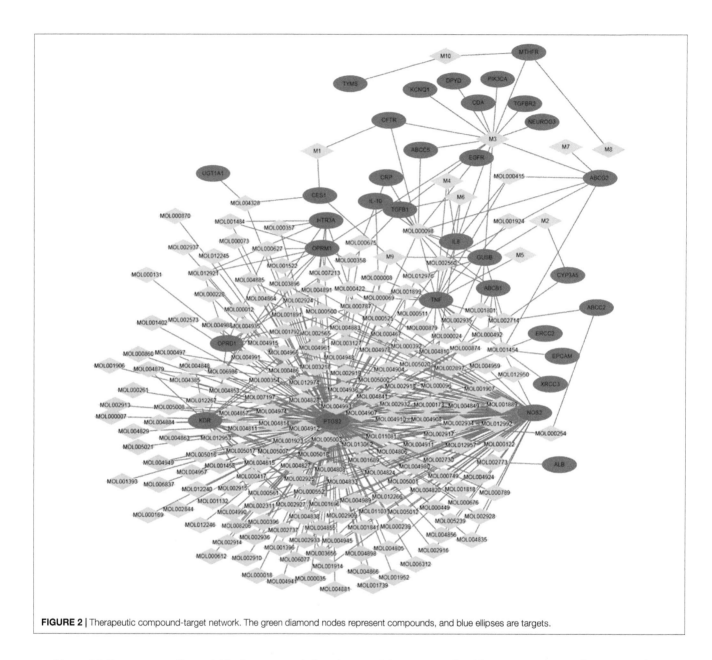

FIGURE 2 | Therapeutic compound-target network. The green diamond nodes represent compounds, and blue ellipses are targets.

notable anti-inflammatory effect, which demonstrated that the anti-inflammatory effect of components combination is superior to that of HQD (**Figure 3C**). Baicalin exerted weak effects and the results were consistent with theory of superimposed effect in TCM.

To further investigate the anti-inflammatory action on macrophages, effects of components combination and HQD on TNF-α and PGE$_2$ production in LPS-activated THP-1 were determined. Differentiated THP-1 was obtained by 48 h treatment with phorbol 12-myristate 13-acetate (PMA). Stimulation of LPS for 8 h increased TNF-α release, whereas preincubation with HQD or components combination notably alleviated the elevation of TNF-α compared with model group. At the optimum concentration 200 µg/mL, components combination showed comparable effect with 100 or 50 µg/mL HQD. An interesting finding is that baicalin showed the best

activity compared with components combination and HQD, which could be used to explain the monarch role of *Scutellaria baicalensis* Georgi in HQD (**Figure 4A**). Stimulation of LPS for 21 h significantly increased PGE$_2$ production, pre-treatment with 200 µg/mL components combination or 100 µg/mL HQD had the same effect to alleviate the LPS-induced increase of PGE$_2$. Baicalin showed some activity but it was inferior to HQD (**Figure 4B**).

DISCUSSION

Traditional Chinese medicine show advantage especially on the treatment of chronic disease, and receive more and more attention. However, the quality control problem of TCM is a major obstacle hindering its modernization and globalization.

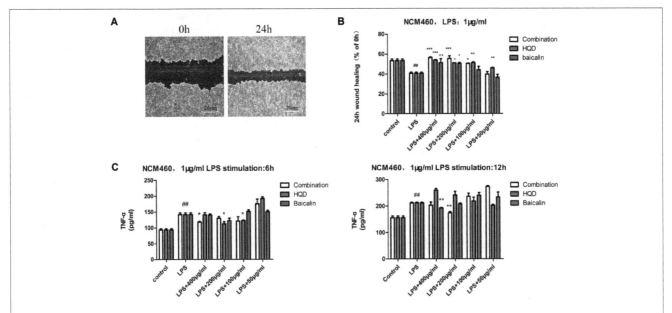

FIGURE 3 | Activity assays of HQD, components combination and baicalin in NCM460. **(A)** Phase contrast microscopy images of two migrating epithelial monolayers of NCM460. **(B)** NCM460 were incubated with vehicle, HQD, the combination and baicalin for 24 h, following cell scratch and 24 h stimulation of LPS. 24 h wound healing was determined as % of 0 h. **(C)** NCM460 were pretreated with vehicle, HQD, the combination and baicalin for 12 h, following 6 or 12 h stimulation of LPS, the accumulated TNF-α in the culture medium were measured using commercial ELISA kits. Results are expressed as mean ± SD of at least three independent experiments. ##$P < 0.01$ versus control group, *$P < 005$, **$P < 0.01$, ***$P < 0.001$ versus model group (One-way analysis of variance with Dunnett's *post hoc* test).

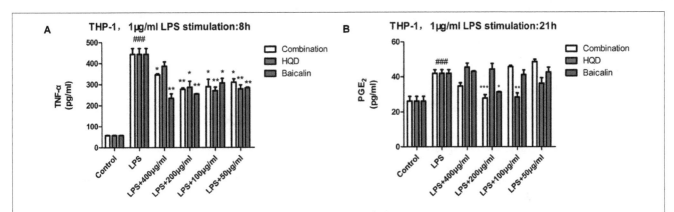

FIGURE 4 | Effects of HQD, components combination and baicalin on TNF-α and PGE$_2$ release in THP-1. **(A)** THP-1 was pretreated with vehicle, HQD, the combination and baicalin for 12 h, following 8 h stimulation of LPS. The accumulated TNF-α in the culture medium were measured using commercial ELISA kit. **(B)** THP-1 was incubated with vehicle, HQD, the combination and baicalin for 12 h, following 21 h stimulation of LPS. Supernatant of THP-1 cells was collected for PGE$_2$ production assay by commercial kit. Results are expressed as mean ± SD of at least three independent experiments. ###$P < 0.01$ versus control group, *$P < 0.05$, **$P < 0.01$, ***$P < 0.001$ versus model group (One-way analysis of variance with Dunnett's *post hoc* test).

Thus the concept of Q-marker was proposed recently to guide the TCM quality investigations. The Q-marker of TCM refers to a group of bioactive constituents that are closely associated with the therapeutic effects. The bottleneck in Q-marker-based quality standard investigation is how to screen out the chemical markers. Zhang et al. (2016a) tried to find the potential Q-markers of *Corydalis* Rhizoma based on biosynthesis, specificity, and pharmacodynamics experiments. Compounds that could be found in the brain tissues were regarded to exert antalgic effect. Non-targeted metabolomics and artificial nerve network were employed to explore the identity markers for five different parts of

P. ginseng (Qiu et al., 2016). But the bioactivity of these markers was not taken into account. A triarchic theory of "property-effect-component" and multidiscipline-based strategies are proposed to discover effect-associated markers. The key steps are to test the effect of the extract or single compounds on multiple models and to determine the pharmacokinetics parameters (Zhang et al., 2016b). It is obvious that the process is time-consuming due to the complex composition of herbs. Although, significant progress has been made for Q-marker discovery, there are some drawbacks in the current studies. There still needs to be a standardized and commonly accepted strategy to follow.

Therefore, in this paper we proposed a systems pharmacology-based Q-marker discovery strategy. This strategy, integrating target prediction databases of Chinese medicine and disease databases, facilitates our understanding of effective components and was successfully applied to the study of HQD. As a result, 9 compounds were filtered out as potential markers, which interacted with 10 diarrhea-related targets including PTGS2, NOS2, and TNF etc. Previous studies have revealed that PHY906, the modified formulation derived from HQD, performed its effect on the intestinal toxicity by inhibiting PTGS2, NOS2, and TNF (Lam et al., 2010). These results proved the feasibility of our strategy to some extent.

Another huge challenge in Q-marker investigation is how to validate whether the selected Q-marker could be responsible for the holistic efficacy of TCM. Thus we borrow the concept of bioactive equivalent combinatorial compounds. Standard references of the selected compounds were pooled together as components combination according to their corresponding concentration in HQD. Irinotecan caused NCM460 damage was chosen as a model to study the bioactive equivalence between components combination and HQD. At the first stage, we only use the cell survival rate as parameter. The result was disappointed and HQD showed no effect on cell survival rate (**Supplementary Figure S3**), which was incompatible with *in vivo* experiment (Wang X. et al., 2017). It was speculated that cell survival rate was not a sensitive parameter and a mechanism based experiment should be designed. According to the C-T network of HQD on the treatment of diarrhea, we found that wogonin, norwogonin, and oroxylin A could affect PTGS2 and NOS2 activity simultaneously, liquiritigenin, baicalin, baicalein, and scutellarein were also associated with PTGS2. Previous studies have revealed that paeoniflorin, baicalin, baicalein, and wogonin could decrease production of tumor necrosis factor-α (TNF-α) (Kwak et al., 2014; Zhai and Guo, 2016). LPS could stimulate intestinal damage and increase the expression of inflammatory factor at the same time (Chen et al., 2001; Huang et al., 2007) in spite of little influence on NCM460 cell survival rate (**Supplementary Figure S4**). Thus, LPS-stimulated NCM460 damage (Bhattacharyya et al., 2008) and LPS-stimulated THP-1-derived macrophage inflammation (Perezperez et al., 1995) were used as cell models to perform the bioactive equivalence assessment using cell mobility, TNF-α and PGE$_2$ release as sensitive parameters.

CONCLUSION

The discovery and validation of Q-marker still face enormous challenges despite the fact that the concept of Q-marker has been presented and great efforts have been made. In this study, a systems pharmacology based strategy was proposed to discover Q-markers of TCM. Compared with other approaches to establish Q-markers, systems pharmacology contributes to finding the effect-associated markers faster and takes full advantage of the existing data. Using this strategy, nine compounds in HQD were screened out to compose components combination. The components combination has been validated

to be almost bioactive equivalent to original decoction and could be deemed as the Q-markers of HQD. It is promising that systems pharmacology could be applied to Q-marker discovery to ensure efficacy and batch-to-batch consistency of TCM. The limitation of this study was that the contribution of each component has not been clarified, which emphasized the value of further research.

AUTHOR CONTRIBUTIONS

X-mD carried out most of the studies, performed the statistical analysis, and wrote the manuscript. D-nC performed the composition identification experiment of HQD. JW and WZ provided professional advice. Z-jZ and F-gX designed the study and revised the manuscript. All authors gave approval to the final version.

FUNDING

This work was supported by the NSFC (Nos. 81773861 and 81302733), Macao Science and Technology Development Fund (FDCT, No. 006/2015/A1), the Program for Jiangsu Province Innovative Research Team, the Program for New Century Excellent Talents in University (No. NCET-13-1036), a project funded by the Priority Academic Program Development of Jiangsu Higher Education Institutions (PAPD), and the Open Project Program of Guangxi Key Laboratory of Traditional Chinese Medicine Quality Standards.

ACKNOWLEDGMENTS

The authors are grateful to Suyun Yu and Xu Wang from Nanjing University of Traditional Chinese Medicine for technical assistance in cell culture and network pharmacology, respectively.

SUPPLEMENTARY MATERIAL

FIGURE S1 | Fingerprint chromatography of HQD.

FIGURE S2 | Quantitative determination results of potential Q-markers.

FIGURE S3 | Influence of CPT-11 and HQD on NCM460 cell survival rate.

FIGURE S4 | Influence of LPS and HQD on NCM460 cell survival rate.

TABLE S1 | Constituents of herbs in HQD.

TABLE S2 | All targets of constituents in HQD.

TABLE S3 | All 64 targets related to diarrhea.

TABLE S4 | Active constituents of herbs in HQD and their corresponding targets related to diarrhea.

TABLE S5 | The degree of compounds and targets.

TABLE S6 | The identified components of HQD in our lab.

REFERENCES

Bhattacharyya, S., Dudeja, P. K., and Tobacman, J. K. (2008). Lipopolysaccharide activates NF-κB by TLR4-Bcl10-dependent and independent pathways in colonic epithelial cells. *Am. J. Gastrointest. Liver Physiol.* 295, G784–G790. doi: 10.1152/ajpgi.90434.2008

Buranasukhon, W., Athikomkulchai, S., Tadtong, S., and Chittasupho, C. (2017). Wound healing activity of *Pluchea indica* leaf extract in oral mucosal cell line and oral spray formulation containing nanoparticles of the extract. *Pharm. Biol.* 55, 1767–1774. doi: 10.1080/13880209.2017.1326511

Chen, Y. C., Shen, S. C., Chen, L. G., Lee, T. J. F., and Yang, L. L. (2001). Wogonin, baicalin, and baicalein inhibition of inducible nitric oxide synthase and cyclooxygenase-2 gene expressions induced by nitric oxide synthase inhibitors and lipopolysaccharide. *Biochem. Pharmacol.* 61, 1417–1427. doi: 10.1016/s0006-2952(01)00594-9

Das, T., Safferling, K., Rausch, S., Grabe, N., Boehm, H., and Spatz, J. P. (2015). A molecular mechanotransduction pathway regulates collective migration of epithelial cells. *Nat. Cell Biol.* 17, 276–287. doi: 10.1038/ncb3115

Huang, G. C., Chow, J. M., Shen, S. C., Yang, L. Y., Lin, C. W., and Chen, Y. C. (2007). Wogonin but not Nor-wogonin inhibits lipopolysaccharide and lipoteichoic acid-induced iNOS gene expression and NO production in macrophages. *Int. Immunopharmacol.* 7, 1054–1063. doi: 10.1016/j.intimp.2007.04.001

Jiang, Y., David, B., Tu, P., and Barbin, Y. (2010). Recent analytical approaches in quality control of traditional Chinese medicines–a review. *Anal. Chim. Acta* 657, 9–18. doi: 10.1016/j.aca.2009.10.024

Kwak, S., Ku, S. K., Han, M. S., and Bae, J. S. (2014). Vascular barrier protective effects of baicalin, baicalein and wogonin *in vitro* and *in vivo*. *Toxicol. Appl. Pharmacol.* 281, 30–38. doi: 10.1016/j.taap.2014.09.003

Lam, W., Bussom, S., Guan, F., Jiang, Z., Zhang, W., Gullen, E. A., et al. (2010). The four-herb Chinese medicine PHY906 reduces chemotherapy-induced gastrointestinal toxicity. *Sci. Transl. Med.* 2:45ra59. doi: 10.1126/scitranslmed.3001270

Liu, C., Chen, S., Xiao, X., Zhang, T., Hou, W., and Liao, M. (2016). A new concept on quality marker of Chinese materia medica: quality control for Chinese medicinal products. *Chin. Tradit. Herb. Drugs* 47, 1443–1457. doi: 10.1016/j.apsb.2017.04.012

Long, F., Yang, H., Xu, Y., Hao, H., and Li, P. (2015). A strategy for the identification of combinatorial bioactive compounds contributing to the holistic effect of herbal medicines. *Sci. Rep.* 5:12361. doi: 10.1038/srep12361

Padilla, A., Keating, P., Hartmann, J., and Mari, F. (2017). Effects of α-conotoxin ImI on TNF-α, IL-8 and TGF-β expression by human macrophage-like cells derived from THP-1 pre-monocytic leukemic cells. *Sci. Rep.* 7:12742. doi: 10.1038/s41598-017-11586-2

Perezperez, G. I., Shepherd, V. L., Morrow, J. D., and Blaser, M. J. (1995). Activation of human THP-1 cells and rat bone marrow-derived macrophages by *Helicobacter pylori* lipopolysaccharide. *Infect. Immun.* 63, 1183–1187.

Qiu, S., Yang, W. Z., Yao, C. L., Qiu, Z. D., Shi, X. J., Zhang, J. X., et al. (2016). Nontargeted metabolomic analysis and "Commercial-homophyletic" comparison-induced biomarkers verification for the systematic chemical differentiation of five different parts of *Panax ginseng*. *J. Chromatogr. A* 1453, 78–87. doi: 10.1016/j.chroma.2016.05.051

Ru, J. L., Li, P., Wang, J. N., Zhou, W., Li, B. H., Huang, C., et al. (2014). TCMSP: a database of systems pharmacology for drug discovery from herbal medicines. *J. Cheminform.* 6:13. doi: 10.1186/1758-2946-6-13

Saif, M. W., Lansigan, F., Ruta, S., Lamb, L., Mezes, M., Elligers, K., et al. (2010). Phase I study of the botanical formulation PHY906 with capecitabine in advanced pancreatic and other gastrointestinal malignancies. *Phytomedicine* 17, 161–169. doi: 10.1016/j.phymed.2009.12.016

Shen, X., Zhao, Z., Luo, X., Wang, H., Hu, B., and Guo, Z. (2016). Systems pharmacology based study of the molecular mechanism of SiNiSan formula for

application in nervous and mental diseases. *Evid. Based Complement. Altern. Med.* 2016:9146378. doi: 10.1155/2016/9146378

Tilton, R., Paiva, A. A., Guan, J. Q., Marathe, R., Jiang, Z., van Eyndhoven, W., et al. (2010). A comprehensive platform for quality control of botanical drugs (PhytomicsQC): a case study of Huangqin Tang (HQT) and PHY906. *Chin. Med.* 5:30. doi: 10.1186/1749-8546-5-30

Wang, E., Bussom, S., Chen, J., Quinn, C., Bedognetti, D., Lam, W., et al. (2011). Interaction of a traditional Chinese Medicine (PHY906) and CPT-11 on the inflammatory process in the tumor microenvironment. *BMC Med. Genomics* 4:38. doi: 10.1186/1755-8794-4-38

Wang, F., Xiong, Z. Y., Li, P., Yang, H., Gao, W., and Li, H. J. (2017). From chemical consistency to effective consistency in precise quality discrimination of Sophora flower-bud and Sophora flower: discovering efficacy-associated markers by fingerprint-activity relationship modeling. *J. Pharm. Biomed. Anal.* 132, 7–16. doi: 10.1016/j.jpba.2016.09.042

Wang, X., Cui, D. N., Dai, X. M., Wang, J., Zhang, W., Zhang, Z. J., et al. (2017). HuangQin decoction attenuates CPT-11-Induced gastrointestinal toxicity by regulating bile acids metabolism homeostasis. *Front. Pharmacol.* 8:156. doi: 10.3389/fphar.2017.00156

Xiang, Z., Sun, H., Cai, X., Chen, D., and Zheng, X. (2015). The study on the material basis and the mechanism for anti-renal interstitial fibrosis efficacy of rhubarb through integration of metabonomics and network pharmacology. *Mol. Biosyst.* 11, 1067–1078. doi: 10.1039/c4mb00573b

Yang, H., Qin, C., Li, Y. H., Tao, L., Zhou, J., Yu, C. Y., et al. (2016). Therapeutic target database update 2016: enriched resource for bench to clinical drug target and targeted pathway information. *Nucleic Acids Res.* 44, D1069–D1074. doi: 10.1093/nar/gkv1230

Yang, W., Zhang, Y., Wu, W., Huang, L., Guo, D., and Liu, C. (2017). Approaches to establish Q-markers for the quality standards of traditional Chinese medicines. *Acta Pharm. Sin. B* 7, 439–446. doi: 10.1016/j.apsb.2017.04.012

Ye, M., Liu, S. H., Jiang, Z., Lee, Y., Tilto, R., and Cheng, Y. C. (2007). Liquid chromatography/mass spectrometry analysis of PHY906, a Chinese medicine formulation for cancer therapy. *Rapid Commun. Mass Spectrom.* 21, 3593–3607. doi: 10.1002/rcm.2832

Yu, G., Zhang, Y., Ren, W., Dong, L., Li, J., Geng, Y., et al. (2017). Network pharmacology-based identification of key pharmacological pathways of Yin-Huang-Qing-Fei capsule acting on chronic bronchitis. *Int. J. Chron. Obstruct. Pulmon. Dis.* 12, 85–94. doi: 10.2147/copd.s121079

Zhai, J. H., and Guo, Y. (2016). Paeoniflorin attenuates cardiac dysfunction in endotoxemic mice via the inhibition of nuclear factor-κB. *Biomed. Pharmacother.* 80, 200–206. doi: 10.1016/j.biopha.2016.03.032

Zhang, T. J., Xu, J., Han, Y. Q., Zhang, H. B., Gong, S. X., and Liu, C. X. (2016a). Quality markers research on Chinese materia medica: nuality evaluation and quality standards of *Corydalis Rhizoma*. *Chin. Tradit. Herb. Drugs* 47, 1458–1467.

Zhang, T. J., Xu, J., Shen, X. P., Han, Y. Q., Hu, J. F., Zhang, H. B., et al. (2016b). Relation of "property-response-component" and action mechanism of Yuanhu Zhitong Dropping Pills based on quality marker (Q-Marker). *Chin. Tradit. Herb. Drugs* 47, 2199–2211.

16

St. John's Wort (*Hypericum perforatum*) Products – How Variable is the Primary Material?

Francesca Scotti[1], Katja Löbel[1], Anthony Booker[1,2] and Michael Heinrich[1]*

[1] *Pharmacognosy and Phytotherapy Group, Pharmaceutical and Biological Chemistry, UCL School of Pharmacy, London, United Kingdom,* [2] *Division of Herbal and East Asian Medicine, Department of Life Sciences, University of Westminster, London, United Kingdom*

*Correspondence:
Michael Heinrich
m.heinrich@ucl.ac.uk

Background: Saint John's wort (*Hypericum perforatum* L., HP) is commonly registered in Europe under the THR scheme (Traditional Herbal Registration) or licensed as a medicine. Nonetheless unregulated medical products and food supplements are accessible through the internet which are often of poor quality. The species' natural distribution stretches through large regions of Europe to China and four subspecies have been distinguished. When compared to the European Pharmacopoeia reference, the presence of additional compounds was linked to so-called Chinese HP.

Aim: In order to obtain an integrated picture of the entire chemoprofile, the chemical composition of HP *materia prima* was studied using a combination of techniques well-established in the relevant industries. The impact of phytogeographic factors on the *materia prima* can shed light on whether the variability of the final products is strongly influenced by these factors of whether they relate to poor processing, adulteration, or other factors linked to the processing of the material.

Methods: Eighty-six *Hypericum* samples (77 *H. perforatum*) were collected from 14 countries. Most were authenticated and harvested in the wild; others came as roughly ground material from commercial cultivations, markets and pharmacies. The samples were analyzed using HPTLC and ^{1}H-NMR-based principal component analysis (PCA).

Results and Discussion: Limited chemical variability was found. Nonetheless, the typical fingerprint of Chinese HP was observed in each specimen from China. Additional compounds were also detected in some samples collected in Spain. Rutin is not necessarily present in the crude material. The variability previously found in the marketed products can be ascribed only partially to the geographical origin of harvested material, but mainly to the plant part harvested, closely related to harvesting techniques, processing and probably time of harvest.

Conclusion: HP can be sourced in a consistent composition (and thus quality) from different geographical sources. However, chemical variability needs to be accounted for when evaluating what is considered authentic good material. Therefore, the processing and good practice are all stages of primary importance, calling for a better (self-)regulation and quality assurance along the value chain of an herbal medical product or botanical.

Keywords: avicularin/guaiaverin, *Hypericum perforatum* (Saint John's wort, SJW), materia prima, natural variability, quality control, subspecies boundaries, value chains

INTRODUCTION

Saint John's wort (*Hypericum perforatum* L. – HP, Hypericaceae) has been used traditionally across Europe for centuries and in contemporary society it plays an important medical role. Its renown ability to treat wounds is being investigated (Oztürk et al., 2007; Süntar et al., 2010, 2011) but, most importantly, it is now widely used as a prescription or over the counter medicine to treat minor to moderate depression (licensed medicines) or 'low mood' (registered products). It was found that its activity is comparable to antidepressants when dealing with mild to moderate depression (Apaydin et al., 2016). In general, it is a licensed drug in many European countries and in the United Kingdom it is registered under the THR scheme. While considerable effort has gone into understanding the chemistry and pharmacology of commercially used materials, little attention has been paid to the biological and chemical complexity of the starting material and specifically to the diversity within the taxon *H. perforatum* (Dauncey et al., 2017). HP could be considered as an umbrella term for different *Hypericum* taxa united by the use as herbal medicines esp. in 'mood disorders.'

The species used medicinally in more recent Western medicine is *Hypericum perforatum*. HP is native to Eurasia, it is found in Europe (excluding the extreme north), the "Levant and western Saudi Arabia to NW India (Uttar Pradesh), Transcaucasia, Turkmenistan to Altai, Angara-Sayan and NW Mongolia; China (W. Xinjiang and from Gansu east to Hebei, south to Jiangxi and west to Yunnan)" (Robson, 2002). It is also found in NW Africa, including Canary Islands, Madeira and Azores. It has been introduced in the American continent, where it can be found from Canada to Argentina, in the Republic of Sudan (Jebel Marra), South Africa, Reunion, Australia, New Zealand, and Japan.

Robson (2002) proposed the distinction of four subspecies, based on minor morphological traits and with a well-defined geographical distribution of two of these subspecies, while the two Central/Western subspecies overlap through a large range of their territories (Dauncey et al., 2017).

Apomictic reproduction is known to give surge to a number of interfertile hybrids, morphologically different but within a continuum, therefore rendering taxonomic identification extremely difficult (Dickinson, 1998; Bicknell and Koltunow, 2004). This tendency, through time, has led to a considerable variability among the morphology of *H. perforatum* species. The state of current knowledge (Robson, 2002) is that these four subspecies possibly originated from a common ancestor (Western Siberia) which, interbred with other *Hypericum* species, gave birth to morphologically distinct, but recurring and geographically restricted, hybrids that are now being recognized as subspecies. According to Robson (2002), from the common ancestor first ssp. *songaricum* and ssp. *perforatum* evolved. Subsequently, ssp. *veronense* and ssp. *chinense*, respectively, evolved. According to Robson ssp. *songaricum* is the closest to the original ancestor. Ssp. *chinense* is seen as particularly distinct from its predecessor, and further away evolutionarily.

This situation raises two distinct but interrelated questions:

(1) What is the quality of the material currently available in different markets and how is this linked to the production of the *materia prima* and the subsequent value chains (Booker et al., 2018).

(2) How does the intrinsic variability of *H. perforatum* impact on the composition of the products available?

Previous investigations have revealed how the quality of food supplements (botanicals) is variable (Zheng and Navarro, 2015; Booker et al., 2016a,b; Barrella et al., 2017; Ruhsam and Hollingsworth, 2018), and studies conducted on the chemical quality of HP products showed problems specific to this species, (Frommenwiler et al., 2016; Booker et al., 2018), including strength and dosage inconsistencies and the presence of food dyes. A chemical pattern previously identified by Huck-Pezzei et al. (2013) and Frommenwiler et al. (2016) was initially labeled "Chinese HP" as it was almost only found in commercial products of Chinese origin. The Chinese material, and, therefore, the ssp. *chinense* has been thought to constitute a specific chemotype differing from the other subspecies. The previously found Chinese HP fingerprint (Frommenwiler et al., 2016; Booker et al., 2018) showcased three main features different from the EP and USP HPTLC standards and raw herbal material analyzed in those studies:

(1) Absence of yellow fluorescent zone at Rf = 0.18, under the blue zone of chlorogenic acid.

(2) Lower intensities of the bands found in the lower third of the chromatogram.

(3) Additional fluorescent band at Rf = 0.49.

As a consequence, it was thought expedient to analyze HP crude drug material collected across the world and evaluate the chemical profiles via nuclear magnetic resonance (NMR) spectroscopy and high performance thin layer chromatography (HPTLC) to verify whether this profile can only be found among Chinese specimens and whether other chemical variation exists in the naturally occurring crude drug material around the globe.

AIMS AND OBJECTIVES

(1) To systematically compare the variability of HP samples originating from diverse geographical locations covering both the main natural range of HP and some selected regions of agricultural production.

(2) To assess what constitutes a good *materia prima*, inclusive of the biodiversity and variability.

(3) To assess whether all accessible subspecies/geographical sources constitute good starting material and to guarantee a good final product.

(4) To find an appropriate method for the evaluation of the *materia prima*.

This has been achieved by analyzing samples from different countries across the world and comparing the data with those provided by the previous study conducted on the finished products available on the market (Booker et al., 2018).

MATERIALS AND METHODS

All solvents were purchased from Merck KGaA, Fisher Scientific Ltd. and VWR International LLC, except of deuterated methanol which was purchased from Cambridge Isotope Laboratories Inc.

Sample Collection

Eighty-six samples (for a detailed description see the **Supplementary Material**) were collected and dried at room temperature and voucher specimens for the unprocessed samples are deposited at UCL School of Pharmacy Herbarium.

Specimens were harvested in the wild or obtained from commercial cultivations, the flowering aerial parts were collected (unless differently stated in the **Supplementary Material**) and dried in the shade.

Commercial processed samples were purchased or donated in the form of roughly ground plant material.

Reference Standards

St. John's wort dry extract (European Pharmacopoeia, EP, Reference Standard 01131, code: Y0001050, batch: 2.0), avicularin and guaiaverin were obtained from Sigma-Aldrich Inc. while rutin (L10815B002) from Adooq Bioscience. Hypericin primary reference standard (batch HWI 01814-1) was purchased from HWI ANALITIK GmbH.

^{1}H-NMR Spectroscopy

Nuclear Magnetic Resonance analysis was carried out using a Bruker Avance Spectrometer featuring a QNP multi-nuclear probe head with z-gradient/5 mm cryoprobe head operating at 500.13 MHz. Spectra were acquired at 298 K, using 64k data points, line broadening factor = 0.16 Hz, pulse width = 30°, relaxation delay d1 = 1 s. Each run was subjected to 256 scans. The acquired data was processed using TopSpin 3.2 software. Chemical shifts were calibrated to the tetramethylsilane (TMS) signal.

Sample Preparation for NMR

The dried material was ground finely using a blender. The solvent choice and the analytical methods followed the outline of the previous study on HP marketed products (Booker et al., 2018) for the purpose of comparability.

Fifty milligrams of powder was extracted in 1 mL deuterated methanol, vortexed for 20 s, sonicated for 5 min at room temperature and finally centrifuged for 5 min at 13,000 rpm. 0.6 mL of supernatant was sent for analysis.

Reference standard pure compounds were simply dissolved in methanol, at the concentration of 1 mg/mL and 0.6 mL was analyzed.

Principal Component Analysis of Data

^{1}H-NMR signals were calibrated to the TMS peak. The spectra acquired were converted to ASCII file using AMIX 3.9.14. Using only positive intensities and no scaling, buckets of 0.04 ppm were created using the multivariate analysis software. Via the use of Excel, the NMR elaborated data was introduced onto SIMCA 14.0, the software utilized for the principal component analysis

(PCA). Sample 22 was analyzed twice and, after different trials, it was established that no scaling in SIMCA gave a statistical model that was to be considered more reliable based on the proximity of the sample 22 repeats in the plot.

HPTLC

HPTLC was performed using a CAMAG setup consisting of a Linomat 5 semi-automated sampler, automatic developing chamber 2 (ADC2), TLC plate heater III and TLC visualizer coupled to visionCATS 2.1 software. The HPTLC plates Silica gel 60 F_{254} used for stationary phase were purchased from Merck KGaA (Darmstadt, Germany).

Sample Preparation for HPTLC Analysis

Five hundred milligrams of powdered material was extracted with 5 mL of methanol, shaken on a rotary mixer for 20 s, sonicated 10 min in at 60°C and filtered using Millex® Syringe filter unit 0.45 µm.

The references hypericin and quercetin were dissolved in methanol, while rutin in acetone, with a concentration of 1 mg/mL then sonicated for 10 min at 60°C. Rutin had to be filtered through a Millex® syringe filter unit 0.45 µm, to remove any residual suspended particle prior to use. The EP standard was prepared in methanol at a concentration of 100 mg/mL.

HPTLC Analysis

The method used reflects the one published by the HPTLC association for the extraction and analysis of HP powdered drug (HPTLC, 2016). Each plate was visualized under white light and UV 254 nm, prior to sample application in order to later correct for the background. 2 µL of sample and standards, were spotted on the plates in bands of 8 mm. The plate was developed in the automatic developing chamber at 33% humidity, with 20 min saturation time, 10 min activation time and 5 min pre-drying. The mobile phase consisted of a freshly prepared mixture of ethyl acetate, dichloromethane, HPLC-grade water, formic acid, glacial acetic acid in the proportion 100:25:11:10:10 (*v/v/v/v/v*). After development, the plate was visualized under white light, UV 254 and 366 nm. Prior to derivatization the plate was heated at 100°C for 3 min and subsequently dipped, while still hot, in NP reagent first (1 g 2-aminoethyl diphenylborinate in 200 mL ethyl acetate) and then PEG reagent (10 g polyethylene glycol 400 in 200 mL dichloromethane), for the detection of flavonoids. The plate was then visualized under white light and UV 366 nm.

RESULTS AND DISCUSSION

With the intention to define the chemical profile of HP, the project embarked on the analysis of samples trying to identify the common as well as the variable chemical components of HPs from different geographical regions. Therefore, our collection of 77 HP samples from 14 different countries covered native Europe extensively (South England, Portugal, Spain, Germany, Switzerland, Italy, Bulgaria, Greece), Lebanon, Tajikistan, China and areas of introduction such as South America (Chile, Argentina) and Australia (**Figure 1**).

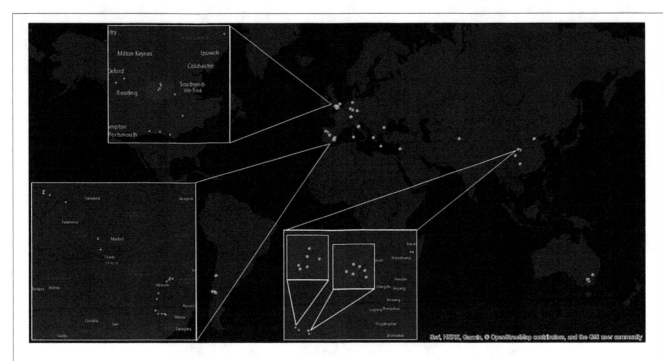

FIGURE 1 | The *H. perforatum* samples used in this project have been collected in 14 countries.

As a first step, the chemical composition of different sections of the aerial parts, the traditionally recommended drug, were analyzed. One single HP specimen from Southern England (nr 53) was cut in 4 parts (sample 53#1 0–18 cm, lower; 53#2 18–37, cm lower intermediate; 53#3 37–54 cm, upper intermediate; 53#4 54–65 cm, flowering tops); in addition, samples containing only leaves (sample 53#5) and only flowers (sample 53#6) were taken from the same specimen.

HPTLC analysis showed, as expected, a variation in the chemical content between parts (**Figure 2**). Material derived to the lower section of the aerial parts was constituted only of woody stems and the methanolic solution obtained was light yellow. The chromatographic fingerprint showed very low levels of detectable components. Samples 53#2 and #3 both contained leaves and slimmer woody stems, the methanolic solution obtained was dark brown in color and the HPTLC fingerprint seemed perfectly acceptable for an HP product.

Sample #4 represented the flowering tops, the part to harvest based on the pharmacopeial requirements ("Whole or fragmented, dried flowering tops of *Hypericum perforatum* L., harvested during flowering time" BP 2018, Ph. Eur. 9.3 Update). In this case the methanolic solution is dark red and the fingerprint is similar to the previous two samples with the addition of a green band at Rf = 0.77 and slightly more concentrated bands of hypericin derivatives (red bands between Rf = 0.54 and Rf = 0.63). As expected, the sample exclusively made of leaves (53 #5) has exactly the same fingerprint of #2 and #3 but the methanolic solution is green in color. Finally, the flower sample, 53 #6, shows a fingerprint with a level of hypericins comparable to #4, the green band at Rf = 0.77, a faint yellow band right above said green band and a much fainter top elution band.

"Chinese HP" with its specific fingerprint characteristics could be adulterated with other species. Therefore, nine samples of other *Hypericum* species growing in China were collected and analyzed by HPTLC including *H. ascyron* (F6), *H. acmosepalum* (F7, 9), *H. uralum* (F8), *H. densiflorum* (F10), *H. beanii* (F11), *H. patulum* (F12), *H. japonicum* (F14), *H. elodeoides* (F15).

The HPTLC (**Figure 3**) and NMR (**Figure 11**) results clearly show that none of the fingerprints features the yellow band at Rf = 0.49 (present in the Chinese *H. perforatum*, **Figure 3**, track 2). The other *Hypericum* species' fingerprints (**Figure 3**, tracks 3–10) are very distinct from *H. perforatum*'s. Except for *H. elodeoides* (**Figure 3**, track 10), they do not contain hypericins and it is unlikely that they could have been added, accidentally or on purpose to boost the products' specifications.

Principal component analysis of NMR data relative to the HP crude drug samples altogether shows a fairly homogeneous spread, without any starkly prominent difference (**Figure 4**). Nonetheless the samples from China and those from the Mediterranean area form separate clusters. Western/Central European samples from Germany and England overlap over both clusters. Analysis of the flavonoid specific area 6–9 ppm failed to show any further difference (see **Supplementary Material**), instead showing an even more homogeneous distribution, with less similarities but without any type of clustering and a broader distribution.

HPTLC analysis of the samples highlighted a few main differences across the collection, namely the presence of the "Chinese HP" fingerprint, the separate presence of the extra yellow band (Rf = 0.49) in other samples, the presence/absence

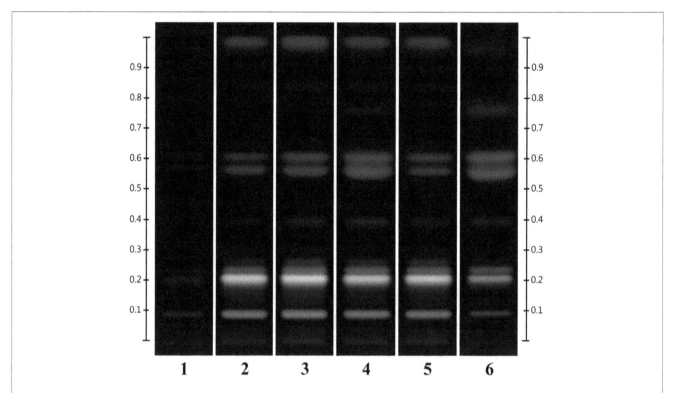

FIGURE 2 | Different parts of *Hyperici herba* (from sample 53) analyzed by HPTLC. Tracks: (1) lower part (0–18 cm); (2) lower intermediate part (18–37 cm); (3) upper intermediate part (37–54 cm); (4) flowering tops (54–65 cm); (5) leaves only; (6) flowers only.

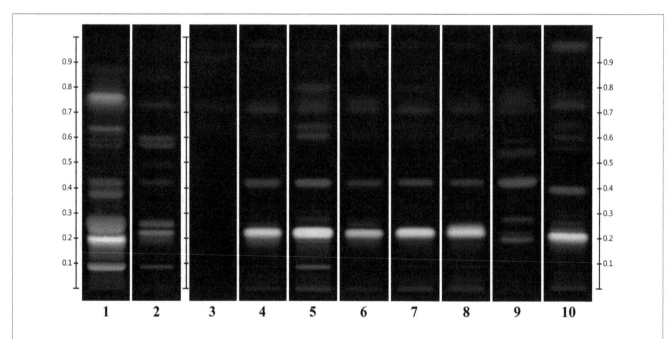

FIGURE 3 | Similarities and differences between EP standard for HP (track 1), Chinese HP (track 2) and other species of *Hypericum*: *H. ascyron* (track 3), *H. acmosepalum* (track 4), *H. uralum* (track 5), *H. densiflorum* (track 6), *H. beanii* (track 7), *H. patulum* (track 8), *H. japonicum* (track 9), *and H. elodeoides* (track 10).

of rutin, low flavonoid concentrations and differences in the hypericins content.

Each of the samples acquired from China showed the "Chinese HP" fingerprint, with, most notably, an extra compound, represented by the yellow band with Rf = 0.49 and the missing yellow band at Rf = 0.18 (**Figure 5**). This seems to define a specific chemotype for specimens belonging to the postulated ssp. *chinense* (also described as geographically restricted to China).

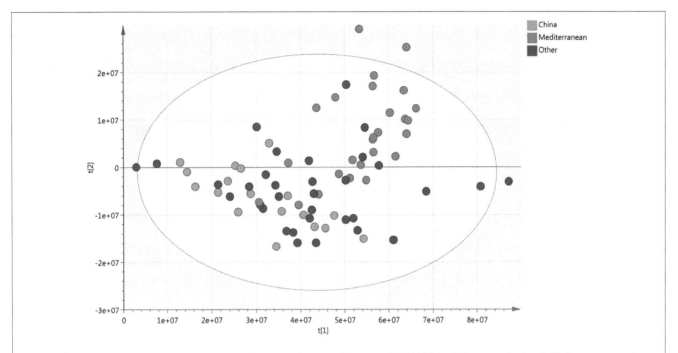

FIGURE 4 | PCA score plot of 77 samples of crude drug of HP coming from 14 different countries, highlighting Chinese samples (green), Mediterranean samples (blue), and all others (red).

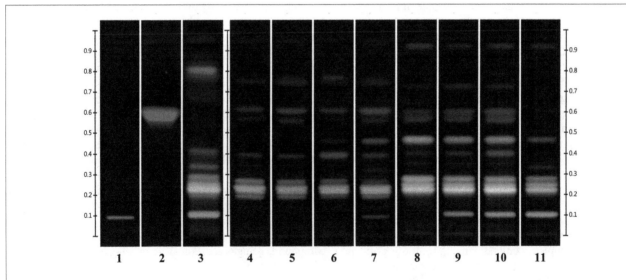

FIGURE 5 | Comparison between Chinese and Spanish samples fingerprints; Tracks: (1) rutin standard; (2) hypericin standard; (3) EP reference standard for HP; (4–7) some samples from Spain (original sample nr 42–45); (8–11) some samples collected in China (original sample nr 59–61 and 64).

Interestingly, a yellow band with Rf = 0.49 was also detected in 50% of the samples collected in Spain (8 out of 16, from two separate regions). In the latter cases though, the persistence of the yellow band with Rf = 0.18 indicates a fingerprint distinct from the Chinese one (**Figure 5**). The compound at Rf = 0.49 was otherwise not detected in any other sample of our collection.

Additionally, rutin is not necessarily found in the crude drug material as 38% (27 out of 71 samples with sufficient flavonoid concentration to be able to read rutin band) of the samples did not show the corresponding band; Chinese samples were always

found to contain rutin, in different concentrations, while the majority (81%) of Spanish material does not contain it. On the other hand, all the marketed products analyzed by Booker et al. (2018) contain rutin.

HPTLC analysis highlighted the presence of lower concentrations of compounds in samples consisting of processed material (purchased or donated in the form of roughly chopped material). Samples 1–5, 22, 23, 24, 65, 66 and 86 were obtained from commercial sources (producers, pharmacies, markets), allegedly being simply roughly processed *materia prima*. Visual inspection revealed roughly chopped herbal material, making it difficult, if not impossible to determine the identity of the plant with the naked eye; in addition, most of them included a high amount of woody material (stems). In the HPTLC analysis samples 1–5 (purchased at herbal markets, in three different regions of China: Yunnan, Hebei, Shanxi) showed an extremely low content of the typical HP compounds at the concentration examined. Samples 22–24 (respectively, purchased as loose material in a pharmacy in Crete, Greece; in a pharmacy in Chile, and acquired through a manufacturer in Chile) and 65–66 (both samples acquired from a manufacturer's cultivation in Bulgaria) show better concentration but still among the lowest across the whole selection. This could be due to the apparent higher amount of woody material present in the mixtures.

This observation could be linked to the results obtained from the HPTLC analysis of the different sections of the aerial parts. The fainter fingerprint of the processed material could be due to the harvesting practice cutting further down the stem and this including a higher percentage of the woody material. Given that the wood itself does contain extremely low quantities of flavonoid compounds, this constitutes a natural bulking agent from the same plant. Whether this was done intentionally or due to a lack of knowledge cannot be ascertained in this study. Of note, for products regulated as botanicals/food supplements, this would not constitute an adulteration, but for herbal medicines it would, if the regulation follows, for example, the European Pharmacopoeia.

Alternatively, the fainter fingerprint could be ascribed to purchasing material from middlemen, implying that little information is available to the processors as to when the material was harvested and handled. Time and conditions of storage can lead to the degradation and oxidation of components, and therefore a lowering of their concentrations.

Based on our analysis, NMR-based PCA is unable to pick up on the composition differences detected via HPTLC. Moreover, the contribution of a single compound on the overall NMR spectra is minimal, especially when considering complex spectra such as those obtained from total plant extracts.

Hypericins, namely hypericin and pseudohypericin, are easily spotted in HPTLC plates treated with NP/PEG as two close red bands at Rf = 0.55–0.60. Their concentration varies across the collection of samples examined, ranging from thick brilliant to faint dark bands. However, no systematic correlations with

regions of origin could be demonstrated. These differences can sometimes be associated with overall low flavonoid content (as in the case of commercial samples), but at times they do not directly correlate. As previously explained their lower content can be due to a lower proportion of flowers and leaves in the samples, the age of the material (often unknown in the case of commercial samples) but can as well be explained by time of the day/season when the material was collected. The failure to find a distinguishable marker peak for hypericin in the NMR spectra reinforces the idea that the NMR-PCA plot would not have taken into consideration the hypericin content differences.

Avicularin Versus Guaiaverin

As previously mentioned, samples of Chinese origin analyzed were found to have a peculiar fingerprint, characterized mainly by the presence of an extra compound at Rf = 0.49. It was initially identified, based on mass spectrometry, as avicularin, or quercetin-3-O-α-arabinofuranose, which had previously been isolated in HP (Wei et al., 2009). Another quercetin-glycoside, guaiaverin (quercetin-3-O-α-L-arabinopyranoside) though, with the same molecular weight and the same fragmentation pattern as avicularin was previously isolated from H. maculatum (Zheleva-Dimitrova et al., 2012), raising doubts relative to the identity of the yellow band at Rf = 0.49 (Booker et al., 2018).

Their molecular structures are similar (**Figure 6**) but their NMR spectra differs and distinct signals can be identified (**Figure 7**). Pure compounds were compared to identify the samples' NMR fingerprints. Peaks at δ (500 MHz, CD$_3$OD) 5.47 (s) and 5.18 (d) ppm, found, respectively, in avicularin and guaiaverin, in an area of low signal crowding, provide a means for distinguishing between the two compounds and were chosen as marker signals. The singlet at 5.47 ppm is found in a representative sample of both Chinese and Spanish samples (No. 59 and 41, respectively), but is missing in another Spanish sample (**Figure 8**, sample 40, yellow) that did not show the extra band at Rf = 0.49. Therefore, the samples with the band at Rf = 0.49 are likely contain avicularin. The doublet at 5.18 ppm seems to be present in all samples' spectra, but as it appears in an area of high signal crowding it did not seem appropriate to derive a clear conclusion solely based on NMR. Next, the possibility of both compounds being present (guaiaverin being present in a very low concentration) was investigated using HPTLC.

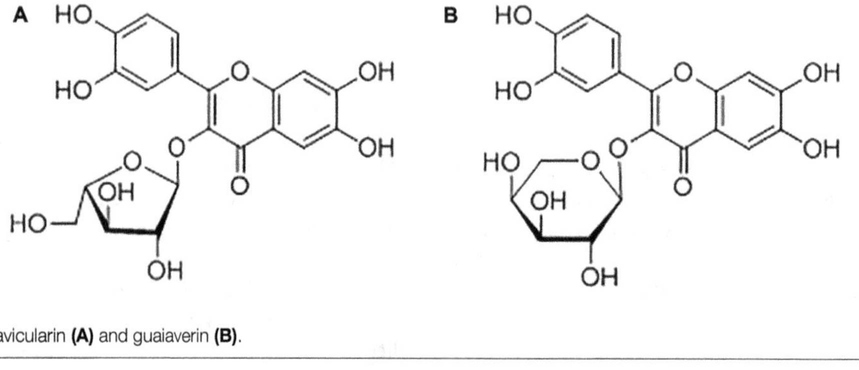

FIGURE 6 | Structures of avicularin **(A)** and guaiaverin **(B)**.

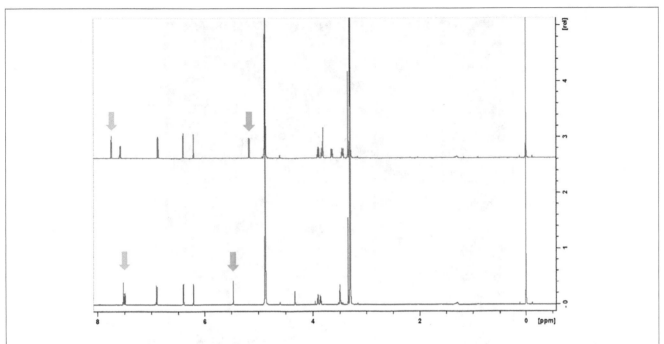

FIGURE 7 | NMR spectra (500 MHz) of avicularin (blue) and guaiaverin (red) in CD$_3$OD, highlighting particularly useful diagnostic features at 7.52 ppm/5.46 ppm (avicularin) and 7.74 ppm/5.16 ppm (guaiaverin).

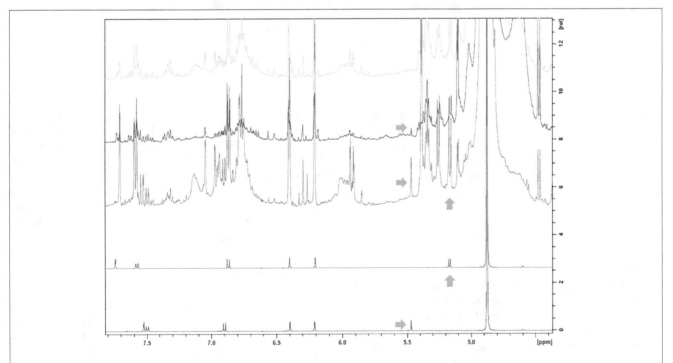

FIGURE 8 | Spectra of avicularin (blue) and guaiaverin (red) compared to sample 59 (from China, green), 41 (from Spain, with extra band, purple) and 40 (from Spain, no extra band, yellow).

HPTLC analysis following the HP protocol showed a significant separation between avicularin and guaiaverin and based on this result the band at Rf = 0.49 represents avicularin (**Figure 9**) but not guaiaverin. Additionally, the band corresponding to guaiaverin (Rf = 0.30) was detected in both Chinese and Spanish samples, indicating the presence of a mixture of the two, with guaiaverin being present in a much lower concentration (**Figure 9**). Guaiaverin was detected also in other HP samples investigated (represented by German sample 51, in **Figure 9**).

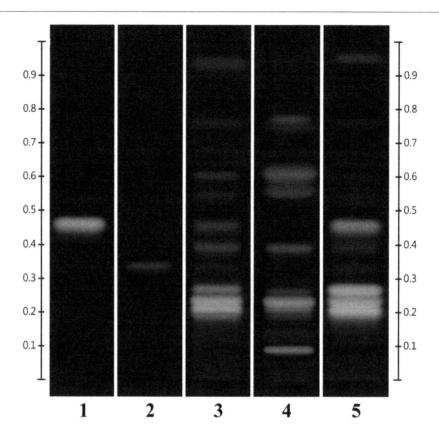

FIGURE 9 | HPTLC detection (366 nm) of avicularin (track 1) and guaiaverin (track 2) in the crude drug material; tracks: (3) sample 41 from Spain; (4) sample 51 from Germany (lacking the extra component at Rf = 0.49); (5) sample 59 from China.

Materia Prima Versus Finished Products

The NMR data obtained from all the 86 samples was plotted against the data collected by Booker et al. (2018) on marketed HP products, excluding products consisting of extracts and/or combination with other plants. The PCA score plot shows that a few marketed products fall far away from the central cluster (**Figure 10**). Due to higher variability found among marketed products, the differences between the crude drug samples disappear. The different chemical fingerprints found in the *materia prima* represent the natural chemovariability, (especially the presence of avicularin) which, however, is minimal compared to the differences found in the finished products. The natural variability cannot explain the marketed products variability. Therefore, the reasons behind it need to be found elsewhere. This demonstrates that unregulated products' significant variation in composition is very heavily influenced by the various processing techniques of the *materia prima*, i.e., the differences in the value chains of these products. This highlights the importance and necessity for a carefully managed and well controlled value chain from the primary material to the finished products.

Comparison of NMR-PCA and HPTLC

Overall, NMR-PCA was able to detect major differences between samples, but has not been useful to discern the much more limited differences between the samples of the *materia prima*.

Of course, it is more affected by total composition than a single compound's variations. It is a useful method for identification of trends and differences between different species, as exemplified in **Figure 11**, and makes evaluation of the results obtained from large pools of samples easier as it provides a general overview.

HPTLC unveils specific chemical differences. The combination of these two methods has helped an all-round evaluation of the chemical profile and differences existing among the HP available in nature.

CONCLUSION

This study demonstrates that the view of 'Chinese HP' containing some unique marker substances cannot be substantiated. The HPTLC profiles have highlighted how the Chinese samples and some of the Spanish samples both contain avicularin. At the same time the Chinese samples carry some extra differences that distinguish them from the Spanish avicularin-containing ones. According to the *Hypericum* monographs (Robson, 2002), the distribution of subspecies *perforatum* and *veronense* overlaps in Mediterranean Europe, with minor morphological differences serving as diagnostic markers. On the other hand subspecies *chinense* is quite isolated geographically. As a consequence, it is possible that these detected anomalies, when compared to the EP standard, represent chemotypes

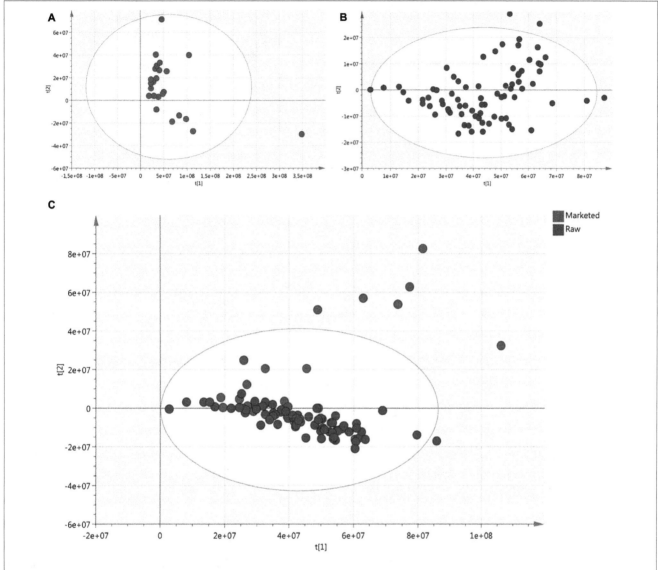

FIGURE 10 | PCA score plots: **(A)** marketed products (no extracts) from data collected in a previous study (Booker et al., 2018); **(B)** crude drug of HP; **(C)** plot comparing crude drug material samples and marketed products.

characteristic for specific geographical regions. Our samples could not be clearly assigned to these subspecies Moreover, this study demonstrates that rutin, though present in the EP standard and found in all the marketed products analyzed previously (Booker et al., 2018), is not necessarily found in the *materia prima*. The hypericins content was not always directly correlated to the overall flavonoid concentration. It was found to be low in commercial material, either due to higher content of woody material, or unknown age of the sample.

It is vital that there is a standard reference representative of good quality crude drug material taking into consideration the natural chemical variability. Pharmacopeial monographs should include a description of such variable characteristics. In the case of HP, this could either result in accepting *H. perforatum* ssp. *chinense* as a source of drug material if it complies with the other

requirements or a new definition of what material is acceptable from a pharmacopeial perspective.

This study for the first time compares a large collection of crude material as a group and also with marketed products, establishing that in the case of HP the naturally occurring chemical differences are not responsible for the poor quality found in the finished commercial products. There is no way of establishing which chemotype has been traditionally used and substantiating that one chemotype is more appropriate than the others. Therefore, these natural differences should not be of major concern. However, in this study all samples were processed using a standard procedure, which is clearly not the case within industry, resulting in inevitable quality variations.

The results regarding the processed material, on the other hand, have highlighted how acquiring material that has been sourced along poorly managed value chains constitutes a concern

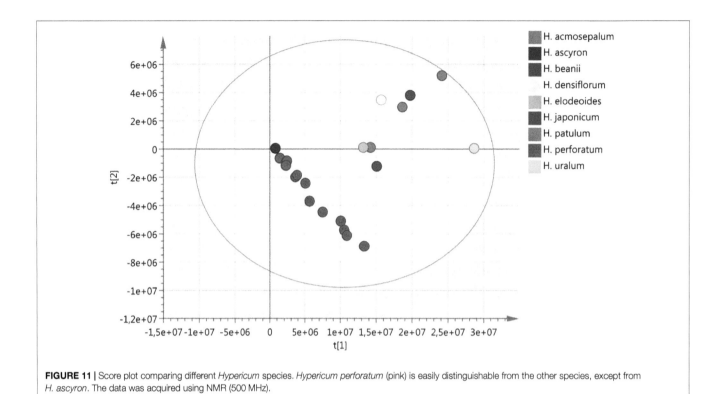

FIGURE 11 | Score plot comparing different *Hypericum* species. *Hypericum perforatum* (pink) is easily distinguishable from the other species, except from *H. ascyron*. The data was acquired using NMR (500 MHz).

that needs to be considered and resolved. In such cases the identity, provenance, collection practices, storage conditions and length of storage are unknown and could lead to poor quality material. This strengthens the importance of minimizing the role of middlemen, who lack the knowledge of how to ascertain good quality, operating between growers/collectors and manufacturers.

This study's findings show the importance of comprehensive investigation and knowledge about crude materials as the foundations for the delivery of quality herbal products on the market. Outreach activities need to target collectors, growers and producers to guarantee that the fundamental steps of cultivating, collecting or acquiring good/acceptable quality material is carried out correctly. If the crude material's natural variation is known the final product's quality will be better defined and more predictable.

AUTHOR CONTRIBUTIONS

FS, AB, and MH contributed to the conception and design of the study. FS gathered the samples and prepared voucher specimens. FS and KL analyzed the samples. FS analyzed the data and drafted the manuscript. All authors contributed to manuscript revision, read and approved the submitted version.

FUNDING

FS's postdoctoral position was funded through a charitable donation by Dr. Willmar Schwabe GmbH and Co. KG, Karlsruhe, Germany, who has had no input into the experimental design and the interpretation of the data.

ACKNOWLEDGMENTS

We would like to thank the Natural History Museum, London, in particular Dr. Norman Robson, for his insight and expertise and Mr. Jacek Wajer for his help and support. The collection of samples would have not been possible without the valuable collaboration of: Dan Zhao (School of Pharmacy, Guiyang University of Chinese Medicine, China), Ziwan Ning (School of Chinese Medicine, Hong Kong Baptist University, Hong Kong), Diego Rivera (Spain), Concepcion Obon De Castro (Spain), Alonso Verde (Spain), Jose Fajardo (Spain), Lixiang Zhai (Hong Kong), Carlos Echiburu Chau (Chile), Roberto Saavedra (Chile), Ivo Pischel (Germany), Sarah Edwards (England), Stephanie Miles (England), Hans Wohlmuth (Australia), Michael Keusgen (Germany), Fabrizio Zara (Italy), Silvia Soldatou (Greece), Zachary Bellman (England), Matthew Traver (England), Nicola Bell (England), Peter Field (England), Marco Leonti (Italy), Ana Maria Carvalho (Portugal), Debora Frommenwiler (Switzerland), and Xiaofei Zhang (China).

REFERENCES

Apaydin, E. A., Maher, A. R., Shanman, R., Booth, M. S., Miles, J. N. V., Sorbero, M. E., et al. (2016). A systematic review of St. John's wort for major depressive disorder. *Syst. Rev.* 5:148. doi: 10.1186/s13643-016-0325-2

Barrella, M. V., Heringer, O. A., Cardoso, P. M. M., Pimentel, E. F., Scherer, R., Lenz, D., et al. (2017). Metals content in herbal supplements. *Biol. Trace Elem. Res.* 175, 488–494. doi: 10.1007/s12011-016-0776-2

Bicknell, R. A., and Koltunow, A. M. (2004). Understanding apomixis: recent advances and remaining conundrums. *Plant Cell* 16(Suppl. 1), S228–S245. doi: 10.1105/tpc.017921

Booker, A., Agapouda, A., Frommenwiler, D., Scotti, F., Reich, E., and Heinrich, M. (2018). St John's wort (*Hypericum perforatum*) products – an assessment of their authenticity and quality. *Phytomedicine* 40, 158–164. doi: 10.1016/j.phymed. 2017.12.012

Booker, A., Frommenwiler, D., Reich, E., Horsfield, S., and Heinrich, M. (2016a). Adulteration and poor quality of *Ginkgo biloba* supplements. *J. Herbal Med.* 6, 79–87. doi: 10.1016/j.chroma.2009.01.013

Booker, A., Jalil, B., Frommenwiler, D., Reich, E., Zhai, L., Kulic, Z., et al. (2016b). The authenticity and quality of *Rhodiola rosea* products. *Phytomedicine* 23, 754–762. doi: 10.1016/j.phymed.2015.10.006

Dauncey, E. A., Irving, J. T. W., and Allkin, R. (2017). A review of issues of nomenclature and taxonomy of *Hypericum perforatum* L. and Kew's Medicinal Plant Names Services. *J. Pharm. Pharmacol.* doi: 10.1111/jphp. 12831

Dickinson, T. A. (1998). Taxonomy of agamic complexes in plants: a role for metapopulation thinking. *Folia Geobot.* 33, 327–332. doi: 10.1007/BF0321 6208

Frommenwiler, D. A., Sudberg, S., Sharaf, M. H., Bzhelyansky, A., Lucas, B., and Reich, E. (2016). St. John's Wort versus Counterfeit St. John's Wort: an HPTLC study. *J. AOAC Int.* 99, 1204–1212. doi: 10.5740/jaoacint. 16-0170

HPTLC (2016). *Identification Method For St John's Wort Herb (SJW), HPTLC Association.* Available at: http://www.HPTLC-association.org [accessed June 20, 2016].

Huck-Pezzei, V. A., Bittner, L. K., Pallua, J. D., Sonderegger, H., Abel, G., Popp, M., et al. (2013). A chromatographic and spectroscopic analytical platform for the characterization of St John's wort extract adulterations. *Anal. Methods* 5, 616–628. doi: 10.1039/C2AY26030A

Oztürk, N., Korkmaz, S., and Oztürk, Y. (2007). Wound-healing activity of St. John's Wort (*Hypericum perforatum* L.) on chicken embryonic fibroblasts. *J. Ethnopharmacol.* 111, 33–39. doi: 10.1016/j.jep.2006.10.029

Robson, N. K. B. (2002). Studies in the genus *Hypericum* L. *(Guttiferae).* 4(2). Section 9. *Hypericum* sensu lato (part 2): subsection 1. *Hypericum* series 1. *Hypericum. Bull. Br. Museum Nat. History* 32, 61–123. doi: 10.1017/ S096804460200004X

Ruhsam, M., and Hollingsworth, P. M. (2018). Authentication of *Eleutherococcus* and *Rhodiola* herbal supplement products in the United Kingdom. *J Pharm Biomed Anal.* 149, 403–409. doi: 10.1016/j.jpba.2017.11.025

Süntar, I. P., Akkol, E. K., Keleş, H., Oktem, A., Başer, K. H., and Yeşilada, E. (2011). A novel wound healing ointment: a formulation of *Hypericum perforatum* oil and sage and oregano essential oils based on traditional Turkish knowledge. *J. Ethnopharmacol.* 134, 89–96. doi: 10.1016/j.jep.2010.11.061

Süntar, I. P., Akkol, E. K., Yilmazer, D., Baykal, T., Kirmizibekmez, H., Alper, M., et al. (2010). Investigations on the *in vivo* wound healing potential of *Hypericum perforatum* L. *J. Ethnopharmacol.* 127, 468–477. doi: 10.1016/j.jep.2009.10.011

Wei, Y., Xie, Q., Dong, W., and Ito, Y. (2009). Separation of epigallocatechin and flavonoids from *Hypericum perforatum* L. by high-speed counter-current chromatography and preparative high-performance liquid chromatography. *J. Chromatogr. A* 1216, 4313–4318. doi: 10.1016/j.chroma.2008.12.056

Zheleva-Dimitrova, D., Nedialkov, P., and Girreser, U. (2012). Benzophenones and flavonoids from *Hypericum maculatum* and their antioxidant activities. *Nat. Prod. Res.* 26, 1576–1583. doi: 10.1080/14786419.2011.582468

Zheng, E. X., and Navarro, V. J. (2015). Liver injury from herbal, dietary, and weight loss supplements: a review. *J. Clin. Transl. Hepatol.* 3, 93–98. doi: 10.14218/JCTH.2015.00006

17

Sequence-Specific Detection of *Aristolochia* DNA – A Simple Test for Contamination of Herbal Products

Tiziana Sgamma[1]*, Eva Masiero[1], Purvi Mali[1], Maslinda Mahat[1,2] and Adrian Slater[1]

[1] Faculty of Health & Life Sciences, Biomolecular Technology Group, De Montfort University, Leicester, United Kingdom,
[2] Natural Product Testing Section, Toxic Compound Detection Unit, National Pharmaceutical Control Bureau, Jalan University, Selangor, Malaysia

Correspondence:
Tiziana Sgamma
tiziana.sgamma@dmu.ac.uk

Herbal medicines are used globally for their health benefits as an alternative therapy method to modern medicines. The market for herbal products has increased rapidly over the last few decades, but this has in turn increased the opportunities for malpractices such as contamination or substitution of products with alternative plant species. In the 1990s, a series of severe renal disease cases were reported in Belgium associated with weight loss treatment, in which the active species *Stephania tetrandra* was found to be substituted with *Aristolochia fangchi*. *A. fangchi* contains toxic aristolochic acids, which have been linked to kidney failure, as well as cancers of the urinary tract. Because of these known toxicities, herbal medicines containing these compounds, or potentially contaminated by these plants, have been restricted or banned in some countries, but they are still available via the internet and in alternate formulations. In this study, a DNA based method based on quantitative real-time PCR (qPCR) was tested to detect and distinguish *Aristolochia* subg. *Siphisia* (Duch.) O.C.Schmidt species from a range of medicinal plants that could potentially be contaminated with *Aristolochia* material. Specific primers were designed to confirm that *Aristolochia* subg. *Siphisia* can be detected, even in small amounts, if it is present in the products, fulfilling the aim of offering a simple, cheaper and faster solution than the chemical methods. A synthetic gBlock template containing the primer sequences was used as a reference standard to calibrate the qPCR assay and to estimate the copy number of a target gene per sample. Generic primers covering the conserved 5.8S rRNA coding region were used as internal control to verify DNA quality and also as a reference gene for relative quantitation. To cope with potentially degraded DNA, all qPCR primer sets were designed to generate PCR products of under 100 bp allowing detection and quantification of *A. fangchi* gBlock even when mixed with *S. tetrandra* gBlock in different ratios. All proportions of *Aristolochia*, from 100 to 2%, were detected. Using standards, associating the copy number to each start quantity, the detection limit was calculated and set to about 50 copies.

Keywords: *Aristolochia*, *Stephania tetrandra*, DNA barcoding, herbal medicines, contamination, gBlock, quantitative real-time PCR

INTRODUCTION

Herbal medicines are often perceived as "good" and "safe" because they are "natural," in contrast to "chemical" drugs. People tend to be more relaxed in using them and ask less questions of producers or practitioners. Unfortunately, it is a well-known fact that many plants are in fact toxic and dangerous (Efferth and Kaina, 2011). In some cases botanical misidentification of plants, deliberately or accidentally, can also play a role in herbal drugs toxic reactions.

In the early '90s, Han Fang Ji (*Stephania tetrandra*) was incorrectly substituted with Guang Fang Ji (*Aristolochia fangchi*) in diet pills probably because of their similar Chinese Pin Yin names (Vanherweghem et al., 1993; Nortier et al., 2000). *Aristolochia manshuriensis* (Guan Mu Tong) has also been reported to have been substituted for other Mu Tong herbal drugs which should have had contained *Akebia* and *Clematis* (Zhu, 2002; Yang et al., 2007). More recently, the substitution of *Solanum lyratum* by *Aristolochia mollissima* in Baiying preparations has been detected by DNA barcoding (Li et al., 2012).

Although *Aristolochia* species are used in Traditional Chinese Medicine (TCM) they are also known for containing nephrotoxic and carcinogenic aristolochic acids (AA) (Nortier et al., 2000; International Agency for Research on Cancer [IARC], 2002). AA have been classified as human carcinogenic class I by the World Health Organization International Agency for Research on Cancer in 2002 (International Agency for Research on Cancer [IARC], 2002). Because of this, herbal mixtures containing *Aristolochia* or plants that could be substituted with it because of similarities in their common names (i.e., *Stephania, Akebia, Asarum, Cocculus,* and *Sinomenium*), have been banned from the market (International Agency for Research on Cancer [IARC], 2002; Medsafe, 2003; Martena et al., 2007; Debelle et al., 2008; Abdullah et al., 2017). In spite of this, some of these species are still available in markets and via the internet and the risk of being contaminated with *Aristolochia* plants is still high (Schaneberg and Khan, 2004; Abdullah et al., 2017). In support of this are the hundreds of cases of renal failure linked to potential contamination by *Aristolochia* species that have been reported over the past two decades (Nortier et al., 2000; Debelle et al., 2008; Michl et al., 2013; Jadot et al., 2017).

There is still a tangible need for development of detection methods to avoid exposure to AA. A reasonable way to decrease this risk should be the systematic quality control of herbal preparations by using reproducible and accurate analytical methods. In the case of *Stephania* pills, herbal drugs are consumed in the form of ground roots. Although there are morphological differences between the roots of the genera described as Fang Ji, they also present many similarities which present the opportunity for mis-identification and substitution especially in powdered and macerated samples (Tankeu et al., 2016). For powdered samples, HPLC methods are used as they are considered to be more reliable (Joshi et al., 2008). Hyperspectral imaging studies that combine both chemical and physical properties have also been conducted in Fang Ji herbal medicines but the accuracy has a 10% limit in terms of prediction

of adulteration (Tankeu et al., 2016). These methods all have limitations such as extensive sample preparation and being correlated to physiological influence, intraspecific differences and storage conditions. Quality control techniques that provide a rapid, inexpensive and accurate discrimination between the Fang Ji herbal medicines are still needed.

The practicality of using DNA barcoding in industrial quality assurance procedures has been recently discussed (Sgamma et al., 2017; Raclariu et al., 2018). Despite controversy around using DNA barcoding for herbal products authentication, DNA-based methods such as quantitative real-time PCR (qPCR), are a valuable addition to the toolkit of industrial quality assurance overcoming many of the limitations of standard DNA barcoding (Yang et al., 2018).

Different DNA-based methods for plants species identification and discrimination have attracted increased interest in recent year in many fields such as commercially processed food ingredients, spices, honey and herbal medicines. Species-specific qPCR assay has been proved to discriminate *Rhodiola rosea* from non-rosea Rhodiola species (Sgamma et al., 2017). Species-specific qPCR assays with Taq Man probes have been successfully used to discriminate several plants species in Corsican honey, while DNA metabarcoding and High Resolution melting analysis have been used to characterize the floral composition of honey in order to investigate honey bee foraging (Laube et al., 2010; Hawkins et al., 2015; Soares et al., 2018). High resolution melting (HRM) has been successfully used to differentiate seven selected *Zingiberaceae* plants (Osathanunkul et al., 2017). Duan et al. (2018) used barcoding coupled with HRM (Bar-HRM) to test the authenticity of *Rhizoma* species used in TCM as compared to their adulterants.

Focusing on the detection of *Aristolochia* species, a number of DNA-based methods, mostly targeting the *matK* and ITS2 regions, have been proved be promising in aiding in species-discrimination. Traditional DNA barcoding, targeting the chloroplast DNA loci *matK*, *rbcL* and *trnH-psbA* showed a different level of polymorphism between the loci with *matK* containing the most variation being able to discriminate genuine herbal medicines from their *Aristolochia* adulterants (Li et al., 2014). Yang et al. (2014) validated the ITS2 region as another DNA barcode region to discriminate *Aristolochia mollissima* from other plants used as herbal medicine including *Menispermi dauricum, Sophora tonkinensis, Stephania tetrandra,* and *Cocculus orbiculatus*. qPCR using TaqMan probes targeting the ITS2 region was also used to authenticate plant species from the Aristolochiaceae family and those from non-Aristolochiaceous substitutes and divide them in groups, but without quantifying the contamination (Wu et al., 2015). Loop-mediated isothermal amplification (LAMP) targeting the ITS2 region has also been proved to be effective in discriminating between Mu-tong, *Akebia caulis*, and its adulterant Guan-mu-tong, *Aristolochia manshuriensis* within 60 min in pure and mixed samples (Wu et al., 2016). More recently, Dechbumroong et al. (2018) developed a low cost and fast species-specific multiplex PCR assay to differentiate three *Aristolochia* species belonging to the subgenus *Aristolochia* (*Aristolochia pierrei, Aristolochia tagala,* and *Aristolochia pothieri*) present in Thailand known as "Krai-Krue."

Here, DNA-based technology is proposed as a complementary approach to identify and quantify adulterant *Aristolochia* subg. *Siphisia* material in herbal formulations providing a reliable quality control for contamination of the plant material.

MATERIALS AND METHODS

Plant Material and Total DNA Extraction

Fresh leaves or dry wood were provided by Dr Ben Gronier (De Montfort University, United Kingdom) and Prof Michael Heinrich (University College London, United Kingdom), respectively (**Table 1**). DNA was extracted from 100 mg of frozen material, previously ground to a fine powder in liquid nitrogen with mortar and pestle, using DNeasy Plant Mini Kit (Qiagen Inc., Germantown, MD, United States) following the manufacturers' guidelines.

DNA Samples

All genomic DNA (gDNA) samples were supplied pre-extracted from the Royal Botanic Gardens, Kew DNA Bank[1] (**Table 1**).

gBlock Fragments

Four double-stranded, sequence-verified gene fragments, or gBlocks (**Table 1**), were ordered from Integrated DNA

---

[1]https://dnabank.science.kew.org/homepage.html

TABLE 1 | Genetic material.

Species	Source	Kew DNA Bank ID	GenBank no. reference sequences
Aristolochia kaempferi	Dry wood- UCL		
Aristolochia californica	gDNA (Kew DNA Bank)	19176	
Aristolochia baetica	gDNA (Kew DNA Bank)	10534.1	
Aristolochia clematitis	gDNA (Kew DNA Bank)	13680	
Stephania tetrandra	gDNA (Kew DNA Bank)	25116	
Stephania glandulifera	Fresh leaves – DMU		
Stephania rotunda	Fresh leaves – DMU		
Cocculus trilobus	gDNA (Kew DNA Bank)	25115	
Cocculus laurifolius	gDNA (Kew DNA Bank)	39431	
Sinomenium acutum	gDNA (Kew DNA Bank)	25382	
Asarum europaeum	gDNA (Kew DNA Bank)	19154	
Asarum arifolium	gDNA (Kew DNA Bank)	198	
Asarum fudsinoi	gDNA (Kew DNA Bank)	21431	
Saussurea alpine	gDNA (Kew DNA Bank)	11885	
Saussurea quercifolia	gDNA (Kew DNA Bank)	44968	
Diploclisia glaucescens	gDNA (Kew DNA Bank)	1318	
Menispermum dahuricum	gDNA (Kew DNA Bank)	24519	
Aristolochia fangchi	gBlocks (IDT)		KP093067.1
Stephania tetrandra	gBlocks (IDT)		FJ609735.1
Cocculus orbiculatus	gBlocks (IDT)		AY864900.1
Sinomenium acutum	gBlocks (IDT)		AB571154.1

Technologies, BVBA (Leuven, Belgium). The gBlocks were designed to cover the 5.8S-ITS2 region within the nuclear ribosomal Internal Transcribed Spacer (nrITS) of the respective species (**Figure 1**). The GenBank accession numbers of the reference sequences are listed in **Table 1**. The gBlocks were resuspended in water at 10 ng/µl concentration. The copy number/µl in each gBlock was calculated converting the concentration from ng/µl to copy number/µl by using the formula provided by IDT guidelines[2] (**Table 2**). After optimisations, the S^{-5} dilution was used as working material.

Phylogenetic Analyses

Phylogenetic analyses were conducted using the MEGA6.06 software package. The evolutionary history was inferred with the Maximum Likelihood method based on the Tamura 3-parameter model (Tamura, 1992).

Primer Design

The NCBI database[3] was accessed to obtain the nrITS sequences of *Aristolochia*, *Stephania*, *Cocculus*, and *Sinomenium*.

Based on all the nrITS sequences obtained, generic and *Aristolochia*-specific primers were designed (**Table 3**). The generic primers were designed to target the 5.8S conserved region while the specific primers were designed to the ITS2 region of selected problematic *Aristolochia* species (**Figure 1**). Primer specificity was determined using Basic Local Alignment Search Tool (BLAST) software[4] and NCBI database (**Supplementary Data Sheet S1**).

Standard PCR and Sequencing (nrITS)

PCR was performed using 1 × MyTaq Red Mix (Bioline), 0.2 µM of each forward (ITS1 TCCGTAGGTGAACCTGCGG) and reverse (ITS4 TCCTCCGCTTATTGATATGC) primers, and 1 µL of gDNA as template. Thermocycling conditions were optimized at 94°C for 2 min, followed by 40 cycles of 94°C for 15 s, 60°C for 30 s and 72°C for 30 s, with a final extension step of 72°C for 2 min. PCR products were run on 2% (w/v) agarose, 1 × TBE gels with 1 µL SYBR® Safe DNA Gel Stain (Invitrogen, Paisley, United Kingdom) at 100 V for 30 min and analyzed in a Gel Doc™ EZ Gel Documentation System (Bio-Rad, Oxford, United Kingdom). Products were submitted for sequence analysis to Macrogen[5] to verify the authenticity of the starting material.

Quantitative Real-Time PCR (qPCR)

Each qPCR reaction contained 1 × Sensifast SYBR green Hi-Rox mix (Bioline), 0.5 µl of gDNA or gBlock, 0.1 µM of each forward and reverse primer (**Table 3**), in a total volume of 10 µl made up with sterilized distilled water (SDW). qPCR was performed using three biological replicates with three technical replicates for each sample. After PCR amplification, all products were sequenced to confirm their identity. *Aristolochia* gBlock serial dilutions

---

[2]https://eu.idtdna.com/pages/education/decoded/article/tips-for-working-with-gblocks-gene-fragments

[3]http://www.ncbi.nlm.nih.gov

[4]http://blast.ncbi.nlm.nih.gov/Blast.cgi

[5]http://www.macrogen.com

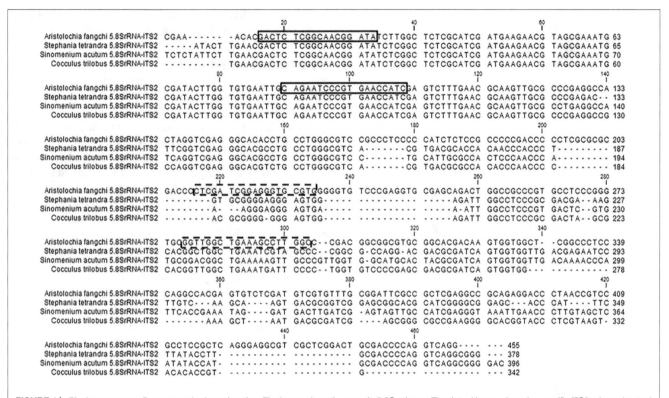

FIGURE 1 | gBlock sequences alignment and primers location. The boxes show the generic 5.8S primers. The dotted boxes show the specific ITS2 primers located on the *Aristolochia fangchi* ITS gBlock sequence.

TABLE 2 | Quantification gBlock Fragments and DNA copy number.

gBlock	fmoles/ng	Calculated copy number/μl in Stock S	Calculated copy number/ μl in working dilution S^{-5}
Aristolochia fangchi	3.56	2.14E + 10	2.14E + 05
Stephania tetrandra	4.28	2.58E + 10	2.58E + 05
Cocculus orbiculatus	4.73	2.85E + 10	2.85E + 05
Sinomenium acutum	4.09	2.46E + 10	2.46E + 05

TABLE 3 | *Aristolochia*-specific and generic primers and annealing temperature (Ta) used in quantitative real-time PCR.

Primer name	Sequence	Ta	Expected size (bp)
Aristolochia-ITS2 F	5'- CTCGATCGGAGGGTGCGTG -3'	62°C	88
Aristolochia-ITS2 R	5'- GCCAAGGCTTTCAGCCAACC-3'		
Generic 5.8 F	5'- GACTCTCGGCAACGGATA-3'	60°C	93
Generic 5.8 R	5'- GATGGTTCACGGGATTCTG-3'		

(from S^{-3} to S^{-7}) were run to generate the standard curve (**Supplementary Data Sheet S2**). Working dilution gBlocks S^{-5}, gDNAs and mixes of *Aristolochia* and *Stephania* gBlocks S^{-5} at different percentages and concentrations (**Table 4**) were used as templates. Water was run as a negative control for each test. A StepOnePlus™ Real-Time PCR thermocycler machine (Applied Biosystem) was used. Thermocycling conditions were

optimized at 95°C for 2 min, followed by 40 cycles of 95°C for 5 s and 30 s at the primer specific Ta (**Table 3**). The melting curve was obtained by melting the amplified template from 65 to 95°C increasing the temperature by 0.5°C per cycle. Analyses were conducted according to MIQE guidelines (Bustin et al., 2009). DNA levels were expressed as a relative proportion of the total DNA by using the generic primers as the "reference gene," and compared to the control sample (*Aristolochia* working dilution gBlocks S^{-5}) using the comparative ($2^{-\Delta\Delta Ct}$) method (Livak and Schmittgen, 2001).

Contamination Testing Using qPCR

A contamination test was performed where the *Aristolochia* gBlock S^{-5} working sample was mixed with the *Stephania* gBlock S^{-5} working sample at different proportions (**Table 4**). Each mix was also diluted 1:10, 1:100, and 1:1000. DNA copy numbers were also calculated (**Table 4**).

RESULTS

Amplification of the gDNA Templates With ITS Generic Primers

To test the quality of the gDNA samples, a standard PCR using ITS1 and ITS4 primers was performed. The expected ITS fragment was detected in most of the samples (**Figure 2**). A very faint band was detected in *Aristolochia californica* (**Figure 2**, lane 4) and no bands were detected in *Aristolochia clematitis*

TABLE 4 | Proportion of *Aristolochia* S^{-5} gBlock mixed with *Stephania* S^{-5} gBlock for contaminations tests and copy number in each dilution.

Aristolochia S^{-5} gBlock %	Stephania S^{-5} gBlock %	Copy number in neat (S^{-5}) mixture		Copy number in 1:10 dilution		Copy number in 1:100 dilution		Copy number in 1:1000 dilution	
		Aristolochia	*Stephania*	*Aristolochia*	*Stephania*	*Aristolochia*	*Stephania*	*Aristolochia*	*Stephania*
100	0	2.14E+05	0	2.14E+04	0	2.14E+03	0	2.14E+02	0
90	10	1.97E+05	2.19E+04	1.97E+04	2.19E+03	1.97E+03	2.19E+02	1.97E+02	2.19E+01
50	50	1.18E+05	1.18E+05	1.18E+04	1.18E+04	1.18E+03	1.18E+03	1.18E+02	1.18E+02
10	90	2.53E+04	2.28E+05	2.53E+03	2.28E+04	2.53E+02	2.28E+03	2.53E+01	2.28E+02
2	98	5.14E+03	2.52E+05	5.14E+02	2.52E+04	5.14E+01	2.52E+03	5.14 E + 00	2.52E+02

sample (**Figure 2**, lane 7) (**Figure 2**). Identification of samples was confirmed by sequencing of the full ITS fragment.

Phylogenetic Analysis

Before designing *Aristolochia* primers the ITS2 regions of *Aristolochia* sequences present on NCBI GenBank database were aligned using the Clustal W MegAlign package of DNAStar (DNAStar Inc.). Evolutionary relationships of the genus members were inferred with the Maximum Likelihood method based on the Tamura 3-parameter model using the MEGA6.06 software package (**Figure 3**). The phylogenetic analysis showed two main clades. Species which have proved particularly problematic with regard to substitution and contamination, including *Aristolochia fangchi, A. manshuriensis* and *A. mollissima* were found to belong to Clade B. These two clades align with the two main *Aristolochia* subgenera (*Aristolochia* and *Siphisia*) supported by morphological and molecular studies (Ohi-Toma et al., 2006; Do et al., 2015; Wu et al., 2015), with the subgenus corresponding to Clade B correctly named as *Aristolochia* subg. *Siphisia* (Duch.) O.C.Schmidt (Ohi-Toma and Murata, 2016).

The clear separation between the two subgenera was apparent from examination of the multiple alignment of *Aristolochia* ITS2 sequences. The divergence between the sequences of the two subgenera was such that it proved difficult to design genus specific-primers that would amplify all members of the genus. This investigation therefore focused on the design of primers to detect the ITS2 sequences of some of the most problematic species, which belong to the subgenus *Siphisia*. These primers were designed to target regions in the ITS2 sequence that are very similar between all members of this subgenus, but differ from members of the subgenus *Aristolochia*. They can therefore be described as "*Aristolochia* subgenus *Siphisia*-specific" primers.

Primers Specificity Testing Using Quantitative Real-Time PCR (qPCR)

Generic and *Aristolochia* subgenus *Siphisia*-specific qPCR primers were designed on the 5.8S and ITS2 region, respectively, within the nrITS sequence (**Figure 1**). Specificity of the developed qPCR reactions was evaluated in triplicate for each sample, including gDNA from various *Aristolochia* species and non-Aristolochiaceous genera including *Stephania, Cocculus, Sinomenium, Asarum, Saussurea, Diploclisia,* and *Menispermum.* Synthetic gBlocks designed to match *Aristolochia fangchi, Stephania tetrandra, Cocculus orbiculatus,* and *Sinomenium acutum* 5.8S and ITS2 regions were used as reference standards (**Figure 1**). The sensitivity of the triplex assay was determined using a serial dilution of *Aristolochia* gBlock DNA fragments representing the synthetic versions of the target genes at concentrations ranging from 0.1 to 1.00E-06 ng/µl per reaction. Linear regressions showed linear relationships (r^2 = 0.999 for all runs) between the quantities of gBlock templates and the cycle threshold (Ct) values across the tested concentration range. The real-time PCR efficiency was 90.1 and 91.8, % for the generic internal control 5.8S and *Aristolochia* subgenus *Siphisia*-specific primers, respectively.

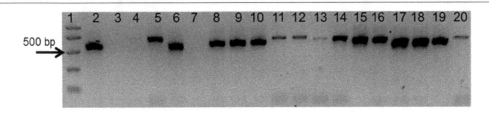

FIGURE 2 | Agarose gel electrophoresis of PCRs using ITS1 and ITS4 generic primers. Gel lanes: (1) Easy Ladder I (Bioline); (2) Positive control; (3) Negative (no template) control; (4) *A. californica*; (5) *A. kaempferi*; (6) *A. baetica*; (7) *A. clematitis*; (8) *S. tetrandra*; (9) *S. glandulifera*; (10) *S. rotunda*; (11) *C. trilobus*; (12) *C. laurifolius*; (13) *S. acutum*; (14) *A. europaeum*; (15) *A. arifolium*; (16) *A. fudsinoi*; (17) *S. alpine*; (18) *D. glaucescens*; (19) *M. dahuricum*; (20) *S. quercifolia*.

As shown in **Figure 4A**, significant amplification signal was obtained in all samples when the generic primers were used. The Ct values in all gBlocks S^{-5} samples and the neat mixtures (*Aristolochia* plus *Stephania*) was between 17.2 and 18.4; the Ct value of the mixture dilutions was on average 20.8, 24.2, and 27.5 for the 1:10, 1:100, and 1:1000 dilutions showing an equivalent pattern when comparing DNA copy numbers. The Ct values of the genomic DNA samples were between 10.8 and 15.8. Primer specificity was assessed by melt curve analysis, with the results showing that just one peak was generated for all samples (**Figure 4B**). The size and uniformity of the product was confirmed visually by running the samples on agarose gel electrophoresis (**Figure 4C**). Interestingly, a product was visible in both *Aristolochia californica* and *Aristolochia clematitis* samples with a Ct value of 14.7 and 14.2, respectively. These two samples showed either a very faint or no band, respectively, when PCR was performed to amplify the full length nrITS fragment (**Figure 2**).

DNA copy numbers and Ct values obtained from qPCR using *Aristolochia* subgenus *Siphisia*-specific primers were used to compare specificity between target and non-target samples. The amplification plots for the *Siphisia*-specific primers showed a clear difference in Ct value (around 15 cycles) between the *Aristolochia* S^{-5} gBlock dilution and the S^{-5} dilution of non-target gBlocks (**Figure 5A**). The melting curve showed the presence of primer dimers and non-specific products with Ct values around and greater than 30 in gDNA non-target samples (**Figure 5B**). The presence of non-specific products in gDNA non-target samples was also confirmed visually running the samples on agarose gel electrophoresis (**Figure 5C**). The expected size product (88 bp) was visible in *Aristolochia* samples belonging to the subgenus *Siphisia* (*Aristolochia californica* and *Aristolochia kaempferi)* while the expected product was not visible in *Aristolochia* samples belonging to the subgenus *Aristolochia* (*Aristolochia baetica* and *Aristolochia clematitis*) or in the non-Aristolochaceous samples.

Relative Quantitative Analysis of *Aristolochia* in Mixed Samples

To verify the feasibility of our method in the detection and quantitation of possible *Aristolochia* contamination in mixed samples, a series of gBlock admixtures containing different amounts of *Stephania tetrandra* (10, 50, 90, and 98% respectively) and model adulterant *Aristolochia fangchi* DNA were prepared

(**Table 4**) starting from the gBlocks S^{-5} dilution. Each of these mixtures was then diluted 1:10, 1:100, and 1:1000 to check detection limits (**Table 4**).

When comparing the relative proportions of *Aristolochia* DNA between the *Aristolochia* gBlock, the other species gBlocks and the mixtures representing the different contamination rates, consistent results were observed for all samples (**Figure 6**). The *Aristolochia* subgenus *Siphisia*-specific primers were able to detect *Aristolochia* DNA down to a 2% contamination level, while no amplification was detected in non-target gBlock samples. DNA copy numbers from the "100% contamination" sample (*Aristolochia* gBlock S^{-5}) were used as the reference for relative DNA copy number calculation. **Figure 7** shows that the serial dilutions showed the same pattern. Putting together this data and the samples melting curve results (**Figure 5B**) it is possible to set a safe detection limit of 2% for the 1:100 dilution which corresponds to a copy number of about 50 copies of *Aristolochia fangchi* nrITS DNA. In contrast, the 2% mixture in the 1:1000 dilution set gave a melting curve profile that indicated possible primer dimer formation. The detection limit is further supported by the detection of the correct amplicon in the 10% contamination mixture of the 1:1000 dilution set which would correspond to about 25 copies of *Aristolochia* nrITS DNA. Although the lowest dilution set of 1:1000 is at the limits of quantitative detection, it is still a useful qualitative indicator of the presence of *Aristolochia* at the lowest % mixtures, but not accurate enough to reliably quantify the amount of contamination.

Testing gDNA

To prove that the detection and quantification test is valid with gDNA, a set of Aristolochiaceous and non-Aristolochiaceous genomic DNA samples were tested. All samples were amplified by the generic primers (**Figure 4**) indicating the absence of plant secondary product PCR inhibitors in the samples. Most of the samples also showed the presence of the full-length nrITS fragment (**Figure 2**), which was then sequenced to confirm the species. Although *Aristolochia californica* and *Aristolochia clematitis* did not show a clear band for the full-length nrITS fragment (**Figure 2**), they both acted as templates for the generic primers (**Figure 4**). None of the non-target species gDNA appeared to be amplified by the *Aristolochia Siphisia*-specific fragment (**Figure 5**), while the expected product was amplified in a range of target species in the *Aristolochia* subgenus *Siphisia* (**Figure 5**). The results were analyzed using the relative

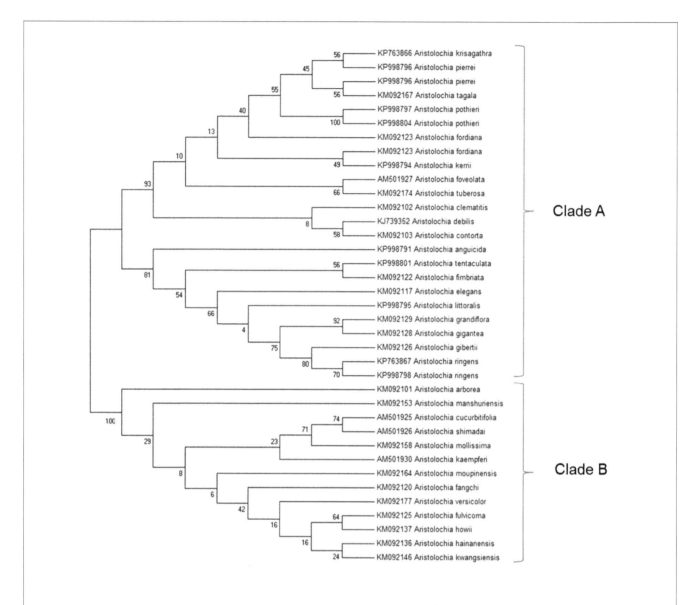

FIGURE 3 | Molecular Phylogenetic analysis by Maximum Likelihood method. The evolutionary history was inferred by using the Maximum Likelihood method based on the Tamura 3-parameter model (Tamura, 1992). The bootstrap consensus tree inferred from 1000 replicates is taken to represent the evolutionary history of the taxa analyzed (Felsenstein, 1985). Branches corresponding to partitions reproduced in less than 50% bootstrap replicates are collapsed. The percentage of replicate trees in which the associated taxa clustered together in the bootstrap test (1000 replicates) are shown next to the branches (Felsenstein, 1985). Initial tree(s) for the heuristic search were obtained by applying the Neighbor-Joining method and BioNJ algorithms to a matrix of pairwise distances estimated using the Maximum Composite Likelihood (MCL) approach, and then selecting the topology with superior log likelihood value. The analysis involved 37 nucleotide sequences. All positions containing gaps and missing data were eliminated. There were a total of 127 positions in the final dataset. Evolutionary analyses were conducted in MEGA6 (Tamura et al., 2013). Accession numbers are given next to the species name.

amplification method to determine the relative quantities of target species DNA compared to the amount of templates for the generic primers (**Figure 8**).

DISCUSSION

Aristolochic acid I and Aristolochic acid II have been identified as potent carcinogens and renal toxins (Arlt et al., 2002). All herbal formulations that contain any *Aristolochia* species have been classified as a Group 1 carcinogen by the International Agency for Research on Cancer (IARC) (International Agency for Research on Cancer [IARC], 2002; Grollman et al., 2007). Despite this classification it has been reported that products containing AA or suspected to contain AA are still in use and available on web sites (Gold and Slone, 2003; Nortier and Vanherweghem, 2007).

A reasonable way to detect the presence of *Aristolochia* contamination and decrease the risk associated with it, would be the systematic quality control of herbal preparations by

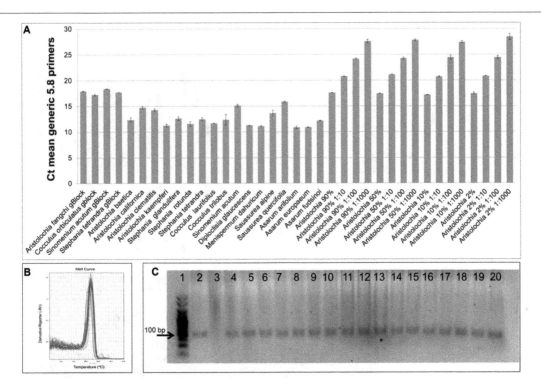

FIGURE 4 | Generic internal control 5.8S quantitative real-time PCR. **(A)** Ct values. qPCR was performed using three biological replicates with three technical replicates for each sample. Error bars represent Standard deviation. **(B)** melting curve for all samples run with the generic 5.8S primers. **(C)** Agarose gel electrophoresis of PCRs using generic internal control 5.8S primers. Expected product size 93 bp. Gel lanes: (1) HyperLadder™ 25 bp (Bioline); (2) Positive control; (3) Negative (no template) control; (4) *A. californica*; (5) *A. kaempferi*; (6) *A. baetica*; (7) *A. clematitis*; (8) *S. tetrandra*; (9) *S. glandulifera*; (10) *S. rotunda*; (11) *C. trilobus*; (12) *C. laurifolius*; (13) *S. acutum*; (14) *A. europaeum*; (15) *A. arifolium*; (16) *A. fudsinoi*; (17) *S. alpine*; (18) *D. glaucescens*; (19) *M. dahuricum*; (20) *S. quercifolia*.

using reproducible and accurate analytical methods. Currently, for industrial quality control, chemical and macro-morphology based analysis are conducted to identify the presence of *Aristolochia* species in herbal medicines (Kite et al., 2002; Lee et al., 2003; Sorenson and Sullivan, 2007; Joshi et al., 2008). These methods have limitations as they may be affected by many factors including growth conditions, environmental factors and post harvesting procedures (Zhang et al., 2012). DNA-based tests have emerged as a powerful, rapid, reliable, robust, and affordable identification system for authentication of medical plants and commercial herbal products that could be incorporated into industrial quality control processes (Sgamma et al., 2017).

Previous work has identified ITS2 as a suitable target to discriminate *Aristolochia* species and used 11 primer/probe combinations in TaqMan qPCR assay to identify herbal material from the Aristolochiaceae family and divide them in groups, but without quantifying the contaminant (Wu et al., 2015). Each combination of primers and probes detected different groups which contained some species from the Aristolochiceae family; for instance group A identified a large number of *Aristolochia* species but also many *Asarum* because they shared sequence similarity (Wu et al., 2015).

In this study, a simpler method was developed for the identification and quantification of the *Aristolochia* subgenus *Siphisia* in pure or mixed samples using DNA-based techniques designed to overcome the limitations of other identification

methods. This was achieved by designing a reliable qPCR test to detect and quantify the presence of very small amounts of *Aristolochia* DNA using an internal control and an *Aristolochia* subgenus *Siphisia*-specific set of primers. qPCR is a simple, fast and sensitive test that could be suited to industrial quality control testing (Sgamma et al., 2017).

One of the limitations of working with banned herbal products is sourcing the samples and this study is not an exception. *Aristolochia fangchi* plant material or gDNA was unavailable. Therefore to overcome this issue, synthetic DNA, a gBlock, was designed based on the reference barcoding regions available in GenBank. The quality and quantity of many samples sourced through DNA banks is similarly a limitation. The amount of gDNA sample provided is usually in the order of few µls. The DNA concentration is also never very high, possibly due to the poor quality of the original plant material. Therefore, having enough material for optimizations and replicates is often an issue. The gDNA samples used in this study were therefore checked through barcoding the nrITS region. The sequence results gave an indication of DNA quality and also a prove of the authenticity of the samples. gBlocks were sourced also for the other plants species used in this study to overcome the problem related to the amount of DNA provided. Another reason for using gBlocks was to develop a quantification assay. Following the MIQE guidelines, when using qPCR for quantification rather than identification, it is necessary

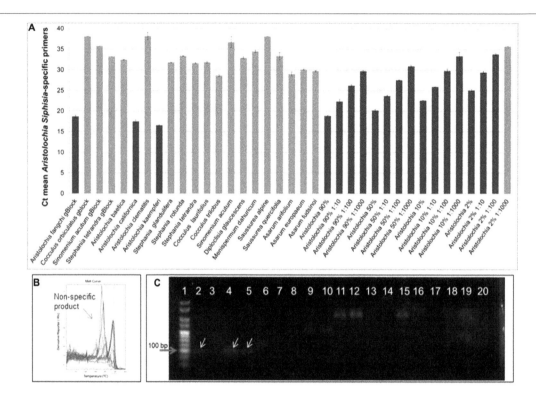

FIGURE 5 | *Aristolochia* subgenus *Siphisia*-specific quantitative real-time **(A)** Ct values. The lighter bars indicate primer dimers or non-specific products as per melting curve data. qPCR was performed using three biological replicates with three technical replicates for each sample. Error bars represent Standard deviation. **(B)** Melting curve for all samples run with *Siphisia*-specific primers. **(C)** Agarose gel electrophoresis of PCRs using *Siphisia*-specific primers. The white arrows point to the products with the expected size (88 bp). Gel lanes: (1) HyperLadder™ 25 bp (Bioline); (2) Positive control; (3) Negative (no template) control; (4) *A. californica*; (5) *A. kaempferi*; (6) *A. baetica*; (7) *A. clematitis*; (8) *S. tetrandra*; (9) *S. glandulifera*; (10) *S. rotunda*; (11) *C. trilobus*; (12) *C. laurifolius*; (13) *S. acutum*; (14) *A. europaeum*; (15) *A. arifolium*; (16) *A. fudsinoi*; (17) *S. alpine*; (18) *D. glaucescens*; (19) *M. dahuricum*; (20) *S. quercifolia*.

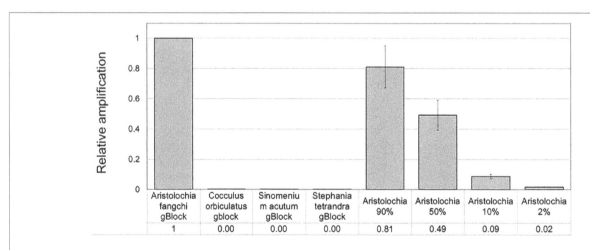

FIGURE 6 | Detection and quantitation of *Aristolochia* subgenus *Siphisia* DNA using the *Siphisia*-specific primers. ΔCt values were calculated as the difference between the mean Ct value of the *Siphisia*-specific amplification and the mean Ct value of the internal control 5.8S amplification. *Aristolochia* S[-5] gBlock was used as calibrator sample. qPCR was performed using three biological replicates with three technical replicates for each sample. Error bars represent Standard deviation.

to generate a standard curve from known quantities of a target (Bustin et al., 2009).

Although quantification kits to be used as validated standards are commercially available, when working with non-human samples they became less reliable (Nielsen et al., 2006;

Conte et al., 2018). Standard templates have been used from a range of sources, including cloned target sequences and PCR products, which require many steps that could potentially contaminate the laboratory and the standard itself. More recently, the use of synthetic gene fragments, such as gBlocks, as a standard

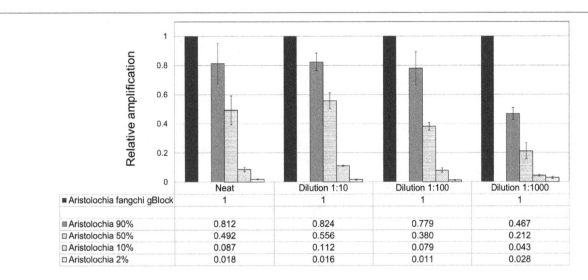

FIGURE 7 | Quantitation of *Aristolochia* subgenus *Siphisia* DNA in admixtures. ΔCt values were calculated as the difference between the mean Ct value of the target *Siphisia*-specific amplification and the mean Ct value of the internal control 5.8S amplification. *Aristolochia* S^{-5} gBlock neat and dilutions 1:10, 1:100, and 1:1000 were used as calibrator samples for the corresponsive dilution mix. qPCR was performed using three biological replicates with three technical replicates for each sample. Error bars represent Standard deviation.

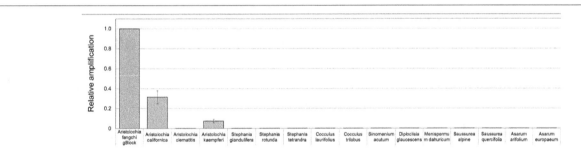

FIGURE 8 | Detection and quantitation of *Aristolochia* subgenus *Siphisia* DNA sequences in genomic DNA samples. ΔCt values were calculated as the difference between the mean Ct value of the target *Aristolochia Siphisia*-specific amplification and the mean Ct value of the internal control 5.8S amplification. *Aristolochia* S^{-5} gBlock was used as calibrator sample. qPCR was performed using three biological replicates with three technical replicates for each sample. Error bars represent Standard deviation.

has becoming an affordable, fast and reliable quantification strategy (Dhanasekaran et al., 2010; Conte et al., 2018).

In this study a gBlock has been used to create a standard curve to overcome the lack of available and reliable material, but also to prove that is possible to create a sensitive and reliable assay which can estimate the copy number of a target gene per sample and could potentially be used in an industrial setting. Reconstitution of the lyophilized gBlocks fragment provided over 2.14E+10 copies of the target. Dilution of the stock standard was done to create a sub-stock that was used to prepare the standard curve for the qPCR assay.

Generic primers were designed to target the conserved 5.8S rRNA coding region to amplify any template DNA. These can be used as an internal control to verify DNA quality and also as a reference gene for relative quantitation of the specific target DNA region. This primer pair was designed to generate a PCR product of under 100 bp which makes them suitable to be used in qPCR and ideal when working with potentially degraded DNA (Sgamma et al., 2017). This "mini-barcode" region proved to be

useful for two of our samples. In fact, *Aristolochia californica* and *Aristolochia clematitis* gDNA samples did not present a clear amplicon for the nrITS fragments but then both of them presented templates for the generic 5.8 primers (**Figure 4**) indicating the presence of possible degraded, but still detectable DNA.

The ITS2 sequences for *Aristolochia* species available in GenBank demonstrated that the ITS2 region can be used to distinguish Aristolochiaceous species from their putative substitutes (non-Aristolochiaceae family) (Wu et al., 2015). In this study the *Aristolochia* species were separated into two clades using the ITS2 region. These two clades were recognized as corresponding to two subgenera previously reported, with Clade A corresponding to *Aristolochia* subgenus *Aristolochia* while Clade B corresponds to *Aristolochia* subgenus *Siphisia* (Ohi-Toma et al., 2006, Do et al., 2015; Ohi-Toma and Murata, 2016). Short "mini-barcode" regions within the ITS2 sequence were targeted for the design of *Siphisia*-specific primers because of the many reports of substitution of non-toxic plants with plants belonging to this subgenus, including *Aristolochia fangchi*, *A. manshuriensis*, *A. kaempferi*, *A. mollissima*, and *A. versicolor* (Debelle et al., 2008). Furthermore, it proved to be difficult to design *Aristolochia* subgenus *Aristolochia* specific primers because the ITS2 sequences within this group are more diverse than those in the *Siphisia* subgenus. Therefore, in this study we chose to work on the subspecies that included Fang Ji and Mu Tong to target the worst known cases of contamination.

Although significantly high DNA copy numbers were present in all of the gBlock and genomic DNA samples, only the target species showed the presence of the *Siphisia*-specific "mini-barcode" regions.

Optimization of qPCR with *Aristolochia Siphisia*-specific primers allowed detection and quantification of this genus in mixed samples containing also *Stephania tetrandra* in different ratios. When *Aristolochia* DNA was mixed with *Stephania* at different rates, it was possible to detect it in 2% ratio *Aristolochia* and 98% of *Stephania*. Using standards associating the copy number to each start quantity this corresponded to about 50 copies. All proportions of *Aristolochia*, from 100 to 2%, were detected. The melting curve data provided confirmation that there was only one amplification product. *Stephania*, *Sinomenium* and *Cocculus* gBlocks or gDNA samples were not amplified by qPCR when using the *Aristolochia* subgenus *Siphisia*-specific primers. Although the amplification curves indicated a small amount of apparent amplification of gDNA samples, it was considered to be negligible because the Ct values were higher than the blank and the melting curves confirmed non-specific product or primer dimer formation. Therefore, it was proved that it is possible to differentiate *Aristolochia* subg. *Siphisia* from the other genera using a DNA-based strategy in pure or mixed samples. The achievement of this study could be utilized by the manufacturers, importers and retailers of herbal products to conduct a preliminary safety test for all of their raw materials. After that stage, only samples that were positively identified to contain *Aristolochia* subg. *Siphisia* species will be further confirmed by chemical analysis. *Cocculus orbiculatus*, *Sinomenium acutum,* and *Stephania tetrandra* have been proven scientifically for their health benefits (Zhao et al.,

2012; Bhagya and Chandrashekar, 2018). This study describes a rapid, sensitive qPCR test for the detection of *Aristolochia* species in the subgenus *Siphisia*. The assay is designed for use by industrial and regulatory quality control laboratories for screening of herbal drugs for contamination by those *Aristolochia* plants that have most frequently been implicated in the toxicity of adulterated medicines. This study represents the first phase of assay development in which the parameters have been optimized using pure components and gBlocks. The next phase will be to trial the assay using DNA extracted from herbal medicines to determine how robust the method is under conditions of PCR inhibitors and low quantities of poor quality fragmented DNA. The qPCR primers sets were in fact designed to generate PCR products of under 100 bp to cope with potentially degraded DNA. The introduction of reliable contamination tests into the supply chains of medicinal plants that are currently banned because of the risk of *Aristolochia* contamination will enhance the quality assurance of the safety of these herbs for consumption. This should help to restore consumer confidence and could eventually lead to the previous bans imposed on these harmless plant species being revoked by the regulatory authorities.

AUTHOR CONTRIBUTIONS

TS and AS conceived the project, designed and supervised the experimental strategy. TS, EM, and AS edited the paper. TS, PM, and MM performed the experiments. TS analyzed the data, and wrote most of the paper.

ACKNOWLEDGMENTS

We greatly appreciate the contribution of Prof Michael Heinrich (University College London, United Kingdom) and Dr. Ben Gronier (De Montfort University, United Kingdom), for the provision of plant material. This project was supported by De Montfort University HEIF funds.

REFERENCES

Abdullah, R., Diaz, L. N., Wesseling, S., and Rietjens, I. M. C. M. (2017). Risk assessment of plant food supplements and other herbal products containing aristolochic acids using the margin of exposure (MOE) approach. *Food Addit. Contam. Part A Chem. Anal. Control Expo. Risk Assess.* 34, 135–144. doi: 10.1080/19440049.2016.1266098

Arlt, V., Stiborova, M., and Schmeiser, H. (2002). Aristolochic acid as a probable human cancer hazard in herbal remedies: a review. *Mutagenesis* 17, 265–277. doi: 10.1093/mutage/17.4.265

Bhagya, N., and Chandrashekar, K. R. (2018). Tetrandrine and cancer – An overview on the molecular approach. *Biomed. Pharmacother.* 97, 624–632. doi: 10.1016/j.biopha.2017.10.116

Bustin, S. A., Benes, V., Garson, J. A., Hellemans, J., Huggett, J., Kubista, M., et al. (2009). The MIQE guidelines: minimum information for publication of

quantitative real-time pcr experiments. *Clin. Chem.* 55, 611–622. doi: 10.1373/clinchem.2008.112797

Conte, J., Potoczniak, M. J., and Tobe, S. S. (2018). Using synthetic oligonucleotides as standards in probe-based qpcr. *Biotechniques* 64, 177–179. doi: 10.2144/btn-2018-2000

Debelle, F. D., Vanherweghem, J., and Nortier, J. L. (2008). Aristolochic acid nephropathy: a worldwide problem. *Kidney Int.* 74, 158–169. doi: 10.1038/ki.2008.129

Dechbumroong, P., Aumnouypol, S., Denduangboripant, J., and Sukrong, S. (2018). DNA barcoding of Aristolochia plants and development of species-specific multiplex PCR to aid HPTLC in ascertainment of Aristolochia herbal materials. *PLoS One* 13:e0202625. doi: 10.1371/journal.pone.0202625

Dhanasekaran, S., Doherty, T. M., and Kenneth, J. (2010). Comparison of different standards for real-time PCR-based absolute quantification. *J. Immunol. Methods* 354, 34–39. doi: 10.1016/j.jim.2010.01.004

Do, T. V., Luu, T. H., Wanke, S., and Neinhuis, C. (2015). Three new species and three new records of Aristolochia Subgenus Siphisia from Vietnam including a key to the Asian species. *Syst. Bot.* 40, 671–691. doi: 10.1600/036364415X689140

Duan, B., Wang, Y., Fang, H., Xiong, C., Li, X., Wang, P., et al. (2018). Authenticity analyses of Rhizoma Paridis using barcoding coupled with high resolution melting (Bar-HRM) analysis to control its quality for medicinal plant product. *Chin. Med.* 13:8. doi: 10.1186/s13020-018-0162-4

Efferth, T., and Kaina, B. (2011). Toxicities by herbal medicines with emphasis to traditional Chinese medicine. *Curr. Drug Metab.* 12, 989–996. doi: 10.2174/138920011798062328

Felsenstein, J. (1985). Confidence-limits on phylogenies – an approach using the bootstrap. *Evolution* 39, 783–791. doi: 10.1111/j.1558-5646.1985.tb00420.x

Gold, L., and Slone, T. (2003). Aristolochic acid, an herbal carcinogen, sold on the Web after FDA alert. *N. Engl. J. Med.* 349, 1576–1577. doi: 10.1056/NEJM200310163491619

Grollman, A. P., Shibutani, S., Moriya, M., Miller, F., Wu, L., Moll, U., et al. (2007). Aristolochic acid and the etiology of endemic (Balkan) nephropathy. *Proc. Natl. Acad. Sci. U.S.A.* 104, 12129–12134. doi: 10.1073/pnas.0701248104

Hawkins, J., De Vere, N., Griffith, A., Ford, C. R., Allainguillaume, J., Hegarty, M. J., et al. (2015). Using DNA Metabarcoding to identify the floral composition of honey: a new tool for investigating honey bee foraging preferences. *PLoS One* 10:e0134735. doi: 10.1371/journal.pone.0134735

International Agency for Research on Cancer [IARC] (2002). *IARC Working Group on the Evaluation of Carcinogenic Risk to Humans. Some Traditional Herbal Medicines, Some Mycotoxins, Naphthalene and Styrene.* Lyon: IARC Monographs on the Evaluation of Carcinogenic Risks to Humans.

Jadot, I., Decleves, A., Nortier, J., and Caron, N. (2017). An integrated view of Aristolochic Acid nephropathy: update of the literature. *Int. J. Mol. Sci.* 18:297. doi: 10.3390/ijms18020297

Joshi, V. C., Avula, B., and Khan, I. A. (2008). Authentication of *Stephania tetrandra* S. Moore (Fang Ji) and differentiation of its common adulterants using microscopy and HPLC analysis. *J. Nat. Med.* 62, 117–121. doi: 10.1007/s11418-007-0200-5

Kite, G., Yule, M., Leon, C., and Simmonds, M. (2002). Detecting aristolochic acids in herbal remedies by liquid chromatography/serial mass spectrometry. *Rapid Commun. Mass Spectrom.* 16, 585–590. doi: 10.1002/rcm.611

Laube, I., Hird, H., Brodmann, P., Ullmann, S., Schoene-Michling, M., Chisholm, J., et al. (2010). Development of primer and probe sets for the detection of plant species in honey. *Food Chem.* 118, 979–986. doi: 10.1016/j.foodchem.2008.09.063

Lee, M., Tsao, C., Iou, S., Chuang, W., and Sheu, S. (2003). Analysis of aristolochic acids in herbal medicines by Lc/Uv and Lc/Ms. *J. Separat. Sci.* 26, 818–822.

Li, M., Au, K., Lam, H., Cheng, L., But, P. P., and Shaw, P. (2014). Molecular identification and cytotoxicity study of herbal medicinal materials that are confused by Aristolochia herbs. *Food Chem.* 147, 332–339. doi: 10.1016/j.foodchem.2013.09.146

Li, M., Au, K., Lam, H., Cheng, L., Jiang, R., But, P. P., et al. (2012). Identification of Baiying (Herba Solani Lyrati) commodity and its toxic substitute Xungufeng (Herba Aristolochiae Mollissimae) using DNA barcoding and chemical profiling techniques. *Food Chem.* 135, 1653–1658. doi: 10.1016/j.foodchem.2012.06.049

Livak, K., and Schmittgen, T. (2001). Analysis of relative gene expression data using real-time quantitative PCR and the 2(T)(-Delta Delta C) method. *Methods* 25, 402–408. doi: 10.1006/meth.2001.1262

Martena, M. J., Van Der Wielen, J. C. A., Van De Laak, L. F. J., Konings, E. J. M., De Groot, H. N., and Rietjens, I. M. C. M. (2007). Enforcement of the ban on aristolochic acids in Chinese traditional herbal preparations on the Dutch market. *Anal. Bioanal. Chem.* 389, 263–275. doi: 10.1007/s00216-007-1310-3

Medsafe (2003). *Director-General's Privileged Statement Under Section 98 of the Medicines Act 1981.* Available at: www.medsafe.govt.nz/hot/media/media2003.asp [accessed October 22, 2018].

Michl, J., Jennings, H. M., Kite, G. C., Ingrouille, M. J., Simmonds, M. S. J., and Heinrich, M. (2013). Is aristolochic acid nephropathy a widespread problem in developing countries? A case study of *Aristolochia indica* L. in Bangladesh using an ethnobotanical-phytochemical approach. *J. Ethnopharmacol.* 149, 235–244. doi: 10.1016/j.jep.2013.06.028

Nielsen, K., Mogensen, H. S., Eriksen, B., Hedman, J., Parson, W., and Morling, N. (2006). Comparison of six Dna quantification methods. *Int. Congr. Ser.* 1288(Suppl. C), 759–761. doi: 10.1016/j.ics.2005.09.095

Nortier, J., Martinez, M., Schmeiser, H., Arlt, V., Bieler, C., Petein, M., et al. (2000). Urothelial carcinoma associated with the use of a Chinese herb (*Aristolochia fangchi*). *N. Engl. J. Med.* 342, 1686–1692. doi: 10.1056/NEJM200006083422301

Nortier, J. L., and Vanherweghem, J. (2007). For patients taking herbal therapy – lessons from aristolochic acid nephropathy. *Nephrol. Dial. Transplant.* 22, 1512–1517. doi: 10.1093/ndt/gfm167

Ohi-Toma, T., and Murata, J. (2016). Nomenclature of Isotrema, Siphisia, and Endodeca, and their related infrageneric taxa of Aristolochia (Aristolochiaceae). *Taxon* 65, 152–157. doi: 10.12705/651.11

Ohi-Toma, T., Sugawara, T., Murata, H., Wanke, S., Neinhuis, C., and Murata, J. (2006). Molecular phylogeny of *Aristolochia sensu* lato (Aristolochiaceae) based on sequences of rbcL, matK, and phyA genes, with special reference to differentiation of chromosome numbers. *Syst. Bot.* 31, 481–492. doi: 10.1600/036364406778388656

Osathanunkul, M., Ounjai, S., Osathanunkul, R., and Madesis, P. (2017). Evaluation of a DNA-based method for spice/herb authentication, so you do not have to worry about what is in your curry, buon appetito! *PLoS One* 12:e0186283. doi: 10.1371/journal.pone.0186283

Raclariu, A. C., Heinrich, M., Ichim, M. C., and De Boer, H. (2018). Benefits and Limitations of DNA barcoding and metabarcoding in herbal product authentication. *Phytochem. Anal.* 29, 123–128. doi: 10.1002/pca.2732

Schaneberg, B., and Khan, I. (2004). Analysis of products suspected of containing Aristolochia or Asarum species. *J. Ethnopharmacol.* 94, 245–249. doi: 10.1016/j.jep.2004.06.010

Sgamma, T., Lockie-Williams, C., Kreuzer, M., Williams, S., Scheyhing, U., Koch, E., et al. (2017). DNA barcoding for industrial quality assurance. *Planta Med.* 83, 1117–1129. doi: 10.1055/s-0043-113448

Soares, S., Grazina, L., Costa, J., Amaral, J. S., Oliveira, M. B. P. P., and Mafra, I. (2018). Botanical authentication of lavender (Lavandula s) honey by a novel DNA-barcoding approach coupled to high resolution melting analysis. *Food Control* 86, 367–373. doi: 10.1016/j.foodcont.2017.11.046

Sorenson, W. R., and Sullivan, D. (2007). Determination of aristolochic acid I in botanicals and dietary supplements potentially contaminated with aristolochic acid I using LC-UV with confirmation by LC/MS: collaborative study. *J. AOAC Int.* 90, 925–933.

Tamura, K. (1992). Estimation of the number of nucleotide substitutions when there are strong transition-transversion and G+c-content biases. *Mol. Biol. Evol.* 9, 678–687.

Tamura, K., Stecher, G., Peterson, D., Filipski, A., and Kumar, S. (2013). MEGA6: molecular evolutionary genetics analysis version 6.0. *Mol. Biol. Evol.* 30, 2725–2729. doi: 10.1093/molbev/mst197

Tankeu, S., Vermaak, I., Chen, W., Sandasi, M., and Viljoen, A. (2016). Differentiation between two "fang ji" herbal medicines, *Stephania tetrandra* and the nephrotoxic *Aristolochia fangchi*, using hyperspectral imaging. *Phytochemistry* 122, 213–222. doi: 10.1016/j.phytochem.2015.11.008

Vanherweghem, J., Depierreux, M., Tielemans, C., Abramowicz, D., Dratwa, M., Jadoul, M., et al. (1993). Rapidly progressive interstitial renal fibrosis in young-women – Association with slimming regimen including Chinese herbs. *Lancet* 341, 387–391. doi: 10.1016/0140-6736(93)92984-2

Wu, L., Sun, W., Wang, B., Zhao, H., Li, Y., Cai, S., et al. (2015). An integrated system for identifying the hidden assassins in traditional medicines containing aristolochic acids. *Sci. Rep.* 5:11318. doi: 10.1038/srep11318

Wu, L., Wang, B., Zhao, M., Liu, W., Zhang, P., Shi, Y., et al. (2016). Rapid identification of officinal akebiae caulis and its toxic adulterant Aristolochiae Manshuriensis Caulis (*Aristolochia manshuriensis*) by loop - mediated isothermal amplification. *Front. Plant Sci.* 7:887. doi: 10.3389/fpls.2016.00887

Yang, F., Ding, F., Chen, H., He, M., Zhu, S., Ma, X., et al. (2018). Dna Barcoding for the identification and authentication of animal species in traditional medicine. *Evid. Based Complement. Altern. Med.* 2018:5160254. doi: 10.1155/2018/5160254

Yang, L., Li, X., and Wang, H. (2007). Possible mechanisms explaining the tendency towards interstitial fibrosis in aristolochic acid-induced acute tubular necrosis. *Nephrol. Dial. Transplant.* 22, 445–456. doi: 10.1093/ndt/gfl556

Yang, P., Li, X., Zhou, H., Hu, H., Zhang, H., Sun, W., et al. (2014). Molecular identification of Chinese materia medica and its adulterants using ITS2 and psbA-trnH Barcodes: a case study on Rhizoma Menispermi. *Chin. Med.* 5, 190–198. doi: 10.4236/cm.2014.54023

Zhang, J., Wider, B., Shang, H., Li, X., and Ernst, E. (2012). Quality of herbal medicines: challenges and solutions. *Complement. Ther. Med.* 20, 100–106. doi: 10.1016/j.ctim.2011.09.004

Zhao, X., Peng, C., Zhang, H., and Qin, L. (2012). Sinomenium acutum: a review of chemistry, pharmacology, pharmacokinetics, and clinical use. *Pharm. Biol.* 50, 1053–1061. doi: 10.3109/13880209.2012. 656847

Zhu, Y.-P. (2002). Toxicity of the Chinese herb Mu Tong (*Aristolochia manshuriensis*). What history tells us. *Adv. Drug. React. Toxicol.* 21, 171–177. doi: 10.1007/BF03256194

18

Mechanism Based Quality Control (MBQC) of Herbal Products

*Wing Lam[1], Yongshen Ren[1], Fulan Guan[1], Zaoli Jiang[1], William Cheng[1],
Chang-Hua Xu[1,2], Shwu-Huey Liu[3] and Yung-Chi Cheng[1]**

[1] *Department of Pharmacology, Yale University School of Medicine, New Haven, CT, United States,* [2] *College of Food Science and Technology, Shanghai Ocean University, Shanghai, China,* [3] *Yiviva Inc., New York, NY, United States*

Correspondence:
Yung-Chi Cheng
yccheng@yale.edu;
yung-chi.cheng@yale.edu

YIV-906 (PHY906), a four-herb Chinese medicine formulation, is inspired by an 1800 year-old Chinese formulation called Huang Qin Tang which is traditionally used to treat gastrointestinal (GI) symptoms. In animal studies, it could enhance anti-tumor activity of different classes of anticancer agents and promote faster recovery of the damaged intestines following irinotecan or radiation treatment. Several clinical studies have shown that YIV-906 had the potential to increase the therapeutic index of cancer treatments (chemotherapy, radiation) by prolonging life and improving patient quality of life. Results of animal studies demonstrated five clinical batches of YIV-906 had very similar *in vivo* activities (protection of body weight loss induced by CPT11 and enhancement of anti-tumor activity of CPT11) while four batches of commercial–made Huang Qin Tang, HQT had no or lower *in vivo* activities. Two quality control platforms were used to correlate the biological activity between YIV906 and HQT. Chemical profiles (using analysis of 77 peaks intensities) obtained from LC-MS could not be used to differentiate YIV-906 from commercial Huang Qin Tang. A mechanism based quality control (MBQC) platform, comprising 18 luciferase reporter cell lines and two enzymatic assays based on the mechanism action of YIV-906, could be used to differentiate YIV-906 from commercial Huang Qin Tang. Results of MBQC could be matched to their *in vivo* activities on irinotecan. In conclusion, the quality control of an herbal product should be dependent on its pharmacological usage. For its specific usage appropriate biological assays based on its mechanism action should be developed for QC. Chemical fingerprints comparison approach has limitations unless irrelevant chemicals have been filtered out. Additionally, using a similarity index is only useful when relevant information is used. A MBQC platform should also be applied on other herbal products.

Keywords: YIV-906, Chinese medicine, mechanism, quality control, chemical fingerprint, herbal products

INTRODUCTION

In human history Herbal Medicine is the oldest medicine. Herbs are the most important elements in different traditional medicines from different cultures around the world including Traditional Chinese Medicine, Ayurveda, Unani and Sidha. Many herbs are widely claimed to help a variety of disease or symptoms. In Asia and certain countries, herbal medicines are used as mainstream medicine for treating diseases. However, in many western countries, most herbal products are still being used as food supplements with low quality control standards. In order to promote herbal medicine as an accepted mainstream medicine in western countries for unmet needs, herbal products need to pass clinical trials with favorable and consistent clinical outcome. So far the FDA has only approved two botanical drugs: Veregen® Ointment and Fulyzaq® (crofelemer). FDA approved Veregen® Ointment, a green tea extract as topical drug for genital warts in 2006. In 2012 the FDA approved Fulyzaq® (crofelemer), an extract of the latex of the South American tree *Croton lechleri* for treating diarrhea in HIV patients in 2012 (Yeo et al., 2013). Quality control for Fulyzaq® is relatively simple because it contains only purified oligomeric procyanidins and proanthocyanidins, which are polymers of (epi)catechin or (epi)gallocatechin.

Many herbal medicines are used as raw extracts with polychemicals because purification may lead to separate active compounds or lose their biological activity. In Traditional Chinese Medicine (TCM) formulations with multiple herbs are commonly used. Due to the chemical complexity of herbal products, it is extremely difficult to reproduce an herbal product with the same biological activity over time without knowing all active ingredients.

We are currently developing YIV-906 (formerly PHY906, KD018) as an adjuvant for cancer therapies. YIV906 is a standardized four-herb formula based on formula "Huang Qin Tang," an 1800-year ago Chinese herbal formulation for numerous gastrointestinal (GI) symptoms, including diarrhea, nausea, and vomiting. These symptoms are common side effects of chemotherapy. YIV906 is composed of four herbs: *Glycyrrhiza uralensis* Fisch (**G**), *Paeonia lactiflora* Pall (**P**), *Scutellaria baicalensis* Georgi (**S**), and *Ziziphus jujuba* Mill (**Z**). YIV-906 was prepared using high-quality herbs selected by highly experienced herbalists and manufactured according to cGMP (current Good Manufacturing Practice) standards. Results from seven Phase (I/II to II) clinical trials with different batches of YIV-906 on 140 evaluable patients in Yale University and other institutions in United States suggested that there was no YIV-906 related toxicity with the used dosage; a clear indication of decreased G3/4 diarrhea, nausea, vomiting, and improved quality of life in those patients who received irinotecan, capecitabine or chemo-radiation were observed (Farrell and Kummar, 2003; Saif et al., 2010; Kummar et al., 2011; Saif et al., 2014). In preclinical studies YIV-906 reduced CPT-11-induced intestinal inflammation by inhibiting NFκB, COX-2, and iNOS while promoting intestinal stem/progenitor cell repopulation by stimulating the Wnt signaling pathway (Lam et al., 2010). YIV-906 also decreased GI toxicity from irradiation (Rockwell et al., 2013). YIV-906 could selectively alternate bacteria population of the intestines dependent on different treatment conditions (Lam et al., 2014). In tumors, YIV-906 was shown to enhance the anti-tumor activity of different classes of anti-cancer agents *in vivo* (Liu and Cheng, 2012). Detailed mechanism studies indicated that YIV-906 increased the anti-tumor activity of CPT-11 and Sorafenib by increasing apoptosis of tumor cells and promoting the polarization of macrophage to M1-like-type that assists tumor rejection in the tumor micro-environment (Wang et al., 2011; Lam et al.,

2015). mRNA array results of colon 38 tumor following CPT-11+YIV-906 treatment suggested that YIV-906 could switch the immune status of tumor from chronic to acute inflammation associated with the up-regulation of IRF5, IFN, and JAK/STAT signaling (Wang et al., 2011). Overall, different batches of YIV-906 manufactured over a period of 15 years appeared to show similar biological activities in clinical and pre-clinical studies.

In this report, we compared different batches of YIV-906 with alternate commercial-made batches of Huang Qin Tang (HQT) for their biological activity on CPT11 of colon 38 tumor bearing BDF1 mice. We also compared correlation analysis based on chemical profiles, which is the most common quality control method used in botanical industry, against biological activities of "mechanism based quality control"(MBQC) could be used to differentiate clinical batches of YIV-906 from the commercial batches of HQT and matched to their biological activity *in vivo*.

MATERIALS AND METHODS

In vivo Mouse Models
Murine Colon 38 cells ($1-2 \times 10^6$ cells in 0.1 ml phosphate-buffered saline, PBS) were transplanted subcutaneously into 4- to 6-week-old female BDF1 mice (Charles River Laboratories). After 10–14 days, mice with tumor sizes of 150–300 mm³ were selected. Unless otherwise indicated, treatment groups each consisted of five mice. Tumor size, body weight, and mortality of the mice were monitored daily. Tumor volume was estimated by using the formula length × width² × π/6. Unless otherwise indicated, treatment groups each consisted of five mice. PHY906 (batches number 6, 7, 8, 10, 11 and F, 38, 39, 40 which are commercial Huang Qin Tang) were given orally (po) for 4 days [twice per day (b.i.d), 500 mg/kg at approximately 10:00 am and 3:00 pm], while CPT-11 (360 mg/kg) was administered intraperitoneal (ip) on Day 1. On Day 1, PHY906 was given 30 min prior to CPT-11 administration. In the control groups, mice were administered a vehicle, either PBS for i.p. administration or water for oral administration. Data was analyzed by two-way ANOVA (GraphPad Prism 6), The difference was considered to be statistically significant when ++ ($P < 0.001$), + ($P < 0.05$) and – ($P > 0.05$).

LC-MS Analysis for Chemical Profiles of the Metabolites of PHY906
10 μl of 10 mg/ml herbal water extract of each sample was subjected to LC-MS analysis. Six times individual experiments were repeated for each sample. The LC-MS analysis was performed on an Agilent 1200 series HPLC coupled with AB SCIEX 4000 QTRAP mass spectrometer. The separation was conducted on an Agilent Zorbax C18HPLC Column (5 μm, 4.6 × 250 mm). The mobile phase is acetonitrile (A) and water with 0.1% formic acid (B) with linear gradient elution: 0 min, 5% A; 10 min, 20% A; 20 min, 25% A; 40 min, 30% A; 45 min, 35% A; 55 min, 45% A; 60 min, 70% A; 62 min, 90% A; 67 min, 90% A; 68 min, 5% A; and 75 min, 5% A. The flow rate is 1.0 mL/min, and the column temperature was set at 30°C, the detection

wavelength was set at 230 nm. The mass spectrometer was operated in the negative modes and equipped with a electrospray ionization (ESI) source. Source parameters were as follow: sheath gas (nitrogen) flow rate and auxiliary gas (nitrogen) flow rate: 60 and 20 arbitrary units, respectively, capillary temperature: 400°C, heater temperature: 30°C, spray voltage was −3.8 kV. The instrument was operated from m/z 120–1000 Da in the full scan mode. Acquisitioning and processing of the data from the mass spectrometer was performed using Analyst 1.4.2® Software, the peaks were compared and a clustering analysis was created by MZmine software.

Mechanism Based Quality Control Platform

18 x Luciferase report cell lines for different signaling pathways were selected. Cells were seeded into half-area 96-well microplate at 20000 cells/well in 40 ul medium for overnight at 37°C 5% CO_2 incubator. Different dosages of PHY906 water extracted from 750 μg/ml to 83 μg/ml were added to the cells and placed in a 37°C 5% CO_2 incubator. After removing medium at 6 h, 10 μl of lysis buffer (Tris-HC 25 mM at pH7.8, DTT 2 mM, CDTA 2 mM, glycerol 10%, Triton X−100 1%) will be used to lyse the cells and 40 μl of luciferase reaction buffer (Tris-HCl 20 mM at pH7.8, $NaHCO_3$ 1 mM, $MgSO_4$ 2.5 mM, DTT 10 mM, Coenzyme-A lithium 60 μM, potassium luciferin 225 μM, ATP 250 μM) will be added for reading luminescence using a luminescence microplate reader. IC50 (concentration required to inhibit 50% of control) or EC50 (concentration required to achieve 50%

of maximum activation) will be determined based on the dos-response curve. IC50 or E50 for each assay were determined from three independent experiments which were done in triplicate with 5 different doses. Methods for determining Cox-2 activity Assay and iNOS activity can be found in reference (Lam et al., 2010).

Algorithm for Determining Correlation Coefficients

Graphpad Prism 6 software will be used to determine the correlation coefficients. Each raw input table represents different genes or different signal pathways. Each column represents different batches. Values of gene expression or IC50 or AC50 were input. "Column analyses" function of the software was selected for correlation analysis. Computing the correlation between each pairs of columns will be performed based on assuming a sample with Gaussian distribution. Pearson coefficients were calculated.

RESULTS

All YIV-906 Batches but Not Commercial Batches of Huang Qin Tang Enhance Antitumor Activity of CPT11 While Reducing the Body Weight Loss Caused by CPT11

We previously showed YIV-906-10 could enhance the action of CPT11 against colon-38 tumor growth while reducing

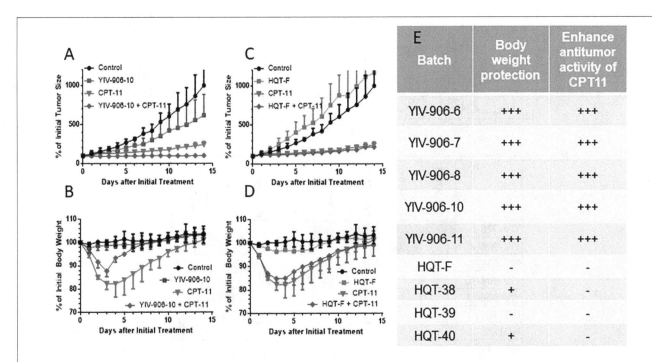

FIGURE 1 | Comparison between *in vivo* activities among different batches of YIV-906 and HQT which is commercial Huang Qin Tang. **(A,B)**. Effect of YIV-906-10 **(A,B)** and HQT-F **(C,D)** on the anti-tumor activity of CPT11 and body weight protection of BDF1 bearing colon 38 tumor. **(E)** Summary of the effect of YIV-906 and HQT on the anti-tumor activity of CPT11 and body weight protection of BDF1 bearing colon 38 tumor. Details of experimental procedures are given in Section "Materials and Methods."

body weight loss caused by CPT11. Here, we compared five different clinical batches (6, 7, 8, 10, and 11) of YIV906 which were manufactured separately over the span of 15 years with commercial batches of Huang Qin Tang, HQT (F, 38, 39, 40) on the biological activities of CPT11 on colon-38 tumor bearing BDF1 mice. Results indicated that YIV-906-10 and other batches YIV-906 enhanced the anti-tumor activity of CPT11 against colon-38 tumor growth (**Figures 1A,E**) while promoted body weight recovery following CPT11 treatment (**Figures 1B,E**). Commercial HQT (F, 38, 39, 40) had no or low *in vivo* activities for enhancing CPT11 action on colon-38 tumor growth (**Figures 1C,E**). Commercial HQT (F, 38, 39, 40) also had no activity in promoting body weight recovery following CPT11 treatment (**Figures 1D,E**). This result confirmed that YIV906 which manufactured apart 15 years could have very similar biological activities.

Chemical Profile and Correlation Analysis for YIV-906 Batches and Commercial Batches of Huang Qin Tang Did Not Match Their Biological Activities on CPT11

Peaks from LC-MS profile were selected once their signals are significantly higher (5 folds higher) than the background (which was roughly about 5×10^4). Totally 77 peaks, which were based on their specific ion pairs in the LC-MS spectra, could be selected from either YIV-906 or HQT. Peaks of the 77 peaks might or might be not commonly found in YIV-906 or HQT (**Figure 2A**). Totally integrated area of the 77 peaks was about 90% of total integrated area of all peaks of chemical profiles. Each corresponding peak of different batches of YIV-906 or HQT were de-noised and aligned using MZmine software (**Figure 2A**).

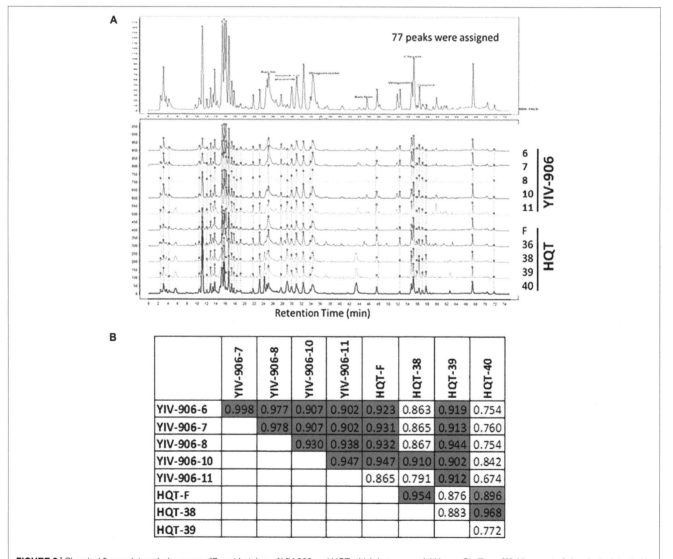

FIGURE 2 | Chemical fingerprint analysis among different batches of YIV-906 and HQT which is commercial Huang Qin Tang. **(A)** Alignment of chemicals detected in LC-MS for YIV-906 and HQT which is commercial Huang Qin Tang. **(B)** Correlation analysis of chemical profiles of YIV-906 and HQT where 1 represents exactly the same and 0 is totally different. Details of experimental procedures are given in Section "Materials and Methods."

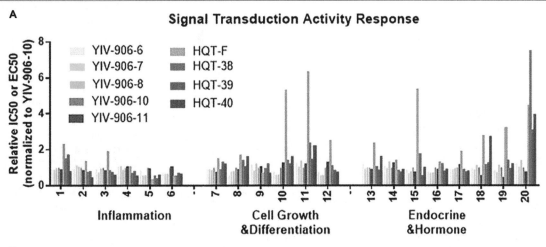

FIGURE 3 | Signal transduction activity response analysis among different batches of YIV-906 and HQT which is commercial Huang Qin Tang. **(A)** Effect of different batches of YIV-906 and HQT on signal transduction activity response using different luciferase reporter cell lines and enzyme assays. **(B)** Correlation analysis of the signal transduction activity response for YIV-906 and HQT where 1 represents exactly the same and 0 is totally different. Details of experimental procedures are given in Section "Materials and Methods."

When all 77 peaks were included for Pearson correlation analysis for each pair of samples, we did find that different pairs of YIV-906 batches demonstrated a strong positive similarity index (R from 0.9 to 0.99, red) (**Figure 2B**). However, based on their chemical profiles, HQT-F and HQT-39, which didn't have any biological activity on CPT11 in animal, also showed a positive similarity to most batches of YIV-906. Therefore, using all detectable chemicals for quality control may lead to a false prediction.

Mechanism Based Quality Control Platform and Correlation Analysis for YIV-906 Batches and Commercial Batches of Huang Qin Tang Matched Their Biological Activities on CPT11

Based on our previous animal and cell culture experiments, we know that YIV-906 had strong impact on inflammatory signaling via inhibiting NFkB, iNOS, COX2, IL6 and could promote tissue recovery by potentiating Wnt signaling. YIV-906 contains flavonoids which are known to have impact on hormone signaling and anti-oxidation property as well. Therefore, we selected 18 relevant luciferase reporter assays and two enzymatic assays, which were relevant to the mechanism action of YIV906,

as our MBQC platform. We may not cover all biological activities for YIV-906 but all selected biological assays for YIV-906 could be used to explain its mechanism action for improving side effect caused by chemotherapy.

We compared the signal transduction activity responses of clinical batches (6, 7, 8, 10, and 11) of YIV906 and commercial batches (F, 38, 39, 40) of HQT across these assays (**Figure 3A**). As compared to YIV-906-10, YIV-906 (6, 7, 8, and 11) showed very similar activities in different assays (**Figure 3A**). However, commercial HQT (F, 38, 39, 40) showed very low activities (with much larger EC50 or IC50) in certain assays when compared with YIV-906 (**Figure 3A**). Biological activities among the HQT batches were also very different (**Figure 3A**). When all these results from the assays of MBQC platform were analyzed using Pearson correlation for each pair samples, we found different batches (6, 7, 8, 10, and 11) of YIV-906 had quite high similarity (R > 0.9) (**Figure 3B**). As expected, HQT (F, 38, 39, 40) batches had lower similarity to YIV-906 (6, 7, 8, 10, and 11) batches (**Figure 3B**) (R < 0.9). Most importantly the correlation analysis based on the MBQC platform fitted results from animal experiments where all YIV-906 showed biological activity on CPT11 but not HQT. This method can be even further simplified using fewer bioassays.

DISCUSSION

In this study, we reported that different batches of YIV-906 manufactured over a period of 15 years had very similar biological activity on CPT11 in animals but not in commercial batches of Huang Qin Tang (HQT). We developed a MBQC platform to differentiate YIV-906 from HQT and predict their biological activities in animals. Chemical profile analysis based on all detectable chemicals of YIV-906 or HQT could not be used to differentiate them and may lead to false predictions for their biological activities.

Here, we showed that the clinical grade YIV-906 had better quality than commercial HQT because different batches of YIV-906 were manufactured according to cGMP protocol in which each manufacturing steps followed standard operation procedure. In addition, herbs for YIV-906 manufacturing were selected by very experience herbalists from defined source and specific season. Other HQT may use different sources of herbs and may not follow cGMP protocol. Some HQT also have different ratio of the four herbs from YIV-906. Therefore, different batches of YIV-906 had better consistency of their biological activities than other HQT.

In 2000, we proposed "phytomics" which covers both chemical and biological fingerprints to characterize herbal mixture (Tilton et al., 2010). However, the relevance of detected chemicals or biological responses to pharmacological activity of herbal mixtures could be an issue. This report highlights that chemical profiles analysis is not the ideal methodology for the quality control of herbal products.

For the past 20 years due to the available of many advanced analytical chemistry technologies, such as HPLC-MS, GC-MS, CE-MS, LC-NMR, NIR, NMR, 2D-IR in the market (Jiang et al., 2010; Song et al., 2013; Wang et al., 2013; Cheng et al., 2014), using chemical profile analysis as quality control became very popular in the botanical industry. People strongly believed that herbal products with similar detected chemical profiles should have similar biological activities. Even herbal pharmacopeia published by some countries heavily rely on one or two so called "key compound(s)" as the quality indication for many herbs. However, quality control dependent on using specific chemical detection can have many drawbacks. There is no single chemical detection method that can cover 100% of the chemicals in a given herbal product: Different chemical detection techniques have their advantages and limitations for detecting certain class chemicals. Many herbs or formulation of herbs have multiple active compounds, without knowing comprehensively all biological activity of all chemicals of these herbal products, including irrelevant chemicals, the analysis will mask the differences and interactions between different herbal preparations.

According to the Botanical Drug Development Guidance for Industry published by FDA in 2016, it is clear that the identification of each constituent of botanical product is impossible and identification of active constituents is not essential. Furthermore, the guidance suggests that biological assays should be developed for the active constituents which are not known or quantifiable before Phase 3 studies. Therefore, future quality control for herbal products should be focusing more on the biological activity of herb product based on their usage rather than their chemical profiles. With enough scientific knowledge on the mechanism action for different claims of a given herbal product, we can select relevant biological assays to establish a specific quality control platform for assessing the quality of the herbal product for the particular usage. The results from the quality control platform *in vitro* should be further validated using *in vivo* experiments.

In conclusion, the quality control of the herb should be depended on its usage. Appropriate biological assays should be developed for the QC of its particular usage. Unless irrelevant chemicals have been filtered out, chemical fingerprint analysis alone has notable shortcomings. Additionally, using a similarity index is only useful when relevant information is used and subject to bias. Unless all the active compounds of an herbal product have been identified, MBQC should always take precedent in the chemical profile analysis and collaboration between academia and industry could help further develop a rigorous MBQC platform. Our novel approach for quality control or CMC could be applied to other herbal medicines in order to ensure their biological activity.

AUTHOR CONTRIBUTIONS

WL did luciferase reporter assays, correlation analysis, and wrote the manuscript. YR did LC-MS analysis. FG did luciferase reporter assays and enzymatic assays. ZJ did animal experiments. WC did correlation analysis and data processing for LC-MS. S-HL provided YIV-906 and wrote the manuscript. C-HX helped setting up LC-MS. Y-CC designed experiments and wrote the manuscript.

FUNDING

This work was supported by grant (1PO1CA154295-01A1) from National Cancer Institute (NCI), NIH, United States. Y-CC is a fellow of National Foundation for Cancer Research (NFCR), United States.

REFERENCES

Cheng, X., Su, X., Chen, X., Zhao, H., Bo, C., Xu, J., et al. (2014). Biological ingredient analysis of traditional Chinese medicine preparation based on high-throughput sequencing: the story for Liuwei Dihuang Wan. *Sci. Rep.* 4:5147. doi: 10.1038/srep05147

Farrell, M. P., and Kummar, S. (2003). Phase I/IIA randomized study of PHY906, a novel herbal agent, as a modulator of chemotherapy in patients with advanced colorectal cancer. *Clin. Colorectal Cancer* 2, 253–256. doi: 10.3816/CCC.2003. n.007

Jiang, Y., David, B., Tu, P., and Barbin, Y. (2010). Recent analytical approaches in quality control of traditional Chinese medicines–a review. *Anal. Chim. Acta* 657, 9–18. doi: 10.1016/j.jep.2009.07.040

Kummar, S., Copur, M. S., Rose, M., Wadler, S., Stephenson, J., O'rourke, M., et al. (2011). A phase I study of the chinese herbal medicine PHY906 as a modulator of irinotecan-based chemotherapy in patients with advanced colorectal cancer. *Clin. Colorectal Cancer* 10, 85–96. doi: 10.1016/j.clcc.2011. 03.003

Lam, W., Bussom, S., Guan, F., Jiang, Z., Zhang, W., Gullen, E. A., et al. (2010). The four-herb Chinese medicine PHY906 reduces chemotherapy-induced gastrointestinal toxicity. *Sci. Transl. Med.* 2:45ra59. doi: 10.1126/scitranslmed. 3001270

Lam, W., Jiang, Z., Guan, F., Hu, R., Liu, S. H., Chu, E., et al. (2014). The number of intestinal bacteria is not critical for the enhancement of antitumor activity and reduction of intestinal toxicity of irinotecan by the Chinese herbal medicine PHY906 (KD018). *BMC Complement. Altern. Med.* 14:490. doi: 10.1186/1472-6882-14-490

Lam, W., Jiang, Z., Guan, F., Huang, X., Hu, R., Wang, J., et al. (2015). PHY906(KD018), an adjuvant based on a 1800-year-old Chinese medicine, enhanced the anti-tumor activity of Sorafenib by changing the tumor microenvironment. *Sci. Rep.* 5:9384. doi: 10.1038/srep 09384

Liu, S. H., and Cheng, Y. C. (2012). Old formula, new Rx: the journey of PHY906 as cancer adjuvant therapy. *J. Ethnopharmacol.* 140, 614–623. doi: 10.1016/j.jep. 2012.01.047

Rockwell, S., Grove, T. A., Liu, Y., Cheng, Y. C., Higgins, S. A., and Booth, C. J. (2013). Preclinical studies of the Chinese Herbal Medicine formulation PHY906 (KD018) as a potential adjunct to radiation therapy. *Int. J. Radiat. Biol.* 89, 16–25. doi: 10.3109/09553002.2012.717733

Saif, M. W., Lansigan, F., Ruta, S., Lamb, L., Mezes, M., Elligers, K., et al. (2010). Phase I study of the botanical formulation PHY906 with capecitabine in advanced pancreatic and other gastrointestinal malignancies. *Phytomedicine* 17, 161–169. doi: 10.1016/j.phymed.2009.12.016

Saif, M. W., Li, J., Lamb, L., Kaley, K., Elligers, K., Jiang, Z., et al. (2014). First-in-human phase II trial of the botanical formulation PHY906 with capecitabine as second-line therapy in patients with advanced pancreatic cancer. *Cancer Chemother. Pharmacol.* 73, 373–380. doi: 10.1007/s00280-013-2359-7

Song, X. Y., Li, Y. D., Shi, Y. P., Jin, L., and Chen, J. (2013). Quality control of traditional Chinese medicines: a review. *Chin. J. Nat. Med.* 11, 596–607. doi: 10.1016/S1875-5364(13)60069-2

Tilton, R., Paiva, A. A., Guan, J. Q., Marathe, R., Jiang, Z., Van Eyndhoven, W., et al. (2010). A comprehensive platform for quality control of botanical drugs (PhytomicsQC): a case study of Huangqin Tang (HQT) and PHY906. *Chin. Med.* 5:30. doi: 10.1186/1749-8546-5-30

Wang, E., Bussom, S., Chen, J., Quinn, C., Bedognetti, D., Lam, W., et al. (2011). Interaction of a traditional Chinese medicine (PHY906) and CPT-11 on the inflammatory process in the tumor microenvironment. *BMC Med. Genomics* 4:38. doi: 10.1186/1755-8794-4-38

Wang, J., Kong, H., Yuan, Z., Gao, P., Dai, W., Hu, C., et al. (2013). A novel strategy to evaluate the quality of traditional Chinese medicine based on the correlation analysis of chemical fingerprint and biological effect. *J. Pharm. Biomed. Anal.* 83, 57–64. doi: 10.1016/j.jpba.2013.04.035

Yeo, Q. M., Crutchley, R., Cottreau, J., Tucker, A., and Garey, K. W. (2013). Crofelemer, a novel antisecretory agent approved for the treatment of HIV-associated diarrhea. *Drugs Today* 49, 239–252. doi: 10.1358/dot.2013.49.4. 1947253

19

Identification of *Ligularia* Herbs Using the Complete Chloroplast Genome as a Super-Barcode

Xinlian Chen[1†], Jianguo Zhou[1†], Yingxian Cui[1], Yu Wang[1], Baozhong Duan[2] and Hui Yao[1]*

[1] *Key Lab of Chinese Medicine Resources Conservation, State Administration of Traditional Chinese Medicine of the People's Republic of China, Institute of Medicinal Plant Development, Chinese Academy of Medical Sciences & Peking Union Medical College, Beijing, China,* [2] *College of Pharmaceutical Science, Dali University, Dali, China*

Correspondence:
Hui Yao
scauyaoh@sina.com

[†] *These authors have contributed equally to this work.*

More than 30 *Ligularia* Cass. (Asteraceae) species have long been used in folk medicine in China. Morphological features and common DNA regions are both not ideal to identify *Ligularia* species. As some *Ligularia* species contain pyrrolizidine alkaloids, which are hazardous to human and animal health and are involved in metabolic toxification in the liver, it is important to find a better way to distinguish these species. Here, we report complete chloroplast (CP) genomes of six *Ligularia* species, *L. intermedia*, *L. jaluensis*, *L. mongolica*, *L. hodgsonii*, *L. veitchiana*, and *L. fischeri*, obtained through high-throughput Illumina sequencing technology. These CP genomes showed typical circular tetramerous structure and their sizes range from 151,118 to 151,253 bp. The GC content of each CP genome is 37.5%. Every CP genome contains 134 genes, including 87 protein-coding genes, 37 tRNA genes, eight rRNA genes, and two pseudogenes (*ycf1* and *rps19*). From the mVISTA, there were no potential coding or non-coding regions to distinguish these six *Ligularia* species, but the maximum likelihood tree of the six *Ligularia* species and other related species showed that the whole CP genome can be used as a super-barcode to identify these six *Ligularia* species. This study provides invaluable data for species identification, allowing for future studies on phylogenetic evolution and safe medical applications of *Ligularia*.

Keywords: *Ligularia* Cass., chloroplast genome, identification, super-barcode, Illumina sequencing

INTRODUCTION

Ligularia Cass., belonging to the Senecioneae tribe of Asteraceae, comprises about 140 species of perennial herbs. These species are distributed in Asia and Europe, with a total of 123 species distributed in China, 89 of which are endemic (Liu and Illarionova, 1989). In China, *Ligularia* species are mainly distributed in mountainous areas in the southwest (Liu and Illarionova, 1989) and more than 30 *Ligularia* species have long been used in folk medicine (Wang, 2007). The roots, stems, leaves, and flowers of them contain various chemical compounds, such as

---

Abbreviations: IR, inverted repeat; LSC, large single-copy; ML, maximum likelihood; SSC, small single-copy; SSRs, simple sequence repeats.

sesquiterpenes (Wang, 2007; Shimizu et al., 2014; Saito et al., 2017) and alkaloids (Asada et al., 1981; Feng, 2016). They are used as herbal medicines for the treatment of bronchitis, coughing, pulmonary tuberculosis, and hemoptysis. These herbal medicines are usually used as substitutes for Asteris Radix et Rhizoma which originates from *Aster tataricus* L. and is recorded in the Chinese Pharmacopoeia (Lin and Liu, 1989; Chinese Pharmacopoeia Commission, 2015). Approximately, 3% of flowering plants (as many as 6,000 species), including *Ligularia* species (Smith and Culvenor, 1981; Stegelmeier et al., 1999), contain pyrrolizidine alkaloids (PAs). It has been reported that various *Ligularia* species contain PAs, including *L. japonica* (Asada et al., 1981), *L. wilsoniana* (Xiong et al., 2016), *L. duciformis*, *L. intermedia*, *L. hodgsonii*, and *L. veitchiana* (Pu et al., 2004). PAs are phytoalexins that function in plant defense systems against herbivores, insects, and plant pathogens. However, they are harmful to human and animal health (Jank and Rath, 2017; Martinello et al., 2017), as they are involved in metabolic toxification in the liver caused by PA poisoning (Bull et al., 1968; Prakash et al., 1999). The German Federal Department of Health stated that the safe total daily dose of PA is less than 1 μg, and doctors do not allow continuous administration of drugs with PA for more than 6 weeks. In addition, all PA-containing products are banned in Australia (Wiedenfeld and Edgar, 2011).

Ligularia has been traditionally classified based on morphological structures, such as the arrangement of inflorescences, leaf shape, leaf veins, and phyllaries (Liu and Illarionova, 1989). Interspecific hybridization of *Ligularia* species is common and their morphological variation is complicated (Hanai et al., 2012; Yu et al., 2014; Saito et al., 2017), making it difficult to correctly identify species. Common DNA barcoding sequences (ITS, *matK*, *psbA-trnH*, and *rbcL*) are also not ideal for identifying *Ligularia* species (He and Pan, 2015). Recently, researchers have screened sequences from the whole chloroplast (CP) genome from numerous plant taxa, such as *Juglans* L. plants and bamboo (Zhang et al., 2011; Hu et al., 2016), or use CP genome as a super-barcode to distinguish species (Xia et al., 2016). The CP genome is highly conserved in plants regardless of the size, structure, or gene content (Tonti-Filippini et al., 2017), and the majority of the retained core genes are involved in the light reactions of photosynthesis or in functions related to transcription or translation (Sato et al., 1999). The CP genome map is a circular DNA molecule that includes a SSC region, a LSC region, and two inverted-repeat (IRa and IRb) regions (Sato et al., 1999). Several CP genomes from Asteraceae have previously been reported, including CP genomes from *Aster* (Choi and Park, 2015), *Ambrosia* (Nagy et al., 2017), *Carthanus* (Lu et al., 2015), and *Taraxacum* (Salih et al., 2017). However, only one CP genome from *Ligularia*, for *L. fischeri*, has previously been published (Lee et al., 2016). In this study, we report the CP genomes of six *Ligularia* species, *L. intermedia*, *L. jaluensis*, *L. mongolica*, *L. hodgsonii*, *L. veitchiana*, and *L. fischeri*, obtained through high-performance Illumina sequencing technology. Our aim is to use the CP genome as a super-barcode for the identification of *Ligularia* species to provide invaluable genetic information for future studies.

MATERIALS AND METHODS

Plant Materials and DNA Extraction

Fresh leaves of *L. intermedia* and *L. fischeri* were collected from Baishan City and Tonghua City, Jilin Province, China, respectively. Fresh leaves of *L. jaluensis* and *L. mongolica* were collected from Yanbian Korean Autonomous Prefecture, Jilin Province. These four species were identified by Prof. Junlin Yu from Tonghua Normal University, Jilin. Fresh leaves of *L. hodgsonii* and *L. veitchiana* were collected from Enshi Tujia and Miao Autonomous Prefecture, Hubei Province, and the Qinling Mountains, Shaanxi Province, respectively. These two samples were identified by Prof. Yulin Lin from the Institute of Medicinal Plant Development (IMPLAD), Chinese Academy of Medical Sciences (CAMS), and Peking Union Medical College (PUMC). The exact GPS coordinates for the collection locations of six *Ligularia* species are listed in Supplementary Table S1. Voucher specimens were deposited in the herbarium at IMPLAD. Collected fresh leaves were stored in a −80°C freezer until further use. DNA extraction was performed using a DNeasy Plant Mini Kit (Qiagen Co., Germany) following the manufacturer's protocol.

Illumina Sequencing and Genome Assembly

Approximately 5–10 μg of high-quality DNA were used to build shotgun libraries with insert sizes of 500 bp and were sequenced in accordance with the protocol for Illumina Hiseq X technology. The total raw data of the six species were produced with 150 bp paired-end read lengths. The software Trimmomatic (Bolger et al., 2014) was employed to filter low-quality reads from the raw data. After filtering for quality sequences, the remaining clean reads were used to assemble the CP genome sequences. The CP sequences of all plants downloaded from the National Center for Biotechnology Information (NCBI) were used to create a reference database. Then, the clean sequences were mapped to the database and the mapped reads were extracted on the basis of coverage and similarity. The extracted reads were assembled into contigs using SOAPdenovo2 (Luo et al., 2012). The scaffold of the CP genome was constructed using SSPACE (Boetzer et al., 2011), and the gaps were filled using GapFiller (Boetzer and Pirovano, 2012).

Validation, Annotation, and Sequence Submission

The accuracy of the assembly of the four boundaries (SSC, LSC, IRa, and IRb regions) of the CP sequences was confirmed through PCR and Sanger sequencing using validated primers (Supplementary Table S2). The thermocycler conditions for the PCR were as follows: 94°C for 5 min; 94°C for 30 s, 56°C for 30 s, 72°C for 1.5 min, and 32 cycles; 72°C for 10 min. The online programs Dual Organellar GenoMe Annotator (DOGMA) (Wyman et al., 2004) and CPGAVAS (Liu et al., 2012) were used for the initial annotation of the CP genomes of the six species, followed by manual correction. The complete data from the study were submitted to NCBI under the BioProject ID PRJNA400300 and BioSample ID SAMN07562669. The assembled complete CP genome sequences of the six *Ligularia* species were submitted to NCBI GenBank with the accession numbers MF539929-MF539933, and MG729822.

Genome Structure Analysis

The software tRNAscan-SE (Schattner et al., 2005) and DOGMA (Wyman et al., 2004) were used to identify tRNA genes. Gene maps were generated using Organellar Genome DRAW v1.2 (Lohse et al., 2007) with default settings and then the gene maps

were checked manually. MEGA 6.0 was used to calculate the GC content (Tamura et al., 2013). REPuter (University of Bielefeld, Bielefeld, Germany) (Kurtz et al., 2001) was used to identify the size and location of repeat sequences in the CP genomes of the six *Ligularia* species. We used the MISA software Misa-Microsatellite Identification Tool, 2017[1] to detect SSRs with the parameter settings the same as those described in Li et al. (2013). All the repeated sequences were manual verified and excess data

[1]http://pgrc.ipk-gatersleben.de/misa/

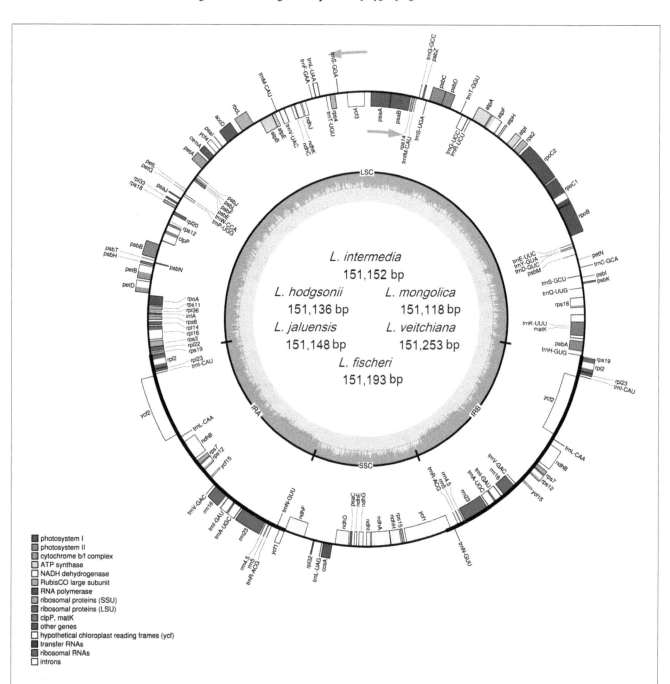

FIGURE 1 | Gene map of the complete CP genomes of the six *Ligularia* species. Genes on the inside of the circle are transcribed clockwise, while those outside are transcribed counter clockwise. The darker gray in the inner circle corresponds to GC content, whereas the lighter gray corresponds to AT content.

TABLE 1 | Summary statistics for assembly of the six CP genomes of *Ligularia* species.

Species names	*L. intermedia*	*L. hodgsonii*	*L. jaluensis*	*L. mongolica*	*L. veitchiana*	*L. fischeri*
Raw reads	53,871,796	42,199,336	43,781,502	37,478,124	36,990,248	36,684,984
Clean reads	52,907,406	41,086,606	42,940,766	36,283,722	35,813,466	35,451,926
Mapped CP reads	434,480	623,388	516,254	378,838	278,424	361,650
Size (bp)	151,152	151,136	151,148	151,118	151,253	151,193
LSC length (bp)	83,258	83,253	83,263	83,244	83,330	83,301
SSC length (bp)	18,232	18,217	18,225	18,214	18,247	18,232
IR length (bp)	24,831	24,833	24,830	24,830	24,838	24,830
Coding (bp)	90,247	90,253	90,247	90,250	90,253	90,247
Non-coding (bp)	60,905	60,883	60,901	60,868	60,000	60,946

TABLE 2 | List of genes found in the six CP genomes of *Ligularia* species.

No.	Group of genes	Gene names	Amount
1	Photosystem I	*psaA, psaB, psaC, psaI, psaJ*	5
2	Photosystem II	*psbA, psbB, psbC, psbD, psbE, psbF, psbH, psbI, psbJ, psbK, psbL, psbM, psbN, psbT, psbZ*	15
3	Cytochrome b/f complex	*petA, petB*, petD*, petG, petL, petN*	6
4	ATP synthase	*atpA, atpB, atpE, atpF*, atpH, atpI*	6
5	NADH dehydrogenase	*ndhA*, ndhB* (×2), ndhC, ndhD, ndhE, ndhF, ndhG, ndhH, ndhI, ndhJ, ndhK*	11
6	RubisCO large subunit	*rbcL*	1
7	RNA polymerase	*rpoA, rpoB, rpoC1*, rpoC2*	4
8	Ribosomal proteins (SSU)	*rps2, rps3, rps4, rps7 (×2), rps8, rps11, rps12** (×2), rps14, rps15, rps16*, rps18, rps19*	12
9	Ribosomal proteins (LSU)	*rpl2* (×2), rpl14, rpl16*, rpl20, rpl22, rpl23 (×2), rpl32, rpl33, rpl36*	9
10	Other genes	*accD, clpP**, matK, ccsA, cemA, infA*	6
11	Proteins of unknown function	*ycf1, ycf2 (×2), ycf3**, ycf4, ycf15*	5
12	Transfer RNAs	*37 tRNAs (6 contain an intron, 7 in the IRs)*	
13	Ribosomal RNAs	*rrn4.5 (×2), rrn5 (×2), rrn16 (×2), rrn23 (×2)*	

One or two asterisks after genes indicate that gene contains one or two introns, respectively.

were removed. The distribution of codon usage was studied using CodonW with the relative synonymous codon usage (RSCU) ratio (Sharp and Li, 1987). The online program Predictive RNA Editor for Plants suite (Mower, 2009) with a cutoff value of 0.8 were used to predict RNA editing sites in the six CP genomes of *Ligularia* species.

Phylogenetic Analysis

For identification purposes and to further phylogenetic research on this genus, we used mVISTA (Thompson et al., 1994) to compare six *Ligularia* species with *L. hodgsonii* as the reference genome. MEGA 6.0 was used to construct the phylogenetic tree with *Platycodon grandiflorus* and *Adenophora remotiflora* included as outgroups based on ML analysis. The details of the selected species (excluding the six *Ligularia* species) are presented in Supplementary Table S3.

RESULTS AND DISCUSSION

CP Genome Structure of Six *Ligularia* Species

The raw data from the six *Ligularia* species is 9.1 Gb for *L. intermedia*, 7.2 Gb for *L. hodgsonii*, 7.4 Gb for *L. jaluensis*, 6.4 Gb for *L. mongolica*, 6.3 Gb for *L. veitchiana*, and 6.2 Gb for

L. fischeri. The sizes of the six CP genomes range from 151,118 bp for *L. mongolica* to 151,253 bp for *L. veitchiana*, which are similar to other Asteraceae CP genomes (Liu et al., 2013; Salih et al., 2017; Wang et al., 2017; Zhang et al., 2017). The investigated genomes showed typical circular tetramerous structure, including an SSC region and an LSC region, separated by two IR regions (**Figure 1**). The corresponding lengths of the four regions from the six species are similar: the SSC lengths range from 18,214 to 18,247 bp, the LSC lengths range from 83,244 to 83,330 bp, and the IR lengths range from 24,830 to 24,838 bp (**Table 1**). The size of the previously published *L. fischeri* CP genome is 151,133 bp, and included an SSC region (18,233 bp), an LSC region (83,238 bp), and two IR regions (24,831 bp apart) (Lee et al., 2016). Our results showed that all six of the newly sequenced CP genomes have a GC content of 37.5%, which is lower than some Asteraceae species (Liu et al., 2013; Salih et al., 2017; Wang et al., 2017; Zhang et al., 2017). The GC content of four homologous regions of the six CP genomes is the same. However, the distribution of the GC content in each region is uneven. The GC content in the IR region is the largest (43.0%), followed by the LSC region (35.6%), and the region with the lowest GC content is the SSC region (30.7%). Our analysis showed that the high GC content in the IR region is attributed to four rRNA genes (*rrn16, rrn23, rrn4.5,* and *rrn5*). The AT content of the first, second, and third position of protein-coding genes in the six CP genomes are 54.5–54.6%, 61.9–62.0%,

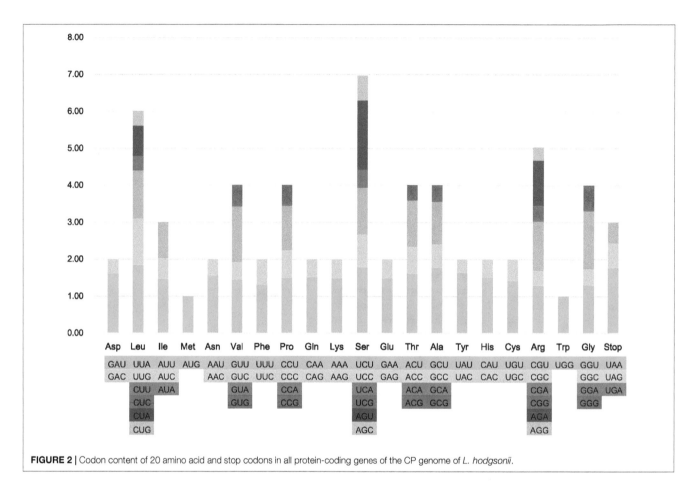

FIGURE 2 | Codon content of 20 amino acid and stop codons in all protein-coding genes of the CP genome of *L. hodgsonii.*

and 70.1%, respectively. The higher AT content in the third site has also been observed in other plants (Yi and Kim, 2012; He et al., 2017; Zhou et al., 2017) and is usually used to distinguish DNA of CP, nucleus, and mitochondria origin (Clegg et al., 1994).

Each of the six CP genomes contains 134 genes, including 87 protein-coding genes, 37 tRNA genes, eight rRNA genes, and two pseudogenes (*ycf1* and *rps19*; **Table 2**). Seven protein-coding genes (*ndhB, rp12, rp123, rps12, rps7, ycf15,* and *ycf2*), seven tRNAs (*trnA-UGC, trnI-CAU, trnI-GAU, trnL-CAA, trnN-GUU, trnR-ACG,* and *trnV-GAC*), and all of the rRNAs (*rrn16, rrn23, rrn4.5,* and *rrn5*) are duplicated in the IR regions, which is similar to *Artemisia annua* (Shen et al., 2017) and *Artemisia frigida* (Liu et al., 2013). The CP genomes of the six *Ligularia* species contain a small 3.4 kb inversion within a large 23 kb inversion in the LSC region, which is a unique feature in Asteraceae (Kim et al., 2005; Liu et al., 2013). The LSC region included 62 protein-coding genes and 22 tRNA genes. The SSC region included 11 protein-coding genes and one tRNA gene (*trnL-UAG*). The CP genomes of each of these six *Ligularia* species did not have an inverted SSC region, which has also been found in the CP genomes of *A. frigida* (Liu et al., 2013), *Scutellaria baicalensis* (Jiang et al., 2017), *Carthamus tinctorius* (Lu et al., 2015), and *Juglans* L. (Hu et al., 2016). In contrast, the SSC regions of *Helianthus annuus, Lactuca sativa* (Timme et al., 2007), and *Aster spathulifolius* (Choi and Park, 2015) are inverted. The functional *ycf1* copy is located in the IRb-SSC boundary and the pseudogene *ycf1* copy is located

in the IRa region. The functional *rps19* copy is on the boundary of LSC and IRa and the pseudogene *rps19* copy is on the IRb region. The coding region occupied 59.67–59.72% of the CP genomes of six *Ligularia* species, including protein-coding genes, tRNA genes, and rRNA genes. Meanwhile, non-coding regions, including introns, pseudogenes, and intergenic spacers occupied 40.28–40.33% of the CP genomes of the six *Ligularia* species.

Codon Usage and RNA Editing Sites

All protein-coding genes in the six *Ligularia* CP genomes are composed of 26,136–26,138 codons. The most and least universal amino acids of the CP genomes of the six *Ligularia* species are leucine (10.8%) and cysteine (1.1%), respectively (**Figure 2**). This is also similar to the CP genome from artichoke (Curci et al., 2015). However, the most universal amino acid from *A. frigida* is isoleucine (Liu et al., 2013). The most and the least abundant amino acids in the *Taraxacum obtusifrons* and *Taraxacum amplum* CP genomes are serine and methionine (Salih et al., 2017), respectively. **Figure 2** shows that with the increase of specific amino acid codes the RSCU increases accordingly. Most of the amino acid codons have preferences, except for methionine and tryptophan. Potential RNA editing sites were predicted for 35 genes from the CP genomes of the six *Ligularia* species. Forty-eight RNA editing sites were identified. S to L of amino acid change appeared most frequently, while R to W and T to I occurred least. Each corresponding gene from

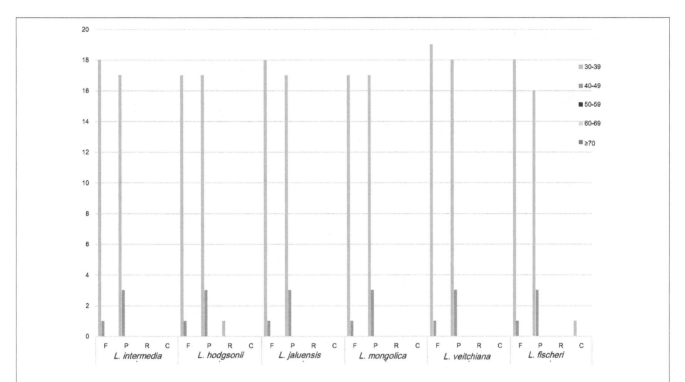

FIGURE 3 | Repeat sequences in six CP genomes. REPuter was used to identify repeat sequences with length ≥30 bp and sequences identified ≥90% in the CP genomes. F, P, R, and C indicate the repeat types F (forward), P (palindrome), R (reverse), and C (complement). Repeats with different lengths are indicated in different colors.

TABLE 3 | The SSR types of the six CP genomes of *Ligularia* species.

SSR type	Repeat unit	Amount					
		L. intermedia	*L. hodgsonii*	*L. jaluensis*	*L. mongolica*	*L. veitchiana*	*L. fischeri*
Mono	A/T	30	29	30	30	37	31
Di	AT/AT	7	6	7	6	7	7
Tri	AAG/CTT	2	2	2	2	2	2
Tri	AAT/ATT	2	2	2	2	3	2
Tri	ATC/ATG	1	1	1	1	1	1
Tetra	AAAG/CTTT	1	1	1	1	1	1
Tetra	AAAT/ATTT	6	6	6	6	6	6
Tetra	AACT/AGTT	1	1	1	1	1	1
Tetra	AATC/ATTG	1	1	1	1	1	1
Tetra	AATT/AATT	1	1	1	1	1	1
Tetra	AGAT/ATCT	1	1	1	1	1	1

the RNA editing sites of the six *Ligularia* species is at the same nucleotide position (Supplementary Table S4).

A total of 18 genes containing introns, including 12 protein-coding genes (*atpF, clpP, ndhA, ndhB, petB, petD, rpl16, rpl2, rpoC1, rps12, rps16*, and *ycf3*), and six tRNA genes (*trnA-UGC, trnG-UCC, trnI-GAU, trnK-UUU, trnL-UAA*, and *trnV-UAC*; Supplementary Table S5), were identified in this study. Nine protein-coding genes contain only one intron and three protein-coding genes (*clpP, rps12*, and *ycf3*) contain two introns. All six tRNAs contain only one intron. *TrnK-UUU* has the longest intron (2,556 bp), which contains *matK*. The *clpP* gene and *ycf3* gene are both located in the LSC region. The *rps12* gene is a

special trans-splicing gene with the 5′ exon located in the LSC region, but the 3′ exon located in the IR region. This condition exists in many species, such as *A. frigida* (Liu et al., 2013), artichoke (Curci et al., 2015), and *Aster spathulifolius* (Choi and Park, 2015).

Long Repeats and SSRs in the CP Genomes From the Six *Ligularia* Species

Repeat sequences, which are related to plastome organization (Salih et al., 2017), are mostly distributed in intergenic regions and intron regions, and only a small fraction is present in the

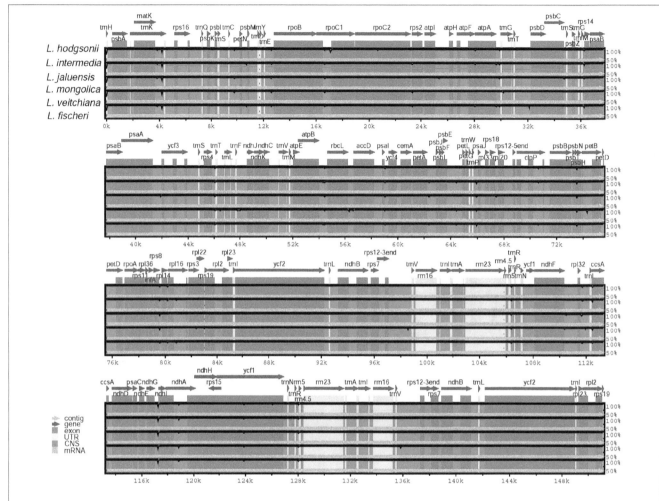

FIGURE 4 | Sequence identity plot comparing six CP genomes with *L. hodgsonii* as a reference using mVISTA. Gray arrows and thick black lines above the alignment indicate genes with their orientation and the position of the IRs, respectively. A cutoff of 70% identity was used for the plots, and the Y-scale represents the percent identity ranging from 50 to 100%.

genetic region. Four types of long repeats were observed in the CP genomes of the six *Ligularia* species, including forward, palindromic, reverse, and complement repeats (**Figure 3**). The length of the repeat unit ranged from 30 to 48 bp. *Ligularia intermedia* and *L. jaluensis* both had 19 forward and 20 palindromic repeats. *Ligularia hodgsonii* had the following repeats: 18 forward, 20 palindromic, and one reverse. *Ligularia mongolica* had 18 forward and 20 palindromic repeats. *Ligularia veitchiana* had 20 forward and 21 palindromic repeats. *Ligularia fischeri* had the following repeats: 19 forward, 19 palindromic, and one complement. The long repeat sequences observed in the CP genomes of the six *Ligularia* species, with *L. hodgsonii* as the reference, are presented in Supplementary Table S6.

Simple sequence repeats, also called microsatellites, exist widely in the genome, and the sequences consist of one to six nucleotide repeat units (Powell et al., 1995). SSRs are widely used in studies on species identification, population genetics, and phylogenetic studies based on polymorphisms (Yang et al., 2011; Jiao et al., 2012; Xue et al., 2012). Four types of SSRs were found in the CP genomes from the six

Ligularia species: mononucleotide (56.6–60.7%), dinucleotide (11.5–13.2%), trinucleotide (9.3–9.8%), and tetranucleotide (18.0–21.6%); the SSRs were mainly distributed in the non-coding region of the LSC and SSC. Of all these SSRs, the number of mononucleotide SSRs (A/T) is the largest, ranging from 29 in *L. hodgsonii* to 37 in *L. veitchiana*, enriching A and T in the CP genomes. The next most common SSR is dinucleotide (AT/AT), six dinucleotide SSRs in CP genomes of *L. hodgsonii* and *L. mongolica* and seven dinucleotide SSRs in other four CP genomes. All of the CP genomes from the six species have two trinucleotide AAG/CTT SSRs, one ATC/ATG trinucleotide SSR, and 11 tetranucleotide SSRs (**Table 3**). The CP genome of *L. veitchiana* has three AAT/ATT trinucleotide SSRs, while the other five species only have two trinucleotide SSRs.

Identification and Phylogenetic Analysis of *Ligularia* Species

The CP genomes from the six *Ligularia* species are highly similar. Among the few variations, non-coding regions exhibited higher

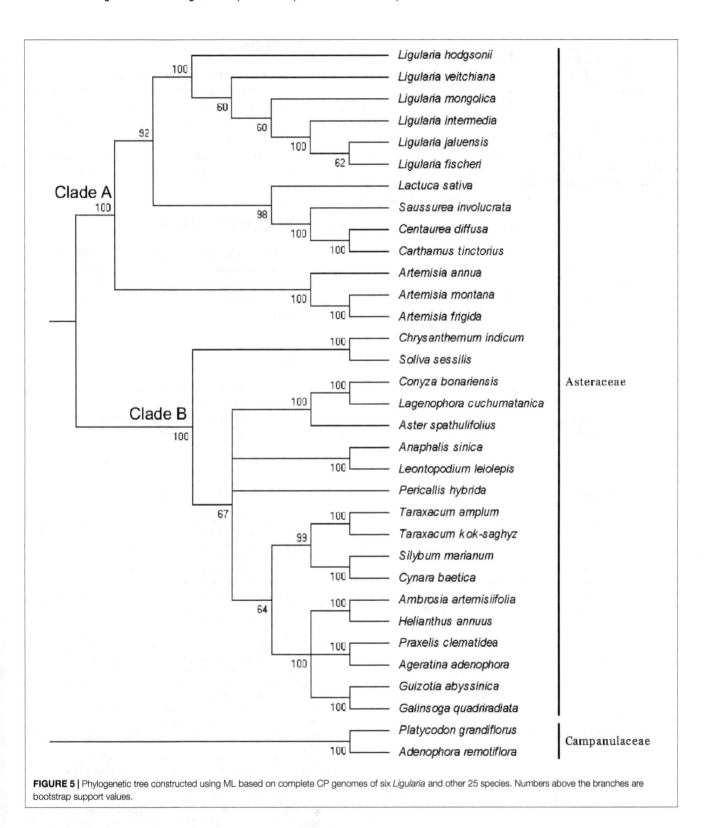

FIGURE 5 | Phylogenetic tree constructed using ML based on complete CP genomes of six *Ligularia* and other 25 species. Numbers above the branches are bootstrap support values.

levels of variability than the coding regions. The largest change in gene length occurred in pseudogene *ycf1*, with 5,097 bp in *L. mongolica*, 5,100 bp in *L. hodgsonii* and *L. veitchiana*, and 5,094 bp in the other three species. This difference led to a divergence in the length of the coding regions of the six species.

The IR regions of the six CP genomes are conservative regardless of the number and order of the genes. Previous research screened highly variable region from CP genomes as the potential DNA barcodes for authenticating species, such as *Dioscorea* (Ma et al., 2018) and *Fritillaria* species (Li et al., 2016).

Sequence homology was investigated compared with the reference CP genome from *L. hodgsonii* using the mVISTA software (**Figure 4**). Our results showed high similarity among all sequences. Differences were observed in the intergenic regions of *matK-trnK* and *ndhG-ndhI* (**Figure 4**). There was only one variable site in the *matK-trnK* region and five variable sites in *ndhG-ndhI* region, but this is not enough to distinguish among the six *Ligularia* species. Because of the highly conservative sequences, the structure, and size of the CP genomes of *Ligularia* species, no obvious hypervariable region was screened. Thus, the complete CP genomes were considered to distinguish *Ligularia* species.

In addition to the six CP genomes sequenced in this study, 25 other CP genomes from Asteraceae were chosen to construct the phylogenetic tree, and *P. grandiflorus* and *A. remotiflora* (Campanulaceae) were included as outgroups (**Figure 5**). In the ML tree, we identified two main clades (clade A and B) excluding outgroup species. Six species of *Ligularia* were a monophyly with well-supported (100%). The support values in clade A were not less than 60%, and *L. fischeri* and *L. jaluensis* have a close relationship. *Ligularia* is most closely related to *L. sativa*, *Saussurea involucrata*, *Centaurea diffusa*, and *Carthamus tinctorius*. The results showed that the CP genomes can be used to identify the six *Ligularia* species.

CONCLUSION

This study reported the CP genomes from six *Ligularia* species, and the structure and composition of the CP genomes are highly similar. Like most Asteraceae species, the CP genomes of the six *Ligularia* species had a small 3.4 kb inversion within a large 23 kb inversion in the LSC region. The ML tree showed that the CP genome can be used to identify the six *Ligularia* species and is expected to become a super-barcode for the identification of *Ligularia* species.

AUTHOR CONTRIBUTIONS

HY conceived the study and acquired the funding. XC, YW, and BD collected samples and conducted the experiment. JZ and YC performed the genome assembly and analysis on the data. XC and JZ wrote the manuscript. All authors have read and approved the final manuscript.

FUNDING

This work was supported by CAMS Innovation Fund for Medical Sciences (CIFMS) (No. 2016-I2M-3-016) and Major Scientific and Technological Special Project for "Significant New Drugs Creation" (No. 2014ZX09304307001).

REFERENCES

Asada, Y., Furuya, T., and Murakami, N. (1981). Pyrrolizidine alkaloids from *Ligularia japonica*. *Planta Med.* 42, 202–203. doi: 10.1055/s-2007-971628

Boetzer, M., Henkel, C. V., Jansen, H. J., Butler, D., and Pirovano, W. (2011). Scaffolding pre-assembled contigs using SSPACE. *Bioinformatics* 27, 578–579. doi: 10.1093/bioinformatics/btq683

Boetzer, M., and Pirovano, W. (2012). Toward almost closed genomes with GapFiller. *Genome Biol.* 13:R56. doi: 10.1186/gb-2012-13-6-r56

Bolger, A. M., Lohse, M., and Usadel, B. (2014). Trimmomatic: a flexible trimmer for Illumina sequence data. *Bioinformatics* 30, 2114–2120. doi: 10.1093/bioinformatics/btu170

Bull, L. B., Culvenor, C. C. J., and Dick, A. T. (1968). *The Pyrrolizidine Alkaloids*. Amsterdam: North Holland Publishing Co.

Chinese Pharmacopoeia Commission (2015). *Pharmacopoeia of the Peoples Republic of China*. China Medical. Ottawa: Science Press, 342–343.

Choi, K. S., and Park, S. (2015). The complete chloroplast genome sequence of *Aster spathulifolius* (Asteraceae); genomic features and relationship with Asteraceae. *Gene* 572, 214–221. doi: 10.1016/j.gene.2015.07.020

Clegg, M. T., Gaut, B. S., Learn, G. H., and Morton, B. R. (1994). Rates and patterns of chloroplast DNA evolution. *Proc. Natl. Acad. Sci. U.S.A.* 91, 6795–6801. doi: 10.1073/pnas.91.15.6795

Curci, P. L., De, P. D., Danzi, D., Vendramin, G. G., and Sonnante, G. (2015). Complete chloroplast genome of the multifunctional crop globe artichoke and comparison with other Asteraceae. *PLoS One* 10:e0120589. doi: 10.1371/journal. pone.0120589

Feng, K. (2016). *Analysis of Alkaloid Component and Toxicity Test in the Aerial Parts of Ligularia rumicifolia*. Ph.D. thesis, Northwest A&F University, Yangling.

Hanai, R., Yamada, H., Suzuki, Y., Nagano, H., Kawahara, T., Yu, J. J., et al. (2012). Chemical constituents of *Ligularia nelumbifolia* and *L. subspicata* hybrid

collected in Shangrila County, Yunnan province of China. *Nat. Prod. Commun.* 7, 1565–1568.

He, L., Qian, J., Li, X., Sun, Z., Xu, X., and Chen, S. (2017). Complete chloroplast genome of medicinal plant *Lonicera japonica*: genome rearrangement, intron gain and loss, and implications for phylogenetic studies. *Molecules* 22, 249–260. doi: 10.3390/molecules22020249

He, W., and Pan, Y. (2015). Study on the DNA barcoding of genus *Ligularia* Cass.(*Asteraceae*). *Plant Divers.* 37, 693–703.

Hu, Y., Woeste, K. E., and Zhao, P. (2016). Completion of the chloroplast genomes of five Chinese *juglans* and their contribution to chloroplast phylogeny. *Front. Plant Sci.* 7:1955. doi: 10.3389/fpls.2016.01955

Jank, B., and Rath, J. (2017). The risk of pyrrolizidine alkaloids in human food and animal feed. *Trends Plant Sci.* 22, 191–193. doi: 10.1016/j.tplants.2017.01.002

Jiang, D., Zhao, Z., Zhang, T., Zhong, W., Liu, C., Yuan, Q., et al. (2017). The chloroplast genome sequence of *Scutellaria baicalensis* provides insight into intraspecific and interspecific chloroplast genome diversity in *Scutellaria*. *Genes* 8:E227. doi: 10.3390/genes8090227

Jiao, Y., Jia, H., Li, X., Chai, M., Jia, H., Chen, Z., et al. (2012). Development of simple sequence repeat (SSR) markers from a genome survey of Chinese bayberry (*Myrica rubra*). *BMC Genomics* 13:201. doi: 10.1186/1471-2164-13-201

Kim, K. J., Choi, K. S., and Jansen, R. K. (2005). Two chloroplast DNA inversions originated simultaneously during the early evolution of the sunflower family (Asteraceae). *Mol. Biol. Evol.* 22, 1783–1792. doi: 10.1093/molbev/msi174

Kurtz, S., Choudhuri, J. V., Ohlebusch, E., Schleiermacher, C., Stoye, J., and Giegerich, R. (2001). Reputer: the manifold applications of repeat analysis on a genomic scale. *Nucleic Acids Res.* 29, 4633–4642. doi: 10.1093/nar/29.22.4633

Lee, J., Lee, H., Lee, S. C., Sang, H. S., Kang, J. H., Lee, T. J., et al. (2016). The complete chloroplast genome sequence of *Ligularia fischeri* (Ledeb.) Turcz. (Asteraceae). *Mitochondrial DNA B* 1, 4–5. doi: 10.1080/23802359.2015.1137793

Li, X., Gao, H., Wang, Y., Song, J., Henry, R., Wu, H., et al. (2013). Complete chloroplast genome sequence of *Magnolia grandiflora* and comparative analysis with related species. *Sci. China Life Sci.* 56, 189–198. doi: 10.1007/s11427-012-4430-8

Li, Y., Yao, H., Song, J., Ren, F., Li, X., and Sun, C. (2016). Screening Fritillaria genus-specific DNA barcodes based on complete chloroplast genome sequences. *Mod. Tradit. Chin. Med. Mater. Med. World Sci. Technol.* 18, 24–28. doi: 10.11842/wst.2016.01.004

Lin, R., and Liu, S. (1989). *Flora Reipublicea Popularis Sinicae*. Ottawa: Science Press, 4–13.

Liu, C., Shi, L., Zhu, Y., Chen, H., Zhang, J., Lin, X., et al. (2012). CpGAVAS, an integrated web server for the annotation, visualization, analysis, and GenBank submission of completely sequenced chloroplast genome sequences. *BMC Genomics* 13:715. doi: 10.1186/1471-2164-13-715

Liu, S., and Illarionova, I. D. (1989). *Flora of China*. Ottawa: Science Press, 20–21.

Liu, Y., Huo, N., Dong, L., Wang, Y., Zhang, S., Young, H. A., et al. (2013). Complete chloroplast genome sequences of Mongolia medicine *Artemisia frigida* and phylogenetic relationships with other plants. *PLoS One* 8:e57533. doi: 10.1371/journal.pone.0057533

Lohse, M., Drechsel, O., and Bock, R. (2007). OrganellarGenomeDRAW (OGDRAW): a tool for the easy generation of high-quality custom graphical maps of plastid and mitochondrial genomes. *Curr. Genet.* 52, 267–274. doi: 10.1007/s00294-007-0161-y

Lu, C., Shen, Q., Yang, J., Wang, B., and Song, C. (2015). The complete chloroplast genome sequence of safflower (*Carthamus tinctorius* L.). *Mitochondrial DNA* 27, 1–3. doi: 10.3109/19401736.2015.1018217

Luo, R., Liu, B., Xie, Y., Li, Z., Huang, W., Yuan, J., et al. (2012). SOAPdenovo2: an empirically improved memory-efficient short-read de novo assembler. *Gigascience* 1, 18–23. doi: 10.1186/2047-217X-1-18

Ma, S., Zhou, J., Li, Y., Chen, X., Wu, M., Sun, W., et al. (2018). Study on complete chloroplast genome of *Dioscorea* opposite and *D. collettii* and screening specific DNA barcodes (in Chinese). *Sci. China Life Sci.* 2018, 48–59. doi: 10.1360/N052017-00160

Martinello, M., Borin, A., Stella, R., Bovo, D., Biancotto, G., Gallina, A., et al. (2017). Development and validation of a QuEChERS method coupled to liquid chromatography and high resolution mass spectrometry to determine pyrrolizidine and tropane alkaloids in honey. *Food Chem* 295–302. doi: 10.1016/j.foodchem.2017.04.186

Misa-Microsatellite Identification Tool (2017). Available at: http://pgrc.ipk-gatersleben.de/misa/ [accessed 16 September 2017]

Mower, J. P. (2009). The PREP suite: predictive RNA editors for plant mitochondrial genes, chloroplast genes and user-defined alignments. *Nucleic Acids Res.* 37, 253–259. doi: 10.1093/nar/gkp337

Nagy, E., Hegedûs, G., Taller, J., Kutasy, B., and Virág, E. (2017). Illumina sequencing of the chloroplast genome of common ragweed (*Ambrosia artemisiifolia* L.). *Data Brief.* 15, 606–611. doi: 10.1016/j.dib.2017.10.009

Powell, W., Morgante, M., Mcdevitt, R., Vendramin, G. G., and Rafalski, J. A. (1995). Polymorphic simple sequence repeat regions in chloroplast genomes: applications to the population genetics of pines. *Proc. Natl. Acad. Sci. U.S.A.* 92, 7759–7763. doi: 10.1073/pnas.92.17.7759

Prakash, A. S., Pereira, T. N., Reilly, P. E., and Seawright, A. A. (1999). Pyrrolizidine alkaloids in human diet. *Mutat. Res.* 443, 53–67. doi: 10.1016/S1383-5742(99)00010-1

Pu, S., Xu, D., Zhang, M., Zhou, H., Wang, Z., and Yu, G. (2004). Detection of hepatotoxic pyrrolizidine alkaloids in Ligularia Cass. with LC/MSn. *Acta Pham. Sin.* 39, 831–835. doi: 10.3321/j.issn:0513-4870.2004.10.014

Saito, Y., Ichihara, M., Takashima, Y., Okamoto, Y., Gong, X., Hanai, R., et al. (2017). Chemical constituents of hybrids of *Ligularia cyathiceps* and *L. lamarum*/*L. subspicata* collected in china: structures of subspicatins M, N, O₁, and O₂, and related compounds. *Phytochemistry* 140, 69–76. doi: 10.1016/j.phytochem.2017.04.015

Salih, R. H. M., Majeský, Ľ., Schwarzacher, T., Gornall, R., and Heslop-Harrison, P. (2017). Complete chloroplast genomes from apomictic *Taraxacum* (Asteraceae): identity and variation between three microspecies. *PLoS One* 12:e0168008. doi: 10.1371/journal.pone.0168008

Sato, S., Nakamura, Y., Kaneko, T., Asamizu, E., and Tabata, S. (1999). Complete structure of the chloroplast genome of *Arabidopsis thaliana*. *DNA Res.* 6, 283–290. doi: 10.1093/dnares/6.5.283

Schattner, P., Brooks, A. N., and Lowe, T. M. (2005). The tRNAscan-SE, snoscan and snoGPS web servers for the detection of tRNAs and snoRNAs. *Nucleic Acids Res.* 33, 686–689. doi: 10.1093/nar/gki366

Sharp, P. M., and Li, W. H. (1987). The codon Adaptation Index–a measure of directional synonymous codon usage bias, and its potential applications. *Nucleic Acids Res.* 15, 1281–1295. doi: 10.1093/nar/15.3.1281

Shen, X., Wu, M., Liao, B., Liu, Z., Bai, R., Xiao, S., et al. (2017). Complete chloroplast genome sequence and phylogenetic analysis of the medicinal plant *Artemisia annua*. *Molecules* 22, 1330–1343. doi: 10.3390/molecules2208 1330

Shimizu, A., Suzuki, Y., Hanai, R., Okamoto, Y., Tori, M., Gong, X., et al. (2014). Chemical and genetic similarity and diversity of *Ligularia anoleuca* and *L. fischeri* collected in the Hengduan Mountains of China. *Phytochemistry* 102, 137–144. doi: 10.1016/j.phytochem.2014.03.019

Smith, L. W., and Culvenor, C. C. J. (1981). Plant sources of hepatotoxic pyrrolizidine alkaloids. *J. Nat. Prod.* 44, 129–152. doi: 10.1021/np50014a001

Stegelmeier, B. L., Edgar, J. A., Colegate, S. M., Gardner, D. L., Schoch, T. K., Coulombe, R. A., et al. (1999). Pyrrolizidine alkaloids plants, metabolism and toxicity. *J. Nat. Toxins* 8, 95–116.

Tamura, K., Stecher, G., Peterson, D., Filipski, A., and Kumar, S. (2013). MEGA6: molecular evolutionary genetics analysis version 6.0. *Mol. Biol. Evol.* 30, 2725–2729. doi: 10.1093/molbev/mst197

Thompson, J. D., Higgins, D. G., and Gibson, T. J. (1994). CLUSTAL W: improving the sensitivity of progressive multiple sequence alignment through sequence weighting, position-specific gap penalties and weight matrix choice. *Nucleic Acids Res.* 22, 4673–4680. doi: 10.1093/nar/22.22.4673

Timme, R., Kuehl, J., Boore, J., and Jansen, R. (2007). A comparative analysis of the *Lactuca* and *Helianthus* (Asteraceae) plastid genomes: Identification of divergent regions and categorization of shared repeats. *Am. J. Bot.* 94, 302–312. doi: 10.3732/ajb.94.3.302

Tonti-Filippini, J., Nevill, P. G., Dixon, K., and Small, I. (2017). What can we do with 1000 plastid genomes? *Plant J.* 90, 808–818. doi: 10.1111/tpj.13491

Wang, Q. (2007). *Cytotoxic Chemical Constituents of Three Ligularia Medicinal Plants*. Ph. D. thesis, Fudan University, Shanghai.

Wang, X., Zhou, Z., Liu, G., and Qian, Z. (2017). Characterization of the complete chloroplast genome of the invasive weed *Galinsoga quadriradiata*, (Asterales: Asteraceae). *Conserv. Genet. Resour.* 10, 89–92. doi: 10.1007/s12686-017-0771-8

Wiedenfeld, H., and Edgar, J. (2011). Toxicity of pyrrolizidine alkaloids to humans and ruminants. *Phytochem. Rev.* 10, 137–151. doi: 10.1007/s11101-010-9174-0

Wyman, S. K., Jansen, R. K., and Boore, J. L. (2004). Automatic annotation of organellar genomes with DOGMA. *Bioinformatics* 20, 3252–3255. doi: 10.1093/bioinformatics/bth352

Xia, Y., Hu, Z., Li, X., Wang, P., Zhang, X., Li, Q., et al. (2016). The complete chloroplast genome sequence of *Chrysanthemum indicum*. *Mitochondrial DNA A* 27, 4668–4669. doi: 10.3109/19401736.2015.1106494

Xiong, A., Yan, A. L., Bi, C. W., Lam, K. Y., Chan, G. K., Lau, K. K., et al. (2016). Clivorine, an otonecine pyrrolizidine alkaloid from *Ligularia* species, impairs neuronal differentiation via NGF-induced signaling pathway in cultured PC12 cells. *Phytomedicine* 23, 931–938. doi: 10.1016/j.phymed.2016.06.006

Xue, J., Wang, S., and Zhou, S. (2012). Polymorphic chloroplast microsatellite loci in *Nelumbo* (Nelumbonaceae). *Am. J. Bot.* 99, 240–244. doi: 10.3732/ajb.1100547

Yang, A., Zhang, J., Yao, X., and Huang, H. (2011). Chloroplast microsatellite markers in *Liriodendron tulipifera* (Magnoliaceae) and cross-species amplification in *L. chinense*. *Am. J. Bot.* 98, e123–e126. doi: 10.3732/ajb.1000532

Yi, D. K., and Kim, K. J. (2012). Complete chloroplast genome sequences of important oilseed crop *Sesamum indicum* L. *PLoS One* 7:e35872. doi: 10.1371/journal.pone.0035872

Yu, J., Kuroda, C., and Gong, X. (2014). Natural hybridization and introgression between *Ligularia cymbulifera* and *L. tongolensis* (Asteraceae, Senecioneae) in four different locations. *PLoS One* 9:e115167. doi: 10.1371/journal.pone. 0115167

Zhang, Y., Iaffaldano, B. J., Zhuang, X., Cardina, J., and Cornish, K. (2017). Chloroplast genome resources and molecular markers differentiate rubber dandelion species from weedy relatives. *BMC Plant Biol.* 17:34. doi: 10.1186/ s12870-016-0967-1

Zhang, Y., Ma, P., and Li, D. (2011). High-throughput sequencing of six bamboo chloroplast genomes: phylogenetic implications for temperate woody bamboos (Poaceae: Bambusoideae). *PLoS One* 6:e20596. doi: 10.1371/journal.pone. 0020596

Zhou, J., Chen, X., Cui, Y., Sun, W., Li, Y., Wang, Y., et al. (2017). Molecular structure and phylogenetic analyses of complete chloroplast genomes of two *Aristolochia* medicinal species. *Int. J. Mol. Sci.* 18, 1839–1853. doi: 10.3390/ ijms18091839

20

Phylogenomic Approaches to DNA Barcoding of Herbal Medicines: Developing Clade-Specific Diagnostic Characters for *Berberis*

Marco Kreuzer[1]*, Caroline Howard[2], Bhaskar Adhikari[3], Colin A. Pendry[3] and Julie A. Hawkins[1]

[1] *School of Biological Sciences, University of Reading, Reading, United Kingdom,* [2] *BP-NIBSC Herbal Laboratory, National Institute for Biological Standards and Control, Potters Bar, United Kingdom,* [3] *Royal Botanic Garden Edinburgh, Edinburgh, United Kingdom*

*Correspondence:
Marco Kreuzer
marco.c.kreuzer@gmail.com

DNA barcoding of herbal medicines has been mainly concerned with authentication of products in trade and has raised awareness of species substitution and adulteration. More recently DNA barcodes have been included in pharmacopoeias, providing tools for regulatory purposes. The commonly used DNA barcoding regions in plants often fail to resolve identification to species level. This can be especially challenging in evolutionarily complex groups where incipient or reticulate speciation is ongoing. In this study, we take a phylogenomic approach, analyzing whole plastid sequences from the evolutionarily complex genus *Berberis* in order to develop DNA barcodes for the medicinally important species *Berberis aristata*. The phylogeny reconstructed from an alignment of ~160 kbp of chloroplast DNA for 57 species reveals that the pharmacopoeial species in question is polyphyletic, complicating development of a species-specific DNA barcode. Instead we propose a DNA barcode that is clade specific, using our phylogeny to define Operational Phylogenetic Units (OPUs). The plastid alignment is then reduced to small, informative DNA regions including nucleotides diagnostic for these OPUs. These DNA barcodes were tested on commercial samples, and shown to discriminate plants in trade and therefore to meet the requirement of a pharmacopoeial standard. The proposed method provides an innovative approach for inferring DNA barcodes for evolutionarily complex groups for regulatory purposes and quality control.

Keywords: DNA barcoding, next-generation sequencing, operational phylogenetic units, herbal medicines, *Berberis*, pharmacopoeia, pharmacopoeial standards, plastome

INTRODUCTION

DNA barcoding has two major objectives: specimen identification, where an unknown sequence is matched to a sequence of a known species, and species discovery, which is equivalent to species delimitation and species description (DeSalle, 2006). DNA barcoding of herbal medicines is mainly concerned with authentication, the identification of specimens for quality assurance (Sgamma et al., 2017). In the last decade, DNA barcoding of herbal medicines has raised awareness of species substitution and adulteration, highlighting issues surrounding the quality of herbal medicines in the global market (Newmaster et al., 2013; Srirama et al., 2017). Regulation of herbal medicines is a pressing issue for regulatory agencies (Directive 2001/83/Ec, 2001; Directive 2004/83/EC, 2004; Vlietinck et al., 2009). Published pharmacopoeial standards for authentication predominantly rely on chemical and anatomical methods (e.g., British Pharmacopoeia, 2016), but DNA barcoding offers new tools for regulatory purposes (de Boer et al., 2015) and DNA barcodes have recently been incorporated into the British Pharmacopoeia for the first time (British Pharmacopoeia Commission, 2017). Here we investigate opportunities and limitations of DNA barcoding using next-generation sequence data of an evolutionarily complex genus. The aim is to design new methodological approaches for producing DNA barcodes for regulatory purposes, pharmacovigilance and quality assurance.

To date, the British Pharmacopoeia has approved 6 annotated DNA barcodes for the individual identification of the following species: *Anethum graveolens* Sowa (ITS2); *Glehnia littoralis* (ITS2); *Ocimum tenuiflorum* (trnH-psbA); *Myristica fragrans* (trnH-psbA); *Phellodendron amurense* (trnH-psbA); and *Phellodendron chinense* (trnH-psbA). The British Pharmacopoeia Commission (2017) have also published guidelines for the use of these barcodes, guiding users through the extraction of DNA, amplification of barcode markers, sequencing and comparison to pharmacopoeial standards. This development of bespoke barcode markers for different species is an approach likely to continue since there is no single, universal DNA barcode for land plants (Hollingsworth et al., 2011). For taxonomic purposes, several propositions have been made (e.g., Kress et al., 2005; Chase et al., 2007; CBOL Plant Working Group et al., 2009). Following Hollingsworth et al. (2011), most studies use a combination of the plastid regions *matK*, *rbcL*, the intergenic spacer *trnH-psbA* and the nuclear ITS2. Advances in sequencing technology have encouraged the barcoding community to augment the standard barcoding approach (Kane et al., 2012; Vaughn et al., 2014; Coissac et al., 2016; Zhang et al., 2017). In the era of next-generation sequencing, some researchers have even argued for the use of whole plastid genomes as barcodes (Kane et al., 2012; Vaughn et al., 2014; Coissac et al., 2016; Zhang et al., 2017; Manzanilla et al., 2018). How whole plastid genomes might be best deployed for pharmacopoeial purposes has hardly been explored yet.

Methodological approaches for specimen identification using DNA barcodes commonly rely on either distance-based measures or phylogenetic methods (Austerlitz et al., 2009). The former are based on the assumption that intra- and interspecific variation do not overlap (e.g., Hebert et al., 2004), also referred to as the barcoding gap (Meyer and Paulay, 2005). Accurate specimen identification using distance-based approaches such as BLAST are highly dependent on a well-curated database in which all members of a group are ideally represented by several individuals (Meyer and Paulay, 2005). The drawbacks of using distance-based approaches are that there is no objective distance threshold criterion and that the nearest neighbor is not always the closest relative (Moritz and Cicero, 2004). Specimen identification using phylogenetic methods is based on membership of a query sequence to a specific clade

(Casiraghi et al., 2010). One difficulty associated with using tree-based barcoding methods is that phylogenies inferred from the barcode sequence might not be resolved sufficiently for an individual to be allocated to a clade, and that clades may exhibit poor support, questioning the robustness of any phylogenetic hypothesis (Moritz and Cicero, 2004). The use of concatenated DNA sequences for species tree inference has been shown to produce more robust phylogenetic hypotheses (Rokas et al., 2003). However, phylogenetic methods of DNA barcoding are not suitable when the underlying system is not based on strictly hierarchical ancestor-descendant relations structures, such as in nested structures (Goldstein and DeSalle, 2005).

Whether specimens of different species can be differentiated depends on the choice of the DNA barcode and the reproductive isolation and evolutionary history of the species under investigation. Although relatively high success rates for the identification of genera has been reported when using common barcodes in plants, limited sequence variation is often the cause of the failure to distinguish between closely related species (Seberg and Petersen, 2009; Parmentier et al., 2013; Braukmann et al., 2017). One incentive for employing genomic approaches for barcoding is that broader genome coverage increases the variation in the barcoding data set (Coissac et al., 2016). However, closely related species may not exhibit a DNA barcoding gap even when the most variable regions are employed. In the case of incipient speciation where lineage sorting is incomplete, species are likely to be paraphyletic (Rieseberg and Brouillet, 1994; Fazekas et al., 2009). Furthermore, cytoplasmic genomes can have different evolutionary histories compared with nuclear genomes because of processes such as chloroplast capture (Rieseberg and Soltis, 1991), and specimens may group geographically rather than taxonomically (Acosta and Premoli, 2010). The success of DNA barcoding may therefore be limited in some plant groups because of their biology and evolutionary history (Percy et al., 2014).

The genus *Berberis* is a case in which DNA barcoding using only a few regions has had limited success (Roy et al., 2010). Similarly, a phylogeny of *Berberis* based on *ndhF* and ITS loci failed to resolve boundaries of several species (Adhikari et al., 2015). *Berberis aristata* is a medicinal plant that has been in traditional use in India for centuries and is nowadays traded throughout the world (Srirama et al., 2017). Local market studies suggest that several species are traded under the same vernacular name (Srivastava and Rawat, 2013), including *B. aristata* and *B. asiatica*. *B. aristata* is described in several pharmacopoeias (Ayurvedic Pharmacopoeia of India, 2001; British Pharmacopoeia, 2016). Chemical and anatomical tests are deficient and conventional macro-morphological and microscopic examination do not distinguish the traded materials (Chandra and Purohit, 1980; Srivastava et al., 2004) therefore there is a strong incentive for the development of a DNA barcoding method for their identification.

The aim of this study is to investigate whole plastid sequences of the genus *Berberis* as a resource for barcode design, utilizing a whole plastid phylogeny of the species in order to better understand the difficulties of using barcoding for pharmacopoeial purposes. In light of the challenges of this complex group, we develop a method for identifying short, informative plastid barcode regions based on diagnostic nucleotides. These barcodes, which are informative of clade membership in a phylogenetic context, are tested on commercial samples, and their utility for regulatory purposes and quality control outlined.

MATERIALS AND METHODS

Sampling
This study includes 85 specimens from 57 species (**Table 1**). The dataset includes sequences from two putative new species (named in this study as B_newsppA and B_newsppB) and one unidentified species (B_spp).

Laboratory Work and DNA Sequencing
DNA Extraction
DNA was extracted using either the Qiagen DNeasy Plant Kit following the manufacturer's protocol or the CTAB method (Doyle and Doyle, 1987). The quality of the extractions was checked for the degree of degradation on 1 or 1.5% agarose gels. Furthermore, we performed PCR amplifications of the *rbcL* gene in different dilutions (1:1, 1:10 and 1:100) and finally we measured the DNA concentration on a Qubit® Fluorometer (Life Technologies, Carlsbad, CA, United States), using the dsDNA High Sensitivity kit. The concentrations after extraction ranged from 1.5 to 34.8 ng/μl.

Library Preparation and Sequencing
The library preparation for the shotgun sequencing was performed according to Meyer and Kircher (2010). The libraries were sequenced in two runs on a MiSeq® and a NextSeq®. Depending on their integrity, the DNA samples were sheared mechanically to a fragment size of approximately 400 bp using a Covaris© sonicator with peak incident power of 75; duty factor of 10%, and 200 cycles per burst. The duration of treatment was chosen according to the observed fragment size on agarose gels and ranged between 30s (medium degradation) and 40s (genomic DNA).

We followed the protocol for blunt-end repair, adapter ligation and adapter fill-in. After each of these steps, the DNA was cleaned-up with AMPure® XP beads (Agencourt®). Before the indexing PCR, the DNA quantity was measured on a Qubit©. Depending on the concentration of adapter-ligated libraries, we aimed to use between 50 and 100 ng of DNA as input for the indexing PCR where possible. Higher concentrations may impair the PCR reaction. In order to avoid high duplication levels, a minimal number of PCR cycles were applied. Libraries with concentrations lower than 40 ng were amplified with 16 PCR cycles. If more than 40 ng of library was used for the PCR, 12 cycles were applied. We used the index sequences ("barcodes") as suggested by the protocol. The final libraries were washed using AMPure® XP beads (Agencourt®). We then measured for concentration with Qubit© and assessed the fragment size using Bioanalyzer® (Agilent). The libraries were diluted to 10 mM and pooled together. The libraries were sequenced in two runs on either an Illumina MiSeq® using the MiSeq v2 reagent kit with the 250 bp paired-end option or a NextSeq® with the NextSeq 500 High Output kit performing 150 bp paired-end sequencing.

Bioinformatics
Raw Read Processing and Quality Control
The adapters of the raw reads were removed either with the built-in Illumina software on sequencers or using cutadapt v. 1.10 (Martin, 2011). Raw reads were trimmed using Trimmomatic v.0.33 (Bolger et al., 2014) with the options LEADING:3, TRAILING:3, SLIDINGWINDOW:4:20. Reads from Illumina NextSeq were discarded when shorter than 30 bp and from MiSeq when shorter than 50 bp. The read quality was checked with FastQC (Andrews, 2010).

Reference Plastid Genome Reconstructions
The reference genome for *B. aristata7* was reconstructed using a hybrid strategy of read mapping and *de novo* assembly. All reads were mapped to the reference plastid genome of *Berberis bealei* (Ma et al., 2013 GenBank reference KF176554), using the Geneious medium-low sensitivity "Map to Reference" function with five iterations. The resulting contig was then checked manually for low coverage and low pairwise identity regions. One read from each of these regions was extracted and all reads were then mapped against these individual reads as a new reference sequence using the same settings as above. The iterations lead to an extension of the read to a contig (typically up to 2,500 bp). The consensus sequences were then mapped to the reference obtained from the first read mapping. This method allowed large indels in the *B. aristata* reference that were not detected by the read mapping algorithm to be identified. The built-in *de novo* algorithm in Geneious 7.1.7 was used for the *de novo* assembly of the plastid genome. We performed the assembly only with reads that matched to the reference sequence of *B. bealei*. The ten largest contigs, ranging in length from 1,132 to 29,132 bp, were then mapped to the *B. aristata* reference and checked for ambiguities. All reads were then mapped again to the new consensus sequence.

Plastid Genome Reconstructions and Alignment
We made our plastid genome reconstructions by mapping to a reference genome, having verified that the levels of variation between B. aristata, our reference, and the chloroplast genome of a member of the distantly related congeneric (B. bealei; Ma et al., 2013 GenBank reference KF176554), were structurally congruent. Reconstructions to a reference permitted a more rapid and cost-effective generation of high quality data than *de novo* assembly. The quality filtered paired-end reads were mapped to a reference genome of *B. aristata7* with Burrows-Wheeler Alignment tool (BWA, ver. 0.7.12, Li and Durbin, 2009). The reference genome was indexed using option "bwa index." Read pairs that survived the quality check were mapped with default options of the command "bwa mem." The resulting SAM file was converted to BAM format with "samtools view" and sorted with "samtools sort" in SAMtools v. 1.2 (Li et al., 2009). Optical read duplicates were removed with Picard tools[1]. We used the single nucleotide

----
[1] http://broadinstitute.github.io/picard, last accessed June 30, 2017

TABLE 1 | Specimen information.

Sample	Species	Locality	Lat.	Long	Collector(s)	Coll. Date	Voucher	Comments
B_angulosa1	B. angulosa Wall. ex Hook.f. & Thomson	Nepal, Illam District	27.11	87.99	Adhikari, B. et al.	14-Jun-07	LKSRB71	
B_angulosa2	B. angulosa Wall. ex Hook.f. & Thomson	Nepal, Rasuwa District	28.21	85.57	Adhikari, B.	03-Aug-07	BL244	
B_angulosa3	B. angulosa Wall. ex Hook.f. & Thomson	Bhutan, Haa	27.27	89.17	Di McNab	01-Jul-05	AS97	Cultivated (J. Harber Coll.)
B_aristata10	Berberis aristata DC.	Nepal, Dhankuta District	27.04918	87.35425	Adhikari, B. et al.	01-Aug-14	WP21.1	
B_aristata11	Berberis aristata DC.	Nepal, Gandaki District	28.39255	83.77315	Adhikari, B.	05-Oct-06	EA109	
B_aristata3	B. aristata DC.	Nepal, Dhankuta District	27.05	87.35	Adhikari, B. et al.	01-Sep-14	WP21.5	
B_aristata4	B. aristata DC.	N/A	N/A	N/A	N/A	N/A	1260210	
B_aristata6	Berberis aristata DC.	Nepal, Koshii District	27.04918	87.35425	Adhikari, B. et al.	01-Aug-14	WP32.5	
B_aristata7	Berberis aristata DC.	Nepal, Koshii District	27.04048	87.31713	Adhikari, B. et al.	01-Aug-14	WP18.2	
B_aristata8	Berberis aristata DC.	Nepal, Dhawalagiri District	28.66222	83.59472	Adhikari, B.	17-Aug-07	EA243	
B_aristata9	Berberis aristata DC.	Nepal, Dhawalagiri District	28.66028	83.59389	Adhikari, B.	17-Aug-07	EA249	
B_asiatica2	B. asiatica Roxb. ex DC.	Nepal, Makwanpur District	27.58	85.16	Adhikari, B. et al.	25-Aug-17	Coll_7.1	
B_asiatica4	B. asiatica Roxb. ex DC.	India, no further details	N/A	N/A	C. Chadwell	N/A	AS82	Cultivated (J. Harber Coll.)
B_asiatica5	Berberis asiatica Roxb. ex DC.	Nepal, Narayani Zone	27.6541	85.09973	Adhikari, B. et al.	01-Aug-14	Coll_38.1	
B_asiatica6	Berberis asiatica Roxb. ex DC.	Nepal, Bagmati Zone	27.77278	85.43166	Adhikari, B. et al.	02-Sep-14	SB1	
B_calliantha	B. calliantha Mulligan	China, Tibet	28.91	89.61	F. Kingdon-Ward, Ex Hillier	21-Nov-24	AS38	Cultivated (J. Harber Coll.)
B_chrysosphaera	B. chrysosphaera Mulligan	China, Tibet	28.65	97.46	F. Kingdon-Ward, Ex Hillier	10-Dec-33	AS39	Cultivated (J. Harber Coll.)
B_con_extensiflora1	B. concinna var. extensiflora Ahrendt	Nepal, Manang District	28.61	84.47	N/A	14-Aug-08	20812277	
B_con_extensiflora2	B. concinna var. extensiflora Ahrendt	Nepal, Myagdi District	28.4	83.69	N/A	04-Oct-06	EA104	
B_con_extensiflora3	B. concinna var. extensiflora Ahrendt	Nepal	N/A	N/A	C. Chadwell	N/A	AS74	Cultivated (J. Harber Coll.)
B_concinna2	Berberis concinna Hook.f.	India, Sikkim	27.83472	88.69944	T D. Atkinson	05-Jul-05	AS102	
B_concolor	B. concolor W. W. Smith	China, Yunnan	28.47	98.91	D. E. Boufford et al.	20-Aug-13	43135	
B_congestiflora	B. congestiflora Gay	Chile, Región IX	N/A	N/A	Gardner et al.	19-Feb-88	1988.0916	Cultivated (RBGE)
B_cooperi	B. cooperi Ahrendt	Bhutan, Timphu	27.47	89.64	J. F. Harber s.n.	01-Aug-97	AS9	Cultivated (J. Harber Coll.)
B_crassilamba	B. crassilamba C. Y. Wu ex S. Y. Bao	China, Yunnan	27.61	99.89	D. E. Boufford et al.	04-Sep-13	43437	
B_darwinii	B. darwinii Hook.	Argentina : Prov. Rio Negro	N/A	N/A	Unknown	N/A	1987.2408	Cultivated (RBGE)
B_derogensis	B. derogensis T. S. Ying	China, Sichuan	29.09	99.38	D. E. Boufford et al.	22-Aug-13	43164	
B_dictyophylla1	B. dictyophylla Franch.	China, Yunnan	27.89	99.68	B & S Wynn-Jones	17-Sep-00	AS93	Cultivated (J. Harber Coll.)
B_dictyophylla2	B. dictyophylla Franch.	China, Yunnan	25.94	100.4	Z. W. Liu s.n.	N/A	AS100	Cultivated (J. Harber Coll.)

(Continued)

TABLE 1 | Continued

Sample	Species	Locality	Lat.	Long	Collector(s)	Coll. Date	Voucher	Comments
B_everestiana1	B. everestiana var. ventosa Ahrendt	Nepal, Solu Khumbu District	27.86	86.64	N/A	23-Sep-05	DNEP3BY156	
B_everestiana2	B. koehneana C. K. Schneid.	Nepal, Mustang District	28.82	83.86	Adhikari, B.	16-Aug-07	EA217	
B_fendleri	B. fendleri A.Gray	N/A	N/A	N/A	N/A	N/A	N/A_2	Cultivated (RBGE)
B_glaucocarpa	B. glaucocarpa Stapf	Nepal, Doti District	29.35	81.06	N/A	01-Jul-09	20918011	
B_graminea	B. graminea Ahrendt	China, Sichuan	28.12	101.18	D. E. Boufford et al.	06-Sep-13	43466	
B_griffithiana1	B. griffithiana C.K.Schneid.	India, Arunachal Pradesh	27.58	91.88	SF 06008	24-Nov-06	AS55	Cultivated (J. Harber Coll.)
B_griffithiana2	B. griffithiana C.K.Schneid.	India, Arunachal Pradesh	27.33	92.31	A Clark 5260	01-Oct-04	AS54	Cultivated (J. Harber Coll.)
B_grodtmanniana	B. grodtmanniana C. K. Schneider	China, Sichuan	27.69	101.22	D. E. Boufford et al.	06-Sep-13	43471	
B_gyalaica1	Berberis gyalaica Ahrendt ex F.Br.	China, Tibet	29.65056	94.36	W. Bentall	27-Jun-05	WB	
B_gyalaica2	Berberis gyalaica Ahrendt ex F.Br.	China, Tibet	28.97444	93.69472	W. Bentall	NA	AS6	Cultivated (J. Harber Coll.)
B_hamiltoniana	Berberis hamiltoniana Ahrendt	Nepal, Bajhang District	29.61553	81.00556	Adhikari, B.	NA	20915095	
B_hookeri2	B. hookeri Lem.	Nepal, Khumbu District	27.76	86.71	N/A	29-Sep-05	DNEP3BY213	
B_hookeri5	Berberis wallichiana DC.	Nepal, Panchthar District	27.10263	87.96897	Adhikari, B. et al.	08-Jun-07	LKSRB28	
B_hookeri6	Berberis hookeri Lem.	Nepal, Myagdi District	28.4014	83.70257	Adhikari, B.	04-Oct-06	EA106	
B_hookeri7	Berberis hookeri Lem.	Nepal, Myagdi District	28.40443	83.69923	Adhikari, B.	13 July 2009	Bajhang0920915095	
B_insignis	Berberis insignis Hook.f. & Thomson	Nepal, Illam District	27.06317	88.01702	Adhikari, B. et al.	16-Jun-07	LKSRB144	
B_jaeschkeana1	B. jaeschkeana var. usteriana C.K.Schneid.	Nepal, Jumla District	29.32	82.18	N/A	03-Jun-08	JRSA12	
B_jaeschkeana2	Berberis jaeschkeana var. usteriana C.K.Schneid.	Nepal, Mustang District	28.71222	83.55889	Adhikari, B.	17-Aug-07	EA238	
B_jamesiana2	B. jamesiana Forrest & W. W. Smith	China, Yunnan	26.11	100.17	D. E. Boufford et al.	14-Sep-13	43530	
B_karnalensis	B. karnalensis Bh.Adhikari	Nepal, Jumla District	29.3	82.18	N/A	03-Jun-08	JRSA5	
B_koehneana	B. koehneana C. K. Schneid.	Nepal, Mustang District	28.68	83.6	N/A	30-Sep-06	EA56	
B_kumaonensis	B. kumaonensis C. K. Schneid.	Nepal, Doti District	29.38	81.12	N/A	02-Jul-09	20915029	
B_leptopoda	B. leptopoda Ahrendt	India, Arunachal Pradesh	28.57	95.06	K. Rushforth		AS103	Cultivated (J. Harber Coll.)
B_levis	B. levis Franch.	China, Yunnan	25.96	100.39	D. E. Boufford et al.	15-Sep-13	43557	
B_mekongensis	B. mekongensis W. W. Smith	China, Yunnan	28.33	99.12	D. E. Boufford et al.	19-Aug-13	43131	
B_micropetala	B. micropetala C.K.Schneid.	India, Manipur	24.67	93.92	N. Macer	04-Jul-05	AS104	Cultivated (J. Harber Coll.)
B_microphylla1	B. microphylla G.Forst.	N/A	N/A	N/A	N/A	N/A	1961.063803	Cultivated (RBGE)
B_montana	B. montana Gay	Chile : Región X	N/A	N/A	Gardner et al.	15-Jun-05	1993.2827B	Cultivated (RBGE)
B_mucrifolia	Berberis mucrifolia Ahrendt	Nepal, Mustang District	28.71194	83.55889	Adhikari, B.	Nov 2009	200404971	Cultivated (RBGE)
B_negeriana	B. negeriana Tischler	Chile, Región VIII	N/A	N/A	Hechenleitner Vega	11-Mar-04	200404971	Cultivated (RBGE)

(Continued)

TABLE 1 | Continued

Sample	Species	Locality	Lat.	Long	Collector(s)	Coll. Date	Voucher	Comments
B_nervosa	B. nervosa Pursh	Canada, British Columbia	N/A	N/A	Halliwell, Brian	23-Aug-78	1978.2559	Cultivated (RBGE)
B_nevinii	B. nevinii A. Gray.	N/A	N/A	N/A	Unknown	Unknown	HC1066	Cultivated (Rancho Santa Ana Botanical Garden)
B_newsppA	Berberis new_speciesA	China Yunnan	27.53	99.64	D. E. Boufford et al.	31-Aug-13	43334	
B_newsppB	Berberis new_speciesB	China Yunnan	28.57	99.83	D. E. Boufford et al.	31-Aug-13	43304	
B_orthobotrys1	B. orthobotrys var. rubicunda Ahrendt	Nepal, Rasuwa District	28.21	85.53	Adhikari, B.	03-Aug-07	BL239	
B_orthobotrys2	B. orthobotrys var. rubicunda Ahrendt	Nepal, Khumbu District	27.79	86.71	N/A	12-Sep-05	DNEP3BY22	
B_pendryi2	Berberis pendryi Bh.Adhikari	Nepal, Mustang District	28.81694	83.87	Adhikari, B.	16-Aug-07	EA29	
B_petiolaris1	B. petiolaris Wall. ex G. Don	Nepal, Mugu District	29.65	82.11	N/A	12-Jun-08	JRSA122	
B_petiolaris2	B. petiolaris Wall. ex G. Don	Nepal, Mugu District	29.65	82.11	N/A	12-Jun-08	JRSA122	Technical Replicate
B_phanera	B. phanera C.K. Schneider	China, Sichuan	28.12	101.18	D. E. Boufford et al.	06-Sep-13	43465	
B_polyodonta	B. polyodonta Fedde	China Yunnan	N/A	N/A	Lijiang et al.	12-Jun-05	1991.1138	Cultivated (RBGE)
B_praecipua	B. praecipua C.K.Schneid.	Bhutan	27.32	89.55	Ruth Liddington	20-Jun-05	AS64	Cultivated (J. Harber Coll.)
B_pruinosa	B. pruinosa Franch.	China, Yunnan	27.46	99.9	D. E. Boufford et al.	04-Sep-13	43442	
B_pseudotibetica	B. pseudotibetica C. Y. Wu	China, Yunnan	28.29	99.16	D. E. Boufford et al.	19-Aug-13	43134	
B_qiaojianensis	B. qiaojianensis S. Y. Bao	China, Yunnan	26.19	103.27	D. E. Boufford et al.	19-Sep-13	43528	
B_spp1	Berberis spp.	Nepal, Panchthar District	27.10389	87.9475	Adhikari, B. et al.	08-Jun-07	LKRSB17	
B_temolaica	Berberis temolaica Ahrendt	China, Tibet	29.2169	94.21528	A. Clark	NA	AS67	Cultivated (J. Harber Coll.)
B_thomsoniana	Berberis thomsoniana C.K.Schneid.	Nepal, Myagdi District	28.40217	83.70247	Adhikari, B.	03-Oct-06	EA101	
B_tibaoshanensis	B. tibaoshanensis S. Y. Bao	China, Yunnan	27.61	99.89	D. E. Boufford et al.	04-Sep-13	43436	
B_tsarica1	Berberis tsarica Ahrendt	Nepal, Khumbu District	27.94111	86.61	Adhikari, B. et al.	20-Sep-05	DNEP3BY132	
B_wallichiana1	B. wallichiana DC.	Nepal, Panchthar District	27.1	87.97	Adhikari, B. et al.	08-Jun-07	LKSRB28	
B_wallichiana2	B. wallichiana DC.	Nepal, Rasuwa District	28.17	85.36	Adhikari, B.	02-Aug-07	BL220	
B_wardii	Berberis wardii C.K.Schneid	India, Assam	26.00472	94.99806	F. Kingdon-Ward	NA	AS66	Cultivated (J. Harber Coll.)
B_wilsoniae1	B. wilsoniae Hemsley	China, Yunnan	27.61	99.72	D. E. Boufford et al.	31-Aug-13	43337	
B_wilsoniae2	B. wilsoniae Hemsley	China, Yunnan	24.96	102.66	Z. W Liu	N/A	AS99	Cultivated (J. Harber Coll.)
B_wilsoniae3	B. wilsoniae Hemsley	China, Yunnan	29.99	101.95	X. H. Li	05-Jul-05	AS98	Cultivated (J. Harber Coll.)

Vouchers are deposited at the Herbarium of the Royal Botanic Garden Edinburgh. Missing information is displayed as N/A.

polymorphism (SNP) calling workflow in GATK (McKenna et al., 2010; Van der Auwera et al., 2013). Regions that contain insertions and deletions are often badly aligned. Therefore, a local realignment process was applied with the command "–T IndelRealigner" in GATK. Variant calling was performed on the realigned BAM files with the "–T HaploTypeCaller" module with haploid settings ("-ploidy 1"). The output is a genomic variant call file (GVCF) that contains base call information for all sites of the markers. The variant calls were then exported with "–T GenotypeGVCFs" to the standard variant call format (VCF). SNP and indel variants were then filtered separately. The first SNP filter applied is quality by depth (QD), which can be considered as the quality of the variant call standardized by the depth of coverage. QD avoids inflation of the Phred quality score for the variant call caused by deep coverage. Variants that had a QD < 2 were filtered out as recommended by Van der Auwera et al. (2013). The FisherStrand (FS) quality filter is a Phred-scaled probability that strand bias exists at a specific site. Specifically, the score is a measure for whether an alternate allele was seen more or less often on either forward or reverse reads. The mapping quality (MQ) in GATK is calculated as the root mean square quality over all reads at a given site. The sites where variance resulted in an MQ score < M 40 were treated as missing data in order to avoid carry-over of reference- specific base pairs. The final sequence was reconstructed with the command "–T FastaAlternateReferenceMaker" in GATK. We checked our pipeline by visual comparison of the final plastid sequence with the BAM file for selected samples.

The plastids were aligned using the MAFFT v7.215 aligner (Katoh and Standley, 2013) with default options. The alignment of repetitive regions such as poly A sequences was not straightforward, therefore two alignment files were created: the first alignment was used for phylogenetic inference, and blocks where no unambiguous alignment could be constructed were removed. Furthermore, the inverted repeats were removed, since SNP calling on these repeats was difficult to address. Reads with polymorphisms in only one region will map to the other repeat as well. Random mapping to inverted repeat regions often results in apparently heterozygous read alignments, precluding unique assignments of SNPs to a specific inverted repeat. The second alignment was used for the barcoding analysis. Regions were masked (coded as "N") where no unambiguous alignment was possible.

Annotation of Plastid Sequence

The online platforms DOGMA (Wyman et al., 2004) and CpGAVAS (Liu et al., 2012) were used for the annotation of the genome of B. aristata7. The full genome sequences were imported into Apollo (Lee et al., 2009). The annotation of B. aristata was compared with the previously published annotation of B. bealei (Ma et al., 2013). Start and stop codons were checked manually. The annotation was visualized using OGdraw.

Universal Barcode Reconstruction

The sequences of matK, rbcL, and trnH-psbA of B. aristata were extracted from the annotated reference B. aristata7. The sequences were then aligned to the plastid genomes using BLAT

(Kent, 2002). The output was parsed to produce a BED file, which denotes the start and end position of an alignment. The respective sequence was then extracted with the "getfasta" option in BEDTools (Quinlan and Hall, 2010).

A two-step pipeline was devised to reconstruct the ITS2 from shotgun sequencing data. Firstly, reads that map to the ITS2 reference were filtered and then a de novo assembly was performed using these reads. Filtering prior to de novo assembly reduces computation time substantially. The reference sequence of ITS2 (Berberis repens, BOLD accession: HIMS1138-12) was indexed with BWA (Li and Durbin, 2009) using the command "bwa index." Trimmed and filtered reads were mapped to the reference with "bwa mem." Mapped reads were then separated from unmapped reads with SAMtools (Li et al., 2009) "samtools view –b –F 4," resulting in a BAM file with only mapped reads. The mapped reads were then extracted to fastq format using Picard tools (see footnote 1) with the command "SamToFastq." The reads were then used for de novo assembly using SPAdes v3.7.0 (Bankevich et al., 2012) and the longest contig extracted.

Barcoding Analysis and Phylogenies

The phylogeny of the plastid alignment was estimated using RAxML v. 8.2.10 (Stamatakis, 2014). The best model of substitution was calculated under the Aikaike Information Criterion in jModeltest2. The ML phylogeny was estimated with 1,000 bootstrap replicates under the GTRGAMMA + I substitution model using the online CIPRES portal (Miller et al., 2010). The whole alignment was considered as a single partition. Members of the compound-leaved Berberis were set as outgroup (B. nervosa, B. polyodonta and B. nevinii).

Potential novel Berberis-specific barcodes were explored by extracting SNP positions of the multiple sequence alignment of whole plastid genomes with the program SNP-sites (Page et al., 2016). The SNPs were summarized in 500 bp windows and their distribution plotted with Circos (Krzywinski et al., 2009). Potential barcodes were selected spanning regions where a 500 bp window had a sequence variability of > 5%, and a maximum amount of missing/masked data <3%. The 500 bp regions were then compared to the annotated plastid genome and the barcodes were constructed to correspond with genomic regions, such as intergenic spacers that are flanked by conservative regions suitable for primer design. These Berberis specific barcodes derived from the whole plastid alignment were evaluated, along with the commonly used barcodes ITS2, rbcL, matK, and trnH-psbA.

TABLE 2 | Commercial samples analyzed in this study.

Sample	Form	Company	Place of Purchase
Market 1	Stem/Bark/Root	UK_1	United Kingdom
Market 2	Stem/Bark/Root	UK_1	United Kingdom
Market 3	Powder	India_1	India, Rajasthan (Internet)

The samples Market1 and Market2 were purchased from the same company. The sample Market3 was purchased from India via the Internet.

The individual barcode regions were aligned using MAFFT v7.215 (Katoh and Standley, 2013) with default options and were then manually trimmed. A first step was to infer a maximum likelihood tree of the barcode with RAxML v.8.2.9 (Stamatakis, 2014) with 1,000 rapid bootstrap replicates ("–f a") under the GTRCAT model. The potential barcodes were sorted according

to the percent variable sites, percent parsimony informative sites, recovery of *B. aristata* and *B. asiatica* groups and the recovery of groups present in the whole plastid phylogeny. The selected barcodes were concatenated and a maximum likelihood phylogeny was built with the same parameters as described above. Phylogenies of the selected barcodes were inferred under

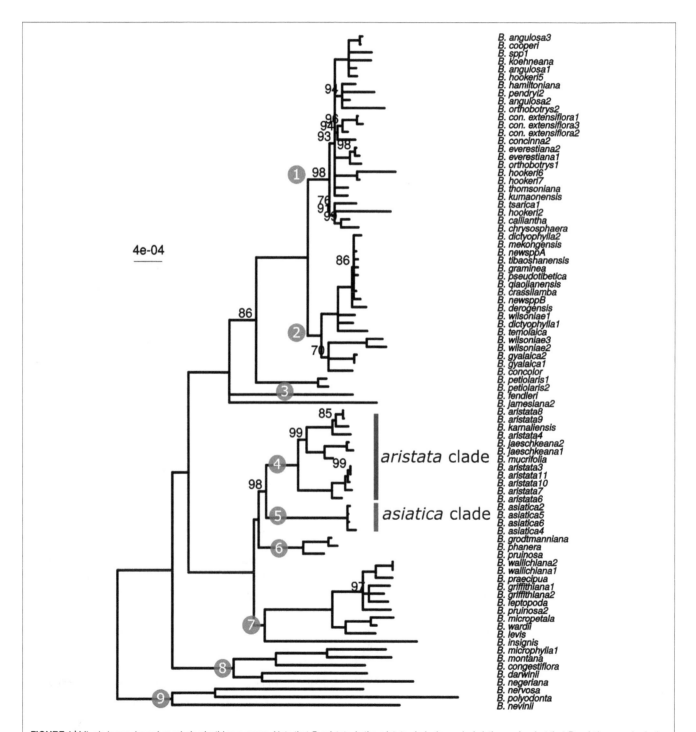

FIGURE 1 | ML phylogeny based on whole plastid sequences. Note that *B. aristata*, in the aristata clade, is a polyphyletic species, but that *B. asiatica* samples in the asiatica group comprise a monophyletic group. Numbers above branches are bootstrap values between 51 and 99. Branches with support <50 were collapsed to polytomies, bootstrap values of 100 are not shown.

the GTRCAT model in RAxML v. 8.2.9 (Stamatakis, 2014). Additionally, haplotype networks were constructed with the function haploNet in the R package pegas (Paradis, 2010). Finally the alignment of each selected barcode was then reduced to SNP sites only and diagnostic polymorphisms were identified for each group in order to delimit a minimal barcode.

Test Data

The first test data consisted of three commercial samples, supposedly of *B. aristata* (**Table 2**). Sequences for the commercial samples were generated and the sequence data used to make identifications according to the diagnostic loci in **Table 4**.

RESULTS

Whole Plastid Phylogeny

The whole plastid phylogeny is shown in **Figure 1**. Nine groups, eight of which are monophyletic, are identified and numbered 1 to 9. The *aristata*, *asiatica* and *Mahonia* clades (numbered 4, 5, and 9 in **Figure 1**) are of most importance in terms of authentication. The plastid phylogeny reveals

that *B. aristata* is not monophyletic since *B. jaeschkeana*, *B. karnaliensis* and *B. mucrifolia* are nested amongst the specimens of this species in clade 4. The topology of the phylogeny is consistent with morphological and biogeographical characters, and with the topology based on nuclear sequence data (Kreuzer et al., in prep.). The annotated plastid sequence of *B_aristata7* is shown in **Supplementary Figure S1** and the corresponding sequence is found on Genbank with reference number MK714340.

Identifying Informative Barcodes

The barcoding analysis aimed to find a set of informative nucleotides that are unique to clades of interest. The topology of the whole plastid genome phylogeny was used to determine evolutionarily meaningful groups, termed Operational Phylogenetic Units (OPUs). Barcodes were then constructed for identifying these OPUs, rather than individual species. A barcoding method based on diagnostic characters was preferred over distance or purely phylogenetic approaches, because of its ease of application to regulatory purposes and to provide an alternative approach in an evolutionarily complex

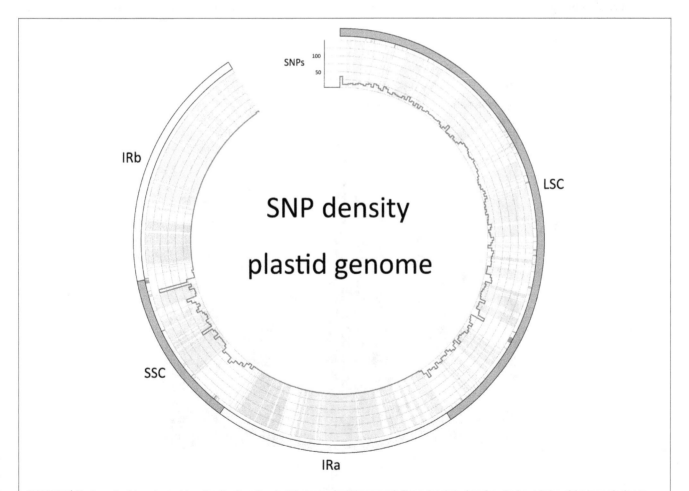

FIGURE 2 | Single nucleotide polymorphism density along the plastid genome (red histograms). The outer circle describes the boundaries of the large single copy, the inverted repeats (IRa and IRb) and the small single copy. Regions that are colored green in the inner circle are coding regions, blue are RNA genes (rRNA and tRNA genes) and white is non-coding sequence. Red color below the outer circle shows regions that have been masked and are thus coded as "N".

group. The density of SNPs in 500 bp windows along the whole plastid alignment is shown in **Figure 2**. The bins contained between 0 and 124 variable sites per 500 bp. The inspection of bins with >25 SNPs (5%) resulted in 21 potential barcode regions. Several of the highly variable bins fell into regions where the alignment was partly masked due to ambiguous alignment, leaving 13 bins for further inspection. Two neighboring bins were combined into a single potential barcode of 1,000 bp, and a set of four bins combined into a 2000 base pair barcode. The barcode of 2,000 bp (SSC_noncoding2) was further examined by partitioning the alignment into 50 bp windows and reducing the barcode size (SSC_noncoding2, **Figure 3**). The *trnH-psbA* intergenic spacer was identified among one of the seven highly variable regions, and together with the *matK*, *rbcL* and ITS2 barcodes, selected because they are commonly used barcode regions, eleven barcode candidates were investigated (**Table 3**). None of the individual barcodes retrieved phylogenies with the same topology as the whole plastid phylogeny. Although the *matK* phylogeny is not well resolved overall, species from the *aristata* and *asiatica* groups were recovered. *B. asiatica* is monophyletic in the non-coding SSC_noncoding2 phylogeny, but species from the *aristata* clade are separated into two groups. The percent variable sites varied

between 2.2 in *rbcL* and 9.85 in the intergenic spacer *ndhI-ndhG* (**Table 3**) and the latter was chosen along with *matK* and SSC_noncoding2 as barcodes for phylogenetic and haplotype analysis (**Figure 4**).

These three barcodes yielded 133 variable positions in total. Nine positions were sufficient to identify seven of the nine groups with clade-specific nucleotide variants. Groups 3 and 8 (**Figure 1**) share a barcode, in other words their barcodes are identical. The phylogeny of the concatenated barcodes *matK*, SSC_noncoding2 and *ndhI-ndhG* barcodes is shown in **Figure 5**. The topology of the tree differs substantially from the total-evidence tree inferred from whole plastid sequences. However, four of the major clades are identified in both trees. Haplotype networks constructed for each of the separate data sets showed variation in the haplotype associated with the *B. aristata* clade (**Figure 4**). There was no haplotype unique to *B. aristata*: for the SSC_noncoding2 region one of the *B. aristata* haplotypes is found also in *B. karnaliensis*; for the matK region there is also a haplotype shared between *B. aristata* and *B. karnaliensis*; for ndhI-ndhG there is a haplotype found in *B. aristata*, *B. jaeschkeana*, *B. karnaliensis* and *B. mucrifolia*. The lack of species-specific haplotypes even in these most variable regions underlines the necessity of a clade-based approach. However, for pharmacopoeial purposes the haplotype

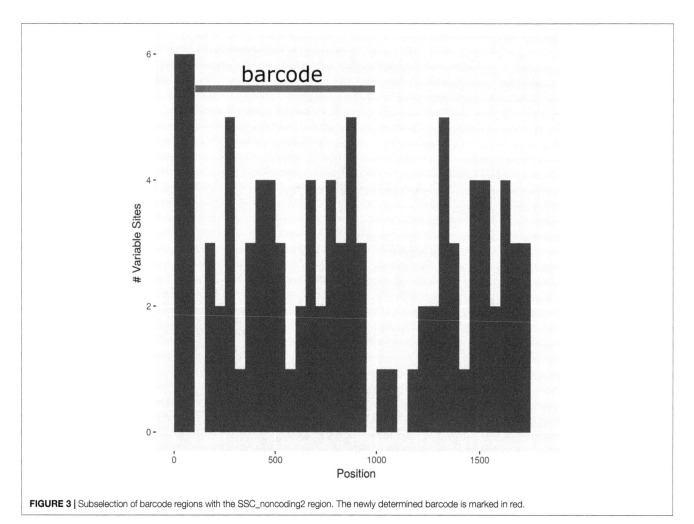

FIGURE 3 | Subselection of barcode regions with the SSC_noncoding2 region. The newly determined barcode is marked in red.

TABLE 3 | Barcode selection resulting from investigating variability patterns across whole plastid alignment.

Barcode	Length (bp)	Var	% Var	PIS	% PIS	*aristata* recovered	*asiatica* recovered
ITS2 (nuclear)	560	45	8.04	24	4.29	No	Yes
matK	**1530**	**39**	**2.55**	**18**	**1.18**	**Yes**	**Yes**
ndhF (partial)	802	40	4.99	23	2.87	No	Yes
ndhI-ndhG	**501**	**48**	**9.58**	**18**	**3.59**	**No**	**Yes**
rbcL	1452	32	2.20	21	1.45	No	Yes
rbcL-atpB	770	32	4.16	19	2.47	No	Yes
rbcL-psaI	626	59	9.42	28	4.47	No	Yes
rpl32-ndhF	1119	80	7.15	40	3.57	Partly	Yes
SSC_noncoding1	741	52	7.02	29	3.91	Partly	No
SSC_noncoding2	**790**	**46**	**5.82**	**27**	**3.42**	**Yes**	**Yes**
trnH-psbA	580	43	7.41	24	4.14	No	Yes

matK and rbcL were not identified as highly variable but included in the study. Var = Variable sites; PIS = parsimony informative sites; "aristata recovered" and "asiatica recovered" indicates whether the clades were recovered in the respective phylogeny. Barcode selection resulting from investigating variability patterns across whole plastid alignment. The DNA barcodes that were selected are highlighted in bold font.

TABLE 4 | *Top*: Matrix of informative barcode positions.

	matK				ndhI-ndhG			SSC_noncoding2	
Position (bp)	755	857	976	1428	151	182	326	47	700
clade. 1	A	G	G	G	C	A	C	A	G
clade. 2	A	G	G	A	C	A	C	A	A
clade. 3	A	G	G	G	A	A	C	A	A
aristata – clade (4)	C	A	G	G	C	A	C	A	A
asiatica – clade (5)	A	G	G	G	C	C	C	A	A
clade. 6	A	G	G	G	C	A	C	A	A
clade. 7	A	G	A	G	C	A	C	A	A
SA clade (8)	A	G	G	G	A	A	C	A	A
Mahonia – clade (9)	A	G	G	G	A	A	A	C	A
					Test Samples				
Market1	A	G	G	G	A	A	N	C	A
Market2	A	G	G	G	A	A	N	C	A
Market3	A	G	G	G	C	C	C	A	A

The positions are relative to the consensus of the multiple sequence alignments of each barcode. "SA clade" stands for South American clade. Bottom: Results of the test samples. Market1, Market2, and Market3 are commercial samples. and Mixture1 and Mixture2 are in silico mixtures. Numbers below multiple base calls represent the ratio of nucleotides in the mapping.

networks reveal separation of the *B. aristata* clade haplotypes and *B. asiatica* haplotypes.

Testing Barcodes

The minimal barcode consists of nine positions and includes barcodes unique to seven groups. No unique SNPs were identified for groups 3, 6, and 8. No individual barcode for groups 6 and 8 could be constructed (**Table 4**). The barcodes were evaluated with the test data set. The commercial samples Market1 and Market2 were identified as belonging to the *Mahonia* clade. The sample Market11 shared the barcode with *B. asiatica* samples.

DISCUSSION

DNA barcoding for quality assurance and pharmacovigilance has great potential and is likely to be implemented as a routine diagnostic method. In this study, we present an approach for barcoding of an evolutionarily complex group of species and demonstrate that these barcodes can identify the species in commercial samples. Our purpose was to provide a barcode for pharmacopoeial purposes that discriminates *B. aristata* and *B. asiatica* since these are the pharmacopoeial species and the main substitute, respectively. We present a solution for barcoding that meets regulatory needs.

With the emergence of new sequencing technologies, whole plastid sequencing has been proposed as an extension of the current barcoding concept (Coissac et al., 2016). It has been shown that whole plastid sequences increase phylogenetic resolution (Parks et al., 2009) and simultaneously increase the effectiveness of discriminating between species. In this study, we show how whole plastid next-generation sequencing can be used to investigate sequence variability patterns for the discovery of informative DNA barcodes. We confirm the difficulty of

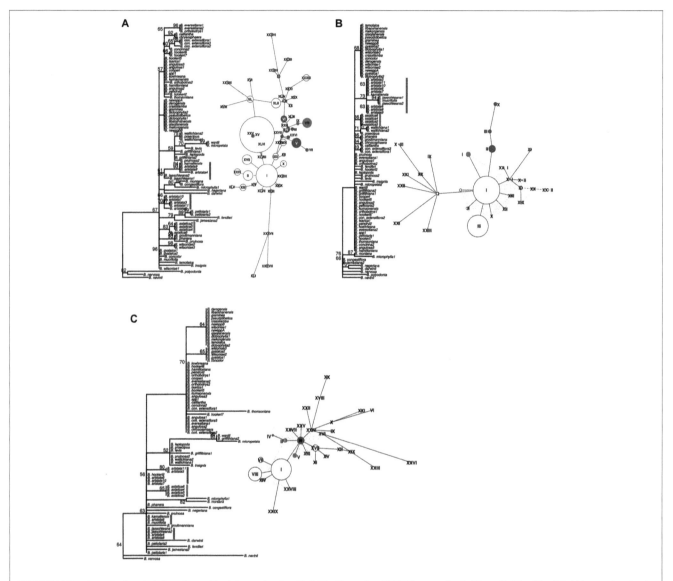

FIGURE 4 | "Maximum likelihood phylogenies and haplotype networks of individual barcodes. **(A)** SSC_noncoding2, **(B)** matK, **(C)** ndhI-ndhG. Values on braches in the phylogeny are ML bootstraps. Species belonging to the *Berberis aristata* clade as recovered from the total plastid phylogeny are identified by green bars, and the *B. asiatica* clades by orange bars on the phylogeny. The same colors are used for the haplotype networks, where Roman numerals indicate different haplotypes and the size of the circles corresponds to the number of samples sharing this haplotype. Species contributing to *B. aristata* clade haplotypes are as follows: SSC_noncoding2 – XXV = *B. mucrifolia* (1 plant), VI = *B. aristata* (2 plants), IV = *B. aristata* (2 plants), III = *B. aristata* (1 plant), XXVI = *B. jaeschkeana* (1 plant), XXVII = *B. jaeschkeana* (1 plant), V = *B. aristata* (2 plants) and *B. karnaliensis* (1 plant), VII = *B. aristata* (1 plant); matK – X = *B. jaeschkeana* (2 plants) and *B. mucrifolia* (1 plant), III = *B. aristata* (3 plants) II = *B. aristata* (5 plants) and *B. karnaliensis* (1 plant); ndhI-ndhG – IV = *B. aristata* (2 plants), II = *B. aristata* (2 plants) and *B. hookeri* (1 plant), III = *B. aristata* (3 plants) and *B. jaeschkeana* (2 plants) and *B. karnaliensis* (1 plant) and *B. mucrifolia* (1 plant)."

barcoding *Berberis* species as suggested by Roy et al. (2010), even when whole plastid sequences are used for comparison. Although the sampling was limited, with only a few of the species represented with multiple samples, the low resolution of the plastid phylogeny at shallow phylogenetic levels and the presence of polyphyletic species (e.g., *B. aristata*) indicates evolutionary reasons for the failure of barcoding this genus to species level (Mutanen et al., 2016). DNA barcoding is challenging in groups where frequent hybridization occurs in conjunction with plastid capture or where lineage sorting has not yet been completed (Fazekas et al., 2009). A salient point

arising from our study is that the pharmacopoeial species, *B. aristata*, is polyphyletic. One explanation for this finding is hybridization, a phenomenon documented in *Berberis* (Adhikari et al., 2012). Low resolution among the closely related species of *Berberis* as reported in the whole plastid phylogeny, could point toward retention of ancestral polymorphism or incomplete lineage sorting (Naciri and Linder, 2015). Misidentification of *B. jaeschkeana*, *B. karnaliensis* and/or *B. mucrifolia* is unlikely, since these have been included in recent revisionary work (Adhikari et al., 2012). Polyphyletic species are likely to persist where they are morphologically robust entities, and

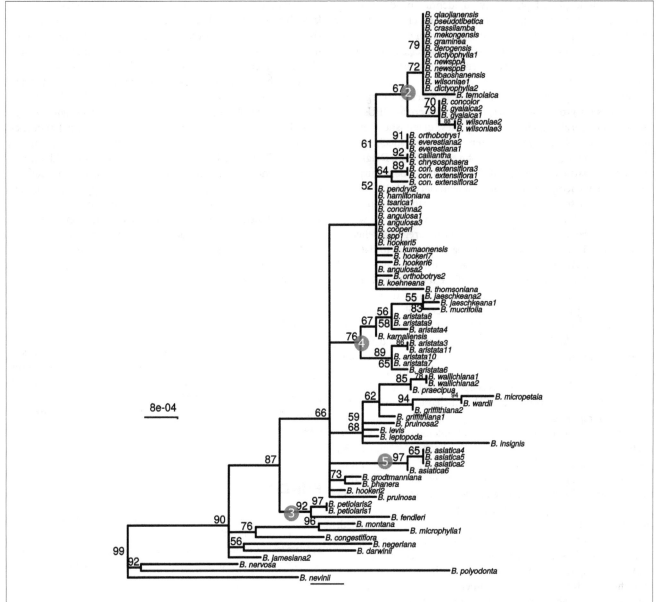

FIGURE 5 | Maximum likelihood tree from the concatenated barcodes *matK*, SSC_noncoding2 and *ndhl-ndhG*. Nodes with bootstrap support <50 were collapsed to polytomies. Bootstrap values between 50 and 99 are shown above branches. No number indicates a bootstrap value of 100. Numbered circles indicate groups that were recovered in the whole plastid phylogeny (see **Figure 1**).

the development of methods for their identification, in this case for pharmacopoeia, benefits from understanding of their evolutionary history. The case of barcoding medicinal *Berberis* species provides an example of how barcoding for regulatory purposes in an evolutionarily complex group can be approached. Phylogenies can be essential for formulating adequate barcoding hypotheses; the whole plastid phylogeny reveals that at least three species are nested in the clade with the main species. The polyphyly of *B. aristata* indicates that universal barcodes are unlikely to delineate these species, and haplotype analysis shows this is the case for three of the most variable regions. Furthermore, several clades show low resolution at terminal branches. We have therefore adapted our classification scheme

and defined meaningful OPUs that do not correspond to existing species limits. OPUs are the entities that can be discriminated by the barcodes put forward. The OPUs in this study are delimited using an integrative approach based on the interpretation of a whole plastid phylogeny, coupled with the detection of diagnostic nucleotides in relatively short barcodes for well-supported groups. These DNA barcodes can be targeted by PCR and Sanger sequencing and therefore offer a simple and fast identification test for regulatory purposes and quality control. Appropriate OPUs would be identified on a case-by-case basis for other evolutionarily complex groups for regulatory purposes. This is because for evolutionarily complex groups barcodes do not confirm species identity. The novelty of our approach lies in using whole plastid phylogeny to identify of short, easily amplified markers that incorporate clade-specific SNPs, and although we expect it to be more widely applicable it is only appropriate when the non-pharmacopoeial species belonging to the OPU are neither candidate adulterants nor substitute species, as is the case here.

The barcode presented in this study is based on diagnostic nucleotides for groups of species, referred to here as OPUs. Like the morphological classification of species, diagnostic methods provide a set of unique characters to assign specimens to species or species groups (Little and Stevenson, 2007). Diagnostic methods are particularly well-suited to pharmacopoeial purposes because a sequence generated from test material can be compared to a published sequence in a way that is comparable to other pharmacopoeial standards. The barcode we propose would require the user to amplify and sequence three regions, whereas the barcodes included in the British Pharmacopoeia to date are single regions (British Pharmacopoeia, 2016). We have limited the number of loci that would be part of the test to three because incorporating more loci would make the test more unwieldy for users. Limiting the number of regions necessarily reduces the number of informative sites. Identifying the most informative regions, as we do here, is therefore important. A deficiency of the diagnostic method is that further samples might show variation that is not present amongst the samples used for barcode design. However, there is scope to modify the published barcodes, perhaps by using the IUPAC nucleotide codes, if novel variants are reported.

The diagnostic method has been implemented in various analysis tools (Sarkar et al., 2008; Weitschek et al., 2013), mainly for specimen identification. Some of the algorithms use logic mining techniques (Bertolazzi et al., 2009). Logic mining for DNA barcoding refers to a two-step process, in which the barcode is first reduced to a set of very informative nucleotides and thereafter a logic mining method is applied, to define a set of formulas for separating the species. More recent approaches, such as BLOG 2.0 (Weitschek et al., 2013), provide a diagnostic, character-based methodology to species identification that is based on supervised machine learning. Character-based approaches circumvents analytical issues such as the nearest-neighbor problem in distance-based methods (DeSalle et al., 2005). Although the in silico mixtures presented in this study were created from the samples that were used for producing the DNA barcode and are therefore not true test samples, the analysis demonstrates the utility of analyzing mixed samples based on diagnostic nucleotides when shotgun sequencing data is available.

We believe that the development of clade-specific DNA barcodes is the way forward when investigating evolutionarily complex species. The barcodes we present are readily understandable and easily applicable for large-scale and routine testing of samples using PCR and Sanger sequencing. DNA barcoding is beyond doubt a powerful method for specimen identification, but its implementation as a routine process for quality assurance (Sgamma et al., 2017) and pharmacovigilance (de Boer et al., 2015) will depend on the ease of application. Neither phylogenetic nor distance methods are appropriate,

since they depend on large databases, sophisticated tools and lack objective criteria. For this reason, the British Pharmacopoeia (BP) approach is to present a sequence which samples must match for authentication. Pharmacopoeias ensure the safe use of pharmaceuticals by defining certain quality standards and DNA barcodes have recently been published in the BP for the first time (British Pharmacopoeia Commission, 2017). The question "does this sample correspond to the pharmacopoeial species?" is addressed by comparison to the pharmacopoeial sequence, since methods based on diagnostic nucleotides provide an easy and straight-forward way to answer the question. Identifying such sequences for inclusion in a pharmacopeia is the challenge addressed by this study. The whole plastid approach described here could become a model that can be applied to species that are difficult to resolve. Success depends on devising a sampling strategy that includes species that are closely related to the target species. Furthermore, the inclusion of distantly related, congeneric species increases the confidence in detected diagnostic nucleotide polymorphisms.

AUTHOR CONTRIBUTIONS

JH, CH, CP, and MK contributed to the conception and design of the study. BA and CP provided samples and made taxonomic identifications. CH and MK conducted the laboratory work. MK performed the data analysis and wrote the first draft of the manuscript. All authors contributed to manuscript revision, read and approved the submitted version.

FUNDING

This work was conducted as part of the MedPlant ITN and received funding from the European Union's Seventh Framework Program for research, technological development and demonstration under grant agreement no. 606895.

ACKNOWLEDGMENTS

We would like to acknowledge the herbal medicines research group, the NGS core facility at the National Institute for Biological Standards and Control (NIBSC) and Edward Mee for help in NGS sequencing. We also would like to thank the group of JH at the University of Reading for facilitating lab work and discussions of the manuscript. Julian Harber has contributed to this study by providing samples from his personal collection.

SUPPLEMENTARY MATERIAL

FIGURE S1 | Gene map of the plastid genome of *Berberis aristata*. Genes on the outside of the circle are transcribed clockwise and genes on the inside anti-clockwise. The dark gray histograms in the inner circle show the GC content.

REFERENCES

Acosta, C. M., and Premoli, A. C. (2010). Evidence of chloroplast capture in south american nothofagus (subgenus nothofagus, nothofagaceae). *Mol. Phylogenet. Evol.* 54, 235–242. doi: 10.1016/j.ympev.2009.08.008

Adhikari, B., Milne, R., Pennington, R. T., Särkinen, T., and Pendry, C. A. (2015). Systematics and biogeography of *Berberis* s. l. inferred from nuclear ITS and chloroplast ndhF gene sequences. *Taxon* 64, 39–48. doi: 10.12705/641.21

Adhikari, B., Pendry, C. A., Pennington, R. T., and Milne, R. I. (2012). A revision of *Berberis* s.s. *(berberidaceae)* in nepal. *Edinburgh J. Bot.* 69, 447–522. doi: 10.1017/S0960428612000261

Andrews, S. (2010). *FastQC: A Quality Control Tool for High Throughput Sequence Data.* Available at: https://www.bioinformatics.babraham.ac.uk/projects/fastqc/ doi: 10.1017/s0960428612000261 (accessed May 2, 2019).

Austerlitz, F., David, O., Schaeffer, B., Bleakley, K., Olteanu, M., Leblois, R., et al. (2009). DNA barcode analysis: a comparison of phylogenetic and statistical classification methods. *BMC Bioinformatics* 10(Suppl. 1):S10. doi: 10.1186/1471-2105-10-S14-S10

Ayurvedic Pharmacopoeia of India (2001). *Ayurvedic Pharmacopoeia of India.* New Delhi: Government of India, Ministry of Health and Family Welfare.

Bankevich, A., Nurk, S., Antipov, D., Gurevich, A. A., Dvorkin, M., Kulikov, A. S., et al. (2012). SPAdes: a new genome assembly algorithm and its applications to single-cell sequencing. *J. Comput. Biol.* 19, 455–477. doi: 10.1089/cmb.2012.0021

Bertolazzi, P., Felici, G., and Weitschek, E. (2009). Learning to classify species with barcodes. *BMC Bioinformatics* 10(Suppl. 14):S7. doi: 10.1186/1471-2105-10-S14-S7

Bolger, A. M., Lohse, M., and Usadel, B. (2014). Trimmomatic: a flexible trimmer for illumina sequence data. *Bioinformatics* 30, 2114–2120. doi: 10.1093/bioinformatics/btu170

Braukmann, T. W. A., Kuzmina, M. L., Sills, J., Zakharov, E. V., and Hebert, P. D. N. (2017). Testing the efficacy of DNA barcodes for identifying the vascular plants of Canada. *PLoS One* 12:e0169515. doi: 10.1371/journal.pone.0169515

British Pharmacopoeia (2016). *British Pharmacopoeia.* London: Medicines and Healthcare Regulatory Agency (MHRA).

British Pharmacopoeia Commission (2017). *British Pharmacopoeia Appendix XI V Deoxyribonucleic Acid (DNA) Based Identification Techniques for Herbal Drugs.* London: TSO.

Casiraghi, M., Labra, M., Ferri, E., Galimberti, A., and de Mattia, F. (2010). DNA barcoding: a six-question tour to improve users' awareness about the method. *Brief. Bioinform.* 11, 440–453. doi: 10.1093/bib/bbq003

Chandra, P., and Purohit, A. N. (1980). Berberine contents and alkaloid profile of *Berberis* species from different altitudes. *Biochem. Syst. Ecol.* 8, 379–380. doi: 10.1016/0305-1978(80)90040-X

Chase, M. W., Cowan, R. S., Hollingsworth, P. M., Berg, C., Van Den Madriñán, S., Petersen, G., et al. (2007). A proposal for a standardised protocol to barcode all land plants published by: international association for plant taxonomy (iapt) linked references are available on jstor for this article: new trends a proposal in plant to barcode all land plants fo. *Taxon* 56, 295–299. doi: 10.1002/tax.562004

Coissac, E., Hollingsworth, P. M., Lavergne, S., and Taberlet, P. (2016). From barcodes to genomes: extending the concept of DNA barcoding. *Mol. Ecol.* 25, 1423–1428. doi: 10.1111/mec.13549

de Boer, H. J., Ichim, M. C., and Newmaster, S. G. (2015). DNA barcoding and pharmacovigilance of herbal medicines. *Drug Saf.* 38, 611–620. doi: 10.1007/s40264-015-0306-8

DeSalle, R. (2006). Species discovery versus species identification in dna barcoding efforts: response to rubinoff. *Conserv. Biol.* 20, 1545–1547. doi: 10.1111/j.1523-1739.2006.00543.x

DeSalle, R., Egan, M. G., and Siddall, M. (2005). The unholy trinity: taxonomy, species delimitation and DNA barcoding. *Philos. Trans. R. Soc. Lond. B Biol. Sci.* 360, 1905–1916. doi: 10.1098/rstb.2005.1722

Directive 2001/83/Ec (2001). On the Community code relating to medicinal products for human use. *Off. J. Eur. Union L* 311, 67–128.

Directive 2004/83/EC (2004). On minimum standards for the qualification and status of third country nationals or stateless persons as refugees or as persons who otherwise need international protection and the content of the protection granted. *Off. J. Eur. Union L* 136, 85–90.

Doyle, J. J., and Doyle, J. L. (1987). A rapid DNA isolation procedure for small quantities of fresh leaf tissue. *Phytochem. Bull.* 19, 11–15.

Fazekas, A. J., Kesanakurti, P. R., Burgess, K. S., Percy, D. M., Graham, S. W., Barrett, S. C. H., et al. (2009). Are plant species inherently harder to discriminate than animal species using DNA barcoding markers? *Mol. Ecol. Resour.* 9 (Suppl. s1), 130–139. doi: 10.1111/j.1755-0998.2009.02652.x

Goldstein, P. Z., and DeSalle, R. (2005). Phylogenetic species, nested hierarchies, and character fixation. *Cladistics* 16, 364–384. doi: 10.1111/j.1096-0031.2000.tb00356.x

Hebert, P. D. N., Stoeckle, M. Y., Zemlak, T. S., and Francis, C. M. (2004). Identification of birds through DNA barcodes. *PLoS Biol.* 2:e312. doi: 10.1371/journal.pbio.0020312

Hollingsworth, P. M., Graham, S. W., and Little, D. P. (2011). Choosing and using a plant DNA barcode. *PLoS One* 6:e19254. doi: 10.1371/journal.pone.0019254

Kane, N., Sveinsson, S., Dempewolf, H., Yang, J. Y., Zhang, D., Engels, J. M. M., et al. (2012). Ultra-barcoding in cacao (Theobroma spp.; *Malvaceae)* using whole chloroplast genomes and nuclear ribosomal DNA. *Am. J. Bot.* 99, 320–329. doi: 10.3732/ajb.1100570

Katoh, K., and Standley, D. M. (2013). MAFFT multiple sequence alignment software version 7: improvements in performance and usability. *Mol. Biol. Evol.* 30, 772–780. doi: 10.1093/molbev/mst010

Kent, W. J. (2002). BLAT—the blast-like alignment tool. *Genome Res.* 12, 656–664. doi: 10.1101/gr.229202

Kress, W. J., Wurdack, K. J., Zimmer, E. A., Weigt, L. A., and Janzen, D. H. (2005). Use of DNA barcodes to identify flowering plants. *Proc. Natl. Acad. Sci. U.S.A.* 102, 8369–8374. doi: 10.1073/pnas.0503123102

Krzywinski, M., Schein, J., Birol, I., Connors, J., Gascoyne, R., Horsman, D., et al. (2009). Circos: an information aesthetic for comparative genomics. *Genome Res.* 19, 1639–1645. doi: 10.1101/gr.092759.109

Lee, E., Harris, N., Gibson, M., Chetty, R., and Lewis, S. (2009). Apollo: a community resource for genome annotation editing. *Bioinformatics* 25, 1836–1837. doi: 10.1093/bioinformatics/btp314

Li, H., and Durbin, R. (2009). Fast and accurate short read alignment with burrows-wheeler transform. *Bioinformatics* 25, 1754–1760. doi: 10.1093/bioinformatics/btp324

Li, H., Handsaker, B., Wysoker, A., Fennell, T., Ruan, J., Homer, N., et al. (2009). The sequence alignment/map format and SAMtools. *Bioinformatics* 25, 2078–2079. doi: 10.1093/bioinformatics/btp352

Little, D. P., and Stevenson, D. W. (2007). A comparison of algorithms for the identification of specimens using DNA barcodes: examples from gymnosperms. *Cladistics* 23, 1–21. doi: 10.1111/j.1096-0031.2006.00126.x

Liu, C., Shi, L., Zhu, Y., Chen, H., Zhang, J., Lin, X., et al. (2012). CpGAVAS, an integrated web server for the annotation, visualization, analysis, and genbank submission of completely sequenced chloroplast genome sequences. *BMC Genomics* 13:715. doi: 10.1186/1471-2164-13-715

Ma, J., Yang, B., Zhu, W., Sun, L., Tian, J., and Wang, X. (2013). The complete chloroplast genome sequence of mahonia bealei (*Berberidaceae)* reveals a significant expansion of the inverted repeat and phylogenetic relationship with other angiosperms. *Gene* 528, 120–131. doi: 10.1016/j.gene.2013.07.037

Manzanilla, V., Kool, A., Nguyen Nhat, L., Nong Van, H., Le Thi Thu, H., and De Boer, H. J. (2018). Phylogenomics and barcoding of panax: toward the identification of ginseng species. *BMC Evol. Biol.* 18:44. doi: 10.1186/s12862-018-1160-y

Martin, M. (2011). Cutadapt removes adapter sequences from high-throughput sequencing reads. *EMBnet J.* 17, 10–12. doi: 10.14806/ej.17.1.200

McKenna, A., Hanna, M., Banks, E., Sivachenko, A., Cibulskis, K., Kernytsky, A., et al. (2010). The genome analysis toolkit: a mapreduce framework for analyzing next-generation DNA sequencing data. *Genome Res.* 20, 1297–1303. doi: 10.1101/gr.107524.110

Meyer, C. P., and Paulay, G. (2005). DNA barcoding: error rates based on comprehensive sampling. *PLoS Biol.* 3:e422. doi: 10.1371/journal.pbio.0030422

Meyer, M., and Kircher, M. (2010). Illumina sequencing library preparation for highly multiplexed target capture and sequencing. *Cold Spring Harb. Protoc.* 2010:pdb.prot5448. doi: 10.1101/pdb.prot5448

Miller, M. A., Pfeiffer, W., and Schwartz, T. (2010). "Creating the CIPRES science gateway for inference of large phylogenetic trees," in *Proceedings of the Gateway Computing Environments Workshop (GCE)*, New Orleans, LA.

Moritz, C., and Cicero, C. (2004). DNA barcoding: promise and pitfalls. *PLoS Biol.* 2:e354. doi: 10.1371/journal.pbio.0020354

Mutanen, M., Kivelä, S. M., Vos, R. A., Doorenweerd, C., Ratnasingham, S., Hausmann, A., et al. (2016). Species-level para- and polyphyly in DNA barcode gene trees: strong operational bias in european lepidoptera. *Syst. Biol.* 65, 1024–1040. doi: 10.1093/sysbio/syw044

Naciri, Y., and Linder, H. P. (2015). Species delimitation and relationships: the dance of the seven veils. *Taxon* 64, 3–16. doi: 10.12705/641.24

Newmaster, S. G., Grguric, M., Shanmughanandhan, D., Ramalingam, S., and Ragupathy, S. (2013). DNA barcoding detects contamination and substitution in north american herbal products. *BMC Med.* 11:222. doi: 10.1186/1741-7015-11-222

Page, A. J., Taylor, B., Delaney, A. J., Soares, J., Seemann, T., Keane, J. A., et al. (2016). SNP-sites: rapid efficient extraction of SNPs from multi-FASTA alignments. *Microb. Genomics* 2:e000056. doi: 10.1099/mgen.0.000056

Paradis, E. (2010). Pegas: an R package for population genetics with an integrated-modular approach. *Bioinformatics* 26, 419–420. doi: 10.1093/bioinformatics/btp696

Parks, M., Cronn, R., and Liston, A. (2009). Increasing phylogenetic resolution at low taxonomic levels using massively parallel sequencing of chloroplast genomes. *BMC Biol.* 7:84. doi: 10.1186/1741-7007-7-84

Parmentier, I., Duminil, J., Kuzmina, M., Philippe, M., Thomas, D. W., Kenfack, D., et al. (2013). How effective are DNA barcodes in the identification of african rainforest trees? *PLoS One* 8:e54921. doi: 10.1371/journal.pone.0054921

Percy, D. M., Argus, G. W., Cronk, Q. C., Fazekas, A. J., Kesanakurti, P. R., Burgess, K. S., et al. (2014). Understanding the spectacular failure of DNA barcoding in willows (Salix): does this result from a trans-specific selective sweep? *Mol. Ecol.* 23, 4737–4756. doi: 10.1111/mec.12837

Plant Working Group, C. B. O. L., Hollingsworth, P. M., Forrest, L. L., Spouge, J. L., Hajibabaei, M., Ratnasingham, S., et al. (2009). A DNA barcode for land plants. *Proc. Natl. Acad. Sci. U.S.A.* 106, 12794–12797. doi: 10.1073/pnas.0905845106

Quinlan, A. R., and Hall, I. M. (2010). BEDTools: a flexible suite of utilities for comparing genomic features. *Bioinformatics* 26, 841–842. doi: 10.1093/bioinformatics/btq033

Rieseberg, L. H., and Brouillet, L. (1994). Are many plant species paraphyletic? *Taxo* 43, 21–32.

Rieseberg, L. H., and Soltis, D. E. (1991). Phylogenetic consequences of cytoplasmic gene flow in plants. *Evol. Trends Plants* 5, 65–84. doi: 10.1007/s00606-006-0485-y

Rokas, A., Williams, B. L., King, N., and Carroll, S. B. (2003). Genome-scale approaches to resolving incongruence in molecular phylogenies. *Nature* 425, 798–804. doi: 10.1038/nature02053

Roy, S., Tyagi, A., Shukla, V., Kumar, A., Singh, U. M., Chaudhary, L. B., et al. (2010). Universal plant DNA barcode loci may not work in complex groups: a case study with Indian *Berberis* species. *PLoS One* 5:e13674. doi: 10.1371/journal.pone.0013674

Sarkar, I. N., Planet, P. J., and Desalle, R. (2008). CAOS software for use in character-based DNA barcoding. *Mol. Ecol. Resour.* 8, 1256–1259. doi: 10.1111/j.1755-0998.2008.02235.x

Seberg, O., and Petersen, G. (2009). How many loci does it take to DNA barcode a crocus? *PLoS One* 4:e4598. doi: 10.1371/journal.pone.0004598

Sgamma, T., Lockie-williams, C., Kreuzer, M., Williams, S., Scheyhing, U., Koch, E., et al. (2017). DNA barcoding for industrial quality assurance. *Planta Med.* 83, 1117–1129. doi: 10.1055/s-0043-113448

Srirama, R., Santhosh Kumar, J. U., Seethapathy, G. S., Newmaster, S. G., Ragupathy, S., Ganeshaiah, K. N., et al. (2017). Species adulteration in the herbal trade: causes, consequences and mitigation. *Drug Saf.* 40, 651–661. doi: 10.1007/s40264-017-0527-0

Srivastava, S., and Rawat, A. K. S. (2013). Quality evaluation of ayurvedic crude drug daruharidra, its allied species, and commercial samples from herbal drug markets of India. *Evid. Based. Complement. Alternat. Med.* 2013:472973. doi: 10.1155/2013/472973

Srivastava, S. K., Rawat, A. K. S., and Mehrotra, S. (2004). Pharmacognostic evaluation of the root of *Berberis* asiatica. *Pharm. Biol.* 42, 467–473. doi: 10.1080/13880200490886256

Stamatakis, A. (2014). RAxML version 8: a tool for phylogenetic analysis and post-analysis of large phylogenies. *Bioinformatics* 30, 1312–1313. doi: 10.1093/bioinformatics/btu033

Van der Auwera, G. A., Carneiro, M. O., Hartl, C., Poplin, R., Del Angel, G., Levy-Moonshine, A., et al. (2013). From fastq data to high confidence variant calls: the genome analysis toolkit best practices pipeline.[GATK]. *Curr. Protoc. Bioinforma.* 43:11.10.1-33

Vaughn, J. N., Chaluvadi, S. R., Tushar Rangan, L., and Bennetzen, J. L. (2014). Whole plastome sequences from five ginger species facilitate marker development and define limits to barcode methodology. *PLoS One* 9:e108581. doi: 10.1371/journal.pone.0108581

Vlietinck, A., Pieters, L., and Apers, S. (2009). Legal requirements for the quality of herbal substances and herbal preparations for the manufacturing of herbal medicinal products in the European union. *Planta Med.* 75, 683–688. doi: 10.1055/s-0029-1185307

Weitschek, E., Van Velzen, R., Felici, G., and Bertolazzi, P. (2013). BLOG 2.0: a software system for character-based species classification with DNA barcode sequences. What it does, how to use it. *Mol. Ecol. Resour.* 13, 1043–1046. doi: 10.1111/1755-0998.12073

Wyman, S. K., Jansen, R. K., and Boore, J. L. (2004). Automatic annotation of organellar genomes with DOGMA. *Bioinformatics* 20, 3252–3255. doi: 10.1093/bioinformatics/bth352

Zhang, N., Erickson, D. L., Ramachandran, P., Ottesen, A. R., Timme, R. E., Funk, V. A., et al. (2017). An analysis of echinacea chloroplast genomes: implications for future botanical identification. *Sci. Rep.* 7:216. doi: 10.1038/s41598-017-00321-6

Permissions

The contributors of this book come from diverse backgrounds, making this book a truly international effort. This book will bring forth new frontiers with its revolutionizing research information and detailed analysis of the nascent developments around the world.

We would like to thank all the contributing authors for lending their expertise to make the book truly unique. They have played a crucial role in the development of this book. Without their invaluable contributions this book wouldn't have been possible. They have made vital efforts to compile up to date information on the varied aspects of this subject to make this book a valuable addition to the collection of many professionals and students.

This book was conceptualized with the vision of imparting up-to-date information and advanced data in this field. To ensure the same, a matchless editorial board was set up. Every individual on the board went through rigorous rounds of assessment to prove their worth. After which they invested a large part of their time researching and compiling the most relevant data for our readers.

The editorial board has been involved in producing this book since its inception. They have spent rigorous hours researching and exploring the diverse topics which have resulted in the successful publishing of this book. They have passed on their knowledge of decades through this book. To expedite this challenging task, the publisher supported the team at every step. A small team of assistant editors was also appointed to further simplify the editing procedure and attain best results for the readers.

Apart from the editorial board, the designing team has also invested a significant amount of their time in understanding the subject and creating the most relevant covers. They scrutinized every image to scout for the most suitable representation of the subject and create an appropriate cover for the book.

The publishing team has been an ardent support to the editorial, designing and production team. Their endless efforts to recruit the best for this project, has resulted in the accomplishment of this book. They are a veteran in the field of academics and their pool of knowledge is as vast as their experience in printing. Their expertise and guidance has proved useful at every step. Their uncompromising quality standards have made this book an exceptional effort. Their encouragement from time to time has been an inspiration for everyone.

The publisher and the editorial board hope that this book will prove to be a valuable piece of knowledge for researchers, students, practitioners and scholars across the globe.

List of Contributors

Jiushi Liu, Xiaoyi Zhang, Haitao Liu and Peigen Xiao
Institute of Medicinal Plant Development, Chinese Academy of Medical Sciences, Peking Union Medical College, Beijing, China
Key Laboratory of Bioactive Substances and Resources Utilization of Chinese Herbal Medicine (Peking Union Medical College), Ministry of Education, Beijing, China

Xueping Wei, Yaodong Qi and Bengang Zhang
Institute of Medicinal Plant Development, Chinese Academy of Medical Sciences, Peking Union Medical College, Beijing, China
Engineering Research Center of Traditional Chinese Medicine Resources, Ministry of Education, Beijing, China

Hao Liu, Xuechun Chen and Yi Wang
Pharmaceutical Informatics Institute, College of Pharmaceutical Sciences, Zhejiang University, Hangzhou, China

Xiaoping Zhao
School of Basic Medical Sciences, Zhejiang Chinese Medical University, Hangzhou, China

Buchang Zhao, Ke Qian and Yang Shi
Shandong Danhong Pharmaceutical Co., Ltd., Heze, China

Mirko Baruscotti
Department of Bioscienze, The PaceLab, University of Milano, Milan, Italy

Jing Zhang, Wen Xu, Peng Wang, Juan Huang, Jun-qi Bai, Zhi-hai Huang, Xu-sheng Liu and Xiao-hui Qiu
Guangdong Provincial Key Laboratory of Clinical Research on Traditional Chinese Medicine Syndrome, The Second Clinical Medical College of Guangzhou University of Chinese Medicine, Guangdong Provincial Hospital of Traditional Chinese Medicine, Guangzhou, China

Xiao-min Dai, Dong-ni Cui, Zun-jian Zhang and Feng-guo Xu
Key Laboratory of Drug Quality Control and Pharmacovigilance, Ministry of Education, China Pharmaceutical University, Nanjing, China
State Key Laboratory of Natural Medicines, China Pharmaceutical University, Nanjing, China

Jing Wang
College of Pharmacy, Shaanxi University of Chinese Medicine, Xianyang, China

Wei Zhang
State Key Laboratory for Quality Research in Chinese Medicines, Macau University of Science and Technology, Taipa, Macau

Manjia Zhao, Yuntao Dai, Qi Li, Pengyue Li and Shilin Chen
Institute of Chinese Materia Medica, China Academy of Chinese Medical Sciences, Beijing, China

Xue-Mei Qin
Modern Research Center for Traditional Chinese Medicine, Shanxi University, Taiyuan, China

Tiziana Sgamma, Eva Masiero, Purvi Mali and Adrian Slater
Faculty of Health & Life Sciences, Biomolecular Technology Group, De Montfort University, Leicester, United Kingdom

Maslinda Mahat
Faculty of Health & Life Sciences, Biomolecular Technology Group, De Montfort University, Leicester, United Kingdom
Natural Product Testing Section, Toxic Compound Detection Unit, National Pharmaceutical Control Bureau, Jalan University, Selangor, Malaysia

Wing Lam, Yongshen Ren, Fulan Guan, Zaoli Jiang, William Cheng and Yung-Chi Cheng
Department of Pharmacology, Yale University School of Medicine, New Haven, CT, United States

Chang-Hua Xu
Department of Pharmacology, Yale University School of Medicine, New Haven, CT, United States
College of Food Science and Technology, Shanghai Ocean University, Shanghai, China

Shwu-Huey Liu
Yiviva Inc., New York, NY, United States

Louise Isager Ahl, Narjes Al-Husseini, Sara Al-Helle and Nina Rønsted
Natural History Museum of Denmark, University of Copenhagen, Copenhagen, Denmark

Dan Staerk
Department of Drug Design and Pharmacology, University of Copenhagen, Copenhagen, Denmark

Olwen M. Grace
Comparative Plant and Fungal Biology, Royal Botanic Gardens Kew, Richmond, United Kingdom

William G. T. Willats
School of Natural and Environmental Sciences, Newcastle University, Newcastle upon Tyne, United Kingdom

Jozef Mravec and Bodil Jørgensen
Department of Plant and Environmental Sciences, University of Copenhagen, Frederiksberg, Denmark

Gopalakrishnan Saroja Seethapathy
Natural History Museum, University of Oslo, Oslo, Norway
Department of Pharmaceutical Chemistry, School of Pharmacy, University of Oslo, Oslo, Norway

Ancuta-Cristina Raclariu-Manolica
Natural History Museum, University of Oslo, Oslo, Norway
Stejarul Research Centre for Biological Sciences, National Institute of Research and Development for Biological Sciences, Piatra Neamt, Romania

Jarl Andreas Anmarkrud and Hugo J. de Boer
Natural History Museum, University of Oslo, Oslo, Norway

Helle Wangensteen
Department of Pharmaceutical Chemistry, School of Pharmacy, University of Oslo, Oslo, Norway

Xiao-yue Wang, Rong Xu, Jun Chen, Jing-yuan Song, Jian-ping Han and Zheng Zhang
Key Laboratory of Bioactive Substances and Resources Utilization of Chinese Herbal Medicine, Ministry of Education, Institute of Medicinal Plant Development, Chinese Academy of Medicinal Science and Peking Union Medicinal College, Beijing, China

Steven-G Newmaster
NHP Research Alliance, Biodiversity Institute of Ontario (BIO), University of Guelph, Guelph, ON, Canada

Shi-lin Chen
Key Laboratory of Beijing for Identification and Safety Evaluation of Chinese Medicine, Institute of Chinese Materia Medica, China Academy of Chinese Medical Sciences, Beijing, China

Mingya Ding, Jin Li, Shuhan Zou, Xiumei Gao and Yan-xu Chang
Tianjin State Key Laboratory of Modern Chinese Medicine, Tianjin University of Traditional Chinese Medicine, Tianjin, China
Tianjin Key Laboratory of Phytochemistry and Pharmaceutical Analysis, Tianjin University of Traditional Chinese Medicine, Tianjin, China

Ge Tang
Department of Nephrology, The First Teaching Hospital, Tianjin University of Traditional Chinese Medicine, Tianjin, China

Sascha Wetters, Thomas Horn and Peter Nick
Molecular Cell Biology, Karlsruhe Institute of Technology, Karlsruhe, Germany

Francesca Scotti, Katja Löbel and Michael Heinrich
Pharmacognosy and Phytotherapy Group, Pharmaceutical and Biological Chemistry, UCL School of Pharmacy, London, United Kingdom

Anthony Booker
Pharmacognosy and Phytotherapy Group, Pharmaceutical and Biological Chemistry, UCL School of Pharmacy, London, United Kingdom
Division of Herbal and East Asian Medicine, Department of Life Sciences, University of Westminster, London, United Kingdom

Mengquan Yang and Wenjing You
CAS Key Laboratory of Synthetic Biology, CAS Center for Excellence in Molecular Plant Sciences, Institute of Plant Physiology and Ecology, Shanghai Institutes for Biological Sciences, Chinese Academy of Sciences, Shanghai, China
University of Chinese Academy of Sciences, Beijing, China

Shiwen Wu and Amit Jaisi
CAS Key Laboratory of Synthetic Biology, CAS Center for Excellence in Molecular Plant Sciences, Institute of Plant Physiology and Ecology, Shanghai Institutes for Biological Sciences, Chinese Academy of Sciences, Shanghai, China

Youli Xiao
CAS Key Laboratory of Synthetic Biology, CAS Center for Excellence in Molecular Plant Sciences, Institute of Plant Physiology and Ecology, Shanghai Institutes for Biological Sciences, Chinese Academy of Sciences, Shanghai, China
University of Chinese Academy of Sciences, Beijing, China
CAS-JIC Centre of Excellence in Plant and Microbial Sciences, Shanghai, China

Martin Fitzgerald
Herbal and East Asian Medicine, School of Life Sciences, College of Liberal Arts and Sciences, University of Westminster, London, United Kingdom

Michael Heinrich
Pharmacognosy and Phytotherapy, UCL School of Pharmacy, London, United Kingdom

Anthony Booker
Herbal and East Asian Medicine, School of Life Sciences, College of Liberal Arts and Sciences, University of Westminster, London, United Kingdom
Pharmacognosy and Phytotherapy, UCL School of Pharmacy, London, United Kingdom

Juan Huang, Lan Guo, Ruixiang Tan, Meijin Wei, Jing Zhang, Ya Zhao, Lu Gong and Zhihai Huang
The Second Clinical College of Guangzhou University of Chinese Medicine, Guangdong Provincial Hospital of Chinese Medicine, Guangzhou, China

Xiaohui Qiu
The Second Clinical College of Guangzhou University of Chinese Medicine, Guangdong Provincial Hospital of Chinese Medicine, Guangzhou, China
Guangdong Provincial Key Laboratory of Clinical Research on Traditional Chinese Medicine Syndrome, Guangzhou, China

Qing Li, Jingxian Feng, Liang Chen, Yun Wang, Ying Xiao, Junfeng Chen, Yangyun Zhou and Wansheng Chen
Department of Pharmacy, Changzheng Hospital, Second Military Medical University, Shanghai, China

Zhichao Xu
Institute of Medicinal Plant Development, Chinese Academy of Medical Sciences, Peking Union Medical College, Beijing, China

Yingjie Zhu
Institute of Chinese Materia Medica, China Academy of Chinese Medical Sciences, Beijing, China

Hexin Tan
Department of Pharmaceutical Botany, School of Pharmacy, Second Military Medical University, Shanghai, China

Lei Zhang
Department of Pharmaceutical Botany, School of Pharmacy, Second Military Medical University, Shanghai, China
State Key Laboratory of Subtropical Silviculture, Zhejiang A & F University, Hangzhou, China

Zhen-wen Liu
CAS Key Laboratory for Plant Diversity and Biogeography of East Asia, Kunming Institute of Botany, Chinese Academy of Sciences, Kunming, China

Yu-zhen Gao and Jing Zhou
School of Pharmaceutical Sciences and Yunnan Key Laboratory of Pharmacology for Natural Products, Kunming Medical University, Kunming, China

Xinlian Chen, Jianguo Zhou, Yingxian Cui, Yu Wang and Hui Yao
Key Lab of Chinese Medicine Resources Conservation, State Administration of Traditional Chinese Medicine of the People's Republic of China, Institute of Medicinal Plant Development, Chinese Academy of Medical Sciences & Peking Union Medical College, Beijing, China

Baozhong Duan
College of Pharmaceutical Science, Dali University, Dali, China

Marco Kreuzer and Julie A. Hawkins
School of Biological Sciences, University of Reading, Reading, United Kingdom

Caroline Howard
BP-NIBSC Herbal Laboratory, National Institute for Biological Standards and Control, Potters Bar, United Kingdom

Bhaskar Adhikari and Colin A. Pendry
Royal Botanic Garden Edinburgh, Edinburgh, United Kingdom

Index

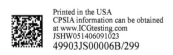

Printed in the USA
CPSIA information can be obtained
at www.ICGtesting.com
JSHW051406091023
49903JS00006B/299